Diagnostic Testing & Nursing Implications

A CASE STUDY APPROACH

Diagnostic Testing & Nursing Implications

A CASE STUDY APPROACH

KATHLEEN DESKA PAGANA, Ph.D., R.N.

Associate Professor
Department of Nursing, Lycoming College,
Williamsport, Pennsylvania

TIMOTHY JAMES PAGANA, M.D., F.A.C.S.

Surgical Oncologist, Williamsport, Pennsylvania

FOURTH EDITION

With 124 *illustrations*

Mosby

St. Louis Baltimore Boston Chicago London Madrid Philadelphia Sydney Toronto

Mosby

Dedicated to Publishing Excellence

Publisher: Alison Miller
Editor-in-Chief: Nancy Coon
Editor: Robin Carter
Editorial Assistant: Jeanne Allison
Project Manager: Linda Clarke
Project Supervisor: Deborah Thorp
Cover: Renee Duenow
Cover Photo: Philippe Sion, The Image Bank
Manufacturing Supervisor: Kathy Grone

FOURTH EDITION

Printed in the United States of America
Composition by The Clarinda Company
Printing/binding by R.R. Donnelley & Sons Company, Crawfordsville

Mosby–Year Book, Inc.
11830 Westline Industrial Drive
St. Louis, Missouri 63146

Library of Congress Cataloging-in-Publication Data

Pagana, Kathleen Deska, 1952-
Diagnostic testing & nursing implications: a case study approach / Kathleen Deska Pagana, Timothy James Pagana.—4th ed.
p. cm.
Includes bibliographical references and index.
ISBN 0-8016-6779-8
1. Diagnosis. 2. Nursing. I. Pagana, Timothy James, 1949- II. Title. III. Title: Diagnostic testing and nursing implications.
[DNLM: 1. Diagnosis, Laboratory—nurses' instruction. 2. Nursing Assessment. QY 4 P128d 1993]
RT48.5.P32 1993
616.07'5'024613—dc20
DNLM/DLC 93-5961
for Library of Congress CIP

95 96 97 98 / 9 8 7 6 5 4 3 2

We lovingly dedicate this book to our three daughters:

Jocelyn Marie Pagana

Denise Kathleen Pagana

Theresa Noel Pagana

PREFACE

With the ever-increasing advances in technology, it remains a major challenge to stay current in the exciting field of diagnostic and laboratory testing. This fourth edition represents another major revision of this widely used textbook. It is still the purpose of this book to make the study of diagnostic and laboratory testing interesting, informative, and enjoyable.

All studies have been updated, and many sections have been completely rewritten. A few of the many new studies include: transesophageal echocardiography, prostate-specific antigen, C-peptide, growth-hormone stimulation test, RBC survival study, and somatomedin C. New case studies address such topics as chronic fatigue syndrome, Lyme disease, tuberculosis, and growth hormone deficiency. The more than 150 illustrations in this text have been further enhanced by photographs such as those of magnetic resonance imaging, fetoscopy, and chorionic villus sampling.

This book is unique in that a concise, yet complete, discussion of anatomy and physiology for each body system starts each chapter. Further, the anatomy, physiology, and pathophysiology as they relate to each diagnostic test are presented in an easy-to-read manner. Many students find this information helpful as a supplement to nursing courses. The practicing nurse will see this information as an excellent and concise review of anatomy, physiology, and pathophysiology.

This edition continues the application of the nursing process with *nursing diagnoses* related to diagnostic testing that was initiated in the third edition. In Chapter 1, a general overview of the nursing process precedes the application of the nursing process to each of the major types of testing—blood, urine, x-ray, nuclear scanning, ultrasound, and endoscopy. Nursing diagnoses and collaborative problems are suggested for each category of laboratory and diagnostic testing. In subsequent chapters, a section on *Nursing Considerations* includes the information on nursing diagnoses and collaborative problems and the information on nursing implications that was included in previous editions. The section on nursing diagnoses/collaborative problems will refer the reader to the related section (e.g., blood, urine, x-ray) in Chapter 1 and will also add additional nursing diagnoses/collaborative problems as needed. This is done in order to avoid writing common nursing diagnoses (such as "possible knowledge deficit") after each study. For example, bronchoscopy is thoroughly described in Chapter 5. The reader is referred to Chapter 1 for the potential nursing diagnoses that generally relate to endoscopic procedures. However, the *specifc* nursing diagnoses and collaborative problems that are pertinent to bronchoscopy are described with the detailed discussion of bronchoscopy in Chapter 5.

Chapter 1 should be interesting for anyone needing a review of the nursing process. The thorough description of each type of diagnostic and laboratory test gives an excellent overview of the major types of studies that are performed. Although this chapter should be invaluable for nursing students, it should also be an excellent review for the practicing nurse.

This book is unique in the field of diagnostic testing because of the organization of information, application of the case study approach, inclusion of nursing diagnoses, use of study questions and answers, and extensive use of illustrations. Nursing implications are comprehensive and clearly stated. The format of this book invites the reader to a full and logical understanding of diagnostic tests and abnormal findings through interesting case studies.

A major feature of the text is its consistent format. Chapters are arranged according to a systems approach (such as cardiovascular, reproductive, and nervous system). The advantage of this feature is that tests relating to a certain system (such as EKG, cardiac catheterization, cardiac enzymes, and cardiac scanning) are all discussed in the same chapter. This systems approach has been beneficial to nurse educators who have selected chapters of this book as required or recommended reading in many of their courses. Although we assume that the reader has a basic knowledge of anatomy and physiology, this information is included in each chapter to provide a general overview of the system to be discussed. This inclusion ensures a better understanding of the related diagnostic procedures.

Case studies precede the discussion of a series of tests and include the following information: the presentation of a commonly seen patient problem, the results (including normal values) of diagnostic studies performed, and a discussion explaining the interpretation of these studies. Patient treatment based on the test results is mentioned. The purpose of the case study is to stimulate the reader's interest by providing an actual patient problem, logical assessment of the problem, and treatment of the problem based on accurate diagnostic testing. These case presentations are commonly seen in the hospital setting. As a result, the nursing student and practicing nurse will more than likely see very similar clinical cases during their hospital experience. Understanding of the logical assessment of the disease and its treatment based on accurate diagnostic testing, as described in this book, no doubt will enhance the nursing care. Case studies appear at the beginning of each section in each chapter to set the stage for the development of succeeding material. However, not all readers will benefit by reading the case study before the remainder of the chapter's content. Based on the reader's prior knowledge of diagnostic testing, he or she may wish to look at the case studies before, after, or both before and after the chapter's contents to have the best opportunity to analyze, integrate, and incorporate the knowledge of diagnostic testing. Also, each diagnostic test may be read independently of the case study. This enables this text to be used for quick reference purposes.

Normal values, possible critical values, rationale, procedure, contraindications, and nursing considerations are discussed for each test. *Normal values* are listed, when appropriate, for the infant, child, adult, and elderly person. Also, where appropriate, values are separated into those for males and females. *Possible critical values* give an indication of results that are well outside the usual range of normal. These results generally require immediate intervention. The *rationale* for a specific study includes specific anatomy and physiology, indications, and complications of the test. The *procedure* describes the actual method of performing the study and includes patient care before, during, and after the study; who performs the study; where the study is performed; the patient's position during the study; the need for anesthesia or sedation; the patient's sensation; and the duration of the procedure. (The procedure for each study may vary somewhat in different hospitals and in different areas of the country.) *Contraindications* are then listed for each study. We have gone to great lengths to exclude clinically irrelevant esoteric information. Yet, in an effort to be complete we have included information that may be uncommonly experienced in a routine clinical nursing practice.

The *nursing considerations* sections include a subsection on potential nursing diagnoses/collaborative problems (thoroughly described in Chapter 1) and also a section on nursing implications. The nursing implications are comprehensive and address the patient's psychologic as well as physiologic needs. Included in this section are interventions (with rationale) describing what the nurse should do before, during, and after the study to ensure both the accuracy of the procedure and the safety of the patient. Potential problems are identified, and key areas of nursing assessment and interventions are described.

Study questions and answers are included at the end of each chapter to ensure comprehension of the diagnostic studies and to describe problems that the nurse commonly faces in caring for patients undergoing diagnostic tests. The study questions challenge the reader to correlate previously presented material with problematic circumstances frequently occurring in nursing practice. These questions stimulate the reader to evaluate a specific problem and to determine appropriate nursing interventions. Answers are provided following each question.

Sections labeled *supplemental information* contain important material not included in the case study for fear of making the section, cumbersome and, therein, losing the reader's interest. This section thus ensures the completeness of the text. Studies that are rarely performed are intentionally excluded from this edition. A bibliography is found at the end of each chapter for the reader who wishes to find additional information on a particular diagnostic procedure.

Over 150 illustrations are included to enhance the reader's understanding of diagnostic procedures. Areas of pathology on x-ray films and nuclear scans are clearly marked by arrows or pointers. In addition to being interesting and helpful to nurses and nursing students, these illustrations have proven to be advantageous in patient teaching.

The table of contents is detailed to assist the reader in easily locating information within the text. Appendix 1 provides a complete list of commonly used abbreviations and symbols. Appendix 2 includes a list of commonly used abbreviations for laboratory and diagnostic testing. This should be extremely useful for the nursing student and practicing nurse who are puzzled reading abbreviations such as: CST, DSA, EGD, HAA, KUB, MRI, RIA, and many others in the patient's chart. Appendixes 3 and 4 list the normal values for blood, plasma, serum, and urine. Studies discussed in this book have the chapter number included in the discussion column of these appendices. Please note that normal values may vary because of different laboratory methods. Since many laboratories are now using the system of International Units (SI units), most common laboratory values are expressed both in conventional and SI units.

Most importantly, the information included in this book is not limited to one specific type of diagnostic testing. All types (such as blood, urine, x-ray, nuclear scanning, ultrasound, endoscopy, noninvasive vascular techniques, and computed tomography) are discussed in detail. This book supplies the information needed to provide thorough and accurate patient teaching in the area of diagnostic testing and to ensure adequate patient preparation so that the test may be performed accurately and safely.

We want to sincerely thank Drs. Gary Lattimer and Leonard Collins for the valuable suggestions to improve this manuscript. We wish to sincerely thank the many people throughout the country who sent in comment cards with recommendations for improving this book. All evaluations and reviews done on this book were most helpful in planning this fourth edition. We sincerely appreciate the efforts of our nursing editors, Don Ladig and Robin Carter, for their help in ensuring the high quality of this book. We also want to sincerely thank Karen M. Olson of Olson Business Services (Williamsport,

Pa.) for her meticulous typing of this manuscript. Finally, we want to thank Lycoming College for the sabbatical leave that was spent on writing this fourth edition. This sabbatical allowed much-needed time to investigate and observe numerous new diagnostic studies and time to thorough update all current studies.

Kathleen Deska Pagana
Timothy James Pagana

CONTENTS

6 Diagnostic Studies Used in the Assessment of the Nervous System, 172

7 Diagnostic Studies Used in the Assessment of the Urinary System, 219

9 Diagnostic Studies Used in the Assessment of the Reproductive System, 322

Diagnostic Testing & Nursing Implications

A CASE STUDY APPROACH

Chapter 1

GENERAL GUIDELINES FOR LABORATORY/DIAGNOSTIC TESTING WITH THE APPLICATION OF THE NURSING PROCESS

Application of the nursing process to diagnostic testing provides a clear framework on which to provide comprehensive nursing care. In this chapter the nursing process is applied directly to laboratory/diagnostic testing. This problem-solving technique is used to equip the nurse with the knowledge necessary to provide comprehensive nursing care before, during, and after these studies. After a general overview of the nursing process as it relates to laboratory/diagnostic testing is presented, each major type of testing (blood, urine, x-ray, nuclear scanning, ultrasound, and endoscopy) will be described using the format of the nursing process. This description will provide an overview of the major types of laboratory and diagnostic testing and include examples of when these tests are indicated and how these test results can be altered by factors such as diet, medications, and other studies. General nursing diagnoses and collaborative problems will be suggested for each type of test. This new approach will help facilitate an increased understanding of diagnostic/laboratory testing.

COMPONENTS OF THE NURSING PROCESS

During the *assessment* phase, the nurse evaluates the need for the specific diagnostic/laboratory test. The nurse should understand the reason for the test and be able to explain it to the patient. For example, telling a patient that a blood test is indicated to evaluate potassium levels because of diuretic therapy is far more professional than simply saying, "the doctor ordered this." Contraindications (such as dye allergies) should be thoroughly assessed.

Nursing diagnoses refer to problems that can be prevented, resolved, or reduced through independent nursing interventions that require no direction or supervision from others. For example, activities such as promoting mobility, assisting with activities of daily living (ADLs), and patient teaching are encompassed within nursing licensure. *Collaborative problems* are potential complications resulting from diagnostic studies, disease, or treatments that can be prevented, resolved, or reduced through collaborative nursing interventions. "Potential complication: infection," "potential complication: bleeding," and "potential complication: phlebitis" are examples of collaborative problems and illustrate the preferred way to write them. These problems are called *collaborative* because collaboration with another professional, most commonly a physician, is required. For example, nurses cannot legally prescribe definitive treatment for phlebitis, but they do prescribe monitoring interventions for early detection. Both nursing diagnoses and collaborative problems should be included in the nursing care plan so that all aspects of patient care may be addressed. Differentiating between nursing diagnoses and collaborative problems is important; nurses should be aware of which problems are treatable by independent nursing interventions and which require collaboration with other health professionals.

Nursing diagnoses/collaborative problems are used to direct the nursing care of the patient. The nurse must decide if the nursing diagnoses/collaborative problems are appropriate to that particular client. Those included in this chapter are general and relate to the general type of diagnostic testing. For example, cleansing bowel preparations are often done for x-ray film studies. If a bowel preparation is not needed, the related nursing diagnoses do not apply. To prevent unnecessary repetition, these general nursing diagnoses are not repeated in the remaining chapters of the book after each particular type of test. Only the nursing diagnoses that are specific or unique to the study will be mentioned after each test in the section "Nursing Considerations."

Many factors are important in *planning* for a diagnostic study. The effect that a test can have on other studies should be considered. For example, a test that uses barium should usually follow other radiologic or ultrasound studies. Inherent in the planning phase are diet restrictions, special preparations (such as bowel prep), and the need for a signed consent.

The *intervention* phase relates to the actual test performance. Patients want to know who will perform the test, where it will be performed, how long it will take, and any sensations they may have. Although nurses do not perform many of these studies, they do coordinate the studies and maintain responsibility for patient preparation and postprocedure care. The nurse must be able to foster a knowledgeable and working relationship with other health care professionals involved in the field of diagnostic testing.

The *evaluation* phase includes postprocedure care of the client and understanding/interpretation of test results. For example, test results of a client who had blood drawn for potassium levels should be used as a guide for other therapy. If the patient is hypokalemic, should potassium be added to an intravenous (IV) drip? Should the patient be given oral potassium? Should the diuretic order be changed, or, should the patient be monitored for cardiac arrhythmias? Test results are also used to determine the need for further studies or if the patient may return to normal activities.

The components of the nursing process will now be applied to the following: blood studies, urine studies, fecal studies, x-ray studies, nuclear scanning, ultrasound studies, and endoscopy procedures.

Blood studies

Assessment. Blood studies are used to assess a multitude of bodily processes or disorders. Common studies include cardiac enzymes, serum lipids, electrolyte levels, red and white blood cell counts, clotting factors, hormone levels, and levels of breakdown products such as urea nitrogen. Blood studies are often done for screening or as part of a routine physical examination.

Nursing Diagnoses/Collaborative Problems for Blood Studies

- Possible knowledge deficit related to test purpose, preparation, and procedure.
- Possible alteration in comfort related to test procedure.
- Possible knowledge deficit related to required dietary modifications.
- Possible anxiety related to possible test results.
- Potential complication: bleeding.

Planning. The key factor regarding planning refers to dietary restrictions. Many studies such as fasting blood sugar (see p. 310) and cholesterol/triglyceride levels (p. 33) require that the patient remain fasting for a designated period of time. Some blood levels, such as cortisol (p. 300), follow a diurnal pattern; this factor must be considered when blood levels are drawn. In general, blood studies are collected when the patient is in a basal or resting state, such as bed rest. Test results on outpatients can be affected by strenuous exercise. Patient posture can also affect certain blood results (for example, albumin) because the vascular compartment is more diluted when one is lying down than when one is standing. With the exception of a glucose tolerance test (see p. 312), most blood tests require only a few minutes to perform.

Intervention. Blood tests are usually drawn by a phlebotomist with a 20-22 gauge needle. However, on many units, nurses perform a large portion of the bloodwork. Gloves should be worn when collecting blood specimens. Blood collection tubes have color-coded stoppers to indicate the presence or absence of different types of additives. Charts are available from the laboratory indicating the type of tube needed for the particular blood tests (for example, blue-top for coagulation studies and gray-top for a glucose determination). Blood should not be drawn from an extremity that is already being used for an IV infusion or for blood administration. If there is no other alternative, the IV drip should be turned off for 3 to 5 minutes before the blood is obtained. This fact should be noted on the laboratory slip.

Blood can also be obtained from an indwelling venous catheter, such as a triple lumen catheter (TLC). Patient unit procedure manuals offer specific guidelines stating the appropriate amount of blood to be drawn from the catheter and discarded before it is collected for laboratory studies. The guidelines also indicate the amount and type of solution needed to flush the catheter to prevent it from being clogged by blood.

Skin punctures can be used for blood tests on capillary blood. Common puncture sites include the fingertips, earlobes, and heel surfaces. Fingertips are often used for small children, and the heel is the most commonly used site for infants. The first drop of blood is discarded, and the blood specimen is collected in capillary tubes or on special filter paper.

Blood cultures should be collected before the initiation of antibiotic therapy. They are usually drawn when the patient manifests a fever. Generally, two or three cultures are taken at 30-minute intervals from different venipuncture sites. The proposed puncture site and the top of tube should be carefully cleansed with an antiseptic solution, such as povidone-iodine solution (Betadine). The culture bottle should be taken immediately to the laboratory.

Evaluation. After a blood specimen is drawn, pressure should be applied to the puncture site and the site should be assessed for bleeding. If venous bleeding persists longer than 5 minutes, a physician should be notified. The laboratory report should be interpreted with caution because error or variations can occur anywhere in the process of patient preparation; specimen collection, handling, and transport; lab analysis; and recording of results. Factors such as diet, activity level, stress, time of day, and drug therapy also affect normal values.

Urine studies

Assessment. Urine tests are easy to obtain and provide valuable information about many areas of the body such as kidney function, glucose metabolism, and various hormone levels. The need for a particular urine test is determined and used to guide patient education. The ability of the patient to obtain specimens appropriately should be assessed to determine necessary nursing interventions.

Nursing Diagnoses/Collaborative Problems for Urine Studies

- Possible knowledge deficit related to test purpose, preparation, and procedure.
- Possible anxiety related to possible test results.

Planning. The type of urine specimen required is important in planning nursing care. Routine urinalysis is best performed using the first morning specimen because it is more concentrated. Random specimens can be collected anytime. Timed or composite specimens are done for chemical quantitative determinations.

A complete specimen must be collected for all timed specimens.

Intervention. For a routine analysis, no special instructions are needed. The patient should be given a urine container the night before so that the morning specimen can be collected. If a culture and sensitivity study is required, the perineal area or penis should be cleansed with an antiseptic. After voiding is initiated, a sterile container is then placed in position to collect a midstream collection. The container is then removed after 5 to 50 ml of urine is obtained; then voiding is completed. Gloves should be worn when assisting the patient with specimen collection.

Timed or composite urine specimens are collected over a period that may range anywhere from 2 to 24 hours. In order to collect a timed specimen, the patient is instructed to void and discard the first specimen. This is noted as the start time of the test. All subsequent urine is saved in a special container for the designated period of time. A preservative is usually used in the collection container. At the end of the specified time period, the patient voids and then adds the urine to the specimen container, thus completing the collection process. The container is then taken to the laboratory.

Evaluation. Because of the noninvasive means of collecting urine specimens, generally no specific nursing interventions are needed after the test. Test results determine the need for a more detailed diagnostic evaluation.

Fecal studies

Assessment. Fecal studies may be used for microbiologic studies, chemical determinations, and parasitic examinations. The type of analysis determines the collection method and proper handling of the specimen. These factors are used to guide patient education.

Nursing Diagnoses/Collaborative Problems for Fecal Studies

- Possible knowledge deficit related to test purpose, preparation, and procedure.

Planning. Although stool collection appears to be a simple procedure, various factors (such as other diagnostic studies, medications, and food) need to be considered in planning the collection. For example, if the patient is also scheduled for x-ray studies using barium sulfate, it is best to collect the stool specimen first. Various medications (for example, tetracyclines and antidiarrheal preparations) affect the detection of intestinal parasites (see p. 80). Stool tests for occult blood (see p. 74) can give false positive results if patients have eaten red meat. It is recommended that the diet be free from meat and fish 2 days prior to testing stools for occult blood. Fecal fat determination (see p. 128) can be collected over a 1 to 5 day range. An accurate and complete collection is vitally important for determining malabsorption syndromes.

Intervention. Stool specimens should be collected in a clean, wide-mouthed container. Urine and toilet paper should not be mixed with the specimen. Both can contaminate the specimen and alter the test results. Generally, stool specimens should be delivered to the laboratory within 30 minutes after passage. As with all types of bodily fluids, the specimen should be handled with care because it represents a potential source of infected material.

Evaluation. Results are assessed to determine appropriate follow-up care of the patient. Since stool collection is noninvasive, no special nursing measures are generally required.

X-ray studies

Assessment. Because of the ability of x-rays to penetrate human tissue, x-rays studies provide a picture of bodily structures which looks like a negative of a photograph. X-ray tests can be as simple as a routine chest x-ray (see p. 136) or as complex as a dye-enhanced cardiac catheterization (see p. 26). With the increasing concern about radiation exposure, it is important to realize that the patient may want to know if the proposed benefit outweighs the risk involved. Rationale for having the test must be clearly addressed in patient education. The patient should also be assessed for any similar or recent x-ray procedures or allergies to iodine dye. Women in their childbearing years should have x-ray examinations during menses or 10 to 14 days after the onset of menses to avoid exposure to a fetus. Pregnant women should not have x-ray procedures because of risk to the fetus.

Nursing Diagnoses/Collaborative Problems for X-Ray Studies

- Possible knowledge deficit related to test purpose, preparation, and procedure.
- Possible anxiety related to unknown sensations of the procedure.
- Possible anxiety related to possible test results.
- Possible alteration in comfort related to test procedure.
- Possible alteration in bowel elimination related to the need for a bowel preparation.
- Possible fluid volume deficit related to nothing by mouth (NPO) status.
- Potential complication: adverse reaction or allergy.

Planning. Several important questions need to be addressed in planning x-ray studies. (1) Are other diagnostic studies ordered? The proper sequencing of radiologic exams is essential. X-ray studies using barium should be scheduled after ultrasonography studies. Barium enemas should follow intravenous pyelograms (IVP). (2) What dietary restrictions are needed? Studies such as the barium enema (see p. 76) and intravenous pyelograms (see p. 232) require that the patient be NPO. (3) Are bowel preparations necessary? Barium enemas and intravenous pyelograms, for example, usually require bowel cleansing regimes to afford appropriate x-ray visualization. (4) Are signed consent forms needed?

Intervention. Most x-ray examinations are performed in the x-ray department by technicians. Metal objects such as necklaces and watches must be removed because they obscure visualization. Since the type of x-ray procedure varies, the patient is instructed regarding proper positioning, holding of breath, or receiving a contrast material such as iodine dye or barium by the oral, intravenous, or rectal route. Shielding of the abdominal organs and testes should be provided.

Evaluation. Patient aftercare is determined by the type of x-ray procedure. For example, a patient having a simple chest x-ray study will not require any special post-procedure care. However, invasive x-ray procedures involving contrast dye, such as cardiac catheterization (see p. 26), require extensive nursing measures to detect potential complications. Results are evaluated to determine when the patient may return to normal diet and activity levels.

Nuclear scanning (radionuclide scanning, scintigraphy)

Assessment. With the administration of a radionuclide and subsequent detection of the measurement of radiation from a particular organ, functional abnormalities of various body areas (such as the brain, heart, lung, and bones) can be detected. Because the half-lives of the radioisotopes are short, only minimal radiation exposure to patients and others occurs. The patient's knowledge and understanding of this information is important in patient education. Although the amount of radioactivity is very small, nuclear scanning is not usually recommended for pregnant or lactating women.

Nursing Diagnoses/Collaborative Problems for Nuclear Scanning

- Possible knowledge deficit related to test purpose, preparation, and procedure.
- Possible anxiety related to fear of radiation.
- Possible anxiety related to possible test results.

Planning. Many of the scanning procedures (for example, cardiac and lung) do not require any special preparations. However, a few have special requirements. For bone scanning (see p. 458), the patient is encouraged to drink several glasses of water between the time of the injection of the isotope and the actual scanning. For some studies, blocking agents may need to be given to prevent other organs from taking up isotopes. For example, Lugol's solution will protect the thyroid from iodine-tagged radionuclides. Several dietary and drug restrictions are also essential before thyroid scanning (see p. 282). Minutes to hours after administration of the isotope, a scintillation camera takes radioactivity readings from the target organ and feeds them to a computer, which produces a two-dimensional scan of the organ. Signed consent forms may be required.

Intervention. A small amount of an organspecific radionuclide is given orally or injected intravenously. After the radioisotope concentrates in the desired area, the area is scanned. The scanning procedure usually takes place in the nuclear medicine department. However, the patient may be administered a radionuclide on the hospital unit and then taken to the nuclear medicine department at the designated time. The patient must lie still during the scanning.

Evaluation. Because little risk is associated with scanning procedures, major nursing assessments are not needed. Patients are usually encouraged to drink extra fluids to enhance excretion of the radionuclide. Although the amount of radionuclide excreted in the urine is very low, rubber gloves are sometimes recommended if the urine must be handled. Some hospitals may advise the patient to flush the toilet several times after voiding.

Ultrasound studies

Assessment. In diagnostic ultrasonography, a harmless high-frequency sound wave is emitted and penetrates the organ being studied. The sound waves bounce back to the sensor and are electronically converted into a picture of the organ. Ultrasonography is used to assess a wide variety of bodily areas including the pelvis, abdomen, heart, and pregnant uterus.

Nursing Diagnoses/Collaborative Problems for Ultrasound Studies

- Possible knowledge deficit related to test purpose, preparation, and procedure.
- Possible anxiety related to possible test results.

Planning. Most ultrasound procedures require little or no preparation. However, the patient having a pelvic sonogram (see p. 358) needs a full bladder, and the patient having an ultrasound examination of the gallbladder (see p. 104) must be kept NPO preprocedure. Signed consent forms may be required.

Intervention. Ultrasound examinations are usually performed in an ultrasound room; however, they can be performed on the patient unit. A greasy paste is applied to the skin overlying the organ. This paste is used to enhance sound transmission and reception by providing an airless buffer; air impedes transmission of sound waves to the body.

Evaluation. Because of the noninvasive nature of ultrasonography, no special nursing measures are needed after the study except for helping the patient remove the ultrasound paste. This procedure may be a preliminary test to some invasive procedure. In that case, nursing interventions will be focused on assessing the patient's need and understanding for the next study.

Endoscopy procedures

Assessment. With the help of a lighted, flexible instrument, internal structures of many areas of the body (such as the stomach, colon, joints, bronchi, urinary system, and biliary tree) can be directly viewed. The specific purpose and procedure should be reviewed with the patient.

Nursing Diagnoses/Collaborative Problems for Endoscopic Procedures

- Possible knowledge deficit related to test purpose, preparation, and procedure.
- Possible alteration in comfort related to procedure.
- High risk for injury related to the effects of sedatives.
- Possible anxiety related to unknown sensations of the test.

- Possible alteration in elimination related to need for bowel prep.
- Possible fluid volume deficit related to need for NPO status.
- Possible anxiety related to possible test results.
- Potential complication: bleeding.
- Potential complication: perforation.

Planning. Preparation for endoscopic procedures varies according to the internal structure to be examined. For example, examination of the stomach (gastroscopy) (see p. 64) will require the passage of an instrument through the esophagus to the stomach. The patient is kept NPO for 8 to 12 hours before the test to prevent gagging, vomiting, and aspiration. For colonoscopy (see p. 78), an instrument is passed through the rectum and into the colon; therefore, the bowel must be cleansed and free of fecal material to afford proper visualization. Arthroscopic examination of the knee joint is usually done under general anesthesia, which necessitates routine preoperative care. Endoscopic examinations should precede barium studies. A signed consent form is required.

Intervention. Endoscopic procedures are preferably performed in a specially equipped endoscopy room or in the operating room by a physician. However, some kinds can safely be performed at the bedside. Air is usually instilled into the bowel during the examination to maintain patency of the bowel lumen and to afford better visualization. This sometimes causes gas pains. In addition to visualization of the desired area, special procedures can be performed. Biopsies can be obtained and bleeding ulcers can be cauterized. Also, knee surgery can be performed during arthroscopy (see p. 429).

Evaluation. Specific postprocedure nursing interventions are determined by the type of endoscopic examination performed. All procedures have the potential complications of perforation and bleeding. Most procedures use some type of sedation. Safety precautions should be observed until the effects of the sedatives have worn off. After gastroscopy (see p. 64) and similar studies, the patient should not eat or drink anything until the gag reflex returns. After colonoscopy (see p. 78) and similar studies, the patient may complain of rectal discomfort. A warm tub bath may be soothing.

The remainder of this book is organized according to body systems. For example, Chapter 2 contains the laboratory and diagnostic studies related to the cardiovascular system. Key information for applying the nursing process to a specific diagnostic study are found in the "rationale," "procedure," "contraindications," and "nursing considerations" sections, which are described for each study. When the nursing diagnosis reads "see blood studies," it refers to the general nursing diagnoses listed with blood studies in this overview chapter. This referral is made to avoid unnecessary repetition throughout the book. Any additional nursing diagnoses are listed with the study in the chapter where they are described. Some special studies, such as cardiac catheterization (see p. 26), have all the nursing diagnoses listed with its description to enhance understanding of complex diagnostic procedures.

BIBLIOGRAPHY

Alfaro R: Application of the nursing process: a step-by-step guide, Philadelphia, 1986, JB Lippincott.

Carpenito LJ: Handbook of nursing diagnosis, ed 2, Philadelphia, 1987, JB Lippincott.

Carpenito L: Nursing diagnosis: application to clinical practice, ed 4, Philadelphia, 1992, JB Lippincott.

Chapter 2

DIAGNOSTIC STUDIES USED IN THE ASSESSMENT OF THE CARDIOVASCULAR SYSTEM

ANATOMY AND PHYSIOLOGY

The heart is located within the mediastinum (the midline cavity between the lungs) and is divided by a septum into the right and left sides. The right side contains unoxygenated (that is, "prepulmonary") blood, and the left side contains the oxygenated (that is, "postpulmonary") blood. Each side is composed of an atrium and a ventricle (Figure 2-1). Unoxygenated venous blood from the venae cavae enters the right atrium and flows into the right ventricle. This ventricle pumps the blood forward into the pulmonary artery leading to the lungs, where it is oxygenated. The oxygenated blood then enters the left atrium, which pumps it into the left ventricle. The left ventricle then pumps the blood into the aorta and through the arteries of the body. The pumping force of the left ventricle pushes the blood through the arterial and venous systems in order to provide the return of blood to the heart.

The flow of blood must be constantly "forward." Valves exist between all chambers of the heart to prevent any backward flow of blood. The tricuspid and mitral (atrioventricular) valves are located between the atria and ventricles on the right and left sides of the heart, respectively. These valves prevent potentially harmful backflow of blood from the ventricles into the atria. The pulmonary valve is located between the right ventricle and the pulmonary artery, and the aortic valve is located between the left ventricle and the aorta. These semilunar valves prevent potentially harmful backflow of the blood from the aorta and pulmonary artery to the ventricles.

The heart wall is made up of three distinct tissue layers in both the atria and the ventricles. The bulk of the heart wall is called the myocar-

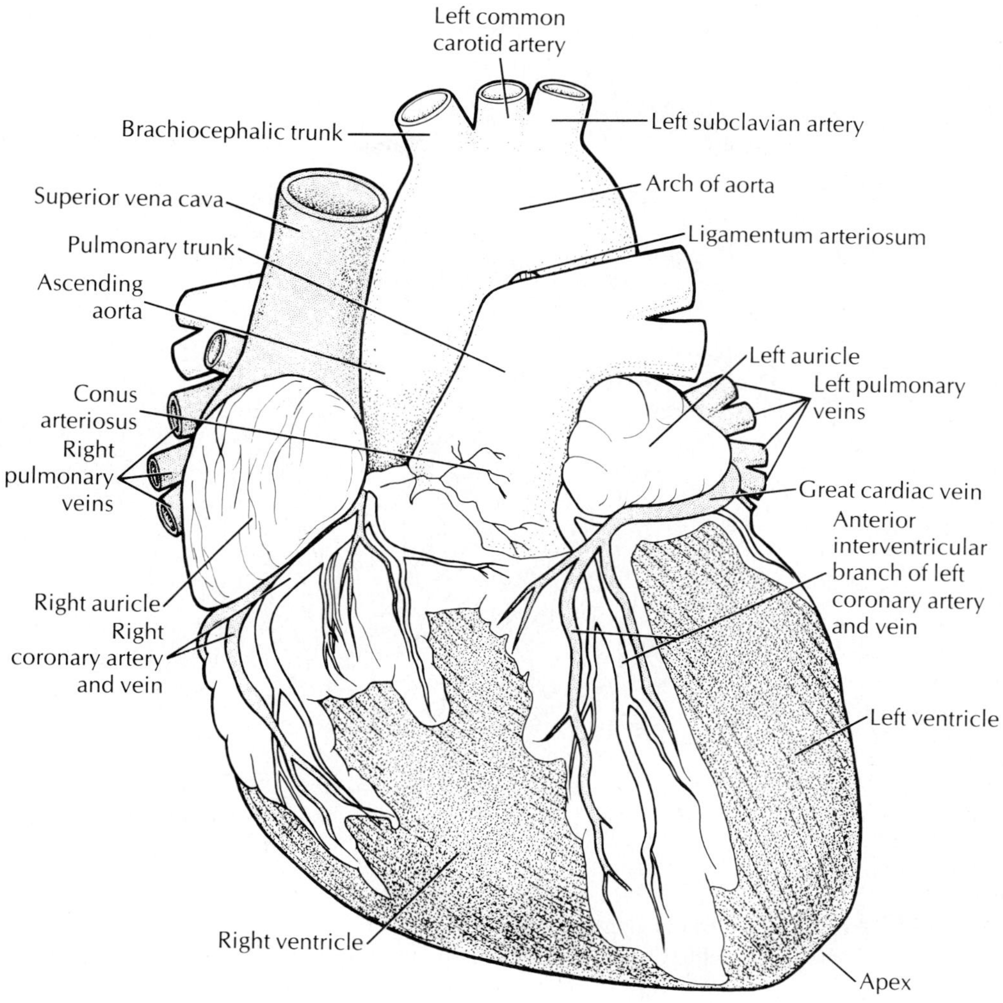

FIGURE 2-1. Anterior view of the heart and great vessels.

dium. The inner lining surface, which comes in contact with the blood, is called the *endocardium.* The outer lining of the heart wall is called the epicardium. The heart is surrounded by a sacklike tissue called *pericardium.* The myocardial cells receive their blood supply from the right and left coronary arteries, which arise from the aorta near its origin (see Figure 2-1).

Specialized cells, located in the superior portion of the atrial wall, form the sinoatrial (SA) node. Here the electrical impulse, which normally stimulates myocardial contraction, begins. The SA node generates about 60 to 100 impulses/minute in the resting state. These impulses are conducted through the atrial muscle cells to the atrioventricular (AV) node, located in the lower part of the right atrium. The AV node then relays the electrical impulses by way of specialized nerve fibers known as the bundle of His, which is located in the septum between the right and the left ventricles. Purkinje fibers then carry the impulses throughout the ventricular walls, stimulating the myocardium to contract (Figure 2-2).

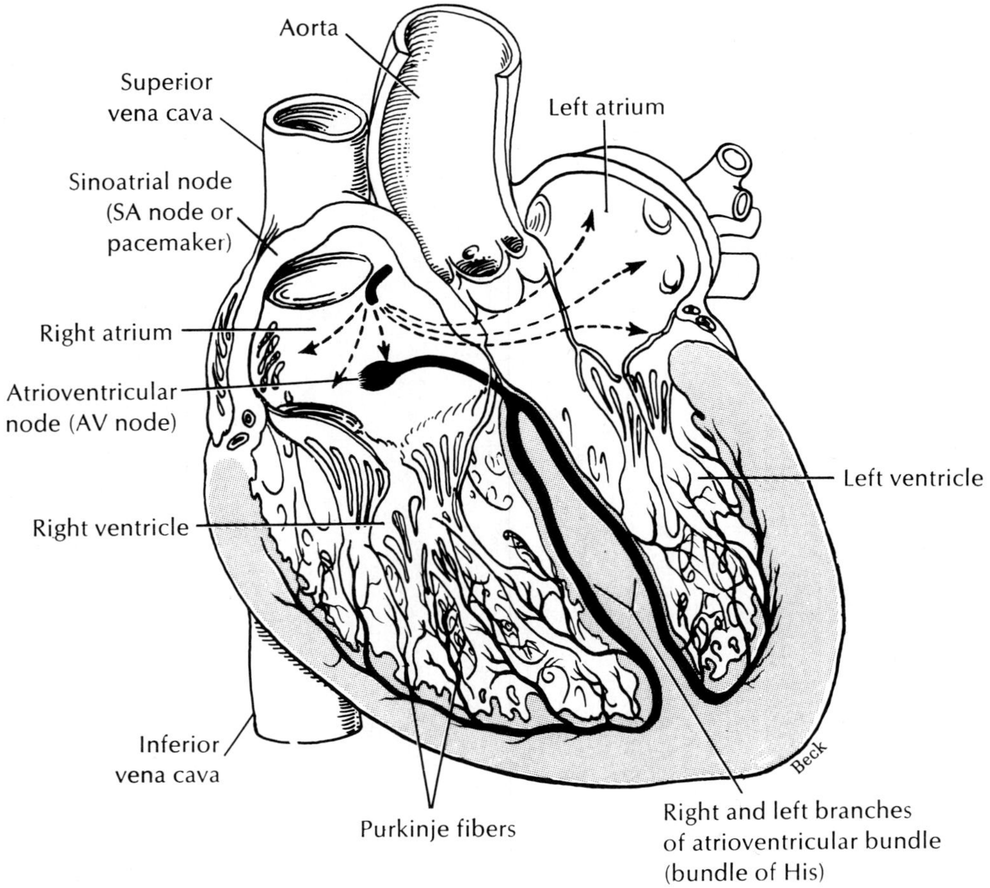

FIGURE 2-2. Electrical conduction system of the heart.

From Anthony CP and Kolthoff NJ: Textbook of anatomy and physiology, ed 9, St Louis, 1975, The CV Mosby Co.

If the SA node fails to generate an electric impulse, the AV node (with an intrinsic rate of 40 to 60 impulses/minute) takes over as impulse generator. If both the SA node and the AV node malfunction, the myocardium will beat at its own ventricular intrinsic rate of 20 to 40 beats/minute.

CASE STUDY 1: ANGINA

Mr. J.P. was a 48-year-old man admitted to the coronary care unit complaining of substernal chest pain. During the 4 months preceding admission, he noted chest pain radiating to his neck and jaw during exercise or emotional upsets. The pain dissipated when he discontinued the activity or relaxed. The results of his physical examination were essentially normal except for a midsystolic murmur heard best over the aortic area of the precordium (second intercostal space on the right sternal border).

Studies	**Results**
Routine laboratory work	Within normal limits (WNL)
Cardiac enzyme studies	

Studies	Results
Creatine phosphokinase (CPK)	20 mU/ml (normal: 5-75 mU/ml)
CPK-MM	100%
CPK-MB	0%
CPK-BB	0%
Lactic dehydrogenase (LDH)	120 ImU/ml (normal: 90-200 ImU/ml)
Serum aspartate aminotransferase (AST; formerly serum glutamic oxaloacetic transaminase, SGOT)	24 IU/L (normal: 5-40 IU/L)
Electrocardiography (EKG)	Evidence of left ventricular hypertrophy
Chest x-ray study	WNL
Exercise stress test	Positive: pain reproduced, ST segment depression noted on EKG (normal: negative)
Echocardiography	Decreased motion of the aortic valve leaflets; remaining valves WNL
Cardiac catheterization	*Pressures* All WNL except: Left ventricular systolic pressure: 180 mm Hg (normal: 90-140 mm Hg) Aortic systolic pressure: 130 mm Hg (normal: 90-140 mm Hg) Ventricular-aortic pressure gradient: 50 mm Hg (normal: 0) *Left ventricular function* Cardiac output: 3.5 L/min (normal: 3-6 L/min) End diastolic volume (EDV): 60 ml/m^2 (normal: 50-90 ml/m^2) End systolic volume (ESV): 22 ml/m^2 (normal: 25 ml/m^2) Stroke volume (SV): 38 ml/m^2 (SV = EDV − ESV) Ejection fraction: 0.63 (normal: 0.67 ± 0.07) *Cineventriculography* Hypertrophy of left ventricle, normal muscle function (normal: normal ventricle) *Analysis of O_2 gas content* No shunting (normal: no shunting) *Coronary angiography (coronary cineangiography)* 90% narrowing of left coronary artery (see Figure 2-9) (normal: no narrowing)
Cardiac radionuclear scanning	Scans normal except for thallium scan, which showed localized area of decreased uptake in the myocardium during exercise
Serum lipids	
Total	1100 mg/dl (normal: 400-1000 mg/dl)
Cholesterol	502 mg/dl (normal: 150-250 mg/dl)
Triglyceride	198 mg/dl (normal: 40-150 mg/dl)
Phospholipids	400 mg/dl (normal: 150-380 mg/dl)

Cardiac radionuclear scanning, EKG, and serial cardiac enzyme studies ruled out the possibility of myocardial infarction. Stress testing and a thallium nucleotide scan indicated that the patient was having exercise-related myocardial ischemia. Echocardiography indicated associated aortic stenosis. Cardiac catheterization (with cineventriculography) demonstrated near-normal ventricular function. The ventricular-to-aortic pressure gradient documented an aortic stenosis, and coronary angiography indicated significant narrowing of the left coronary artery. The patient's angina was then thought to be caused by a combination of coronary artery disease, aortic stenosis, and ventricular hypertrophy. Open heart surgery was performed. His aortic valve was replaced with a prosthesis, and an aortocoronary artery bypass graft was performed. Postoperatively, Mr. J.P. did well. Because his serum lipids study showed type IIa hyperlipidemia, a low-cholesterol diet was prescribed. Six months later he was asymptomatic and jogging 5 miles per day.

DISCUSSION OF TESTS

Cardiac enzyme studies

Creatine phosphokinase (CP, CPK) or creatine kinase (CK)

Normal values:

Total CPK

Adult/elderly: male, 12-70 U/ml or 55-170 U/L (SI units) female, 10-55 U/ml or 30-135 U/L (SI units)

Values are higher after exercise.

Newborn: 68-580 U/L (SI units)

Isoenzymes

CPK-MM: 100%

CPK-MB: 0%

CPK-BB: 0%

Serum aspartate aminotransferase (AST), formerly serum oxaloacetic transaminase (SGOT)

Normal findings:

Adult: 8-20 U/L, 5-40 IU/L, or 8-20 U/L (SI units); females tend to have slightly lower values than men.

Elderly: values slightly higher than adult

Child: values similar to adult

Newborn/infant: 15-60 U/L

Lactic dehydrogenase (LDH)

Normal values:

Adult/elderly: 45-90 U/L (30° C), 115-225 IU/L, or 0.4-1.7 μmol/L (SI units)

Isoenzymes in adult/elderly values

LDH-1: 17%-27%

LDH-2: 27%-37%

LDH-3: 18%-25%

LDH-4: 3%-8%

LDH-5: 0%-5%

Child: 60-170 U/L (30° C)

Infant: 100-250 U/L

Newborn: 160-450 U/L

Rationale. When the heart muscle is damaged, enzymes contained within the muscle cells are released into the bloodstream, causing increased serum levels. Studies of cardiac enzymes (CPK, AST, LDH) are useful in confirming a myocardial infarction (MI) when they are viewed in relation to the EKG and the clinical picture. The rate of liberation of specific enzymes varies following infarction, and the temporal pattern of enzyme elevation is of diagnostic importance. Enzyme determinations are also useful in following the course of a myocardial infarction and in detecting an extension of it. (See Table 2-1.)

TABLE 2-1. Time Frame for Cardiac Enzyme Changes after Myocardial Injury

Enzyme	Begins to rise (within X hours)	Peaks	Returns to normal
CPK	6	18 hr	2-3 days
CPK-MB	3-6	12-24 hr	12-48 hr
AST (formerly SGOT)	6-10	12-48 hr	3-4 days
LDH	24-72	3-4 days	14 days

CPK. The enzyme CPK (or CK, as it is now often called) is found predominantly in the heart muscle, skeletal muscle, and brain. The serum CPK level rises within 6 hours after damage to myocardial cells, peaks in approximately 18 hours, and returns to normal in 2 or 3 days. Levels of CPK are generally measured until they peak and decline. Prolonged elevated CPK levels indicate ongoing heart muscle injury. Generally, the higher the CPK levels, the greater the size of the infarction. Because minor insults to skeletal muscle (such as vigorous exercise, a fall, or an intramuscular injection) can elevate total CPK levels, it is not reliably specific as an indicator for myocardial damage. For example, potential sources of total CPK elevation include myopathy associated with chronic alcoholism, electrical cardioversion, cardiac catheterization, hypothyroidism, stroke, surgery, or clofibrate therapy. Fractionation of CPK into isoenzymes to quantitate the cardiac component of the total enzyme provides a much more specific index of cardiac muscle damage.

Creatine phosphokinase can be fractionated into three isoenzymes: CPK-BB (CPK_1), CPK-MB (CPK_2); and CPK-MM (CPK_3). The isoenzyme MB provides a unique marker for damaged myocardial cells. The CPK-MB level begins to rise 3 to 6 hours after the onset of infarction, peaks in 12 to 24 hours, and returns to normal in 12 to 48 hours. Since small infarcts may not elevate the MB fraction dramatically, it is important to note the time the blood specimen is drawn. Some physicians recommend four specimens, one obtained every 6 hours after the onset of the symptoms. The CPK-MB level does not rise after angina without myocardial infarction, pulmonary embolism, or congestive heart failure.

The CPK-BB isoenzyme is found predominately in the brain and lungs, and the CPK-MM isoenzyme is found primarily in skeletal muscle. The CPK-MM is the isoenzyme that comprises almost all of the circulatory enzymes in healthy people. When isoenzyme levels are reported, percentage levels of each are recorded. Normally CPK levels consist of 100% of the CPK-MM isoenzyme. After a myocardial infarction one may find a 60% elevation of CPK-MB and a 40% elevation of CPK-MM. After a stroke there may be an 80% elevation of CPK-BB and a 20% elevation of CPK-MM.

More cardiologists are now accepting positive CPK and CPK-MB levels as diagnostic of a myocardial infarction if the patient was admitted for chest pain within 24 hours. (The LDH and AST levels are not routinely measured.) This approach allows the cardiologist to prove or disprove the diagnosis of an MI within 24 hours without having the patient unnecessarily occupy a bed in the coronary care unit (CCU) for additional days.

The total CPK level is being increasingly used to time and quantify the infarction. This timing is important because of efforts to reverse or prevent infarctions with *thrombolytic therapy*. When a cardiologist considers a patient a candidate for thrombolytic therapy, the CPK level is measured stat. If the CPK level is already elevated, the suggestion that the infarct has already occurred dictates that thrombolytic therapy should not be used. If the CPK is not elevated, thrombolytic therapy may be used.

Besides myocardial infarction, CPK-MB levels are elevated in patients with myocarditis, rhabdomyolysis, and Reye's syndrome.

CPK-BB levels are increased in patients who have experienced a stroke, seizure, pulmonary infarction, or intestinal ischemia.

CPK-MM levels indicate muscular dystrophy, myositis, or skeletal muscle injury.

AST. The enzyme AST is found in very high concentrations in the heart and liver and in moderately large amounts in the skeletal muscle, kidneys, and pancreas. After myocardial injury the AST level rises within 6 to 10 hours, peaks at 12 to 48 hours, and returns to normal in approximately 3 to 4 days. A characteristic rise in the AST level occurs in about 90% to 95% of patients with clinically proven MIs. The AST level does not usually rise in unstable angina, pericarditis, or rheumatic carditis. Liver disease (Chapter 4) will also cause elevation of the AST level and complicate enzyme diagnosis in the cardiac patient. Other conditions that may cause elevations of the AST level include administration of salicylates, opiates, or coumarin-type anticoagulants; primary muscle disease; cardiac operations; acute pancreatitis; extensive central nervous system damage; hemolytic crisis; eclampsia; crush injuries or burns; hypothyroidism; and infarction of the kidneys, spleen, or intestine. Drugs such as warfarin, digoxin, erythromycin, oral contraceptives, opiates, and salicylates can cause fictitiously high blood levels of AST.

LDH. The enzyme LDH is found in many body tissues, especially the heart, liver, kidneys, skeletal muscle, brain, red blood cells, and lungs. The serum LDH level rises within 24 to 72 hours after an MI, peaks in 3 to 4 days, and returns to normal in approximately 14 days. This makes the serum LDH level especially useful for a delayed diagnosis in myocardial infarction (for example, in cases where the patient reports having had severe chest pain 4 days ago). Because LDH is widely distributed through the body, the total LDH level is not a specific indicator of myocardial disease. LDH, like CPK, is more useful diagnostically when fractionated into isoenzymes. Five LDH isoenzymes, called LDH-1 through LDH-5, may be separated by electrophoresis. Isoenzyme LDH-1 predominates in the heart and red blood cells, while LDH-2 comes mostly from the reticuloendothelial system; LDH-3 comes from the lungs and other tissues; LDH-4 comes from the kidney, placenta, and pancreas; and LDH-5 is mainly from the liver and striated muscle. Serum levels of LDH-2 are higher than that of the other four isoenzymes.

In patients with MIs, the LDH-1 level is a more sensitive and specific indicator of myocardial infarction than total LDH level. Its sensitivity is greater than 95%. Most physicians consider myocardial infarction the diagnosis when LDH-1 activity is greater than LDH-2 activity (LDH-1/LDH-2 > 1). This is referred to as a *flipped* LDH because the typical LDH-1/LDH-2 ratio of <1 is reversed. In an acute myocardial infarction the flipped LDH ratio usually appears between 12 and 24 hours and is present within 48 hours in about 80% of patients. When LDH-2 is greater than LDH-1 (a normal LDH-1/LDH-2 ratio), it is considered reliable evidence against the myocardial infarction. The patient may have had a severe ischemic episode in the remote past or only minimal recent heart damage. Drugs that may cause increased LDH levels include alcohol, narcotics, anesthetics, aspirin, mithramycin, and procainamide.

Some laboratories measure only the LDH-1 level. An elevated LDH level with greater than 40% LDH-1 is considered diagnostic of myocardial damage.

Procedure. Peripheral venipuncture is performed, and one red-top tube of blood is drawn. Usually the CPK, LDH, and AST enzymes are drawn daily for 3 days and then again 1 week after the patient's admission. However this varies as hospitals attempt to economize. Hemolysis of blood should be avoided. Isoenzymes are separated by electrophoresis.

Contraindications. None.

Nursing considerations

Nursing Diagnoses/Collaborative Problems

See Blood studies, p. 2.

Nursing Implications with Rationale

- Discuss with the patient the need for frequent venipuncture. Allow the patient to discuss his or her fears.
- Rotate the venipuncture sites. Apply pressure to the venipuncture site after the procedure is completed. Observe the site for bleeding.
- Avoid hemolysis of blood because the red blood cells have high LDH levels and will produce falsely elevated LDH levels when hemolyzed.
- Avoid giving the patient with cardiac disease intramuscular (IM) injections, because the CPK level may be elevated from minor muscle trauma. If the patient did receive an IM injection in the emergency room before admission to your unit, indicate the date and time of the injection on the lab slip.
- On each lab slip for cardiac enzyme studies include the date and time when the blood was drawn. This record enables a more accurate interpretation of the temporal pattern of enzyme level rise.

Electrocardiography

(EKG, ECG)

Normal values: normal rate (60-100 beats/minute), rhythm, and wave deflections.

Rationale. The electrocardiogram (EKG) is a graphic representation of the electric impulses the heart generates during the cardiac cycle. The electric impulses are conducted to the body's surface, where they are detected by electrodes placed on the patient's limbs and chest to reflect activity from a variety of spatial perspectives. The EKG lead system is composed of five electrodes. Electrodes are placed on the four extremities and on varying sites on the chest. Each combination of electrodes is called a lead.

A 12-lead EKG provides a comprehensive view of the flow of the heart's electric currents in two different planes. There are six limb leads (combination of electrodes on the extremities) and six chest leads (corresponding to six sites on

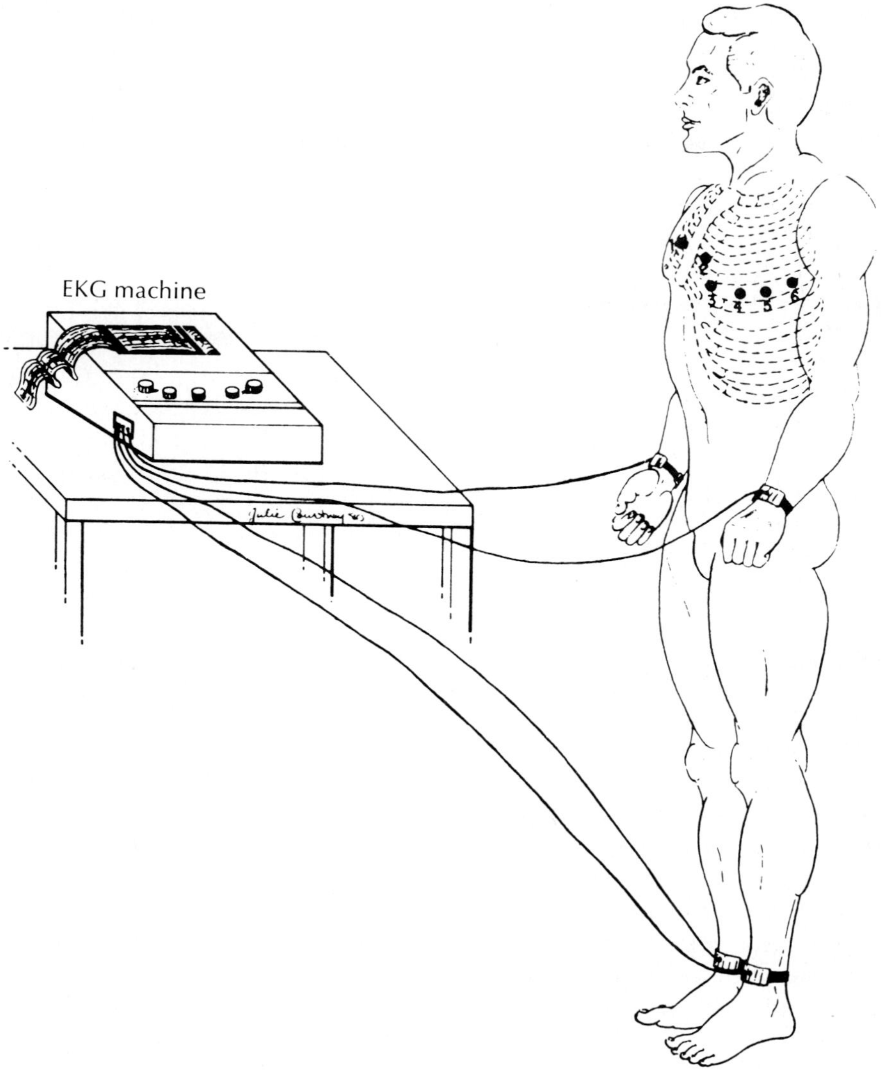

FIGURE 2-3. Placement of EKG electrodes.

the chest). Leads I, II, and III are considered the "standard" limb leads. Lead I records the difference in potential between the left arm (LA) and the right arm (RA). Lead II records the electric potential between the RA and the left leg (LL). Lead III reflects the difference between the LA and the LL. The right leg (RL) electrode is an inactive ground in all leads. There are three "augmented" limb leads: aV_R, aV_L, aV_F (a, augmented; V, vector [unipolar]; R, right arm; L, left arm; F, left foot or leg). The augmented leads measure the electrode potential between the center of the heart and the right arm (aV_r), the left arm (aV_L), and the left leg (aV_F). The six standard chest, or "precordial," leads (V_1 to V_6) are recorded by placing electrodes at six different positions on the chest, surrounding the heart (Figure 2-3).

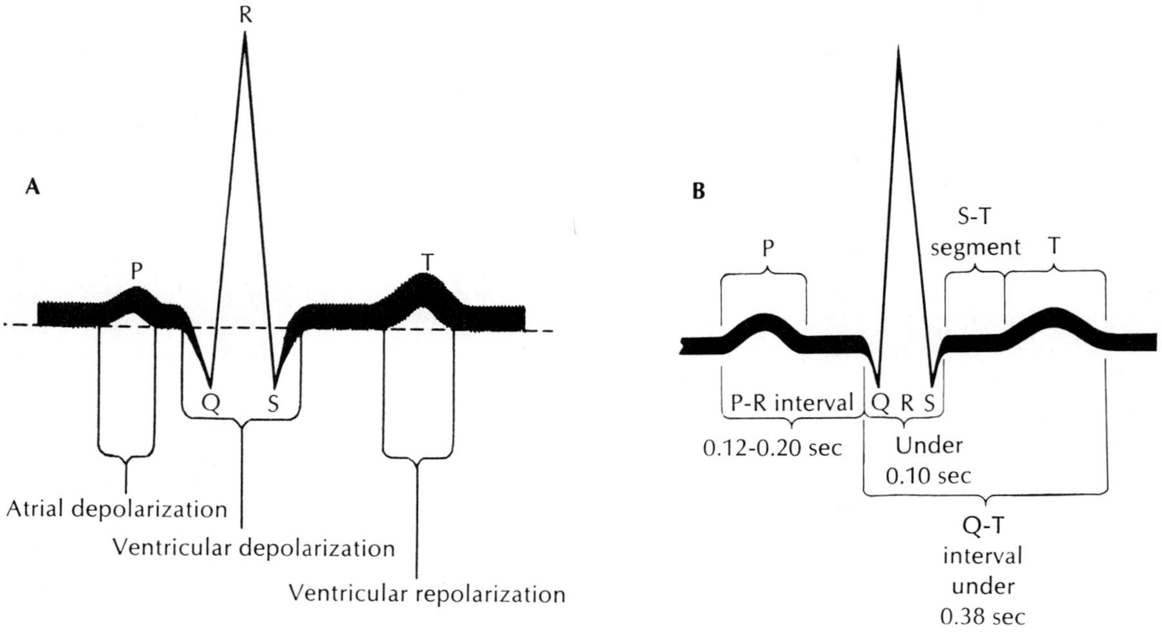

FIGURE 2-4. **A,** Normal EKG deflections during depolarization and repolarization of the atrium and ventricles. **B,** Principal EKG intervals between P, QRS, and T waves.
A From Anthony CP and Kolthoff NJ: Textbook of anatomy and physiology, ed 9, St Louis, 1975, The CV Mosby Co.

Electrocardiograms are recorded on special paper with a graphic background of horizontal and vertical lines for rapid measurement of time intervals (*X* coordinate) and voltages (*Y* coordinate). Time duration is measured by vertical lines 1 mm apart, each representing 0.04 second. Voltage is measured by horizontal lines 1 mm apart. Five small squares are equal to 0.5 mV.

The normal EKG pattern is composed of waves arbitrarily designated by the letters P, Q, R, S, and T. The Q, R, and S waves are grouped together and described as the QRS complex. The typical EKG pattern and normal time intervals are shown in Figure 2-4. The significance of the waves and time intervals is as follows:

P wave—represents atrial depolarization that indicates atrial contraction. It represents electrical activity associated with the spread of the original impulse from the SA node through the atria (see Figure 2-2). If the P waves are absent or altered, the cardiac impulse originates outside the SA node.

P-R interval—represents the time required for the impulse to travel from the SA node to the AV node (see Figure 2-2). If this interval is prolonged, a conduction delay exists in the AV node (such as a first-degree heart block). If the P-R interval is shortened, the impulse must have reached the ventricle through a "short-cut" (as in Wolff-Parkinson-White syndrome).

QRS complex—represents ventricular depolarization. This complex consists of an initial downward (negative) deflection (Q wave), a large upward (positive) deflection (R wave), and a small downward deflection (S wave). A widened QRS complex indicates abnormal or prolonged ventricular depolarization time (such as in a bundle branch block).

ST segment—represents the period between the completion of depolarization and the beginning of repolarization of the ventricular muscle. This segment may be elevated or depressed in transient muscle ischemia (such as angina) or in muscle injury (such as in the early stages of myocardial infarction).

T wave—represents ventricular repolarization (that is, return to neutral electrical activity).

Through the analysis of these waveforms and time intervals valuable information about the heart may be obtained. The EKG is used primarily to identify abnormal heart rhythms (arrhythmias) and to diagnose acute myocardial infarction, conduction defects, and ventricular hypertrophy. It is important to note that the EKG may be normal even in the presence of heart disease if the heart disorder does not affect the electrical activity of the heart.

The EKG should be studied in an orderly manner. The five basic steps to the identification of cardiac arrhythmias are as follows:

1. *Calculate the heart rate.* This can be done easily by counting the number of complete cycles (R wave to R wave is one cycle) in a 6-inch strip (6 seconds) of EKG paper and multiplying this number by 10 to get the rate/minute. The normal rate should be 60 to 100 beats/minute. *Bradycardia* describes a rate below 60, and *tachycardia* describes rates over 100 (see Figure 2-5). Several other methods are also used to calculate heart rate.
2. *Measure the rhythm of the R waves.* R waves that occur at regular intervals constitute "regular rhythm." When the difference between two R waves is greater than 0.12 second, the ventricular rhythm is "irregular."
3. *Examine the P wave.* A normally positioned P wave (see Figure 2-4) preceding each QRS complex indicates a "sinus rhythm." If P waves are absent or abnormally shaped, the cardiac impulse is originating outside of the SA node (ectopic pacemaker).
4. *Measure the P-R interval.* An increase or decrease in this interval is an indication of a defect in the conduction system between the atria and the ventricles (see Figure 2-4).
5. *Measure the QRS complex.* A widened QRS complex indicates an intraventricular conduction defect (such as premature ventricular contractions, PVCs). See Figures 2-5 and 2-6 for a sample of normal sinus rhythm and some of the more common arrhythmias. A more thorough and comprehensive discussion of EKG interpretation may be found elsewhere and is beyond the scope of this chapter.

Procedure. The patient is placed in the supine position on a table or bed. The machine is turned on so that it will be ready to use after the electrodes are applied. The skin areas designated for electrode placement (see Figure 2-3) are prepared by using alcohol swabs or sandpaper to remove skin oil or debris. Sometimes the skin is shaved if the patient has a large amount of hair. Electrode paste is applied to ensure electrical conduction between the skin and the electrodes. The four limb leads are usually held in place by straps that encircle the extremity. Newer machines have clamps (much like a clothespin) that can easily be opened and applied. Many cardiologists recommend that arm electrodes be placed on the upper arm, because fewer muscle tremors are detected there. The chest leads (suction cups) are applied either one at a time, three at a time, or all six at once, depending on the type of EKG machine. These leads (Figure 2-3) are positioned as follows:

V_1: in the fourth intercostal space (4ICS) at the right sternal border
V_2: in 4ICS at the left sternal border
V_3: midway between V_2 and V_4
V_4: in 5ICS at the midclavicular line
V_5: at the left anterior axillary line at the level of V_4 horizontally
V_6: at the left midaxillary line on the level of V_4 horizontally

Although this procedure entails no discomfort for the patient, he or she must lie still without talking while the EKG is recorded. Cardiac

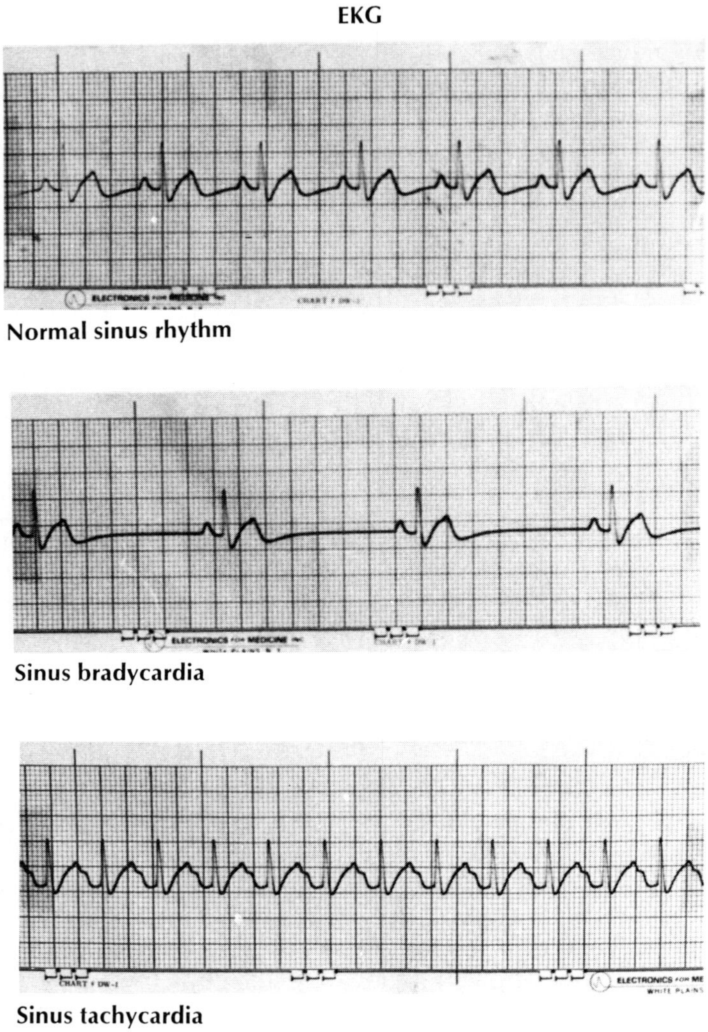

FIGURE 2-5. Common EKG rhythm strips. *Top,* Normal sinus rhythm (NSR) (rate, 80 beats/minute); *middle,* sinus bradycardia (rate, 40 beats/minute); *bottom,* sinus tachycardia (rate, 140 beats/minute).

technicians and nurses perform the procedure in less than 5 minutes in the "heart station" or at the bedside.

For some patients at high risk for malignant ventricular dysrhythmias, a *signal-averaged EKG (SAE)* can be performed. This test works by averaging several hundred QRS waveforms to detect late potentials that are likely to lead to ventricular dysrhythmias. SAEs have been a useful precursor to electrophysiologic studies (see page 37) because they can identify patients with unexplained syncope who may have ventricular tachycardias induced by the electrophysiologic study. SAEs can be performed at the bedside in approximately 15 to 20 minutes. This test must be ordered separately from a standard EKG.

If a continuous recording of the electrical ac-

EKG

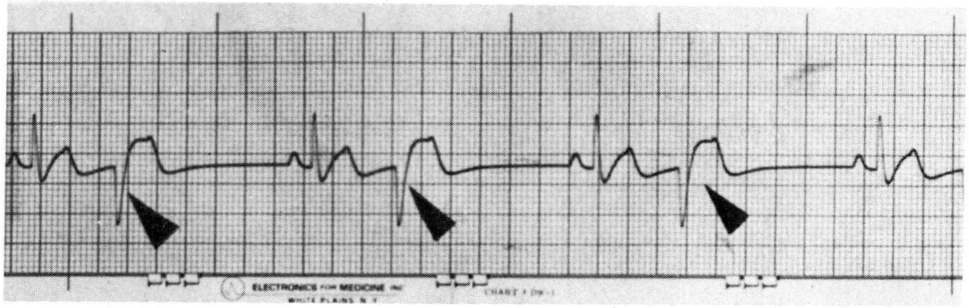

PVCs

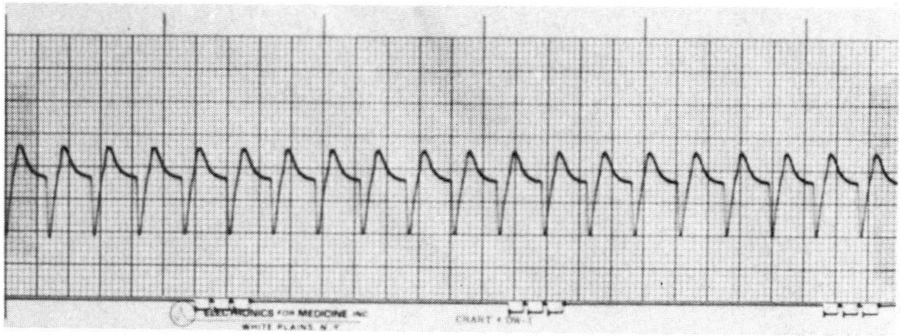

Ventricular tachycardia

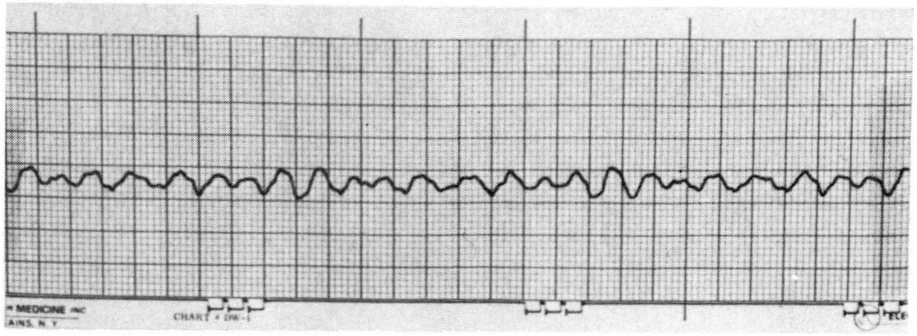

Ventricular fibrillation

FIGURE 2-6. Serious arrhythmias. *Top,* Multiple premature ventricular contractions (PVCs) (black pointers indicate PVCs); *middle,* ventricular tachycardia; *bottom,* ventricular fibrillation.

tivity of the heart is desired, a small, portable *Holter monitor* can be attached to the leads and carried by the patient in a sling around the chest or abdomen for up to several weeks. This is often referred to as *ambulatory monitoring* or *ambulatory electrocardiography.* With Holter monitoring, an EKG is recorded continuously on magnetic tape during unrestricted activity, rest, and sleep. The tape recorder is also equipped with a time clock permitting accurate time monitoring. The patient carries a diary and records daily activities to see if there is a correlation between the symptoms and EKG findings. Most units also have an "event marker," so that if the patient has any pain, syncope, or palpitations, the event marker will identify the symptom clearly on the tape. Holter monitoring is used primarily to identify suspected cardiac rhythm disturbance. It is also used to correlate rhythm disturbances with symptoms of dizziness, syncope, palpitations, or chest pain, and to assess pacemaker function, effectiveness of medications, and the mechanisms by which rhythm disturbance occurs. At the completion of the test period the tape is scanned for abnormalities.

Event recorders are now being used to follow patients with periodic "spells" or near-syncope. Event recorders are small recorders the patients may carry and attach to themselves if they feel symptoms or dysrhythmias. The recorders have electrodes that the patients simply hold to their chest to record the EKG. Some recorders are capable of storing the information, which can later be relayed over the phone to the physician's office. (This is convenient if patients have short spells of symptoms or dysrhythmias while driving, for instance.) Other recorders require that patients call the physician's office during the event so the EKG is directly transmitted. In the near future, event recorders will be small enough to be worn as a wristwatch.

Contraindications. This test is contraindicated in the uncooperative patient.

Nursing considerations

Nursing Diagnoses/Collaborative Problems

- Possible knowledge deficit related to test purpose, preparation, and procedure.
- Possible anxiety related to test results.

Nursing Implications with Rationale

- Explain the procedure to the patient. Assure him or her that the flow of electric current is *from* the patient. He or she will feel nothing during this procedure.
- Expose only the patient's chest and arms. Keep the abdomen and thighs adequately covered.
- Prepare the patient's skin and apply only a small amount of electrode gel. A large amount may produce a wandering baseline by allowing movement of the electrode. The gel will usually feel cold.
- Apply the electrodes and wires so that tension on the electrodes is avoided. Do not put the rubber straps on tightly. If the chest suction cup electrode will not remain in place by suction alone, instruct the patient to hold it in place.
- After the EKG is recorded, remove the electrodes from the patient's skin and wipe off the electrode gel.
- If *Holter monitoring* is being used, explain the procedure carefully to the patient. Instruct the patient in the use of the diary and event monitor. Inform the patient that the monitor cannot get wet; therefore, bathing, swimming, and showering must be avoided. Tell the patient that electric gadgets such as electric toothbrushes can cause artifacts on the EKG tape. Therefore, their use should be noted in the diary.

Exercise stress testing

(stress testing, exercise testing, electrocardiographic stress testing)

Normal value: negative (no significant symptoms or EKG abnormalities).

Rationale. Exercise stress testing is a noninvasive study that provides valuable cardiovascular information that cannot be obtained by examination of a patient in the resting state. The EKG, heart rate, and blood pressure are recorded while the patient engages in some type of physical activity (stress). The three methods of stress testing include climbing stair steps (Master's two-step test), pedaling a stationary bicycle, and walking a treadmill (Figure 2-7). The treadmill test is most frequently used today because it is the most standardized and reproducible.

The usual goal of the testing is to increase the heart rate either to just below maximum levels or until the patient attains a "target heart rate," which is 80% to 90% of the maximum heart rate.

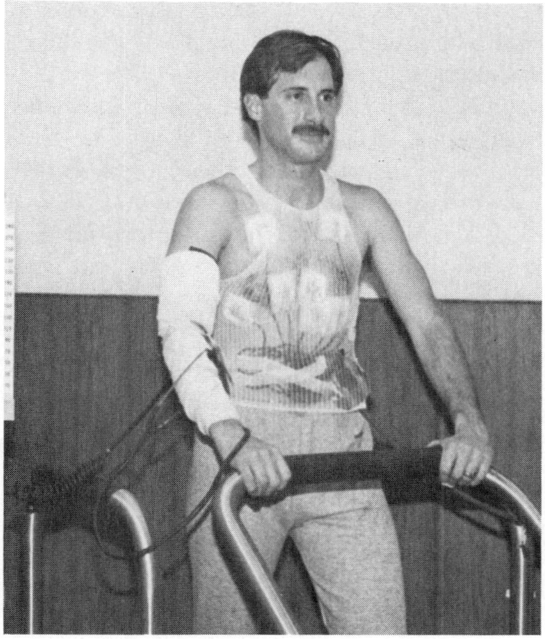

FIGURE 2-7. Exercise stress testing. Patient is walking on a treadmill while blood pressure, EKG, and other parameters are being monitored.

The test is stopped if the patient develops symptoms (symptom limited). Maximum heart rates are determined according to age and sex. The maximum heart rate for adults is about 150 to 200 beats/minute. Tables are available for predicted rates. The expected maximum heart rate should be adjusted if the patient is taking medications such as beta-blockers or calcium channel blockers, as well as any other drugs that affect heart rate.

All stress testing is *symptom limited.* This testing is used to evaluate the functional capacity of the heart or the result of therapy such as an exercise program, medication, or surgery. With this type of test, the exercise continues until symptoms develop or until the patient feels exhausted and can no longer continue. The study can also be stopped when 80% to 90% of the maximum heart rate is reached. This test provides valuable information regarding a specific exercise prescription for cardiac patients after a myocardial infarction.

Patients who are recovering from an acute myocardial infarction or from coronary artery bypass graft surgery may have a *limited-stress test.* The object of limited-stress testing is to determine if the patient may begin to increase activities after a heart attack. The heart rate chosen for the end point of this testing is the rate necessary to achieve usual activities after discharge, such as stair climbing, driving, or having sexual intercourse. Usually this rate is about 110 to 130 beats/minute.

Exercise stress testing can be done in single or multiple stages. With single-stage testing, the workload is held constant. An example of this is the Master's two-step test, which is seldom conducted today. In multistage testing (for example, pedaling a stationary bike or walking a treadmill) the workload is increased at regular intervals until a desired level is met. For example, the speed and incline of a treadmill may be increased at 2- to 5-minute intervals or the resistance that the patient must pedal on a bicycle is increased. Multistage testing is commonly referred to as graded exercise stress testing (GEST or GEX).

Exercise stress testing is based on the principle that occluded arteries are unable to meet the heart's increased demand for oxygen during the stress testing. This may lead to chest pain, fatigue, dyspnea, excessive tachycardia, or a fall in blood pressure—all reasons to discontinue the test. When the test is terminated prematurely for any other reason, the results are considered incomplete. ST segment displacement, which is most reliable characteristic of myocardial ischemia, may occur during or immediately after the stress test. The stress test is considered positive when the recording paper shows a depression of the ST segment of 1 mm (0.1 mV) below the baseline. The test is negative when there are no EKG abnormalities and the patient has no significant symptoms and attains the expected heart rate (see Procedure).

The indications for stress testing are the following:

1. To evaluate chest pain in a patient who is suspected of having coronary artery disease. If the pain can be reproduced during the exercise, then one may infer that the pain is caused by ischemic coronary artery disease.
2. To determine the limits of safe exercise during cardiac rehabilitation and to evaluate patients with cardiac disease before they start physical fitness programs.
3. To detect labile or exercise-related hypertension.
4. To detect exercise-related leg cramps indicative of peripheral vascular disease (intermittent claudication).
5. To evaluate the effectiveness of antiarrhythmic or antianginal treatment.
6. To stratify patients with lesions or suspected coronary artery disease into high risk or low risk categories.

Stress testing entails some risks, although they are uncommon. Complications include fatal cardiac arrhythmias and myocardial infarction.

Several new forms of stress testing have been developed for use with the patient in the recumbent position. These are generally used for patients unable to perform the usual exercise stress tests because of conditions such as severe arthritis, paralysis, or claudication. The heart can be stressed by having the patient perform leg exercises with a bicycle or squeeze isometric hand grips. The cardiologist may also decide to use an electric pacer to increase the heart rate or to infuse a controlled amount of cardiac stimulants that induces cardiac stress.

Exercise stress testing may also be combined with myocardial perfusion imaging (gated nuclear ventriculography or angiography) to improve the diagnostic accuracy of this procedure. This type is often called *thallium stress testing* (p. 31). This combination helps decrease the frequency (approximately 10% to 15%) of false positive and false negative results. For some unknown reason, stress testing is much more accurate for men than for women.

Procedure. The patient reports to the cardiology clinic, usually after 4 hours of abstinence from eating, drinking, and smoking. The EKG electrodes are placed on the patient and attached to a monitor. A pre-stress test EKG is recorded. Vital signs are taken for baseline values. During stress testing the EKG and heart rate are recorded continuously by monitoring devices; blood pressure is recorded intermittently. The test is terminated when there are increasingly frequent PVCs, spurts of ventricular tachycardia, ST segment depression, drop in blood pressure, or worsening patient complaints of chest pain, exhaustion, generalized fatigue, dyspnea, or dizziness.

After the stress test, EKGs and vital signs are recorded at intervals during a 5- to 10-minute recovery period. A cardiologist performs a stress test in approximately 30 to 45 minutes.

Contraindications. Stress testing is contraindicated in patients with unstable angina, in patients with aortic valve diseases and often in patients who have had a myocardial infarction within the preceding few weeks. However, limited-stress testing may be performed with little or no risk in post-MI patients. The policy about stress testing patients with "fresh" myocardial infarctions often varies.

Nursing considerations

Nursing Diagnoses/Collaborative Problems

- Possible knowledge deficit related to test purpose, preparation, and procedure.
- Possible anxiety related to unknown sensations during the procedure.
- Possible anxiety related to test results.
- Potential complication: cardiac arrhythmias.
- Potential complication: myocardial infarction.

Nursing Implications with Rationale

- Explain the procedure to the patient. Describe the type of exercise testing that will be used. Many patients are anxious and require considerable emotional support.

- Ensure that the physician has obtained the written informed consent for this procedure.
- Instruct the patient to eat a light meal, without coffee or tea (stimulants) or alcohol (a depressant), 4 hours before the test. Heavy meals divert blood to the gastrointestinal tract; and, when exercise is begun, a large portion of the remaining blood goes to skeletal muscle. A heavy meal before stress testing may cause signs of ischemia much earlier than if no meal had been taken.
- Instruct the patient that smoking is not permitted for at least 4 hours before the test. Nicotine causes transient coronary artery spasm, which may last up to 12 hours.
- Instruct the patient to get adequate sleep the night before the test.
- Instruct the patient to wear loose-fitting clothes with a shirt that buttons down the front. This facilitates application of monitoring devices. Most clinics will have the patient put on a hospital gown because of the possibility of cardiac arrest. Women should wear a bra.
- Inform the patient that he or she will need to wear comfortable, well-fitting shoes with rubber soles. This will ensure safety and stability on the inclined treadmill or stairs. Slippers are not permitted.
- Some physicians may want their patients to discontinue certain drugs (such as beta-blockers like propranolol [Inderal], which limit the heart rate) before the stress testing. Some patients taking digoxin may have drug-induced ST segment changes related to exercise.
- Patients taking coronary vasodilators like nitroglycerine may perform at a higher level of exercise and may have fewer arrhythmias, thus masking an ischemic response.
- Instruct the patient to report, during the test, any signs of chest pain, exhaustion, shortness of breath, or generalized fatigue. Observe safety precautions (stand next to the patient) in case dizziness or falling occurs.
- Ensure that appropriate emergency equipment, including a defibrillator, an Ambu bag, and antiarrhythmia drugs, is available in the testing room. Those in attendance during the study should know how to use the emergency equipment.
- After the study advise the patient to rest for several hours and to avoid stimulants or extreme temperature changes.
- After the study advise the patient not to take a hot shower for at least 2 hours. A hot shower may cause an increase in cutaneous vasodilation and lead to orthostatic hypotension. This is especially hazardous for patients whose blood pressure dropped during the stress test.
- If the stress test's results are positive, encourage the patient to verbalize his or her feelings, and provide emotional support.

Echocardiography

(cardiac echo, transthoracic echocardiography [TTE])

Normal values: normal position, size, and movements of cardiac valves and chambers.

Rationale. Echocardiography is a noninvasive ultrasound procedure used to evaluate the structure and function of the heart. In diagnostic ultrasonography, a harmless high-frequency sound wave is emitted from a transducer and penetrates the organ being studied. For transthoracic echocardiography, the transducer is placed over the heart, and sound waves are bounced off the heart structures and reflected back to the transducer as a series of echoes. The echoes are amplified and displayed on an oscilloscope. The data appear as lines and spaces representing bone, cardiac chambers, valves, septum, and muscle (Figure 2-8). The tracings are recorded on moving graph paper and on videotape.

It is now possible to perform echocardiography via the esophagus using a probe mounted on an endoscope. This is referred to as transesophageal echocardiography (TEE, see p 35).

A complete echocardiographic study usually

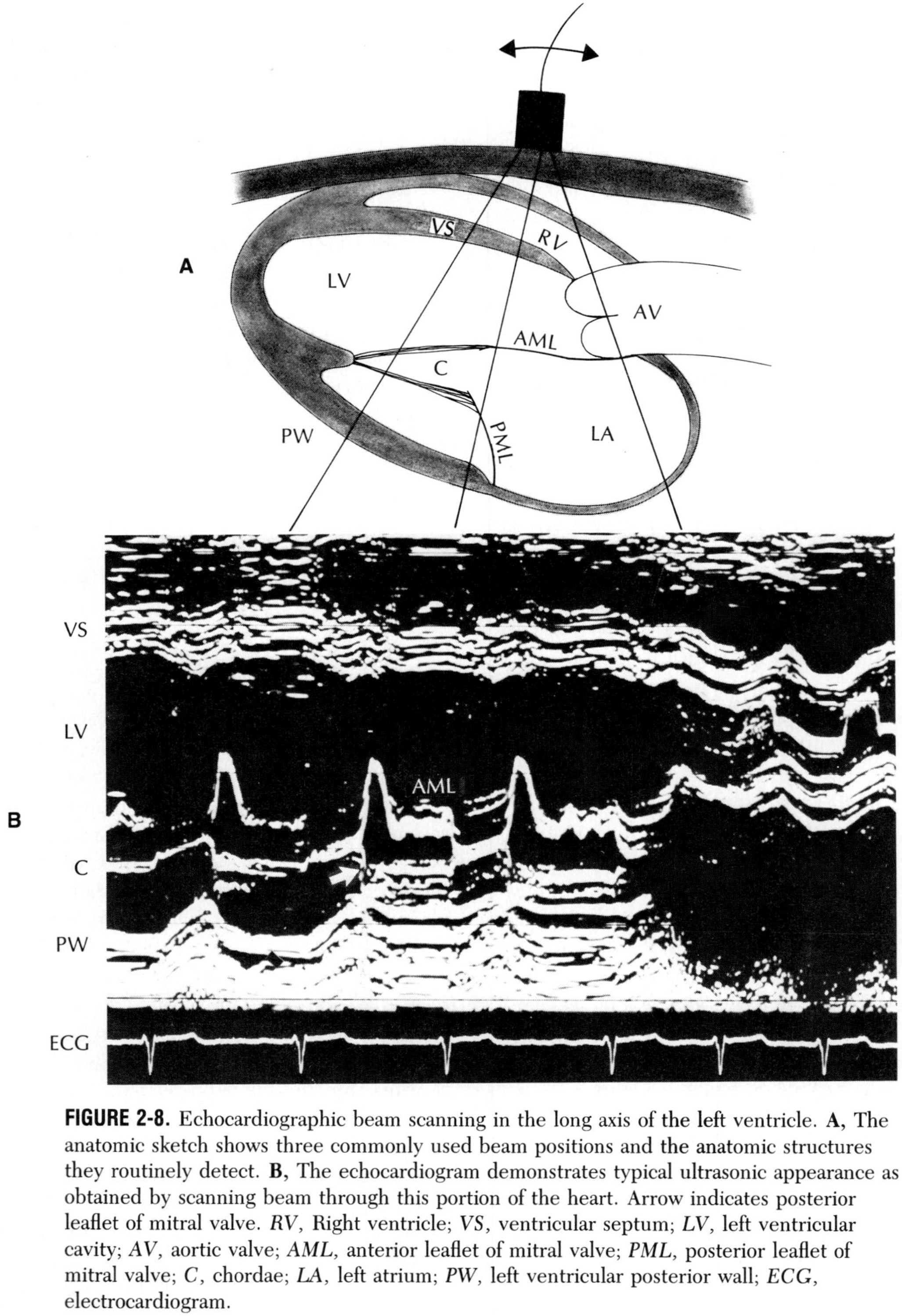

FIGURE 2-8. Echocardiographic beam scanning in the long axis of the left ventricle. **A,** The anatomic sketch shows three commonly used beam positions and the anatomic structures they routinely detect. **B,** The echocardiogram demonstrates typical ultrasonic appearance as obtained by scanning beam through this portion of the heart. Arrow indicates posterior leaflet of mitral valve. *RV,* Right ventricle; *VS,* ventricular septum; *LV,* left ventricular cavity; *AV,* aortic valve; *AML,* anterior leaflet of mitral valve; *PML,* posterior leaflet of mitral valve; *C,* chordae; *LA,* left atrium; *PW,* left ventricular posterior wall; *ECG,* electrocardiogram.

From Nanda NC and Gramiak R: Clinical echocardiography, St Louis, 1978, The CV Mosby Co.

includes M-mode recordings, two-dimensional (2-D) recordings, and a Doppler study. *M-mode echocardiography* provides a time-motion study of the heart (hence, the *M* for motion) by tracking the motion of various cardiac structures over a period of time. This unidimensional technique allows the movements and dimensions of various cardiac structures to be located and studied. *Two-D echocardiography* represents further development of this ultrasound technique. For 2-D, or cross-sectional, echocardiography the angle of the ultrasonic beam is moved rapidly within a sector and produces a sector scan. This enables the 2-D echocardiogram to produce spatial anatomic relationships, which make this test much more versatile than M-mode echocardiography. Two-D echocardiographic machines have the capability of simultaneously performing M-mode echocardiography.

A new and exciting addition to routine 2-D and M-mode echocardiography is Doppler and color Doppler echocardiography. Doppler echocardiography detects patterns of blood flow and measures changes in the velocity of blood flow within the heart and great vessels. The Doppler system allows the examiner to hear sound waves moving toward or away from the examination point as different frequencies; therefore, the Doppler has different sounds. By assigning a computerized weighted number to these sounds based on their frequency, one is able to map and determine the origin of these sounds.

Sound waves inside the heart come from normal flow through the chambers or from turbulent flow across abnormal valves or through septal wall defects. By mapping the sounds with Doppler, one can determine the origin of the sounds and the amount of blood causing them. In this way, cardiologists can accurately determine and quantify noninvasively (for the first time) the site and the functional severity of a heart murmur caused by narrowed leaky valves or septal defects. Doppler echocardiography is specifically indicated to assist in the examination of murmurs, while regular 2-D echocardiography will better evaluate heart wall motion in patients with an injured myocardium caused by heart attacks. Furthermore, 2-D echocardiography can detect mural thrombi, which may occur following MI.

For color flow imaging, the colors blue and red represent the direction of a given jetstream of blood. The various hues from dull to bright represent varying blood velocities. These variants result in a color map of a given jetstream of blood with readily identifiable quantity and direction. Thus, the Doppler information provides spacial orientation that makes the flow information more readily understood when compared to conventional approaches. The most useful application of color flow imaging is in the detection of valvular regurgitation, where reversed flow of blood is easily seen and quantitated. Doppler color flow imaging also allows for the identification of certain valvular stenotic jets (such as mitral stenosis) and may also be of help in assessing proper functioning of prosthetic valves.

Echocardiography is used in the diagnosis of pericardial effusion, valve disease, subaortic stenosis, cardiomyopathy, cardiac tumor, congenital heart disease, aortic root disease, prolapse, and mural thrombosis. No complications are associated with this study.

Procedure. No patient sedation or fasting is required. The patient must undress to the waist. The patient lies on a bed, first in the supine position and then later in the left lateral decubitus position. The ultrasonographer (a trained technician or cardiologist) applies mineral oil or glycerine to the skin over the fourth left intercostal space. This paste is used to enhance transmission and reception of sound waves. The technician places a pencil-like probe (transducer) on the skin, and then tilts or rocks it into various positions (see Figure 2-8) to inscribe an arc that will demonstrate several areas of the heart sequentially. An EKG is recorded simultaneously during echocardiography to time the events demonstrated by ultrasound with the cardiac cycle. During this study a drug such as amyl nitrate may be inhaled to increase the contractility of the heart and to provide additional information about the valves.

Echocardiography is usually performed in a darkened room in a cardiology clinic or in the cardiologist's office. It can be performed at the bedside or in the emergency room in an emergency situation (for example, if needed to rule out pericardial effusion or evaluate a patient who is having myocardial infarction). The duration of this study is approximately 15 to 45 minutes. Most patients will not feel any discomfort during this procedure although some may complain of pressure from the probe pressing against the chest.

Contraindications. This test is contraindicated in the uncooperative patient. It may be difficult to perform in obese patients or in patients with chronic lung disease because the increased airspace does not conduct ultrasound waves well.

Nursing considerations

Nursing Diagnoses/Collaborative Problems

- Possible knowledge deficit related to test purpose, preparation, and procedure.
- Possible anxiety related to unknown sensations of the procedure.
- Possible alteration in comfort related to test procedure.

Nursing Implications with Rationale

- Explain the procedure to the patient. Assure him or her that this is a painless study. Provide as much privacy and draping as possible.
- Explain to the patient that a gel will be applied to the skin over the heart to enhance the transmission of sound waves. Tell the patient that an EKG is normally run continuously during the study. Limb EKG leads will be applied (see EKG study).
- Make sure that the request form for echocardiography includes the patient history and the specific problem that the referring physician suspects.
- After the study remove the gel from the patient's chest.

Cardiac catheterization

(coronary angiography, angiocardiography, ventriculography)

Normal values: normal heart, blood vessels, pressures, and volumes (see definition of terms in Supplemental Information section).

Rationale. Cardiac catheterization is a procedure that allows the heart and the major blood vessels surrounding it to be studied. During the study a catheter is passed through a peripheral vein or artery and into the heart and surrounding vessels. Through the catheter, pressures are recorded, radiopaque dye is injected for angiography, and cardiac output and other measurements of cardiac function are determined (see Supplemental Information). Cardiac catheterization is performed for the reasons enumerated below:

1. To identify, document, locate, and quantitate the severity of atherosclerotic plaques within the coronary arteries.
2. To evaluate the severity of acquired and congenital cardiac valve disorders.
3. To determine the severity of nonvalvular congenital disorders such as ventricular or atrial septal defects, transposition of the great vessels, patent ductus arteriosus, and anomalous venous return to the heart.
4. To evaluate the success of previous heart surgery or balloon angioplasty.
5. To evaluate cardiac muscle function (that is, its ability to pump the blood contained within the heart).
6. To identify ventricular aneurysms, which may follow a myocardial infarction.
7. To identify and locate acquired diseases of the great vessels entering and leaving the heart (such as atherosclerosis or aneurysms of the aortic arch or superior

vena caval obstruction secondary to malignancy).

8. To identify and locate congenital disorders of the great vessels leaving the heart (such as coarctation of the aorta, patent ductus arteriosus, or right-sided aortic arch).
9. To insert a catheter to measure the pulmonary artery pressure, the pulmonary wedge pressure, and the cardiac output (see Supplemental Information, p. 40).
10. To evaluate an acute myocardial infarction and to facilitate infusion of streptokinase into the occluded artery to reopen the artery and prevent or limit the myocardial infarction size.

Possible complications of cardiac catheterization include the following:

1. Cardiac arrhythmias, leading to ventricular fibrillation.
2. Perforation of the heart by the catheter.
3. Stroke or myocardial infarction caused by dislodging an atherosclerotic plaque or thrombus.
4. Peripheral arterial complications such as thrombosis, embolism, aneurysm, or bleeding.
5. Allergic reaction to iodine dye, causing hives or anaphylactic shock.
6. Infection.
7. Pneumothorax if subclavian vein is used for access.

As with any procedure, the incidence of these complications is greatly reduced when competent and experienced personnel perform the procedure in a well-equipped cardiac catheterization laboratory.

Procedure. The patient is kept fasting from solid food for 6 to 8 hours before catheterization. Fluids are often permitted until 3 hours before the study. The patient is often sedated with midazolam (Versed) and either meperidine (Demerol) or morphine 30 to 60 minutes before the study. Young children require general anesthesia.

Cardiac catheterization is performed under sterile conditions. The catheter insertion site is prepared and anesthetized with a local anesthetic (such as lidocaine). EKG leads are placed on the four extremities. A peripheral intravenous (IV) needle is inserted to allow venous access in the event that antiarrhythmic drugs are needed.

To study the *right side* of the heart, a sterile radiopaque catheter is inserted into the antecubital, femoral, or subclavian vein and then into the superior or inferior vena cava. The catheter is then advanced through the right atrium and ventricle and into the pulmonary artery. The course of the catheter is followed by fluoroscopy. Radiopaque dye may be injected and x-ray films may be taken at any time. The heart is constantly monitored during the procedure. PVCs (premature ventricular contractions) may occur as the catheter is passed into the ventricle. An increase in PVCs may necessitate the IV administration of lidocaine (Xylocaine) or the withdrawal of the catheter. Routine blood pressures are checked at regular intervals during the procedure. As the catheter is passed through the heart, pressures within the superior vena cava, the right atrium, the right ventricle, and the pulmonary artery are recorded. Blood samples are drawn for analyses of oxygen content. Radiopaque dye may be injected at selected sites to permit opacification of the right heart chambers with cinegraphic recording. Catheterization of the right side of the heart is usually performed in the cardiac catheterization lab, but it may also be performed at the bedside in the CCU or Intensive Care Unit (ICU).

For *left-sided* heart catheterization, the catheter is usually passed retrogradely from the femoral or brachial artery into the aorta and then into the left ventricle. Left-side catheterization can also be achieved transseptally by puncturing the atrial septum during right-sided catheterization with a needle and passing the catheter from the right atrium into the left atrium. The EKG and blood pressure readings are mon-

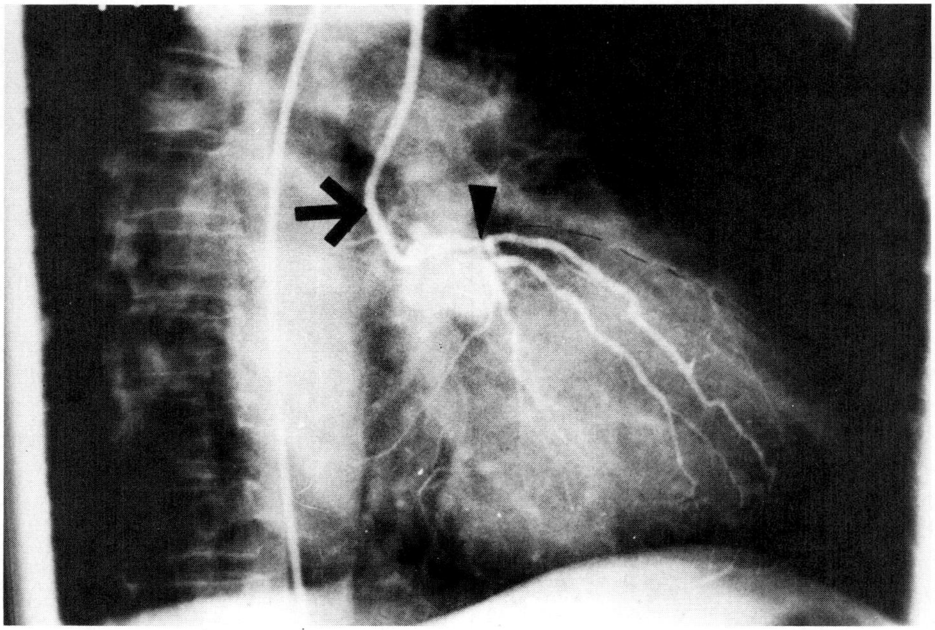

FIGURE 2-9. Coronary angiogram, lateral view. Black arrow indicates angiocatheter; black pointer indicates narrowing of the left coronary artery. Dotted line indicates what would have been the normal course of the anterior descending artery had proximal narrowing not occurred. Dye-filled vessels represent collateralization.

itored closely during the procedure. Once the catheter is correctly positioned by fluoroscopy, pressure readings are measured and blood samples are drawn for oxygen content. Radiopaque dye is injected into the left ventricle and movie-type x-ray films are taken (cineventriculography).

Angiographic visualization of the coronary arteries is one of the most commonly applied diagnostic procedures in the cardiac catheterization laboratory. For the visualization of the coronary arteries, special catheters are placed at the orifice of the arteries, dye is then injected, and the coronary arteries are visualized (coronary cineangiography, Figure 2-9). In some cases, when coronary artery spasm is suspected and obstructive coronary artery disease is absent, intravenous ergonovine maleate may be given to induce coronary artery spasm. This spasm can be promptly reversed by sublingual, intravenous, or intracoronary administration of nitroglycerine. During the injection of dye into the coronary arteries, the table is moved from side to side or tilted. The patient may feel as if he or she is falling. Left-sided catheterization is usually performed in the cardiac catheterization laboratory.

Transluminal coronary angioplasty is a therapeutic procedure that can be performed during coronary angiography in medical centers where open-heart surgery can be done in case of complications. For this procedure a specially designed balloon catheter is introduced via the coronary catheter and placed across a stenotic area of the coronary artery. This area can then be dilated by controlled inflation of the balloon catheter. The coronary arteriogram is repeated to document the effect of the forceful dilatation of the stenotic area of the coronary artery.

After the study of either side of the heart, the cardiac catheter is removed. If access to the peripheral vessel required a cutdown, this is then sutured and covered with a dry, sterile pressure dressing. The catheter insertion site is immobilized for several hours. Pressure is applied to the site. Vital signs are monitored frequently over the next 4 to 6 hours. The puncture site is assessed for signs of bleeding. Peripheral pulses, color, temperature, and neurologic status are evaluated in the involved extremity every hour.

For most patients, cardiac catheterization is an anxiety-producing experience. The patient must lie still on a hard, x-ray examination table that may rotate in several positions. The room is usually darkened to allow for visualization of the fluoroscopic screen. The patient's arm may feel as though it is going to sleep if the brachial artery is used for access. As the catheter touches the ventricles, the patient may feel palpitations (that is, the heart skipping a beat) because of PVCs. When the radiopaque dye is injected, the patient may feel a warm flush. This feeling of warmth frequently is so strong that it simulates being thrown into a fire. Although transient (4 to 10 seconds), it is very uncomfortable. Some patients have a tendency to cough as the catheter is passed into the pulmonary artery. Patients may be asked to cough during the procedure to increase the heart rate. Cardiologists perform catheterization in approximately 1 to 3 hours. Because of tremendous improvements in safety, cardiac catheterization can now be performed on an outpatient basis as well as an inpatient basis.

Contraindications. Cardiac catheterization is contraindicated in the following patients:

1. Uncooperative patients.
2. Patients who would refuse surgery if the lesion found were amenable to surgery. (This is not meant to imply that this study is done solely as a prerequisite to surgery.)
3. Patients with iodine-dye allergies who have not received the appropriate preventive treatment (see p. 30). In many hospitals, non-ionic dyes (such as omnipaque and hyapaque) are being used.
4. Patients who are pregnant. Studies requiring radiation exposure should be delayed until completion of the pregnancy.
5. Patients with poor renal function. Iodine can further injure the kidneys.

Nursing considerations

Nursing Diagnoses/Collaborative Problems

- Possible knowledge deficit related to test purpose, preparation, and procedure.
- Possible anxiety related to unknown sensations of the procedure.
- Possible anxiety related to possible test results.
- High risk for alteration in comfort related to test procedure.
- Possible injury related to the effects of sedatives.
- Potential complication: adverse reaction/allergy.
- Potential complication: cardiac arrhythmias.
- Potential complication: perforation.
- Potential complication: stroke or myocardial infarction.
- Potential complication: peripheral arterial problems.
- Potential complication: infection.

Nursing Implications with Rationale

- The physician who obtains the written permission for this study should thoroughly explain the procedure to the patient. Ask the patient to verbalize his or her understanding of the test and then reinforce the patient's understanding. Explain the sensations that the patient is likely to have (see Procedure). Allow the patient ample time to verbalize apprehensions or fears regarding this test.

- Locate the catheter insertion site for the patient and explain that a local anesthetic will be used. Inform the patient that the insertion site will be shaved and prepared with an antiseptic scrub to avoid infection.
- Withhold food and fluid for 6 to 8 hours before the procedure to prevent the patient's vomiting and aspirating the vomitus during the study.
- Determine whether the patient has any dye allergies. If so, he or she should be given a regimen to prevent allergic reaction. A commonly used regimen is prednisone, 5 mg four times daily, and diphenhydromine (Benadryl), 25 mg four times daily, for 3 days before and after the test.
- Mark the patient's peripheral pulses with a pen before catheterization. This will permit quicker assessment of the pulses after the procedure. Note and record the quality of the pulses as baseline data.
- Tell the patient that he or she will be lying still on a hard table for the duration of this procedure and that the room will be darkened at intervals.
- Make sure that emergency equipment (defibrillator, airway, Ambu bag, EKG monitor, antiarrhythmic drugs) is present in the catheterization room. The nurse in attendance should be knowledgeable in the use of this equipment.
- Administer the preprocedure drugs as ordered before catheterization.
- Most patients are very tired after this procedure, and the physician often orders bed rest for several hours to allow for complete sealing of the arterial puncture. In such cases, enforce safety measures (such as elevated side rails) until the effect of the preprocedure medications has worn off.
- Keep the extremity in which the catheter was placed straight and immobilized for several hours after catheterization to prevent bleeding and discomfort. Apply ice to the site if ordered. The physician may order a sandbag for femoral arterial access sites.
- Monitor the patient's vital signs at frequent intervals (usually every 15 minutes for four times, then every 30 minutes for four times, then every hour for four times, and then every 4 hours) for arrhythmias and hypotension. Report any abnormalities to the physician.
- After the procedure, observe the arterial puncture site for hemorrhage, inflammation, hematoma, or absence of pulse. Check the peripheral pulses and compare the quality of the pulses with the preprocedure baseline values. Assess the extremity for signs of ischemia (numbness, tingling, pain, absence of peripheral pulses, and loss of function). The color and temperature of the extremity are compared with the color and temperature of the uninvolved extremities.
- Encourage fluids after the procedure to aid in eliminating the contrast medium.
- Encourage the patient to verbalize his or her experience with cardiac catheterization. The patient should be advised when sexual intercourse can be resumed (usually 1 to 2 weeks) after the procedure.

Cardiac nuclear scanning

(myocardial scan, cardiac, scan, nuclear cardiac scanning, heart scan, thallium scan, dipyridamole-thallium scan, multigated acquisition scan [MUGA], radionuclide ventriculography [RVG], nitro test, heart shunt study)

Normal value: normal myocardial cells, normal ejection fractions and velocities.

Rationale. Cardiac radionuclear scanning is a noninvasive and safe method of recognizing cardiac disease. Many different radiocompound materials can be used (such as technetium-99m pertechnetate, thallium-201, technetium-99m pyrophosphate, and isonitrile). These compounds are injected intravenously into the patient. With the use of a radiation detector placed over the heart, an image of the heart can be recorded and photographed.

TABLE 2-2. Myocardial Scanning

Disease	Technetium-99m pyrophosphate*	Thallium-201†
None (normal)	No uptake	Diffuse and even uptake
Acute myocardial infarction	"Hot" spot	"Cold" spot
Myocardial ischemia	"Warm" spot	Normal at rest "Cold" spot during exercise‡
Old myocardial infarction	No uptake	"Cold spot"§

*And related compounds, such as mercury-203, gallium-67, or any technetium-99m labeled compound.
†And related compounds, such as potassium-43, cesium-131, or rubidium-86.
‡Such as stress testing.
§Unable to differentiate "acute" from "old" myocardial infarction.

Basically, radionuclide scanning is used to evaluate coronary artery perfusion or to evaluate ventricular function. In evaluations of the patency of the coronary arteries, the picture characteristic of abnormality varies according to the type of radiocompound used. When thallium is used, all normal myocardial cells take up the substance and show up (or light up) on the photoscan. Ischemic or infarcted cells do not take up the substance and appear as dark spots (cold spots) surrounded by normal cells on the photoscan. Many institutions are switching from thallium to isonitrile or sestamibi because its shorter half-life permits much quicker testing. Technetium pyrophosphate, on the other hand, is taken up only by ischemic or infarcted cells. Therefore an acute myocardial infarction will show up as a "hot spot" on this kind of cardiac photoscan (see Table 2-2).

Thallium-201 can be injected intravenously during exercise stress testing (see p. 20) when the patient is at the peak level of stress. The thallium-201 accumulates in the myocardium in direct proportion to regional myocardial blood flow and extraction of thallium by the myocardial cells. Therefore, a normal myocardium has much greater thallium activity than an abnormal one. Scanning is performed and repeated several hours (usually 4) later, and the images are compared to detect exercise-induced ischemia. For patients unable to achieve an adequate heart rate increase during the stress test, thallium-201 imaging at rest and during exercise is more accurate than exercise stress testing alone in diagnosing coronary artery disease. *Exercise stress testing with thallium scanning* or *thallium stress testing* is also used to assess more accurately the extent of coronary artery disease and to assess postoperative patency of a coronary bypass graft. Serial thallium imaging may also be used to evaluate the progression of disease.

When exercise is not advisable or possible during myocardial scanning, the *dipyridamole-thallium scan* can be used as a substitute for exercise thallium stress testing. Dipyridamole (Persantine) is a coronary vasodilator, which simulates the exercise portion of this test. For this reason, the procedure may be referred to as "chemical stress testing." Persantine is given to the patient who is unable to exercise to see if there is a uniform change in flow. If there is a significant obstruction in one coronary, there will be a discrepancy in flow, which can be visualized with a thallium gamma-ray detector camera. Because the vascular dilatation can rob blood from other areas of the heart and precipitate angina or myocardial infarction, the test must be performed with a cardiologist in attendance. Intravenous aminophylline reverses this effect. Persantine-thallium scanning may be indicated for patients with orthopedic, arthritic, neurologic, or pulmonary limitations that preclude evaluation with exercise testing. Other candidates include those with morbid obesity and those taking beta-blockers. Recently, *adenosine* has been used in some medical centers in place of Persantine to save a step because Persantine is converted in the body to adenosine.

For the evaluation of ventricular performance, technetium-99m is usually used. Radionuclide ventriculography (RVG) uses an intravascular indicator to delineate heart chambers and large vessels. RVG may be performed using two different methods. In the *first-pass technique,* a radiotracer is injected intravenously. As the substance passes through the right heart, lungs, and left heart the first time (called the "first pass-through"), the function of the heart valves can be determined. The amount of radionuclide ejected with each heartbeat can be calculated to determine the ejection fraction. The shape of the ventricles can be recorded on a film called a *ventriculogram.*

The second method of performing RVG is called the *gated method.* Computer-assisted cardiac scanning allows the myocardial wall to be photographed in motion. This procedure, called *gated blood pool imaging, gated pool ejection fraction (GPEF),* or multigated acquisition scan (MUGA), is similar to fluoroscopic ventriculography performed during cardiac catheterization, yet it is noninvasive, unlike catheterization. Gated scans are frequently obtained after first-pass scans, since no additional radionuclide injection is needed. This test analyzes the left ventricular function by assessing systole and diastole and by calculating the ejection fraction (EF). Cardiac images are synchronized with the EKG. The term *gated* refers to this synchronization. A series of images of blood flow through the heart can be studied in sequence. Counts are recorded from several hundred cardiac cycles following distribution of the radiotracer throughout the blood pool. Computers are used to provide images of the spatial distribution and density of counts over time. Serial measurement of EF and wall motion abnormalities (such as akinesias, dyskinesias, and hypokinesias) may be used to evaluate the presence of cardiac disease, follow the deterioration or improvement of cardiac function with or without medical/surgical therapy, and measure the effect of potentially cardiotoxic medications (such as adriamycin).

Gated imaging performed during stress testing may be referred to as a stress-MUGA. For this test, the patient uses an exercise bike in either the upright or supine position. Nitroglycerine can be given sublingually during gated and stress-MUGA studies to evaluate the effect of nitroglycerine on heart performance and blood pressure. This procedure may be called a "nitro-MUGA" or "nitro test."

Assessment of left-to-right heart shunts can be called a *shunt scintigraphy* or *heart shunt study.* This test is valuable in detecting atrial septal defects. For this angiographic test, the radiotracer is rapidly injected into the right external jugular vein. Serial images are taken and the blood flow through the heart and lungs is visualized. A left-to-right shunt causes a reappearance of radioactivity within the lung.

The technetium *pyrophosphate heart scan* (PYP scan) is used to identify the location, extent, and size of a recent myocardial infarction. Pyrophosphate binds to calcium in irreversibly damaged myocardial cells. Acute infarction is associated with an area of increased radioactivity or a "hot spot" on imaging. Scans are most likely to be positive when injections are performed 2 to 3 days after a suspected infarction when the elevated creatine kinase has often returned to normal. This test may be referred to as *acute infarct scintigraphy.*

The computer-driven display analysis for nuclear coronary perfusion studies has recently been significantly improved by the addition of single photon emission computed tomography (SPECT). SPECT is a noninvasive technique that greatly improves the resolution of images and the quantification of ischemia. In this technique, images are obtained from many different angles and reconstructed using tomographic techniques. SPECT involves the use of single photon-emitting radionuclides (such as thallium). It provides a three-dimensional image (transaxial, sagittal, and coronal) of physiologic processes with greater image contrast and resolution than traditional imaging. It also has the capability of quantification.

Specific indications for cardiac scanning include the following:

1. Assessment of systolic and diastolic ventricular function.
2. Identification and quantification of intracardiac shunts.
3. Assessment of myocardial perfusion.
4. Detection of acute myocardial infarction.
5. Screening of adults for old infarction (especially before surgery).
6. Evaluation of medical or surgical therapy.
7. Evaluation of precoronary and postcoronary bypass surgery for myocardial perfusion.
8. Evaluation of patients with chest pain and uninterpretable or equivocal EKGs because of drug effects, bundle branch block, or left ventricular hypertrophy.
9. Ruling out of acute or old MI in patients who have bundle branch blocks. (An EKG is not diagnostic of acute myocardial infarction in patients with bundle branch blocks.)
10. Quantification and surveillance of myocardial infarction.

These studies are free of complications. The era of noninvasive myocardial radioscanning is just beginning; these tests will undoubtedly be a vital part of the evaluation of many patients with myocardial disease.

Procedure. The unsedated patient is given an IV injection of the appropriate radionuclide. Most injections use a peripheral vein, except shunt studies which use the jugular vein. Fasting requirements vary with the type of procedure indicated. Shortly thereafter (but in less than 4 hours) a gamma-ray detector is placed over the precordium. The patient is first placed in the supine position, then in the lateral position, and then in both oblique positions. The detector records the image of the heart, and a Polaroid photo of that image is taken. During testing with isonitrile, the patient may be given milk and muffins to enhance the scan results. The only part of the test that is at all uncomfortable is the venous puncture required for the injection. A nuclear medicine technician performs the myocardial scan in less than 30 minutes. Repeat films may be taken later in the day.

Contraindications. This test is contraindicated in the uncooperative patient. It is also contraindicated in the pregnant patient because of the possibility of the radiopaque dye causing damage to the developing fetus.

Nursing considerations

Nursing Diagnoses/Collaborative Problems

See Nuclear scanning, p. 5.

Nursing Implications with Rationale

- Explain the procedure to the patient. Encourage verbalization of the patient's fears.
- Smoking is usually prohibited for several hours before the test.
- Give the patient specific instructions regarding fasting and taking medications preceding the test. Instructions will vary according to the different types of cardiac scans.
- Reassure the patient that this procedure is safe and noninvasive. Provide emotional support.

Serum lipids study

(blood lipids; lipid profile; cholesterol, triglycerides, phospholipids)

Total lipids

Normal values: 400-1000 mg/dl

Cholesterol

Normal findings: vary with age and testing center

Adult/elderly: 150-200 mg/dl or 3.90-6.50 mmol/L (SI units)

Child: 120-200 mg/dl

Infant: 70-175 mg/dl

Newborn: 53-135 mg/dl

Triglycerides (TGs)
Normal findings:
Adult/elderly:
Male: 40-160 mg/dl or 0.4-1.6 g/L (SI units)
Female: 35-135 mg/dl or 0.35-1.35 g/L (SI units)

Child	Male	Female
0-5 years:	30-86 mg/dl	32-99 mg/dl
6-11 years:	31-108 mg/dl	35-114 mg/dl
12-15 years:	36-138 mg/dl	41-138 mg/dl
16-19 years:	40-163 mg/dl	40-128 mg/dl

Phospholipids
Normal values: 150-380 mg/dl
Cholesterol lipoproteins
HDL
Normal values: >45 mg/dl (men)
>55 mg/dl (women)
VLDL
Normal values: 25% to 50%
LDL
Normal values: 60-180 mg/dl

$$\text{LDL} = \text{total cholesterol} - \left(\text{HDL} - \frac{\text{triglycerides}}{5}\right)$$

Rationale. Determination of serum lipid levels provides quantitative data useful in the diagnosis and management of atherosclerotic disease. When lipids (such as cholesterol, triglycerides, and phospholipids) are transported in the bloodstream, they are combined with proteins and are therefore called lipoproteins. Hyperlipoproteinemia refers to elevation of these lipoprotein complexes in the blood. The lipoproteins can be separated into six types, determined by the major lipid elevation and the major lipoprotein elevation (Table 2-3).

Types II and IV are important in cardiac disease. The typing of the hyperlipoproteinemias is useful, because the dietary treatment varies with the type. For example, type IV is treated primarily with a low-carbohydrate diet.

The lipoproteins can be separated by electrophoresis and fractionated into high-density lipoprotein (HDL), which is predominately composed of protein; low-density lipoprotein (LDL), which is composed primarily of cholesterol; and very low-density lipoprotein (VLDL), consisting mainly of triglycerides and of chylomicrons which are primarily triglycerides. LDL has a strong association with coronary artery disease, and HDL is inversely associated with risk of coronary artery disease. It is suspected that HDL is cardioprotective because it removes the cholesterol from peripheral tissues and prevents cellular uptake.

HDL has a protective role for the cardiac patient because high levels of this lipoprotein class are statistically associated with a decreased risk of myocardial infarction. The HDL/total cholesterol ratio should be at least 1:5, with the ideal ratio of 1/3. The ideal LDL should be <160 in people with coronary artery disease and <180 in those without it.

Since the liver makes cholesterol from ingested fats, liver disease and malnutrition are associated with low cholesterol levels. Many drugs (e.g., steroids, beta-adrenergic blockers, oral contraceptives, thiazides, and vitamin D) can raise cholesterol levels. Cholesterol inhibi-

TABLE 2-3. Patterns of Hyperlipoproteinemia

Lipoprotein type	Major lipoprotein elevation	Major lipid elevation
I (rare)	Chylomicrons	Triglycerides
IIa (common)	LDL	Cholesterol
IIb	LDL and VLDL	Cholesterol and triglycerides
III (uncommon)	Remnants	Triglycerides and cholesterol
IV (common)	VLDL	Triglycerides
V (uncommon)	VLDL and chylomicrons	Triglycerides and cholesterol

tors (e.g., lovastatin, niacin, bile salt binding agents, and some antihypertensives) can lower cholesterol.

Although genetics is the main determinant of cholesterol and lipoprotein levels, other factors can affect lipid blood level. For example, regular vigorous exercise can raise HDL levels, and binge eating or ingesting foods high in fat content raise LDL levels.

Procedure. The patient must fast for at least 12 to 14 hours after eating a normal diet for at least 2 weeks. Water is permitted. Alcohol should be avoided because its sugar content causes the triglyceride level to rise and remain elevated for several hours. If possible, thyroid medication, steroidal contraceptives, and lipid-lowering drugs should be avoided for at least 3 weeks. A peripheral venipuncture is performed; two tubes (red and lavender top) of blood are drawn. Fractionation into lipoproteins is done by either ultracentrifugation or electrophoresis.

Contraindications. None.

Nursing considerations

Nursing Diagnoses/Collaborative Problems

See Blood studies, p. 2.

Nursing Implications with Rationale

- Explain the purpose of the study to the patient. Instruct the patient about diet and fasting.
- After the venipuncture is performed, apply pressure or a pressure dressing to the site.
- Observe the site for bleeding.

SUPPLEMENTAL INFORMATION

Transesophageal echocardiography

(TEE)

Normal values: Normal position, size, and movement of heart valves and heart chambers.

Rationale. Transesophageal echocardiography (TEE) ultrasonically images the heart from a retrocardiac vantage point, thereby avoiding interference from interposed ribs, lungs, and subcutaneous tissue (see Figure 2-10). For this procedure, a high-frequency ultrasound transducer mounted on an endoscope provides better resolution than that of images obtained with routine transthoracic echocardiography (see page 23). For TEE, the distal end of the endoscope is advanced into the esophagus, and the transducer is positioned behind the heart. Controls on the handle of the endoscope permit the transducer to be rotated 360° and also flexed in both the anteroposterior and right-left lateral planes.

TEE images have better resolution than those obtained transthoracically because of the higher frequency and closer proximity of the transducer to the cardiac structures. TEE is performed only on patients who have already had the transthoracic examination.

TEE has both intraoperative and nonoperative applications. The primary nonsurgical indication is evaluation of structures inaccessible or poorly visualized transthoracically. Examples include patients who are obese or patients with chronic obstructive pulmonary disease (COPD).

Nonsurgical or ambulatory TEE is performed for the following reasons:

1. To visual the mitral valve.
2. To differentiate intracavity from extracardiac masses and tumors.
3. To visualize the atrial septum (such as for septal defects).
4. To diagnose thoracic aortic dissection.
5. To detect valvular vegetation indicative of endocarditis.
6. To determine cardiac sources of embolism.
7. To detect coronary artery disease.

Intraoperative applications of TEE are used primarily to monitor the high-risk patient for ischemia. Patients undergoing major abdominal, peripheral vascular, and carotid artery procedures are at high risk for intraoperative ischemia because of the high prevalence of coronary artery disease. TEE is more sensitive than the EKG for detecting ischemia. TEE is also used intraoperatively to evaluate the surgical results

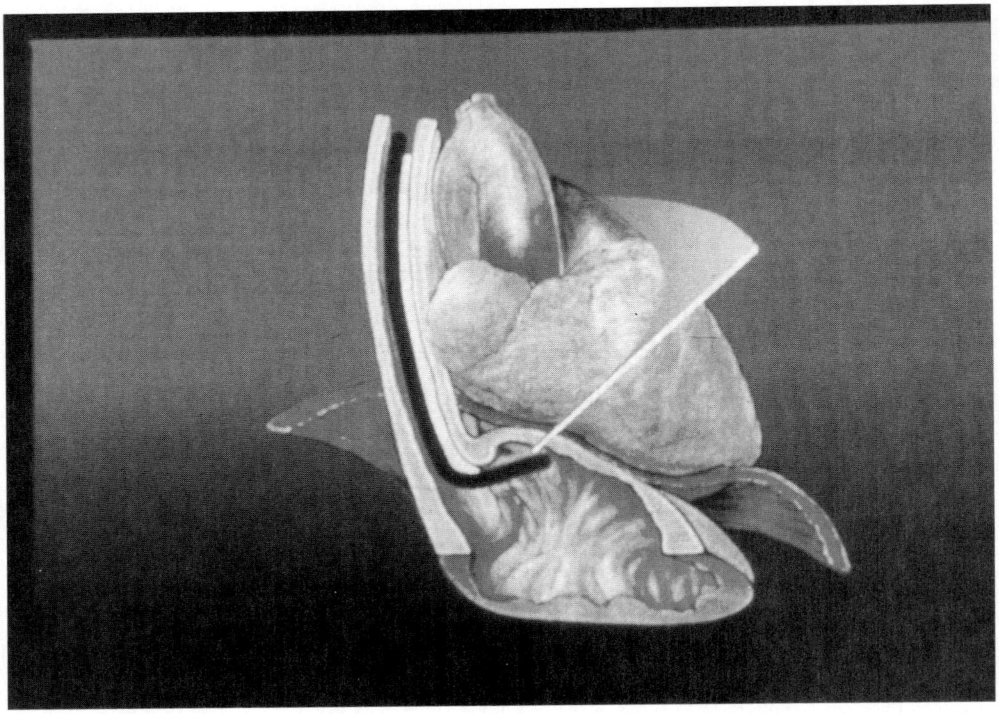

FIGURE 2-10. Diagram illustrating location of the transesophageal endoscope within the esophagus. The probe is in the fundus of the stomach and is anteflexed for imaging the transgastric short-axis view of the left ventricle.
Courtesy Advanced Technology Laboratory.

of valvular or congenital heart disease. TEE is also the most sensitive technique for detecting air emboli—a serious complication of neurosurgery performed in the upright position.

Complications of TEE are rare. Esophageal trauma, bleeding, and arrhythmias rarely occur.

Procedure. The patient is kept fasting for 4 to 6 hours before TEE is performed. Oral prostheses are removed, and intravenous access is established. Intravenous sedation is commonly provided with the short-acting benzodiazepine midazolam (Versed) along with meperidine (Demerol) or stadol to reduce patient anxiety, provide antegrade amnesia, and improve compliance. This is often referred to as "conscious sedation." EKG leads are applied, and a rhythm strip is continually displayed on the EKG machine. A blood pressure cuff is monitored periodically, and pulse oximetry is used to determine oxygen saturation.

The pharynx is anesthetized with Cetacaine or lidocaine to depress the gag reflex. For intubation, the patient is placed in the left lateral decubitus position. Intubation can also be performed with the patient in the supine or upright sitting position. A bite guard protects the endoscope from the patient's teeth. The transducer is slowly introduced into the throat. The patient is asked to swallow, and the transducer is advanced into position behind the heart. The room is darkened, and the ultrasound images are displayed on the monitor. After the desired images are visualized, the endoscope is removed. This procedure is performed by a cardiologist and endoscopist in approximately 20 minutes in an endoscopy suite or in the ICU or

CCU. After the procedure, naloxone or mazicon may be administered to reverse the effect of the narcotics. Patients are observed closely for approximately one hour after the procedure until the effects of the sedatives have worn off.

Contraindications. TEE is contraindicated in the following patients.

1. Patients with esophageal abnormalities such as stricture, varices, diverticuli, scleroderma, and esophagitis.
2. Patients with a bleeding disorder.
3. Patients with a history of prior esophageal surgery may be at risk.
4. Patients who cannot cooperate during the procedures.

Nursing considerations

Nursing Diagnoses/Collaborative Problems

- Possible knowledge deficit related to test purpose, preparation, and procedure.
- Possible alteration in comfort related to procedure.
- Possible injury related to the effects of sedatives.
- Possible anxiety related to unknown sensations of the test.
- Potential complication: bleeding
- Potential complication: perforation
- Potential complication: aspiration of gastric contents

Nursing Implications with Rationale

- Explain the procedure to the patient. Patients may be apprehensive about this study. Provide emotional support.
- Obtain the patient's written consent.
- Keep the patient NPO for the designated time before the test (usually 4 to 6 hours). This is done to prevent regurgitation when the scope is passed.
- Tell the patient that the test is not painful but may cause discomfort when the gag reflex is initiated. Inform the patient that the throat will be anesthetized to minimize this discomfort.
- Remove the patient's dentures and eyeglasses before the test. Since the tube is passed through the mouth, oral hygiene procedures should be performed before and after the test.
- Explain to the patient that he or she will be unable to speak when the endoscope is passed.
- After the patient's throat has been anesthetized, do not allow the patient to eat or drink anything until the gag reflex returns (usually in about 2 hours).
- After the test, inform the patient that he or she may be hoarse or complain of a sore throat for several days. Drinking cool fluids and gargling may help to relieve some of the soreness.
- Observe safety precautions until the effects of the sedatives have worn off.
- Monitor the vital signs as ordered.

Electrophysiologic study

(EPS, cardiac mapping, EP)

Normal values: normal electrical conduction of the heart

Rationale. An electrophysiologic study (EPS) is an invasive procedure (similar to cardiac catheterization) whereby electrode catheters are placed within the heart to record cardiac activity. An EPS is useful in diagnosing diseases of the heart's conduction system and in directing their treatment. This study has greatly enhanced understanding of the mechanisms of tachyarrhythmias. The electrode catheters can be used to pace the heart to induce arrhythmias. If the patient is on an antiarrhythmic medication (such as lidocaine, phenytoin, or quinidine), the EPS can determine the efficacy of the medication by seeing how easily arrhythmias can be induced. Arrhythmias can also be treated by *catheter ablation,* which involves delivery of energy through a catheter to induce closed-chest electroablation of cells that induce arrhythmias. Catheter ablation of the AV junction has been used to control refractory supraventricular arrhythmias.

Possible complications for EPS include the following:

1. Cardiac arrhythmias, leading to ventricular fibrillation.
2. Perforation of the heart by the catheter.
3. Stroke or myocardial infarction caused by dislodging an atherosclerotic plaque or thrombus.
4. Peripheral arterial complications, such as thrombosis, embolism, aneurysm, or bleeding.
5. Infection.

Procedure. The patient is usually kept fasting for 6 to 8 hours before the EPS. (Fluids are often permitted until 3 hours before the test.) EKG leads are attached. A peripheral IV needle is inserted to allow the administration of medications. The catheter insertion site is prepared and anesthetized with a local anesthetic (such as lidocaine). Catheters are inserted into a vein or artery (usually femoral) and threaded via fluoroscopy to the right and left heart, respectively. Baseline surface and intracardiac EKGs are recorded. Various parts of the conduction system are stimulated by atrial or ventricular pacing. Mapping, or locating the site of origin of a recurrent ventricular tachycardia, can be done. Drugs are administered via the IV line to assess the efficacy of certain drugs for arrhythmias.

For most patients, this is an anxiety-producing experience. The patient must lie still on a hard x-ray table in a darkened room. He or she may have sensations of palpitations and light-headedness or dizziness. These sensations should be reported to the doctor.

After completion of the test, the catheters are removed and direct pressure is applied to the insertion site. Occasionally, a catheter may be left in place for follow-up studies the next day. A cardiologist performs this procedure in 1 to 4 hours. After the procedure, vital signs are monitored frequently over the next 4 to 6 hours. The puncture site is assessed for bleeding. The patient is kept on bed rest for several hours. Peripheral pulses, color, temperature, and neurologic status are evaluated in the involved extremity.

Contraindications. EPS is contraindicated in the uncooperative patient.

Nursing considerations

Nursing Diagnoses/Collaborative Problems

- Possible knowledge deficit related to test purpose, preparation, and procedure.
- Possible anxiety related to unknown sensations of the procedure.
- Possible anxiety related to test results.
- Possible alteration in comfort related to test procedure.
- Potential complication: bleeding.
- Potential complication: cardiac arrhythmia.
- Potential complication: perforation.
- Potential complication: stroke or myocardial infarction.
- Potential complication: peripheral vascular problems.
- Potential complication: infection.

Nursing Implications with Rationale

- The physician who obtains the permission for the study should thoroughly explain the procedure to the patient. Ask the patient to verbalize his or her understanding of the test and then reinforce the patient's understanding.
- Explain the sensations that the patient is likely to have (see Procedure). Allow the patient ample time to verbalize apprehensions or fears regarding this test.
- Locate the catheter insertion site for the patient and explain that a local anesthetic will be used. Inform the patient that the insertion site will be shaved and prepped with an antiseptic scrub to avoid infection.
- Withhold food or fluid for 6 to 8 hours before the procedure to prevent the patient's vomiting and aspirating during the study.
- Mark the patient's peripheral pulses with a pen before catheterization. This will permit

quick assessment of the pulses after the procedure. Note and record the quality of the pulses as baseline data.

- Tell the patient that he or she will be lying still on a hard table for the duration of this procedure and that the room will be darkened at intervals.
- Make sure that emergency equipment is present in the catheterization room where EPS is performed.
- After the procedure, the patient is usually kept on bed rest for several hours to allow complete sealing of the puncture site.
- Keep the extremity in which the catheter was placed straight and immobilized for several hours to prevent bleeding and discomfort. Apply ice to the site if ordered.
- Monitor the patient's vital signs at frequent intervals (usually every 15 minutes for four times, then every 30 minutes for four times, then every hour for four times, then every 4 hours) for arrhythmias and hypotension. Any abnormalities should be reported to the physician.
- After the procedure, observe the puncture site for hemorrhage, inflammation, hematoma, or absence of pulse. Check the peripheral pulses and compare the quality of the pulses with the preprocedure baseline values. Assess the extremity for signs of ischemia (numbness, tingling, pain, absence of peripheral pulses, and loss of function). The color and temperature of the extremity are compared with the uninvolved extremity.
- After the procedure, additional monitoring may be needed for any medications that the patient received during the procedure. For example, a patient receiving quinidine should be monitored for hypotension and for abdominal cramping.
- If an electrocatheter is left in place for subsequent studies, it is sutured in place and covered with a sterile dressing.
- If the patient has an adverse reaction to a drug administered during EPS, the EKG should be carefully monitored until the drug is eliminated from the body.

Tilt table testing

Normal values: no vasopressor syncope.

Rationale. Tilt table testing is a provocative technique used to diagnose vasopressor syncope. Patients with this syndrome usually demonstrate symptomatic hypotension or syncope within a few minutes of being tilted upright approximately 60° to 80°. Patients without vasopressor syncope usually demonstrate a small decrease in systolic blood pressure and an increase in diastolic blood pressure and heart rate. Recently, tilt table testing has been used in conjunction with electrophysiologic studies (see page 37) to assess the efficacy of prophylactic pacing in some patients with vasopressor syncope and to evaluate the impact of posture with some tachyarrhythmias.

Procedure. For this test, the nonfasting and nonsedated patient is usually taken to the cardiology clinic or any other room where a tilt table is located. An arterial line is usually inserted for accurate monitoring of the blood pressure. The patient then lies in the supine position on a horizontal tilt table. After strapping the patient in place, the table is raised 60° to 80°. The patient's blood pressure and pulse are monitored before and during this test. There is no discomfort associated with this test, and it is usually performed by a cardiologist in approximately 30 minutes.

Contraindications. None.

Nursing considerations

Nursing Diagnoses/Collaborative Problems

- Possible knowledge deficit related to test purpose, preparation, and procedure.
- Possible anxiety related to test results.

Nursing Implications with Rationale

- Explain the procedure to the patient.

- Inform the patient if the physician wants any medications held before the test.
- Obtain the patient's blood pressure and pulse as baseline values before the test.
- Monitor the patient's blood pressure and pulse throughout the testing.
- During the test instruct the patient to report any signs of dizziness or light-headedness.
- After the test, monitor the arterial and intravenous site for bleeding. A pressure dressing should be firmly secured to the site.

Definition of terms used in invasive cardiac monitoring and catheterization

Pressures

Routine blood pressure—routine brachial artery pressure (normal: 90-140/60-90 mm Hg).

Systolic left ventricular pressure—peak pressure in the left ventricle during systole (normal: 90-140 mm Hg).

End diastolic left ventricular pressure—pressure in the left ventricle at the end of diastole (normal: 4-12 mm Hg).

Central venous pressure (CVP)—pressure in the superior vena cava (normal: 2-14 cm H_2O).

Pulmonary wedge pressure—pressure in the pulmonary venules, an indirect measurement of left atrial pressure (normal: 6-15 mm Hg).

Pulmonary artery pressure—pressure in the pulmonary artery (normal: 15-28/5-16 mm Hg).

Aortic artery pressure—same as routine blood pressure.

Volumes

End diastolic volume (EDV)—amount of blood present in the left ventricle at the end of diastole (normal: 50-90 ml/m^2).

End systolic volume (ESV)—amount of blood present in the left ventricle at the end of systole (normal: 25 ml/m^2).

Stroke volume—amount of blood ejected from the heart in one contraction (SV = EDV − ESV).

Ejection fraction (EF)—proportion (fraction) of EDV that is ejected from the left ventricle during systole (EF = SV/EDV) (normal: 0.67 ± 0.07).

Cardiac output (CO)—amount of blood ejected by the heart in 1 minute (normal: 3-6 L/min).

Cardiac index (CI)—amount of blood ejected by the heart in 1 minute per square meter of body surface (CI = CO/body surface area) (normal: 2.8 to 4.2 L/min/m^2 for a patient with 1.5 m^2 of body surface).

Pericardiocentesis

(pericardial fluid analysis)

Normal value: clear, straw-colored pericardial fluid without evidence of pathogens, blood, or malignant cells.

Rationale. Pericardiocentesis, which involves the needle aspiration of fluid from the pericardial sac, may be performed for therapeutic or diagnostic purposes. Therapeutically, it is conducted as an emergency measure to relieve cardiac tamponade by removing fluid and relieving pressure surrounding the heart. Diagnostically, pericardiocentesis is performed to remove a small sample of the pericardial fluid for laboratory examination. Pericardial fluid analysis confirms a diagnosis and helps to identify the cause of pericardial effusion.

This procedure should be performed cautiously because of the risk of complications, which include laceration of a coronary artery or the myocardium; ventricular fibrillation and other arrhythmias; vasovagal arrest; pleural infection; pneumothorax; and inadvertent puncture of the lung, liver, or stomach. These complications are minimized when an experienced physician who pays careful attention to proper technique performs the procedure. To minimize complications an echocardiography is done before pericardiocentesis to determine the appropriate site.

Procedure. No fluid or food restrictions are necessary before this procedure. (However, for an elective procedure the patient is often kept fasting for 4 to 6 hours.) Pericardiocentesis is usually performed with the patient in a supine position with the head of the bed elevated 60°. A peripheral IV is started and maintained at keep-vein-open (KVO) rate of about 20 ml/hour to administer preprocedure medications and to

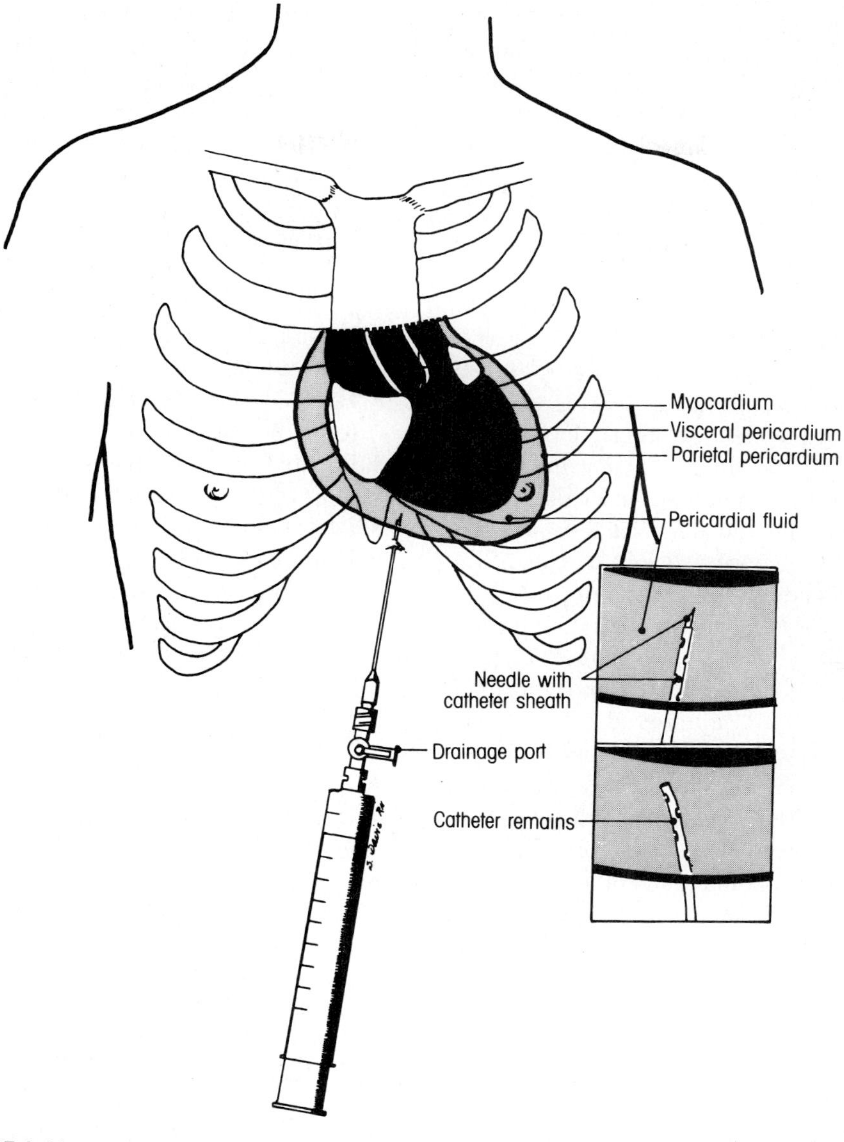

FIGURE 2-11. Pericardiocentesis procedure and aspiration of pericardial fluid. Needle is inserted between xiphoid process and left lower costal margin and advanced toward clavicle. Needle makes a 20- to 30-degree angle with abdominal wall. For recurrent cardiac tamponade and large pericardial effusion, indwelling pericardial catheter may remain.
From Guzzetta CE and Dossey BM: Cardiovascular nursing: bodymind tapestry, St Louis, 1984, The CV Mosby Co.

have venous access in the event of any complications. Atropine is usually given intravenously or intramuscularly to prevent the vasovagal reflex of bradycardia and hypotension, which may occur when the pericardium is punctured. An area in the fifth to sixth intercostal space at the left sternal margin (or subxyphoid) is antiseptically prepared with povidone-iodine solution and injected with a local anesthetic (such as 1% lidocaine without epinephrine). A large-bore, short-beveled pericardiocentesis needle attached to a three-way stopcock with a 50 ml syringe is introduced at a 20- to 30-degree angle with the frontal plane. An EKG lead wire is then attached by an alligator clamp to the hub of the needle. As the needle is inserted through the chest wall into the pericardial sac (Figure 2-11), the EKG is observed for changes in the ST segment. The ST segment is normal if the needle is in the pericardial sac, and it is elevated if the needle touches the epicardium. The pericardial fluid is then aspirated, and specimen tubes are labeled and numbered. The pericardial fluid is evaluated for color, turbidity, blood, white blood cell (WBC) and differential counts, hemoglobin, cultures, cytology, glucose, cholesterol, and protein.

Some patients with recurrent cardiac tamponade may need an indwelling pericardial catheter (see Fig. 2-11) for continuous drainage. With certain types of pericarditis, medications (antibiotics, antineoplastics, or corticosteroids) may be instilled during the procedure. Occasionally, a catheter may be left in situ for 1 to 3 days. When the needle is removed, pressure is immediately applied to the site with a sterile gauze pad for about 3 to 5 minutes. A bandage is then applied. A physician performs this procedure in approximately 10 to 20 minutes. Although the test is not considered painful, most patients will feel pressure as the needle is introduced into the pericardial sac.

Contraindications. Pericardiocentesis is contraindicated in the following patients:

1. Uncooperative or uncontrollable patients because the risk of laceration is increased.
2. Patients with a bleeding disorder or those receiving anticoagulant therapy because an inadvertent puncture of a cardiac chamber could precipitate uncontrollable bleeding into the pericardial sac and result in cardiac tamponade.

Nursing considerations

Nursing Diagnoses/Collaborative Problems

- Possible knowledge deficit related to test purpose, preparation, and procedure.
- High risk for alteration in comfort related to test procedure.
- Possible anxiety related to unknown sensations of the procedure.
- Potential complication: bleeding
- Potential complication: cardiac arrhythmias.
- Potential complication: vasovagal arrest.
- Potential complication: pleural infection.
- Potential complication: pneumothorax.
- Potential complication: perforation.

Nursing Implications with Rationale

- Explain the procedure to the patient. Pericardiocentesis is a very frightening experience for most patients.
- Ensure that the physician has obtained written and informed consent before the procedure.
- Assist the physician as necessary during the procedure. Observe the EKG for evidence of ST elevation, which would indicate if the needle touched the epicardial wall. If this occurs, the needle should then be slightly retracted.
- Observe the aspirate for blood. Gross blood indicates inadvertent puncture of a cardiac chamber. The blood should not clot if it is from the pericardial space.
- Carefully label and number the specimen tubes of pericardial fluid and send them to the laboratory immediately after the procedure. The specimen tubes usually contain an additive. If the proper additives are not used, the test results may be inaccurate.
- If bacterial culture and sensitivity tests are

scheduled, record any antibiotic therapy that the patient is receiving on the lab slip.

- After the procedure observe the puncture site for bleeding and hematoma formation.
- After the procedure monitor the vital signs closely (normally every 15 minutes for four times, then every 30 minutes for four times, then every hour for four times, and then every 4 hours). A falling blood pressure and a rising pulse may indicate bleeding. An increase in temperature may indicate infection.
- If a catheter remains in place for continual drainage, it is usually sutured to the skin and a sterile dressing is applied. The catheter is connected to a sterile drainage bag and secured safely below the level of the patient's midchest to prevent return of the drainage into the pericardial sac.
- Catheters are usually removed within 24 to 48 hours because of the risk of infection. After the sutures are cut, the catheter is withdrawn with a firm continuous pull. A sterile dressing is applied to the puncture site.

Serum myoglobin

Normal values: 0-85 ng/ml

Rationale. Myoglobin is an oxygen-binding protein found in cardiac tissue as well as in skeletal muscle. Measurements of myoglobin are used as an index of damage in myocardial infarction or in reinfarction. Increased levels indicate muscular injury or death. This test is more sensitive than CPK isoenzymes, but not as specific because injury, inflammation, or ischemia to noncardiac skeletal muscles can also cause elevations.

Procedure. Peripheral venipuncture is performed and approximately 5 ml of blood is placed in a red-top tube. No fasting is required.

Contraindications. None.

Nursing considerations

Nursing Diagnoses/Collaborative Problems

See Blood studies, p. 2.

Nursing Implications with Rationale

- Apply pressure to the venipuncture site after the procedure is completed. Observe the site for bleeding.

CASE STUDY 2: THROMBOPHLEBITIS

Mrs. N. was a 32-year-old nursing assistant who was admitted to the hospital complaining of a painful, swollen right leg. She was otherwise in good health. On physical examination, her right leg was seen to be one and one half times the size of her left leg. The right calf was tender and there was a 3+ pitting edema in that leg.

Studies	Results
Routine laboratory work	WNL
Doppler ultrasound and plethysmographic venous study	Occlusion of the deep venous system in the right thigh and calf (normal: no occlusion)
Venography	Same as above
^{125}I fibrinogen uptake test	Increased nuclear activity in right thigh and calf compatible with thrombophlebitis (normal: no increased uptake)

The diagnosis of acute deep-vein thrombophlebitis was made. Heparin therapy was prescribed. After full anticoagulation, she was switched to warfarin (Coumadin) (see Heparin and Warfarin Monitoring, pp. 406-409). She was discharged and continued receiving warfarin therapy and prothrombin time monitoring. After 4 months, the warfarin was discontinued.

DISCUSSION OF TESTS

Doppler ultrasound and plethysmographic venous study

Normal values: normal venous patency and venous volume.

Rationale. This combination study is used to diagnose venous thrombosis by means of two noninvasive, harmless, and painless techniques. *Doppler ultrasound* is used to determine venous patency by detecting moving red blood

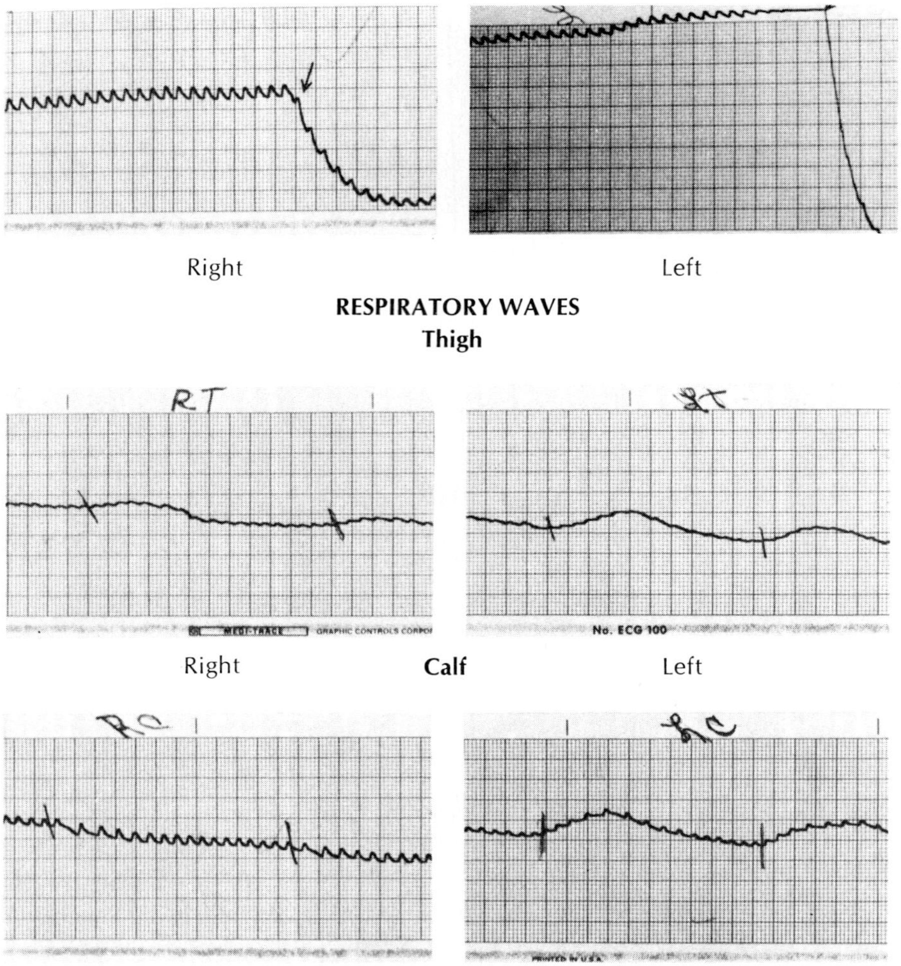

FIGURE 2-12. Venous plethysmography demonstrating chronic venous thrombosis of the right leg. *Upper frames* are recordings from the monitor cuff. Arrows indicate release of the proximal occlusion cuff. Note the decreased slope of "release waveforms" in the right leg. *Middle and lower frames* are recordings from the monitor cuff at the thigh and calf, respectively, during respiration. Vertical marks indicate respiration. Note, in the right leg, the lack of venous pressure variations associated with respiration.

cells within a vein. A transducer directs an ultrasound beam at a vein. Moving red blood cells reflect the beam back to the transducer, which then transforms the flow velocity into a "swishing" noise that is augmented by an audio speaker. If the vein is occluded, no swishing sound will be detected. *Plethysmography* measures changes in venous volume of the leg. The plethysmograph is placed on the leg and the venous volume is recorded. The venous system is then occluded proximally to the plethysmograph with a tourniquet. The sudden increase in venous volume is then displayed on a pulse-volume recorder. When the proximal tourniquet is released, the venous volume should rapidly return to the preocclusion level. In patients

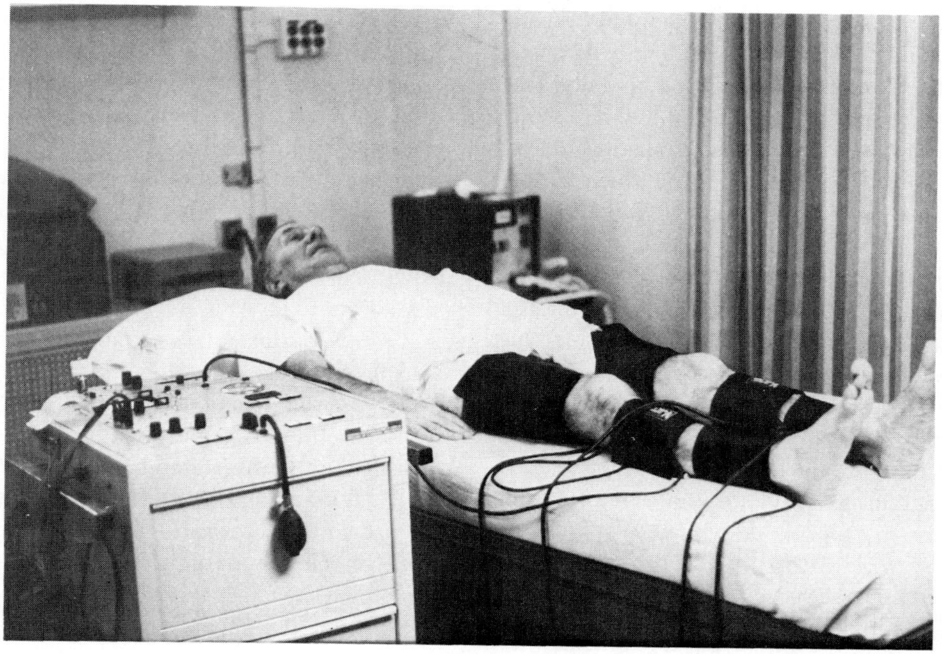

FIGURE 2-13. Placement of "occlusion cuffs" for plethysmography.

with venous thrombosis, the venous outflow is obstructed and the volume cannot dissipate quickly (Figure 2-12). Although the results of the Doppler ultrasound and plethysmographic venous study are less accurate than those of venography (see Venography, p. 46), no complications are associated with this study, and it can be performed easily and quickly on any patient with suspected venous occlusion.

Procedure. No fasting or sedation is required. The tests that make up the study can be performed equally well at the bedside or in the noninvasive vascular studies laboratory. The patient is placed in the supine position. Plethysmography is performed first. A large, inflatable "occlusion cuff" (Figure 2-13) is placed high on the patient's thigh. A second, smaller plethysmographic "monitor cuff" is placed on the calf and inflated to 10 mm Hg to facilitate recognition of small changes in the leg's venous volume. Normally, as the patient takes a sustained deep breath, the venous volume increases because of the decreased venous return from the legs caused by increased intraabdominal and thoracic pressures. As the patient exhales, the venous volume decreases. These respiratory waves are displayed on a pulse-volume recorder. Diminished respiratory waves indicate venous thrombosis (Figure 2-12).

The occlusion cuff is then inflated to 50 mm Hg. As the cuff is occluded, the monitor cuff records the rising venous volume and displays this on the recorder (Figure 2-12). After the highest volume is recorded, the occlusion cuff is rapidly deflated, and the leg should return to its preocclusion volume within 1 second. If the return to normal volume is delayed for a prolonged period of time (for example, 10 seconds), acute thrombosis exists. If the return to normal volume is partially delayed (for example, 2 to 5 seconds), the venous thrombosis is said to be chronic, and venous collateralization has already formed.

Next, the Doppler ultrasound test is performed. A conductive paste is applied to the skin overlying the vein to be studied. The paste is used to enhance sound transmission. The transducer "probe" is placed on the skin, and characteristic swishing sounds indicating movement of blood within an unoccluded and nonthrombosed vein are sought. Both the superficial and deep venous systems are evaluated by placing the sound detector on the ankle, calf, thigh, and groin. Failure to detect any sound indicates the lack of free-flowing blood within the venous system (thrombosis).

No complications or discomfort is associated with this study. A trained technician performs the study in approximately 15 minutes.

Contraindications. This study is contraindicated in the uncooperative patient.

Nursing considerations

Nursing Diagnoses/Collaborative Problems

See Ultrasound studies, p. 6.

- Possible anxiety related to unknown sensations of the procedure.
- Possible alteration in comfort related to procedure.

Nursing Implications with Rationale

- Explain the procedure to the patient. Reassure the patient that no discomfort is associated with this study.
- Tell the patient that he or she must lie still during the procedure.
- Gently remove any occlusive dressings or stockings from the leg. The patient's leg may be tender to the touch.
- After the study gently remove the conduction lubricant from the patient's extremities. Massaging the legs is contraindicated because it may dislodge thrombi.

Venography

(phlebography, venogram)

Normal value: negative (no venous thrombosis).

Rationale. Venography is an x-ray study designed to identify and locate thrombi within the venous system of the lower extremities. During this study, radiopaque dye is injected into the venous system of the affected extremity, and x-ray films are taken. Obstruction of the flow of the dye column or filling defects within the dye-filled vein indicate that thrombosis exists. A positive study confirms the diagnosis of venous thrombosis (Figure 2-14). A normal study (negative) makes the diagnosis of venous thrombosis very unlikely (Figure 2-15).

Complications in venography, though rare, include the following:

1. Allergic reaction to iodinated dye. This reaction can be prevented by using a steroid-antihistamine preparation (see p. 30, fourth nursing implication under Cardiac Catheterization).
2. Subcutaneous infiltration of dye, causing pain, swelling, and cellulitis.
3. Induction of venous thrombophlebitis (that is, the dye injection itself may cause thrombophlebitis even in a normal extremity).
4. Bacteremia, if there is compromised sterile technique.
5. Embolism, caused by dislodgement of a thrombus.

Procedure. No sedation or fasting is required. The patient is taken to the x-ray department and placed in the supine position on the x-ray table. Catheterization of a superficial vein on the foot is performed. This may require a surgical cutdown. The radiologist then injects an iodinated, radiopaque dye into the vein and takes x-ray films to follow the course of the dye up the leg. Frequently a tourniquet is placed on the leg to prevent filling of the superficial saphenous system. This study takes approximately 30 to 90 minutes. Often, both extremities are studied even though only one leg is suspected to contain deep venous thrombosis. The normal extremity is used for comparison with the involved extremity. The venous catheterization is only as uncomfortable as any cutaneous needle stick. The dye itself may cause a warm flush, but this is not as severe as with arteriography.

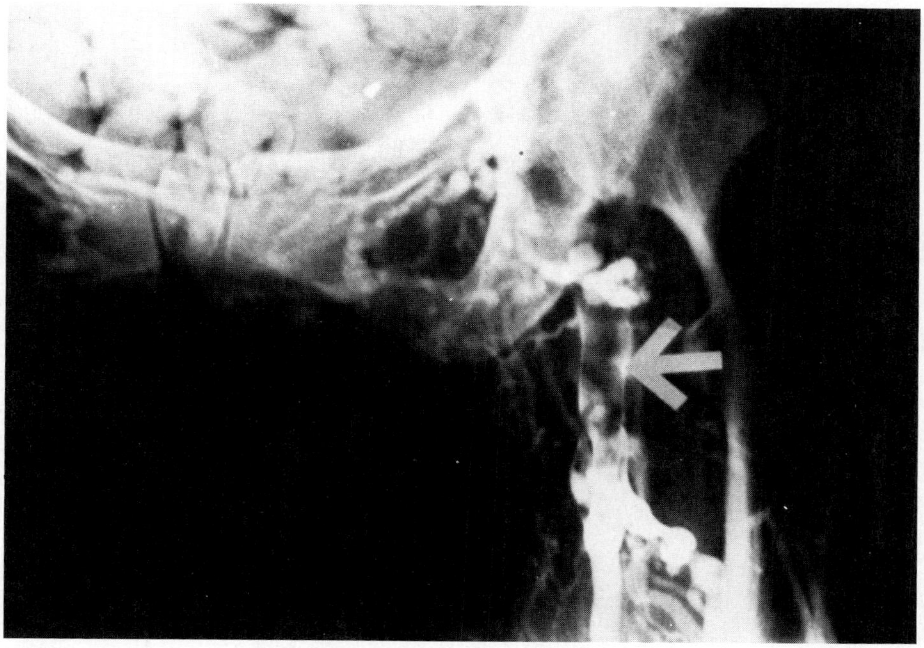

FIGURE 2-14. Abnormal venogram. Arrow indicates clot within the proximal femoral vein.

Contraindications. This study is contraindicated in the uncooperative patient, the patient allergic to iodinated dye, the patient with severe edema of the legs making venous access impossible, and the patient with renal failure because iodinated dye is nephrotoxic.

Nursing considerations

Nursing Diagnoses/Collaborative Problems

See X-ray studies, p. 5.

- Potential complication: cellulitis.
- Potential complication: thrombophlebitis.
- Potential complication: bacteremia.
- Potential complication: embolism.

Nursing Implications with Rationale

- Explain the procedure to the patient and allay the patient's fears regarding venography.
- Assess the patient for allergies to dye. Administer a steroid-antihistamine preparation if ordered for the patient allergic to the dye (p. 30).
- Ensure that the patient is adequately hydrated before testing. Iodinated dye can further impair renal function, especially if it is already compromised by dehydration or chronic renal disease.
- See that patients in a considerable amount of pain are medicated so that they can lie still during this procedure. Handle the affected extremity very gently.
- After the study assess the patient for cellulitis (redness, swelling, pain, tenderness), indicative of subcutaneous infiltration of dye.
- After the study assess the patient for signs of bacteremia (increased temperature, tachycardia, cutaneous flush, or chills).

^{125}I fibrinogen uptake test

(FUT, radioactive fibrinogen scanning)

Normal value: negative (no deep-vein thrombosis).

Rationale. ^{125}I fibrinogen uptake is a noninvasive radionuclear test used to identify thrombi

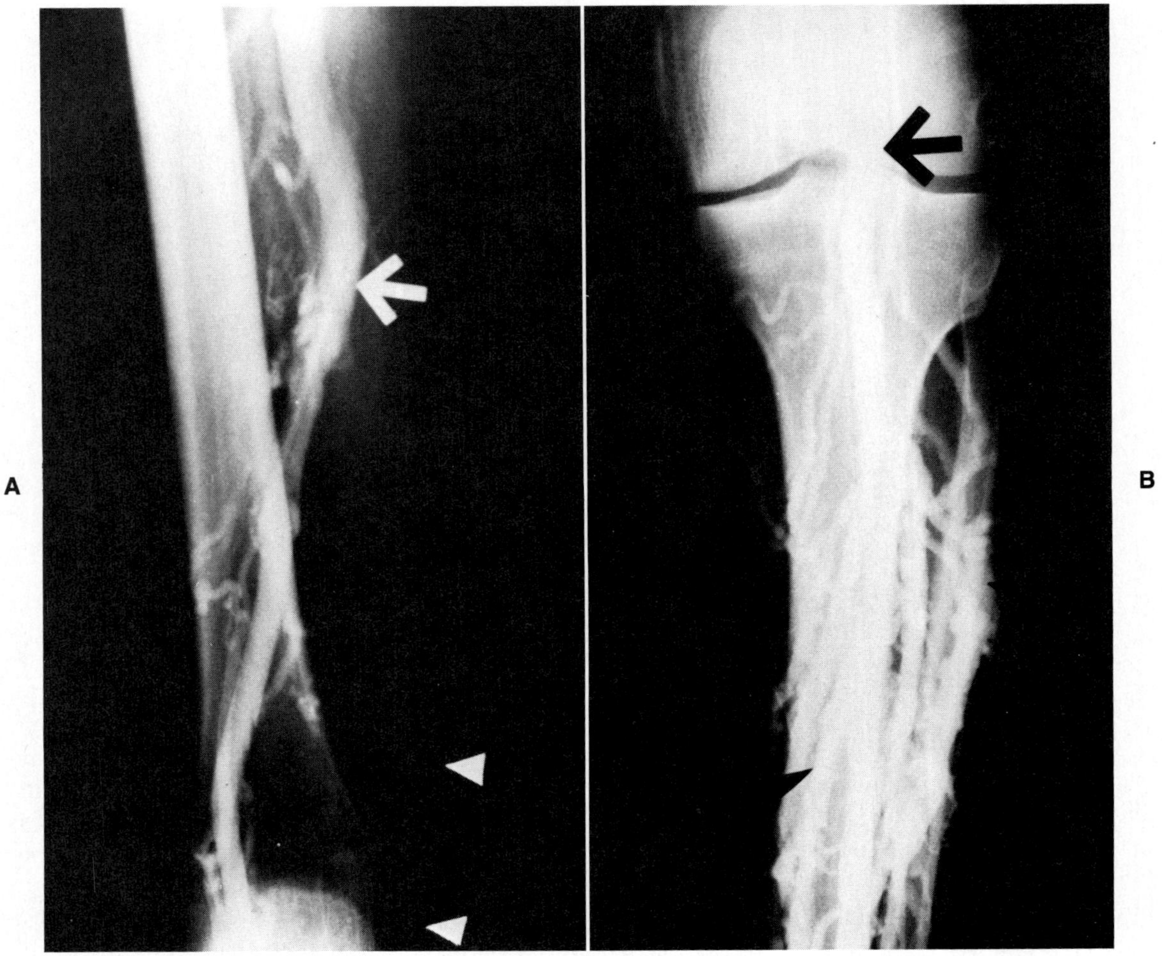

FIGURE 2-15. **A**, Normal venogram of the upper half of the leg. White arrow indicates normal deep femoral vein. Small white pointers indicate poorly visualized superficial saphenous vein. **B**, Normal venogram of lower leg. Black arrow indicates normal popliteal vein. Small black pointer indicates one of many normal unnamed deep veins in the calf.

in the veins of the extremities. Large amounts of fibrinogen are normally present at the site of clot formation because of the importance of fibrinogen (factor I) in hemostasis (see page 386). When an external source of fibrinogen is tagged with ^{125}I and given intravenously to the patient, one can detect the iodinated fibrinogen in the bloodstream by means of a gamma-ray detector. At areas where clot formation is occurring (such as venous thromboses), the ^{125}I count is markedly increased. The test is about 80% to 90% accurate in the diagnosis of deep-vein thrombophlebitis. Although it was once thought to be able to recognize only "forming" clots, it is now known that established clots can be detected by the FUT. Not only is this test useful in the study of established deep-vein thromboses, but it is also useful in the detection of subclinical, early thromboses in patients at high risk of deep-vein thrombosis. There are several disadvantages to

FUT testing as compared with conventional venography:

1. FUT cannot detect deep-vein thrombosis in the upper thigh. Because a high quantity of fibrinogen normally occurs in this area, an increase caused by thrombosis will not be recognized.
2. It is necessary to wait 24 hours between giving ^{125}I fibrinogen and testing the leg for increased uptake. This is a major disadvantage when one needs to know if deep-vein thrombosis exists so that anticoagulation therapy can be instituted.
3. Because the fibrinogen used for ^{125}I labeling is obtained from donated blood, the possibility of hepatitis transmission exists.

Procedure. The nonfasting, unsedated patient is taken to the nuclear medicine department, and an intravenous injection of ^{125}I-labeled fibrinogen is administered. The patient is returned to the nuclear medicine department 24 hours later, and a geigerlike detector is placed over the patient's ankles, calf, and lower thighs. The amount of ^{125}I present at these sites is recorded and compared with the amount present at the opposite leg or at the precordium. If the amount of ^{125}I detected at any area is 15 times greater than that found at the area used for comparison, the test is considered positive for deep-vein thrombosis. This test causes no discomfort, other than that associated with the injection of fibrinogen. Thyroid gland uptake of the radioiodine should be blocked by giving Lugol's solution or potassium iodine before injection. The scanning takes about 1 hour to complete and is usually performed by a radionuclear technician. The test is interpreted by a nuclear medicine physician.

Contraindications. This test is contraindicated in the following patients:

1. Patients in whom the diagnosis of deep-vein thrombosis is needed in less than 24 hours.
2. Patients with ongoing inflammation of the leg (such as superficial phlebitis, cellulitis, and active arthritis), because fibrinogen will also go to areas of inflammation and give a false-positive result.
3. Patients with primary lymphedema, because fibrinogen is increased in the legs of patients afflicted by lymphedema praecox (primary lymphedema characterized by diffuse swelling of the lower extremities).
4. Patients who are allergic to iodine.

Nursing considerations

Nursing Diagnoses/Collaborative Problems

See Nuclear scanning, p. 5.

Nursing Implications with Rationale

- Explain the procedure to the patient. Provide emotional support.
- Before the study assess the patient's legs for evidence of inflammation, which will cause a false positive result.
- Caution nursing mothers to refrain from breast-feeding for 24 to 48 hours after injection of ^{125}I.

CASE STUDY 3: PERIPHERAL VASCULAR DISEASE

Mr. R. was a 52-year-old man who complained of pain and cramping in his right calf while walking two blocks. The pain was relieved with cessation of activity. The pain had been increasing in frequency and intensity. Physical examination findings were essentially normal except for decreased hair on the right leg. The patient's popliteal, dorsalis pedis, and posterior tibial pulses were markedly decreased in comparison to those of his left leg.

Studies	Results
Routine laboratory work	WNL
Doppler ultrasound systolic pressures	Femoral: 130 mm Hg Popliteal: 90 mm Hg Posterior tibial: 88 mm Hg Dorsalis pedis: 88 mm Hg (normal: same as brachial systolic blood pressure)

Studies	Results
Arterial plethysmography	Decreased amplitude of distal femoral, popliteal, dorsalis pedis, and posterior tibial pulse waves (see Figure 2-16)
Femoral arteriography of right leg	Obstruction of the femoral artery at the midthigh level (see Figure 2-17)

With the clinical picture of classic intermittent claudication, the noninvasive Doppler and plethysmographic arterial vascular study merely documented the presence and location of the arterial occlusion in the proximal femoral artery. Most vascular surgeons require arteriography to document the location of the vascular occlusion. Mr. R. underwent a bypass from the proximal femoral artery to the popliteal artery. After surgery he was asymptomatic.

DISCUSSION OF TESTS

Doppler ultrasound and plethysmographic arterial study

(noninvasive arterial studies)

Normal value: negative (no arterial occlusion).

Rationale. With the use of this painless and harmless noninvasive study, one can identify and locate peripheral arteriosclerotic occlusive disease. By placing blood pressure cuffs on the thigh, calf, and ankle, the systolic pressure in the various arteries of an extremity can be measured by ultrasound. The extremely sensitive Doppler ultrasound detector can detect even minimal blood flow. Normally, there is less than a 20 mm Hg drop in systolic pressure from the arm to the arteries of the leg. If the pressure in the arteries of the leg is less than the arm's systolic blood pressure by 20 mm Hg or more, arterial occlusion exists immediately proximal to the area where the decreased pressure was noted.

By attaching these blood pressure cuffs to a plethysmograph (that is, a pulse-volume recorder), each arterial pulse can be displayed as a pulse wave. Reduction in amplitude of a pulse wave in any of the three cuffs indicates arterial occlusion immediately proximal to the area where the decreased amplitude was noted (Figure 2-16). A positive result is reliable evidence of arteriosclerotic peripheral vascular occlusion. A negative result, however, does not definitely exclude this diagnosis, because extensive vascular collateralization can compensate for even a complete arterial occlusion. No complications are associated with this test.

Procedure. The patient is placed in a supine position. The tests involved in this study can be performed at the bedside or in the noninvasive vascular studies laboratory. No fasting or sedation is required for this painless study. The Doppler ultrasound test is performed first. Blood pressure cuffs are placed around the thigh, calf, and ankle. A conductive paste is applied to the skin overlying the arteries to be studied. The proximal cuff is inflated to a level above systolic pressure. The Doppler ultrasound blood flow detector is placed immediately distal to that of the inflated cuff. The pressure is slowly released. The highest pressure at which the blood flow is heard (as a swishing noise) is recorded as the systolic pressure of the artery located under the detector. The procedure is then repeated at the calf and ankle level.

Next the cuffs are attached to a plethysmograph. The cuffs are minimally inflated to 65 mm Hg to increase their sensitivity to pulse waves. The pulse waves are recorded on the plethysmographic tape. The amplitudes of the wave at each cuff are measured and compared. This study requires about 15 minutes to perform and is usually done by a trained technician. No discomfort is associated with it.

Contraindications. This test is contraindicated in the uncooperative patient.

Nursing considerations

Nursing Diagnoses/Collaborative Problems

See Ultrasound studies, p. 6.

- Possible anxiety related to unknown sensations of the procedure.
- Possible alteration in comfort related to test procedure.

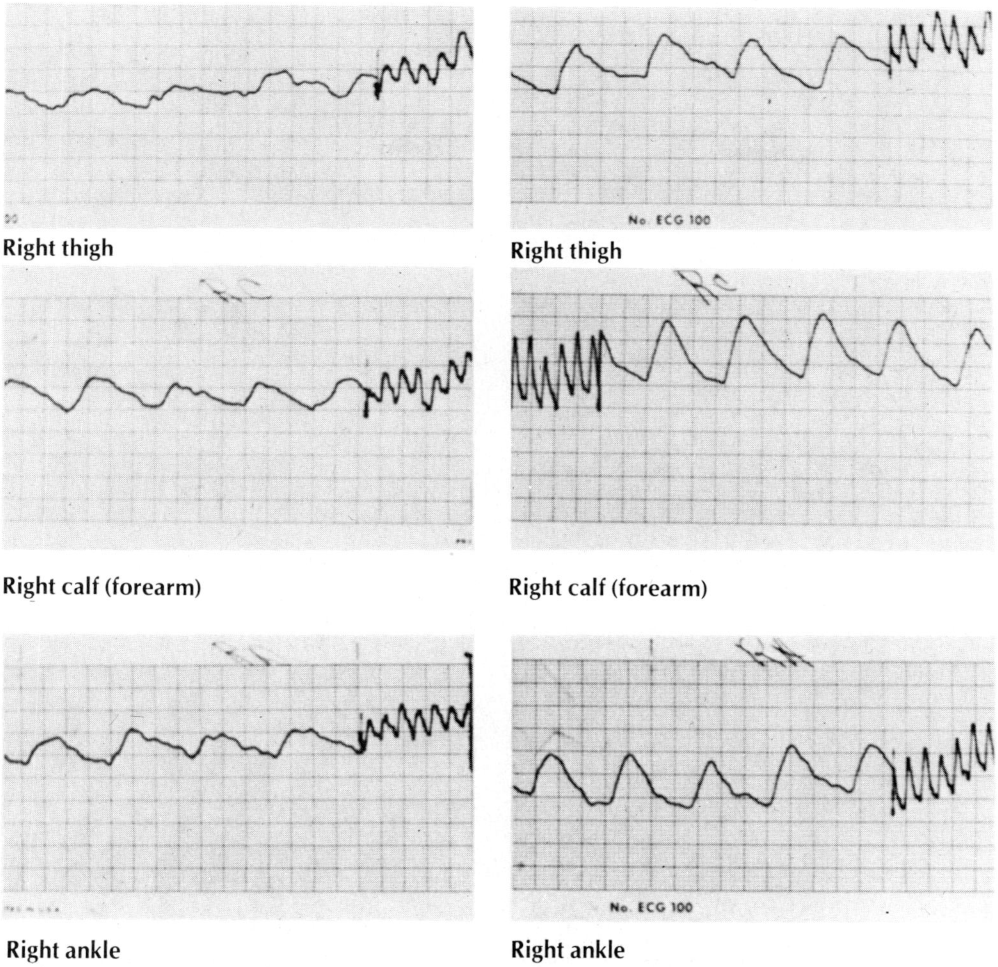

FIGURE 2-16. Arterial plethysmography. Pulse pressure waves of a patient with femoral arterial occlusive disease *before* arterial reconstruction *(left frames)* and *after* arterial reconstruction *(right frames)*. Upper, middle, and lower frames are recordings of the thigh, calf, and ankle, respectively.

Nursing Implications with Rationale

- See Doppler ultrasound and Plethysmographic Venous Study.
- Instruct the patient to avoid smoking for at least 30 minutes before the Doppler study. Nicotine causes constriction of the peripheral arteries and alters the Doppler ultrasound test's results.

Femoral arteriography

(femoral angiogram)

Normal value: normal femoral arterial vasculature.

Rationale. Femoral arteriography allows for accurate identification and location of occlusions within the femoral arterial system. After a catheter is placed in the femoral artery, radiopaque

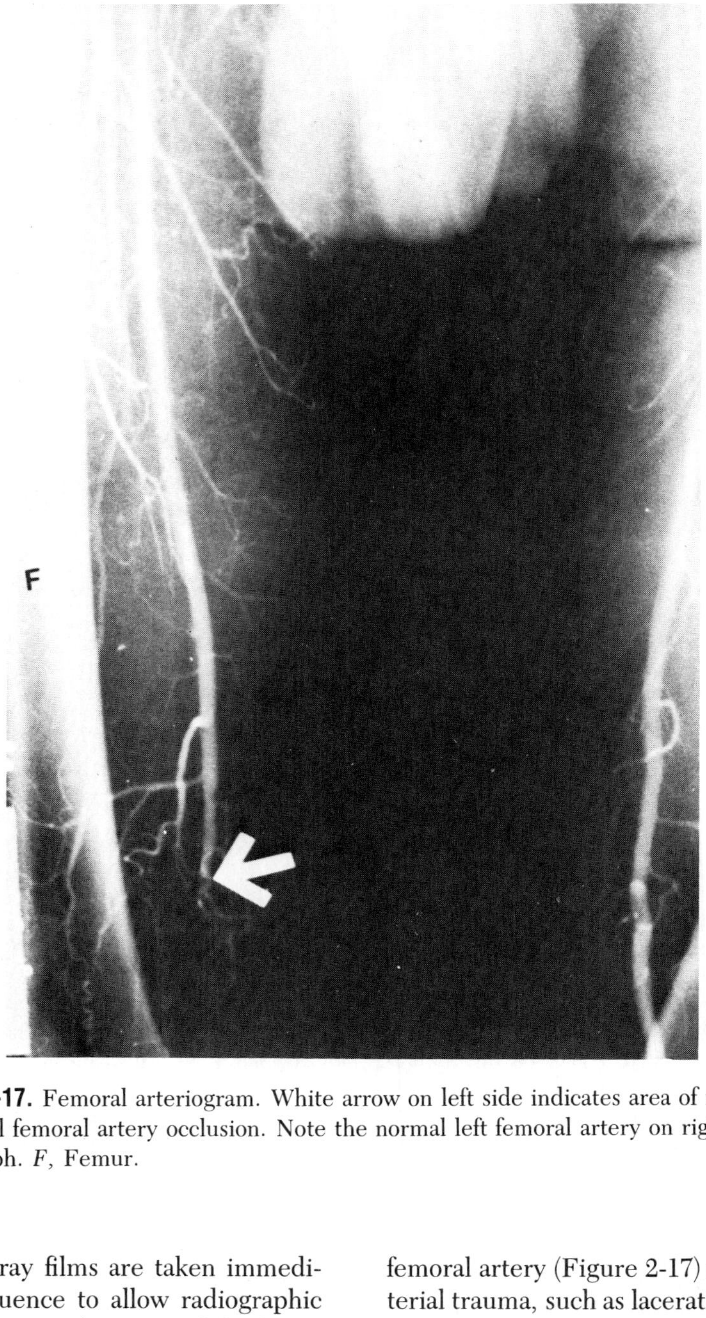

FIGURE 2-17. Femoral arteriogram. White arrow on left side indicates area of right superficial femoral artery occlusion. Note the normal left femoral artery on right side of photograph. *F*, Femur.

dye is injected. X-ray films are taken immediately in timed sequence to allow radiographic visualization of the arterial system of the lower extremity. Total or near-total occlusion of the flow of dye is seen in arteriosclerotic vascular occlusive disease. Arterial emboli or acute thrombosis will be seen as total occlusions of the femoral artery (Figure 2-17) or its branches. Arterial trauma, such as lacerations or intimal tears (laceration of the inner lining), are likewise seen as total or near-total obstructions to the flow. Fusiform dilatation of the femoral artery or its branches is indicative of aneurysm. Unusual arterial disorders such as Buerger's disease and fibromuscular dysplasia have pathognomonic arteriographic findings.

Femoral arteriography is usually done electively on patients who have symptoms and signs of peripheral vascular disease. However, emergency arteriography is needed when blood flow to an extremity has ceased suddenly. Immediate surgical therapy is needed, and that surgery is most effective when the surgeon has knowledge of the etiology and location of the sudden occlusion. This knowledge can be obtained only by arteriography.

Complications of this study include hemorrhage at the site of the arterial puncture; disruption of an arteriosclerotic plaque, leading to sudden occlusion of the femoral vessel, catheter dissection of the intimal lining of the artery from the remaining wall; allergic reaction to the dye; pseudoaneurysm formation; and embolism to the distal extremity.

Procedure. Preferably, the patient is kept fasting for 8 hours, although this is not necessary. Usually sedation (meperidine) is ordered, if needed, for arteriography. The patient is taken to the "special studies" arteriography laboratory (usually in the radiology department) and placed on a special, moveable x-ray table. He or she is asked to lie still in the supine position. To decrease the possibility of spasm or emboli, the femoral artery on the side opposite to the involved extremity is catheterized after the groin is prepared and draped in a sterile manner. A radiopaque catheter is guided under x-ray visualization into the proximal iliac artery, through the aorta, and down the leg to be studied. Once the catheter is positioned in the involved femoral vessel, radiopaque dye is injected, and x-ray films of the thigh, calf, and ankle are taken immediately at a timed sequence. This allows visualization of the femoral artery and its branches. After the x-ray films are taken, the catheter is removed and a pressure dressing is applied to the puncture site.

As with all arteriograms, the patient will feel an uncomfortable and sometimes painful heat flash, which usually lasts less than 10 seconds. This, along with the initial arterial puncture, is the only discomfort the patient will feel. A radiologist performs this study in approximately 40 minutes.

Contraindications. This study is contraindicated in the uncooperative patient and in the patient allergic to dye. The test must be considered risky for those who have compromised renal function. The iodine contrast may cause further deterioration of renal function, especially in dehydrated patients. The use of a nonionic iodinated contrast medium can minimize the effect on the kidneys.

Nursing considerations

Nursing Diagnoses/Collaborative Problems

See X-ray studies, p. 5.

- Possible injury related to sedatives.
- Potential complication: adverse reaction or allergy.
- Potential complication: bleeding.
- Potential complication: perforation.
- Potential complication: stroke.
- Potential complication: peripheral arterial problems.
- Potential complication: infection.

Nursing Implications with Rationale

- Explain the procedure to the patient. Tell the patient where the catheter will be inserted. Inform the patient that he or she will feel a warm flush when the dye is injected. Provide emotional support.
- Assess the patient for allergies to iodine dye.
- Keep the patient NPO from midnight on the day of the study.
- Ensure that informed, written consent for this procedure is obtained before administering the preprocedure medications.
- Generally, keep the patient on bed rest for about 8 hours after the procedure to allow complete sealing of the puncture site.
- After the procedure observe the catheter insertion site for inflammation, hemorrhage, hematoma, or the absence of peripheral

pulses. Usually, apply a pressure dressing and sandbag to the catheter site. Assess the involved extremity for numbness, tingling, pain, or loss of function. The color and temperature of the involved extremity are compared with the color and temperature of the uninvolved extremity.

- Assess the vital signs for evidence of bleeding (decreased blood pressure and increased pulse). Vital sign measurements are usually ordered every 15 minutes for four times, then every 30 minutes for four times, then every hour for four times, and then every 4 hours. Of course, one may take these more frequently.
- Apply cold compresses to the puncture site if these are needed to reduce discomfort and swelling. Administer mild analgesics, if these have been ordered. If the patient is having continuous, severe pain, the physician should check the site, because a hematoma may be forming.

SUPPLEMENTAL INFORMATION

Carotid duplex scanning

(ultrasonic duplex scanning)

Normal value: normal carotid artery; absence of plaques and stenosis.

Rationale. Since stroke is a common cause of death, a number of noninvasive tests have been developed to evaluate arterial occlusive disease of the extracranial carotid arteries. Indirect tests (such as oculoplethysmography, see Chapter 6) evaluate hemodynamic changes at some point removed from the site of occlusion, and direct tests provide anatomic or hemodynamic information concerning the carotid artery itself. Ultrasonic duplex scanning is a direct type of noninvasive procedure used to detect extracranial carotid artery disease. The duplex concept is based on the ability to define the walls in the vessel within a two-dimensional image and uses the pulse Doppler to evaluate blood velocities, pulse wave amplitude and configuration within the artery visualized.

With the development of the Fast Fourier Transform (FFT) spectrum analyzer, it became obvious that velocity patterns recorded from the common carotid artery could be of additional use in detecting high grade stenosis or total occlusion of the internal carotid artery. This is a great advantage of Duplex scanning since indirect studies have two major disadvantages. (1) Indirect studies cannot detect minimal disease, which may not markedly affect flow or pressure. (It is now known that disease of the carotid bifurcation, which may produce transient ischemic attacks and strokes, can vary from minimal lesions to total occlusion.) (2) Indirect studies cannot differentiate high-grade stenosis from complete obstruction. Thus, a great benefit of duplex scanning is that it is a noninvasive technique that can identify both normal vessels and those within the entire spectrum of disease involvement.

Procedure. No special patient preparation is required before carotid Duplex scanning. The study is done with the patient in the supine position with the head supported to prevent lateral movement. A water-soluble gel is used to couple the sound from the scanner to the skin surface. Images of the vessel wall and the arterial wave form as well as amplitude are obtained. This study is done by a technologist and is interpreted by a radiologist, cardiologist, or vascular surgeon. It takes about 15 to 30 minutes.

Contraindications. None.

Nursing considerations

Nursing Diagnoses/Collaborative Problems

- Possible knowledge deficit related to test purpose, preparation, and procedure.
- Possible anxiety related to test results.

Nursing Implications with Rationale

- Explain the procedure to the patient. Assure him or her that this is a painless study.
- Explain to the patient that a gel will be applied to the skin over the area to enhance transmission of sound waves.

- After the study, remove the gel from the patient's neck area.

QUESTIONS AND ANSWERS

1. **QUESTION:** Why is an electrocardiogram referred to as either an EKG or an ECG?
   ANSWER: *EKG* is an abbreviation of the German word *Electrokardiogram. ECG* is the abbreviation of the English word *electrocardiogram.* Many people prefer the abbreviation *EKG* to avoid confusion with the abbreviation for *electroencephalogram* (EEG).
2. **QUESTION:** The physician has requested an EKG on a 6-week-old infant. What may be an appropriate method of quieting your patient during this procedure?
   ANSWER: Plan to record the EKG at a time when the infant usually receives a bottle feeding. If necessary, distract the infant's attention with toys or keys. If it is necessary for anyone to hold or touch the child, that person should wear rubber gloves to avoid electrical interference.
3. **QUESTION:** You are the nurse in the coronary care unit. While observing the cardiac monitors, you see a straight line for one of the patients. What should be your immediate reaction?
   ANSWER: Sometimes mechanical failure causes the equipment used for cardiac monitoring to display a straight or flat line on the cardiac monitor instead of the patient's normal heartbeat. Nevertheless, the possibility exists that the patient's heart has indeed stopped. Therefore, before notifying the appropriate personnel involved in cardiac resuscitation, you should go immediately to the patient's room and assess the patient for signs of cardiac arrest.
4. **QUESTION:** Your patient has had a cardiac arrest and is being resuscitated. The EKG machine is attached to the patient to monitor cardiac rhythm. It is decided to attempt defibrillation of the heart. What precautions should be taken concerning the EKG machine?
   ANSWER: During defibrillation, 400 mV of electric power is delivered. This power will be transformed from the patient to the EKG machine if the patient is not detached from it. This reversed electrical flow may damage the machine. It is important to detach the lead wires from the EKG machine to protect it from any harm during defibrillation.
5. **QUESTION:** Your patient has returned from the operating room after having a radical mastectomy of the left breast. Your assessment indicates that the patient's vital signs are stable and that the dressings covering the entire left chest are dry and intact. Because of the patient's history of coronary artery disease, the surgeon has requested an EKG. How should you perform this test?
   ANSWER: Obviously, the dressings applied to a patient who has had either a left-breast mastectomy or left-sided chest surgery will prevent you from adequately placing the precordial leads for the EKG. You should notify the physician that it is impossible to perform this study unless the dressings are removed. At the physician's discretion, you may leave the dressings in place and do the EKG using only the six limb leads, or you may remove the dressings and obtain a complete 12-lead EKG.
6. **QUESTION:** Your patient has returned from femoral arteriography performed through the right groin. The patient begins to complain of right-leg pain, weakness, and tingling. You assess the patient and find a small hematoma in the groin. You note that the right leg is pale, pulseless, and cooler than the left. What are the appropriate nursing interventions?
   ANSWER: It appears as though your patient has suffered an arteriocclusion of the right femoral vessels. The arterial puncture most probably dislodged an intimal (inner arterial lining) atherosclerotic plaque, causing an embolus or dissection of the vessel. You should reassure the patient and do the following:
   1. Notify the physician of your present findings.
   2. Not elevate the leg, because elevation will exacerbate the arterial ischemia.
   3. Prepare the patient for surgery, if this is directed by the physician.
      a. Shave and prepare both sides of the groin.
      b. Start an IV line.
      c. Keep the patient NPO.
      d. Obtain two red-top tubes for typing and cross-matching blood.
      e. Assist in obtaining an informed consent for arterial embolectomy or arterial intimal repair.

      (This routine may vary from hospital to hospital.)
   4. Make the appropriate arrangements if a second femoral arteriogram is ordered before surgery.

7. **QUESTION:** Your patient is admitted for an evaluation of increasingly frequent chest pains. In a review of other system complaints, you find that the patient has bilateral calf pain when walking two blocks (intermittent claudication). One of the studies ordered for this patient is a stress test. Can you expect that this test will be completed reliably?

   ANSWER: No. The patient's peripheral vascular occlusive disease will cause the patient to have calf pain. This calf pain will probably precede exercise-induced chest pain or EKG changes and thus cause the stress test to be terminated prematurely. This patient may be a candidate for the dipyridamole-thallium myocardial perfusion study.

8. **QUESTION:** What is the purpose of determining oxygen content in the blood obtained from the various heart chambers and arteries during cardiac catheterization?

   ANSWER: Abnormal shunting of blood from one heart chamber to another can be diagnosed by the abnormal oxygen content of the blood withdrawn from a particular chamber. For example, in a patient with an atrial septal defect, the oxygen content of the blood in the right atrium is much higher than that of blood drawn from the superior vena cava. Normally, these areas have the same oxygen content. The elevated oxygen content in the right atrium is caused by the mixing of blood from the left atrium with the blood contained in the right atrium.

BIBLIOGRAPHY

Bierman EL: Atherosclerosis and other forms of arteriosclerosis. In Wilson J and others, editors: Harrisons's principles of internal medicine, ed 12, New York, 1991, McGraw-Hill.

Biagine A and others: Early assessment of coronary reserve after bypass surgery by dipyridamole transesophageal echocardiographic stress test, Am Heart J 120 (5):1097-1101, 1990.

Braunwald E, editor: Heart disease: a textbook of cardiovascular medicine, ed 3, Philadelphia, 1991, WB Saunders.

Come PC and others: Noninvasive methods of cardiac examination. In Wilson J and others, editors: Harrison's principles of internal medicine, ed 12, New York, 1991, McGraw-Hill.

Daniel WG, Erbel R, and others: Safety of transesophageal echocardiology: a multicenter survey of 10,419 examinations, Circulation 83:817-821, 1991.

DiLucente L, Gorcsan J: Transesophageal echocardiography: application to the postoperative cardiac surgery patient, Dimens Crit Care Nurs 10 (2):74-80, March-April, 1991.

Docker CS and others: Intraoperative echocardiography: an essential tool in cardiac surgery . . . epicardial echocardiography . . . transesophageal echocardiography, AORN 55 (1):167, 169-173, 1992.

Fisher EA, Stahl JA, and others: Transesophageal echocardiography: procedures and clinical applications, J Am Coll Cardiol 18 (5):1338-1348, 1991.

Gibler WB and others: Chest pain: how many tests are enough? Patient Care 25 (1):18-33, 1991.

Higgins CB: Newer cardiac imaging techniques. In Braunwald E, editor: Heart disease, ed 4, Philadelphia, 1992, WB Saunders.

Kisslo J, Adam DB, Belkin RN: Doppler color flow imaging, New York, 1988, Churchill Livingstone.

Lam J and others: Safety and diagnostic accuracy of dipyridamole-thallium imaging in the elderly, J Am Coll Cardiol 11:585-589, 1988.

Myerburg RJ: Electrocardiography. In Wilson J and others, editors: Harrison's principles of internal medicine, ed 12, New York, 1991, McGraw-Hill.

Pasternak RC and others: Acute myocardial infarction. In Wilson J and others, editors: Harrison's principles of internal medicine, ed 12, New York, 1991, McGraw-Hill.

Pinner J: Patient teaching for x-ray and other diagnostics, RN 54 (3):32-36, 1991.

Robie BH: Cardiovascular technology: noninvasive diagnosis of cardiovascular disease using ultrasound imaging, J Cardiovasc Nurs 6 (2):36-42, January, 1992.

Selwyn AP, Braunwald E: Ischemic heart disease. In Wilson J and others, editors: Harrison's principles of internal medicine, ed 12, New York, 1991, McGraw-Hill.

Sergi NA: When your patient needs a stress test. RN 54 (3):26-30, 1991.

Seward JB, Khanderia BK, and others: Biplane transesophageal echocardiography: anatomic correlations, image orientation, and clinical applications, Mayo Clin Proc 65:1993-2213, 1988.

Skalaroff HJ: Preoperative evaluation of patients with cardiac disease, Mt Sinai J Med 58 (1):48-57, January 1991.

Stevens L, Redd R, and Buchingham T. Emergency catheter ablation of refractory ventricular tachycardia. Crit Care Nurs 9:5, 1989.

Taylor DC: Duplex ultrasound in assessment of vascular disease in clinical hypertension, Am J Hypertension, 4 (6):550-556, 1991.

Velos JC: A review of cardiac modalities, Nurse Pract Forum 2 (4):231-238, December 1991.

Zaret BL and others: Nuclear cardiology. In Braunwald E, editor: Heart disease, ed 4, Philadelphia, 1992, WB Saunders.

Chapter 3

DIAGNOSTIC STUDIES USED IN THE ASSESSMENT OF THE
GASTROINTESTINAL SYSTEM

ANATOMY AND PHYSIOLOGY

The primary function of the gastrointestinal (GI) tract (Figure 3-1) is to provide the body with water, electrolytes, and nutrients. To accomplish this, food must be moved through the system while digestive enzymes are secreted to break down the food to a form that can easily be absorbed by the GI tract's lining cells.

The *esophagus* is a long muscular tube that, by successive and synchronized contractions, moves food from the pharynx (posterior mouth) through the lower esophageal sphincter and into the *stomach.* The stomach is a J-shaped structure that lies between the esophagus and the duodenum. In the stomach food is stored. Here the parietal and chief cells, located in the lining of the proximal stomach, secrete hydrochloric acid and pepsinogen, respectively. The acid and enzymes mix with the food, and the digestive process is begun. Intrinsic factor, essential to the absorption of vitamin B_{12}, is also secreted by the parietal cells.

Partially digested food (chyme) is expelled through the pyloric sphincter and into the *duodenum.* Here the pancreas and biliary tract enter the GI tract. The pancreas secretes proteolytic enzymes (trypsin and chymotrypsin), lipolytic enzymes (lipase), and amylatic enzymes (amylase). Because all digestive enzymes work best in an alkaline environment, water and bicarbonate also are secreted by the pancreas to provide an optimum basic pH. Water and bicarbonate are also secreted by the biliary system, along with bile salts, bilirubin, cholesterol, and phospholipids. The bile salts mix with the fatty acids and speed absorption of the fats. Bil-

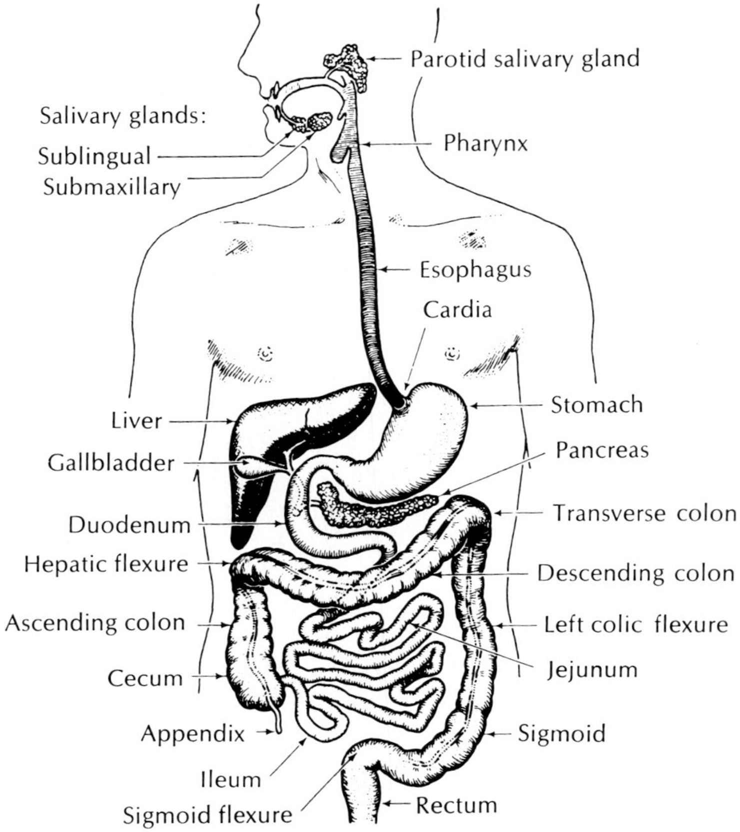

FIGURE 3-1. Anatomy of the gastrointestinal tract.
From Schottelius BA and Schottelius DD: Textbook of physiology, ed 18, St Louis, 1978, The CV Mosby Co.

irubin, cholesterol, and phospholipids have little or no digestive function and are merely excreta.

As the chyme moves through the *small bowel* (jejunum and ileum), further digestion and nutrient absorption occur. Finally, water and electrolytes (sodium, potassium, chloride, and bicarbonates) are absorbed in the *colon*. Undigested material (feces) is moved into the *rectum*. The rectum is a vault at the end of the GI tract where the feces are stored until evacuation.

The entire GI system is regulated by a neurohormonal feedback system. Gastrin (secreted in the mucosa of the distal stomach), along with the vagus nerve, stimulates hydrochloric acid secretion and propulsive muscular action of the stomach and intestines. The acid load in the duodenum stimulates the secretion of cholecystokinin and secretin from the duodenal mucosa. These in turn stimulate, respectively, secretions of biliary and pancreatic products of digestion. After digestion is completed, secretin and enterokinase (made by the intestinal mucosa) inhibit gastrin release and thereby slow the digestive process to its "between meal" activity.

CASE STUDY 1: PEPTIC ULCER DISEASE

A 35-year-old male executive had a 6-month history of epigastric discomfort that occurred 2 hours after meals and frequently awoke him at night. The pain was relieved by antacids or food. The physical examination results were negative.

Studies	**Results**
Routine laboratory studies	Negative
Upper gastrointestinal series (UGI)	Large gastric ulcer on lesser curvature of stomach
Gastric analysis	
Basal acid output (BAO)	4 mEq/hr (normal: 2-5 mEq/hr)
Maximal acid output (MAO)	12 mEq/hr (normal: 10-20 mEq/hr)
BAO/MAO	0.3 (normal: <0.6)
Gastroscopy	Confirmed presence of ulcer
Biopsies of ulcer through gastroscope	Benign
Gastric washings for cytology	Negative for malignant cells
Serum gastrin study	90 pg/ml (normal: 40-150 pg/ml)

The results of the UGI clearly demonstrated that this man's symptoms were caused by an ulcer. Because gastric analysis showed him not to be achlorhydric, the etiology of the ulcer was suspected to be peptic rather than neoplastic. No malignant cells were seen in the gastric washings or in the biopsy specimens taken through the gastroscope. Because the possibility of malignancy was excluded, a conservative medical regimen that included antacids (such as Maalox), cimetidine (Tagamet), and rest was prescribed. Repeat UGI series that were performed 6 weeks later demonstrated near total healing of the ulcer.

DISCUSSION OF TESTS

Upper gastrointestinal study

(upper GI series, UGI)

Normal values: normal size, contour, patency, filling, positioning, and transit time of barium.

Rationale. The upper GI study consists of a series of x-ray films of the lower esophagus, stomach, and duodenum using barium sulfate as the contrast medium. The purpose of this examination is to detect ulcers (Figure 3-2), tumors, inflammations, or anatomic malposition (e.g., hiatal hernia). Also, repeat UGIs allow one to follow the healing process of ulcers. Generally if a 50% reduction in the size of the ulcer within 3 weeks does not occur, malignancy must be ruled out as the cause of a gastric ulcer.

Procedure. To examine the upper GI tract, the fasting patient is required to swallow approximately 8 ounces of barium. Barium is a white, chalky, radiopaque substance that is ingested in a suspension much like a milk shake. It is usually flavored to increase palatability. After drinking the barium, the patient is moved through several positional changes, such as prone, supine, and lateral, to promote barium flow by gravity through the upper GI tract. Small spot films are taken at the discretion of the radiologist. Large films are taken in certain standard, specified positions.

As this contrast medium descends, the lower esophagus is examined for position, patency, and filling defects (which would indicate tumors, scarring, or varices (see barium swallow, p. 69). As the barium fills the stomach, the gastric wall is examined for ulcers (both benign and malignant), filling defects (tumors, most commonly malignant), and anatomic abnormalities such as hiatal hernia (Figure 3-3). As the barium leaves the stomach, the patency of the pyloric valve is evaluated. Benign ulcers are the most common pathologic condition seen in the duodenum. The duration of this study is about 30 minutes. The patient may be uncomfortable lying on the hard, x-ray table.

If a contrast is requested, the patient is asked to swallow CO_2 powder. The CO_2 gas acts to create a contrast to the barium and provides more accurate visualization of the mucosa of the esophagus, stomach, and duodenum.

If desired, a *small bowel follow-through study* may be performed by instructing the patient to drink additional barium mixed with saline solution. Films are then taken at timed in-

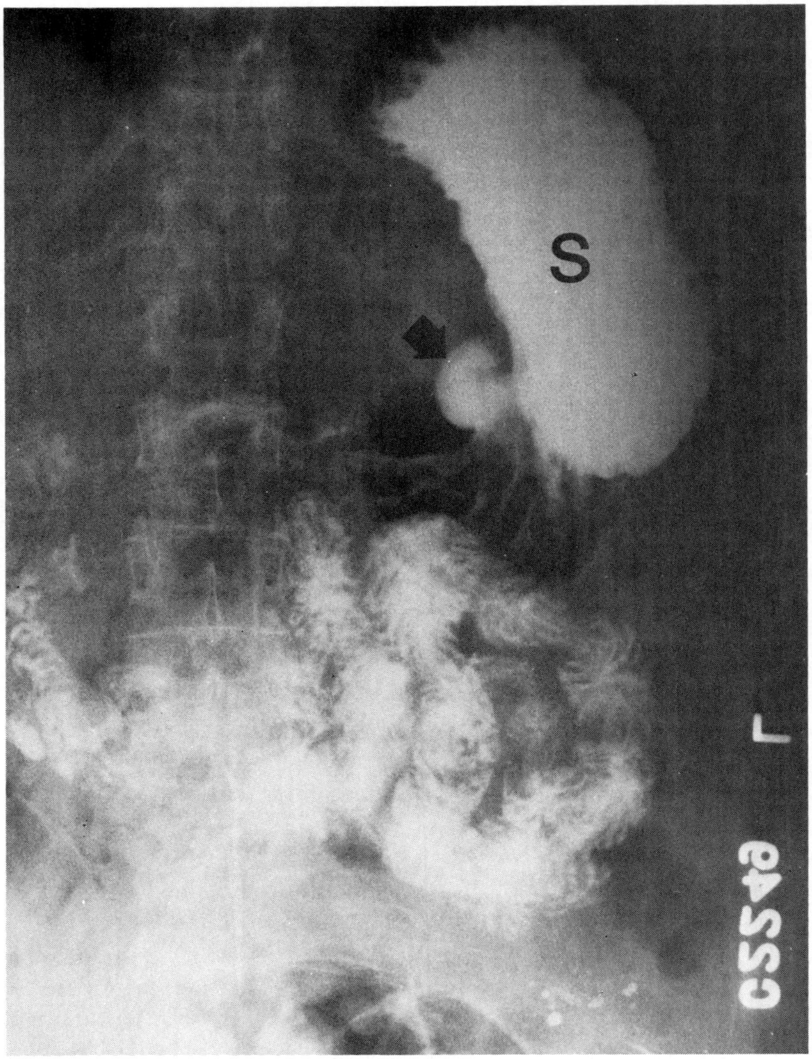

FIGURE 3-2. Upper gastrointestinal series demonstrating an ulcer *(black arrow)* on the lesser curvature of the stomach *(S)*.

tervals to follow the progression of the barium through the small intestine. A significant delay in the transit time of barium may occur with benign or malignant obstruction. The flow of barium is faster in patients with hypermotility of the bowel (as in malabsorption). Sometimes transit time is so delayed (as in partial bowel obstruction) that x-ray films must be taken 24 hours later to see complete progression of the barium meal.

Small bowel follow-through studies are also helpful in identifying and defining the anatomy of small bowel fistulas (abnormal connections between the small bowel and other abdominal organs or skin).

A more accurate radiographic evaluation of

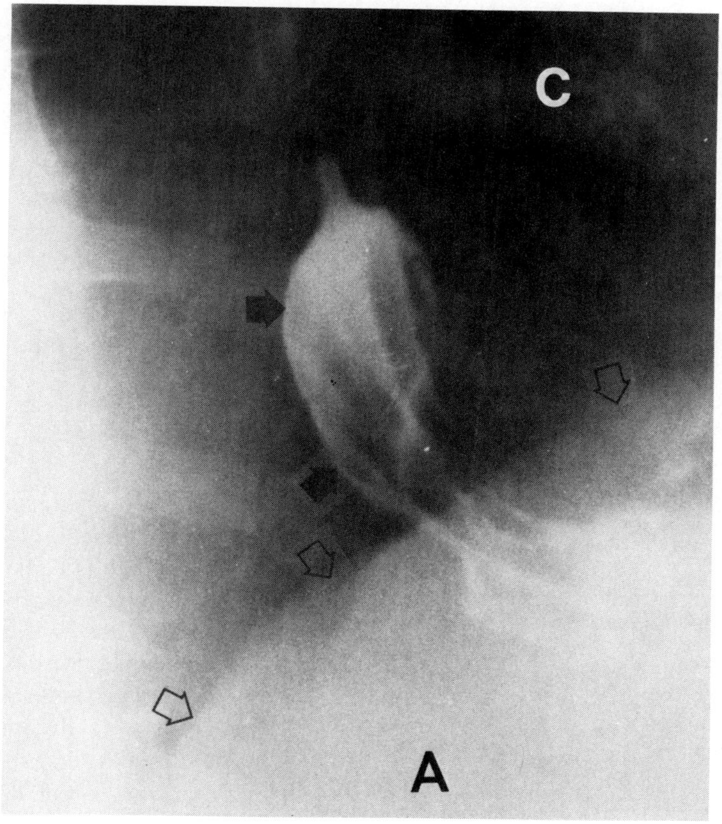

FIGURE 3-3. Upper gastrointestinal series demonstrating hiatal hernia. Note that proximal portion of the stomach *(solid black arrows)* is above the diaphragm *(arrow outlines)* and lying within the chest *(C)*. *A*, Abdominal cavity.

the small intestine is provided by the *small bowel enema.* Unlike the small bowel follow-through study where the barium is swallowed by the patient, during a small bowel enema a tube is placed through the mouth, esophagus, stomach, and duodenum and into the small intestine. Through this tube, barium is injected and allowed to flow through the small intestine. The small bowel enema affords an improved visualization because the barium injected through the tube is concentrated and not diluted by gastric and duodenal juices as it is during UGI and small bowel follow-through studies. The small intestine is, therefore, more accurately outlined by the dye and more easily evaluated radiographically. This test is especially useful in the evaluation of patients with partial small bowel obstruction of unknown etiology. Tumors, inflammatory bowel disease, ulcers, and small bowel fistula may be more easily identified and defined with this procedure.

The tube can be placed transorally with the use of a weighted tip. However, having the endoscopist deliver the tube to the upper small bowel via enteroscopy (p. 65) is easier. After the barium has been injected through the tube, the small bowel enema is carried out as described in the discussion concerning UGI and small bowel follow-through studies.

Contraindications. Although the UGI is a relatively benign examination, it is contraindicated in certain patients. These include the following:

1. Patients with complete bowel obstruction.
2. Patients with perforated viscera (such as stomach, duodenum, or small bowel); if barium were to leak out of a perforated organ, an intense inflammatory reaction and abscess could occur. To avoid this complication, these patients should have an UGI using a water-soluble agent (such as Gastrografin).
3. Patients with unstable vital signs, who should not be unsupervised during the length of time required for this test.
4. Uncooperative patients, because of the necessity of frequent position changes.

Nursing considerations

Nursing Diagnoses/Collaborative Problems

See X-ray studies, p. 5.

- Possible alteration in elimination related to barium retention.
- Potential complication: bowel obstruction or fecal impaction.

Nursing Implications with Rationale

- Explain the procedure to the patient. Encourage verbalization of the patient's questions or fears.
- Keep the patient NPO after midnight. Food and fluid in the stomach prevents the barium from accurately outlining the GI tract, and the radiographic results may be misleading.
- Explain to the patient that the test may take several hours and that during that time he or she cannot eat or drink. The patient may eat as soon as the radiology department determines that the series is completed.
- Assure the patient that the test will not cause any discomfort other than that of lying on a hard table.
- Explain to the patient the importance of rectally expelling all of the barium. Stools will be light in color until all of the barium is expelled. Eventual absorption of fecal water may cause a hardened barium impaction. Increasing fluids is usually effective. Occasionally a mild laxative (such as magnesium citrate) or an enema may be needed to prevent this complication.

Gastric analysis

(tube gastric analysis, tubeless gastric analysis/ Diagnex Blue Test)

Normal values:
Tube gastric analysis: BAO, 2-5 mEq/hr; MAO 10-20 mEq/hr.
Tubeless gastric analysis: detectable dye in the urine.

Rationale. The contents of the stomach are aspirated to determine the amount of acid produced by the parietal cells within the stomach during the resting state (BAO) and during the stimulated (MAO) state. This information is useful for the following reasons:

1. To determine the location and type of ulcer (Table 3-1). Because benign peptic ulceration requires the presence of acid, ulcerations that occur in an environment of

TABLE 3-1. Basal and Betazole Hydrochloride (Histalog)–stimulated* Gastric Secretions in Normal Subjects and in Patients with Peptic Ulcer or with Gastric Cancer

Condition	Basal acid output (mEq/1 hour)	Maximal acid output (mEq/1 hour)
Normal: Male	2-5	10-20
Female	1-4	7-15
Duodenal ulcer: Male	5-10	15-30
Female	3-8	10-20
Gastric ulcer: Male	1-5	10-20
Female	1-3	5-15
Gastric cancer: Male	0-3	0-10
Female	0-3	0-5

*Betazole hydrochloride given in dose of 1.5 mg/kg of body weight.

achlorhydria (that is, the absence of hydrochloric acid (HCl) in the gastric juice) can only be malignant in origin. No ulcer can be considered "peptic" without the presence of acid. Also, the location of benign peptic ulcers can be predicted by the quantity of acid produced. Normal or low-normal acid levels are thought to indicate a gastric location, whereas increased acid levels are indicative of duodenal ulcers.

2. To determine Zollinger-Ellison syndrome (ZE syndrome). In this disease, a pancreatic islet-cell tumor secretes abundant gastrin, which then stimulates the stomach to secrete acid. Therefore, the stomach is never found in the resting state. This causes the value of the BAO to approach that of the MAO. The BAO/MAO ratio would then be greater than 0.6 in this syndrome. This persistently high level of acidity causes the serious and complicated peptic ulcer disease characteristic of ZE syndrome.
3. To determine the efficacy of therapy. To be therapeutic, medical or surgical treatment of peptic ulcer disease must substantially decrease the acid output of the stomach. Baseline values are determined by a pretreatment gastric analysis. The study is repeated during treatment. Effective therapy is indicated by a 50% reduction in the quantity of acid produced.

Procedure. To reliably assess gastric acid secretion, a nasogastric (NG) tube must be inserted into the dependent portion of the fasting patient's stomach. A syringe is attached to the NG tube, and all gastric contents aspirated are discarded. Four samples are then aspirated at 15-minute intervals, placed in clean specimen containers, numbered, and sent to the chemistry laboratory for analysis. The BAO (measured in milliequivalents per hour) is determined by multiplying the number of mEq in the highest basal measurements by four. For example, if the highest basal measurement were 0.8 mEq/15 min, the BAO would be 3.2 mEq/hr.

After the fasting specimens are collected, the patient receives histamine phosphate (0.04 mg/kg) or betazole hydrochloride (1 to 2 mg/kg) subcutaneously. This maximally stimulates acid production in the stomach. Eight specimens are then aspirated at 15-minute intervals. The MAO is determined by multiplying the number of mEq in the highest stimulated measurement by four. The duration of this procedure is about 3 hours. Except for the initial gagging associated with the insertion of the NG tube, this test is not uncomfortable.

A *tubeless gastric analysis (Diagnex Blue Test)* can also be performed on an empty stomach to determine the presence or absence of hydrochloric acid. This test will not indicate the amount of free acid in the stomach. The procedure is begun by asking a patient to empty the bladder and then ingest a gastric stimulant (such as a tablet of caffeine) and a glass of water, followed by a resin dye (such as Diagnex Blue or Azuresin) in a glass of water. If the gastric contents contain free hydrochloric acid, the stomach acid displaces the dye from the resin base. The dye is then absorbed by the bowel mucosa and excreted into the urine. The bladder is emptied at the end of the test (approximately 2 hours). The urine may be blue or blue-green for several days. Absence of blue color in the urine usually indicates the absence of hydrochloric acid in the stomach. By analyzing the amount of dye excreted in the urine, the amount of acid in the stomach can be estimated. Absence of the dye in the urine is indicative of achlorhydria.

Contraindications. In patients with cardiac disease, carcinoid syndrome, and hypertension, the dose of betazole or histamine should be decreased. Patients with allergies are not given histamine.

Nursing considerations

Nursing Diagnoses/Collaborative Problems

- Possible knowledge deficit related to the test purpose, preparation, and procedure.
- Possible alteration in comfort related to test procedure.

Nursing Implications with Rationale

- Explain the test to the patient. Most patients are very apprehensive about this study. Encourage verbalization of the patient's fears. Provide emotional support.
- Keep the patient NPO after midnight. Food and fluid alters gastric acid secretion.
- Do not give the patient any anticholinergic medications for 24 hours before the test. Anticholinergics inhibit the histamine stimulation of gastric acid secretion. Artificially low acid measurements will result.
- Inform the patient that smoking is prohibited before the test because it stimulates secretion of the gastric cells.
- After measuring the distance from the tip of the ear to the tip of the nose and to the tip of the sternum, lubricate the end of the NG tube (Levin #12, #14, or #16) and insert the tube into the dependent portion of the stomach. When the second marker of the Levin tube is at the nares, the tip of the tube should usually be well within the stomach. Then securely tape the NG tube to the patient's nose or cheek, making sure that the tube does not press or pull against the nares.
- Attach a 50 ml syringe to the NG tube for aspiration. Aspirate and discard the first specimen. At the appropriate time interval, aspirate the entire gastric contents and place them in the specimen container.
- Instruct the patient to expectorate saliva, because saliva may buffer the acid content of the stomach.
- After the histamine is administered, monitor the patient for side effects. The three principal actions of histamine are (1) contraction of smooth muscle (uterine, intestinal, and bronchial), (2) dilatation of capillaries, and (3) promotion of gastric acid secretion. The dilatation of the capillaries produces the side effects most bothersome to the patients: flushing, increase in skin temperature, itching, and a drop in blood pressure. The fall in blood pressure is usually transient.
- After the subcutaneous injection of histamine, take the patient's pulse and blood pressure immediately. Usually the pulse rate increases and blood pressure decreases slightly. Symptoms of overdose include a drop in blood pressure, intense headache, dyspnea, flushing, vomiting, diarrhea, and shock. Epinephrine will prevent or quickly counteract these symptoms.
- When the test is completed, clamp and withdraw the NG tube. Give mouth and nose care. The patient can usually resume a normal diet.
- If the *tubeless gastric analysis* is performed, inform the patient about this screening test. Administer the stimulant and resin dye at the designated times, and collect the urine specimen. Tell the patient that the urine may be blue or blue-green for several days.

Esophagogastroduodenoscopy

(UGI endoscopy, gastroscopy)

Normal value: normal GI tract.

Rationale. Endoscopy enables direct visualization of the upper GI tract by means of a long, fiber-optic, flexible scope. The esophagus, stomach, and duodenum are examined for tumors, varices, mucosal inflammations, hiatal hernias, polyps, ulcers, and obstruction. The gastroscope has several channels through which cable-activated instruments can be passed to extract biopsy specimens. Also, the endoscopist can remove polyps and coagulate sources of active gastrointestinal bleeding through these accessory channels. Areas of narrowing can be dilated by the endoscope itself or by passing a dilator with the scope. Camera equipment may be attached to the viewing lens and the existing pathologic condition can be photographed. Without a doubt, fiber-optic visualization is one of the most important advancements in the diagnosis and therapeutics of gastrointestinal problems.

Not only can the esophagus, stomach, and duodenum be evaluated by endoscopy, but by the use of a longer fiber-optic scope the upper small intestine can also be evaluated. This is referred to as *enteroscopy*. Abnormalities of the small bowel that can be evaluated using enteroscopy include arteriovenous (AV) malformation, tumors, enteropathies (such as celiac and Crohn's disease), and ulcers.

A rare complication of this procedure is perforation of the esophagus, stomach, and duodenum. That complication is rare unless dilatation of an obstruction is required. Other complications include bleeding from the site of extraction of the biopsy specimen, aspiration of gastric contents into the lungs, and respiratory arrest resulting from diazepam overdose.

Procedure. This examination is usually performed in an endoscopy room, with the patient in the left-lateral decubitus (Sim's) position. The fasting patient is sedated with midazolam (Versed) before the examination. Atropine is given to decrease secretions. The patient's posterior pharynx is anesthetized with lidocaine to inactivate the gag reflex and to lessen the discomfort caused by the passage of the scope. The scope is then passed slowly into the mouth, esophagus, stomach, and duodenum. Air is insufflated to maintain patency of the lumen. A gastroenterologist usually performs this procedure in 30 minutes.

Contraindications. This study should not be performed on:

1. Patients who cannot cooperate fully. As in all studies that require technical finesse, patient cooperation is essential for successful completion.
2. Patients who have severe UGI bleeding. The viewing lens may be covered with blood clots and prevent good visualization. The stomach should be lavaged and aspirated clear of clots before this procedure is attempted.
3. Patients with esophageal diverticula. The scope can, too easily, fall into the diverticulum and perforate its wall.
4. Patients who are suspected of having a perforated viscus.

Nursing considerations

Nursing Diagnoses/Collaborative Problems

See Endoscopic procedures, pp. 6-7.

- Possible injury related to sedation.
- Potential complication: respiratory arrest from overdose of sedatives.
- Potential complication: aspiration of gastric contents.

Nursing Implications with Rationale

- Explain the procedure to the patient and obtain written permission for this test. Tell the patient what drugs will be prescribed and what their effects will be.
- Keep the patient NPO after midnight to provide optimum visualization of the GI tract and to prevent regurgitation when the gastroscope is passed.
- Tell the patient that the test is not painful but may cause discomfort and vomiting when the gag reflex is initiated. Encourage verbalization of the patient's fears. Provide emotional support.
- Remove the patient's dentures and eyeglasses before the test. Since the tube is passed through the mouth, oral hygiene procedures should be performed before and after the test.
- Explain to the patient that he or she will be unable to speak when the scope is positioned in the GI tract.
- Place any tissue specimens into an appropriate specimen container and label the container correctly.
- Have an Ambu bag ready in case of respiratory arrest from Versed overdose. Physostigmine (Antilirium) should be available to counteract serious respiratory depression.
- After the patient's throat has been anesthetized with lidocaine, do not allow the patient to eat or drink anything until the gag reflex returns (usually about 2 to 4 hours).
- Inform the patient that after the anesthesia wears off, he or she may be hoarse and complain of a sore throat for several days. Drinking cool fluids and gargling will help relieve some of this soreness.

- Observe the patient for bleeding, fever, abdominal pain, dysphagia, and dyspnea. Monitor the vital signs as ordered.
- Observe safety precautions until the effects of the sedatives have worn off.

Examination for gastric cytology

Normal values: no malignancy.

Rationale. Gastric cells can be examined microscopically to detect malignancy. Tumor cells are often shed into the lumen from a cancerous lesion. These cells can be collected by a gastric aspiration and examined. It is important to realize that the value of this test depends totally on the ability of the cytologist to read the slides accurately. By itself, a negative cytology report does not rule out malignancy; it reinforces the assumption of benignancy. A positive cytology report indicates malignancy.

Procedure. Gastric aspiration for cytology can be obtained during gastroscopy (p. 64) or with the insertion of an NG tube. Approximately 100 ml of saline solution is instilled through the tube. The patient is asked to turn 360 degrees several times. The fluid is aspirated and sent to the cytology laboratory in a covered container. The NG tube or gastroscope is removed. The fluid obtained is centrifuged, and the precipitate containing the cells is smeared on a microscopic slide. It is then stained and read by the cytologist.

Contraindications. If using gastroscopy to obtain a specimen, refer to contraindications stated for that study.

Nursing considerations

Nursing Diagnoses/Collaborative Problems

- Possible knowledge deficit related to test purpose, preparation, and procedure.
- Possible alteration in comfort related to procedure.

Nursing Implications with Rationale

- Explain the procedure to the patient.
- Keep the patient NPO after midnight.
- Tell the patient that the discomfort associated with this test is caused by the passage of the NG tube or gastroscope. Encourage verbalization of the patient's questions or fears.
- See the discussion of gastroscopy.

Serum gastrin level determination

Normal values: 40-150 pg/ml.

Rationale. Gastrin, a hormone normally produced by the G cells located in the distal part of the stomach (called the antrum), is a potent stimulator of gastric acid. Gastrin release is stimulated by distention of the antrum with food or by an alkaline environment within the stomach. The gastric acid is then released by the parietal cells located in the proximal stomach mucosa, and the pH of the stomach is reduced. By a negative feedback mechanism, the acid production halts further gastrin secretion.

In patients with plain duodenal ulcers, gastrin levels are normal. Gastrin levels are mildly increased in patients with pernicious anemia or gastric ulcers and those who have had an antiulcer surgical procedure. This increase is because of a persistent alkaline environment that exists in their stomach and causes constant gastrin stimulation. The gastrin level is extremely high in patients with Zollinger-Ellison syndrome or G-cell hyperplasia (increased size and activity of G cells in the distal stomach).

Zollinger-Ellison syndrome can be differentiated from the other causes of hypergastrinemia by the *calcium infusion test* or the *secretin stimulation test.*

For the *calcium infusion test,* calcium gluconate is administered intravenously for 3 hours. A preinfusion blood sample is then compared to specimens taken every 30 minutes up to 4 hours. The *secretin stimulation test* is performed by administering secretin intravenously for 1 hour with blood specimens drawn before and at 15-minute intervals afterward.

During calcium or secretin infusion, patients with ZE syndrome have a marked increase in gastrin production, whereas a decrease is noted in patients who have hypergastrinemia from other causes.

Not all ZE syndrome patients exhibit increased levels of gastrin. Some may have "top" normal gastrin levels, a situation that makes these patients difficult to differentiate from those with routine ulcer disease. However, if during calcium or secretin infusion the patient exhibits a marked increase in serum gastrin levels, it is safe to conclude that he or she has ZE syndrome.

Procedure. After the patient fasts for 12 hours, blood is withdrawn from a peripheral vein and placed in a red-top tube that contains no anticoagulant.

Contraindications. None.

Nursing considerations

Nursing Diagnoses/Collaborative Problems

See Blood studies, p. 2.

Nursing Implications with Rationale

- Apply pressure or a pressure dressing to the venipuncture site after the procedure is completed. Observe the site for bleeding.

SUPPLEMENTAL INFORMATION

Gastric emptying scan

Normal values: depend on the test meal provided.

Rationale. A gastric emptying scan is a nuclear medicine study that involves providing the patient with a solid or liquid test meal containing a radionuclide and then scanning until the stomach is empty. This study is used to assess the ability of the stomach to empty solids or liquids and to evaluate disorders that may cause a delay in gastric emptying, such as obstructing peptic ulcers, gastric malignancies, or following gastric surgery. The study is also used as a noninvasive method of estimating the acid-secretory ability of the stomach without performing gastric aspiration.

Procedure. After remaining NPO after midnight, the patient ingests the test meal. In the solid-emptying study, a cooked egg white containing technetium-99m is eaten. In the liquid-emptying study, the patient drinks orange juice containing technetium-99m. After ingestion of the test meal, the person lies supine under a gamma ray detector camera that records images until gastric emptying has been completed. The procedure is finished in approximately 1½ hours and is performed in the nuclear medicine department. There is no discomfort associated with the study other than lying on a hard table.

Contraindications. The study is contraindicated in the pregnant or lactating patient.

Nursing considerations

Nursing Diagnoses/Collaborative Problems

See Nuclear scanning procedures, p. 5.

Nursing Implications with Rationale

- Explain the procedure to the patient. Assure the patient that no pain is associated with this study.
- Make sure the patient understands that only a small dose of nuclear material is eaten. Reassure the patient that this procedure is safe and noninvasive.

D-Xylose absorption test

Normal values:

Adults: Blood levels of xylose equal to 25-40 mg/dl in 2 hours after ingestion; 80% to 95% excreted in urine in 5 hours.

Children: Blood levels of xylose equal to 30 mg/dl in 1 hour after ingestion; 16% to 33% excreted in the urine in 5 hours.

Rationale. The D-xylose absorption test is used to determine the cause of malabsorption syndrome and to aid in the differential diagnosis of malabsorption. Absorption is normal in pancreatic steatorrhea (caused by pancreatic exocrine insufficiency) but impaired in enterogenous steatorrhea. For this test, xylose (which the body does not metabolize) is administered orally. Its absorption levels are subsequently checked in both the blood and the urine. Levels of D-xylose in the blood and urine help evaluate the absorptive qualities of the small intestines. Decreased amounts imply malabsorption for D-xylose. Abnormal results are most frequently seen in nontropical and tropical sprue.

Procedure. For the D-xylose absorption test, the patient is kept fasting at least 8 hours, usually from midnight before the test. Before the monosaccharide D-xylose is administered, a peripheral venipuncture is performed and approximately 7 ml of venous blood is placed in a red-top tube. A first voided morning urine specimen is also collected.

The adult patient then receives 25 g D-xylose dissolved in 8 ounces of water, followed by another 8 ounces of water. For children, a calibrated dose of D-xylose is based on the body weight. The patient should remain on bed rest during the test since activity can affect the test results by altering digestive activity. The peripheral venipuncture is then repeated in 2 hours for an adult and in 1 hour for a child. All urine is collected for the designated time period, usually 5 hours.

Contraindications. The test is contraindicated in patients with abnormal kidney functions and those who are dehydrated.

Nursing considerations

Nursing Diagnoses/Collaborative Problems

See Blood studies, p. 2 and Urine studies, p. 3.

Nursing Implications with Rationale

- Explain the procedure to the patient. Instruct the patient to drink the designated amount of D-xylose and not to eat or drink anything else until the study is completed.
- Observe the patient for nausea, vomiting, and diarrhea, which may occur as side effects of D-xylose.
- Explain to the patient that bed rest is necessary during the test since activity can alter the digestive process and affect test results.
- Draw the blood at the appropriate time, and apply pressure or a pressure dressing to the venous puncture site after the blood is drawn. Observe the site for bleeding.
- Explain the procedure for collecting the urine, and continue the collection for the indicated time period.
- After the study is completed, provide the patient with food or fluids and inform the patient that normal activity can be resumed.

Lactose tolerance test

Normal values: plasma glucose levels rise >20 mg/dl.

Rationale. This test is performed to detect lactose intolerance. Lactose is the disaccharide commonly found in milk products. During the digestive process, lactose is broken down to glucose and galactose by the intestinal enzyme lactase. In the absence of this enzyme, lactose is not broken down and absorption does not occur. Abdominal cramps, blotting, flatus and diarrhea result from bacterial metabolism of the increased lactose in the bowel. Since lactose is not broken down to glucose and galactose, the plasma glucose levels do not rise as expected. Therefore, levels below the designated amount suggest an intestinal lactase deficiency. This test can be followed by a monosaccharide tolerance test such as glucose or galactose tolerance test.

Procedure. The patient is instructed to fast and to avoid strenuous exercise for 8 hours before the test. After a fasting blood sugar is obtained, the patient receives a specified dose (approximately 100 g) of lactose orally in 200 ml of water. Blood is then withdrawn from a peripheral vein and placed in a gray-top tube at 30, 60, and 120 minutes after the loading dose of lactose. Plasma glucose levels are then determined on that blood (see p. 310).

Contraindications. None.

Nursing considerations

Nursing Diagnoses/Collaborative Problems

See Blood studies, p. 2.

Nursing Implications with Rationale

- Explain the procedure to the patient. Instruct the patient to drink the entire amount of lactose and not to eat anything else until the blood is drawn. Inform the patient that smoking is also prohibited since it may increase the blood sugar level.

- Draw the blood at the appropriate time, and apply pressure or a pressure dressing to the venous puncture site after the blood is obtained. Observe the site for bleeding.

CASE STUDY 2: ESOPHAGEAL REFLUX

Ms. K. was a 45-year-old woman who complained of heartburn and frequent regurgitation of "sour" material into her mouth. The results of her physical examination were negative.

Studies	**Results**
Routine laboratory studies	Negative
Barium swallow (BS)	Hiatal hernia (Figure 3-3)
Esophageal function studies (EFS)	
Lower esophageal sphincter (LES) pressure	4 mm Hg (normal: 10-20 mm Hg)
Acid reflux	Positive in all positions (normal: negative)
Acid clearing	Cleared to pH 5 after 20 swallows (normal: <10 swallows)
Swallowing waves	Normal amplitude and normal progression
Bernstein test	Positive (normal: negative)
Esophagoscopy (see Gastroscopy)	Reddened, friable, and hyperemic esophageal mucosa seen, indicating esophagitis

The barium swallow indicated a hiatal hernia. Although many patients with a hiatal hernia have no reflux, this patient's symptoms of reflux necessitated esophageal function studies. She was found to have a hypotensive LES, along with severe acid reflux into her esophagus. The abnormal acid clearing and the positive Bernstein test result indicated esophagitis caused by severe reflux. The esophagitis was directly visualized during esophagoscopy.

Although most patients with such severe symptoms do not respond to medical therapy, conservative management is usually attempted first. Ms. K. was given antacid (Maalox) and cimetidine (Tagamet). She was told to avoid the use of tobacco and caffeine. Her diet was limited to small, frequent, bland feedings. She was instructed to sleep with the head of her bed elevated at night.

Because Ms. K. had only minimal relief of her symptoms after 6 weeks of medical management, she was admitted to the hospital for a surgical antireflux procedure. A Nissen fundoplication was performed. She had no further symptoms.

DISCUSSION OF TESTS

Barium swallow

Normal values: normal size, contour, filling, patency, and positioning of the esophagus.

Rationale. This barium contrast study is a more thorough study of the esophagus than that provided by most UGIs. As in most barium contrast studies, defects in luminal filling and narrowing of the barium column indicate tumor (Figure 3-4), scarred stricture, or varices. With a barium swallow, anatomic abnormalities such as hiatal hernia are easily recognized (see Figure 3-3). Left atrial dilatation, aortic aneurysm, and paraesophageal tumors (such as bronchial or mediastinal tumors) may cause extrinsic compression of the barium column within the esophagus.

In patients with esophageal reflux, the radiologist may detect return of gastric barium into the esophagus. This is best seen during fluoroscopy (a motion-picture x-ray study).

Procedure. The fasting patient swallows a flavored barium solution similar to that used in a UGI. The patient is secured to a tilt table and placed in various positions as x-ray films are taken.

The radiologist follows the barium column through the entire esophagus. Both frontal and lateral views are taken. This procedure takes about 15 minutes to perform and is not uncomfortable.

Contraindications. Again, as in all barium contrast studies, if a suspicion of gastrointestinal perforation exists, the study is not performed. If barium were to leak out of a perforated organ, an intense inflammatory reaction and abscess could occur. To avoid this complication

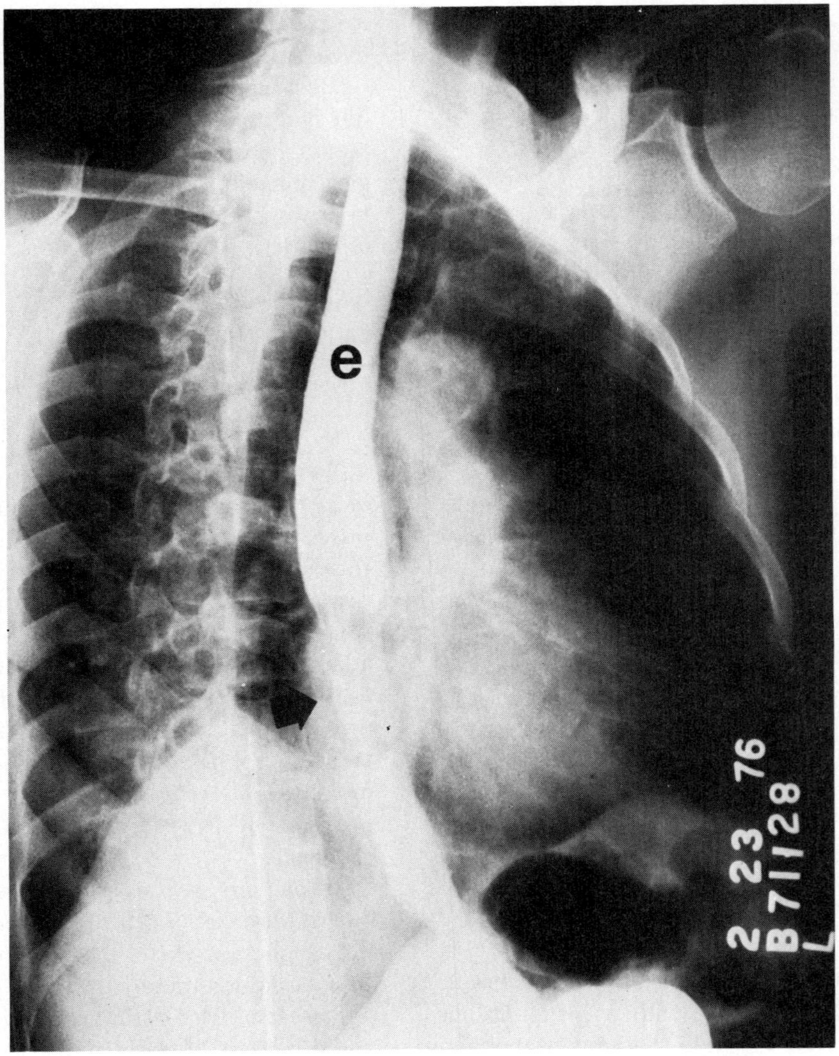

FIGURE 3-4. Barium swallow demonstrating an esophageal cancer *(black arrow)* within the esophagus *(e)*.

when perforation is suspected, a water-soluble contrast medium (such as Gastrografin) is used. Any extravasated Gastrografin is absorbed by the capillaries and eventually excreted in the urine.

Nursing considerations

Nursing Diagnoses/Collaborative Problems

See X-ray studies, p. 5.

- Possible alteration in elimination related to barium retention.
- Potential complication: bowel obstruction or fecal impaction.

Nursing Implications with Rationale

- Explain the procedure to the patient.
- Make sure that the patient evacuates the barium. (See nursing implications for UGI, p. 62.)

Esophageal function studies

LES pressure
Normal values: 10-20 mm Hg
Swallowing pattern
Normal value: normal peristaltic waves
Acid reflux
Normal value: negative
Acid clearing
Normal value: <10 swallows
Bernstein test
Normal value: negative

Rationale. Esophageal function studies (EFS) include the following: determination of the lower esophageal sphincter (LES) pressure; graphic recording of esophageal swallowing waves; detection of reflux of gastric acid back into the esophagus; detection of the ability of the esophagus to clear acid; and finally an attempt to reproduce symptoms of heartburn. Each is discussed separately.

Manometry studies. Two manometry studies are used in assessing esophageal function: measurement of LES pressure and graphic recording of swallowing waves (motility). The LES is the valve between the esophagus and stomach. Free reflux of gastric acid occurs when the sphincter is unable to maintain a pressure greater than the tension within the stomach. Examples of such disorders are gastroesophageal reflux in the adult and chalasia (incompetent or relaxed LES) in the infant. Increased sphincter pressures, as found in patients with achalasia (failure of the LES to relax normally with swallowing), will not permit food to pass through into the stomach. These patients complain of dysphagia (difficulty in swallowing).

Normal swallowing requires synchronous and propulsive peristaltic waves in the esophagus. The pattern of these waves can be recorded on a graph. In achalasia few, if any, swallowing waves are detected. In contrast, diffuse esophageal spasm is characterized by strong, asynchronous, nonpropulsive waves.

Acid reflux with pH probe. Acid reflux is the primary component of gastroesophageal reflux. Patients who have an incompetent LES regurgitate gastric acid into the esophagus, causing a drop in pH there.

Acid clearing. Normal subjects can completely clear hydrochloric acid from their esophagus in less than 10 swallows. Patients with decreased esophageal motility (frequently caused by severe esophagitis) require a greater number of swallows to clear the acid.

Bernstein test (acid perfusion). The Bernstein test is simply an attempt to reproduce the symptoms of gastroesophageal reflux. If the patient suffers pain with the instillation of hydrochloric acid into the esophagus, the test is positive and indicates reflux esophagitis. If the patient has no discomfort, a cause other than esophageal reflux must be sought to explain the patient's complaints.

Procedure. Esophageal studies are usually performed in a room specially equipped with appropriate instruments. The fasting, unsedated patient is asked to swallow three very thin tubes, the ends of which are 5 cm apart (Figure 3-5). The other ends of the tubes are attached to transducers for pressure recordings. All tubes are passed into the stomach.

The three tubes are slowly pulled back into the esophagus. A rapid and extreme increase in the pressure readings indicates the high-pressure zone of the LES. The *LES pressure* is recorded as each of the three tubes reaches this point.

With all tubes in the esophagus, the patient is asked to swallow. With normal *motility* the proximal tube registers a rapid rise and fall in pressure. This pattern is successively and graphically recorded through the transducer of the middle and then of the distal tube (if three tubes are used). The tubes are then replaced into the stomach, a fourth tube (pH indicator) is passed into the esophagus. The stomach is filled with approximately 100 ml of 0.1 N hydrochloric acid. If a drop in esophageal pH occurs, this indicates *acid reflux* from the stomach into the esophagus.

Next the tubes are returned to the esophagus. Hydrochloric acid is instilled through

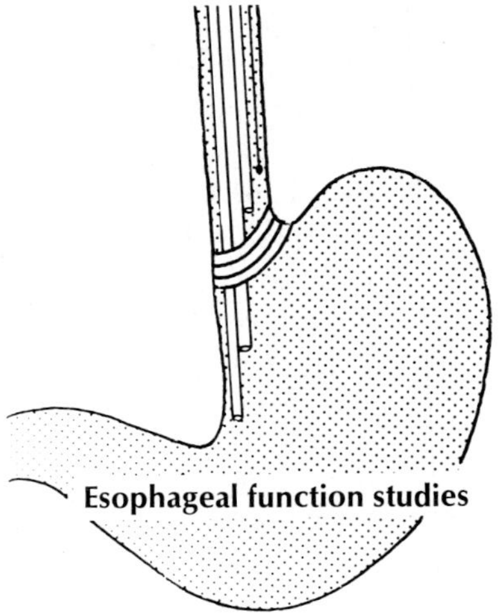

FIGURE 3-5. Esophageal function studies demonstrating placement of manometry tubes and pH probe within the esophagus.

them. *Acid clearing* is determined by counting the number of swallows required to clear the acid completely.

Finally 0.1 N hydrochloric acid and saline solution are alternately instilled into the esophagus for the *Bernstein test*. The patient is not told which solution is being infused. If the patient volunteers symptoms of discomfort while the acid is running, the test is positive. If no discomfort is recognized, the test is negative.

Surprisingly, the entire study is not uncomfortable despite some initial gagging. No significant complications have been reported. The duration of the study is approximately 30 minutes.

Contraindications. This test should not be attempted with uncooperative or unstable patients.

Nursing considerations

Nursing Diagnoses/Collaborative Problems

- Possible knowledge deficit related to test purpose, preparation, and procedure.
- High risk for alteration in comfort related to test procedure.
- Possible anxiety related to unknown sensations during the procedure.
- Potential complication: aspiration of gastric contents.

Nursing Implications with Rationale

- Explain the procedure to the patient and describe the initial gagging associated with the study. Most patients are very apprehensive about this test. Provide emotional support.
- Keep the patient NPO after midnight to prevent aspiration of gastric contents into the lungs during the study.
- Avoid sedating the patient, because sedation causes a false decrease in LES pressure. Also, the patient's participation is essential for swallowing the tubes, swallowing during acid clearance, and describing any discomfort during the instillation of hydrochloric acid.

SUPPLEMENTAL INFORMATION

Gastroesophageal reflux scan

(GE reflux scan)

Normal values: negative; no evidence of reflux.

Rationale. This nuclear medicine procedure is used to evaluate suspected gastroesophageal reflux in patients with symptoms such as heartburn, regurgitation, vomiting, and dysphagia. This study is also indicated to evaluate esophageal motility, assess response of reflux to therapy, and detect the aspiration of gastric contents into the lungs.

Procedure. For this procedure the patient eats a full meal just before the study. The patient assumes a supine position while images are taken over the chest. The patient then swallows a mouthful of a tracer cocktail (such as orange juice, dilute hydrochloric acid, or Technetium-99m–labeled protein such as sulphur colloid), and images are taken. Then after drinking the remainder of the cocktail and some water, the patient assumes an upright position and images of the chest are taken. A large binder (similar to a blood pressure cuff) is then placed around the abdomen to increase intraabdominal pressure, which stresses the sphincter at the gastroesophageal junction. The patient is placed in the supine position while under the gamma ray detector camera. Esophageal activity is determined by taking images with no pressure applied to the abdomen and then with gradual increments in pressure up to 100 mm Hg. The entire procedure is completed in approximately 30 minutes in the nuclear medicine department. The only discomfort associated with the study is that of lying on a hard table and the application of some abdominal pressure from the binder.

Aspiration scans can also be performed by adding a radionuclide to the evening meal and then keeping the patient in a supine position until the next morning. Images are then made over the lungs to detect esophageal-tracheal aspiration of the tracer. Infants are evaluated for chalasia by adding the tracer into the formula and then taking films over the next hour with delayed films as needed.

Contraindications. This procedure is not performed on patients who are pregnant or lactating or those with any contraindications to increasing abdominal pressure.

Nursing considerations

Nursing Diagnoses/Collaborative Problems

See Nuclear scanning procedures, p. 5.

Nursing Implications with Rationale

- Explain the procedure to the patient. Assure the patient that no pain is associated with this study.
- Make sure the patient and/or family understand that only a small dose of nuclear material is used.

CASE STUDY 3: COLON CANCER

An 85-year-old man with previously normal bowel function began to complain of constipation, rectal bleeding, and pencil-like stool. The results of a physical examination were negative.

Studies	Results
Routine laboratory studies	Normal, except hemoglobin (10 g/dl) and hematocrit (29%) (normal hemoglobin: 12-13 g/dl) (normal hematocrit: 36-42%)
Examination of stool for occult blood	Positive (normal: negative)
Carcinoembryonic antigen (CEA) test	33 ng/ml (normal: <2 ng/ml)
Sigmoidoscopy	No tumor seen
Barium enema (BE) study	Stricture in left side of colon
Colonoscopy	Tumor in left side of colon, no other synchronous lesion found
Colonoscopic biopsy	Adenocarcinoma

The elevated CEA level and the occult (hidden) blood in the stool indicated serious colorectal disease. Because the sigmoidoscopy was normal, the disease was suspected to be beyond the reach of the 25 cm sigmoidoscope. The barium enema study demonstrated a narrowing in the left side of the colon, which could have been caused by infection, infestation, or neoplasm. Adenocarcinoma of the colon was diagnosed by means of a colonoscopic biopsy. The patient had surgery to resect the left side of his colon. Postoperatively, his CEA level was 1.8 ng/ml. On examination 3 years later, no evidence of disease was found. Five years after surgery, his CEA had risen to 38 ng/ml. He was found to have liver metastasis from his primary tumor in the colon. He died 18 months later.

DISCUSSION OF TESTS

Examination of stool for occult blood

Normal value: negative.

Rationale. Tumors of the large intestine grow into the lumen and are subjected to repeated trauma by the fecal stream. Eventually the tumor ulcerates and bleeding occurs. Most times the bleeding is so slight that gross blood is not seen in the stool. If this occult blood is detected in the stool, a benign or malignant gastrointestinal tumor should be suspected; however, false positives do occur.

Occult blood in the stool may also occur in ulceration and inflammation of the upper or lower gastrointestinal system. Other causes include hematobilia (bleeding from the liver) and the swallowing of oral or nasopharyngeal blood.

Procedure. The preparation for collecting a stool for occult blood varies. Often the preparation involves prescribing a high-fiber diet and abstinence from red meats for 48 to 72 hours before the test. Medications such as iron preparations, iodides, colchicine, salicylates, steroids, and ascorbic acid may be withheld for 48 hours before testing. Eliminating meat decreases the incidence of weak false-positive test results. The high-residue diet increases detection of significant lesions. If patients on an unrestricted diet who are screened for occult blood manifest a weak positive result, they are usually studied again later on a restricted diet.

Stool is obtained by digital retrieval by the nurse or physician. Alternatively, the patient can be asked to save his or her stool in a container or to smear a specimen on a card/paper which can then be sent to the laboratory. There are several methods of examining the stool for occult blood. The two most common ones are as follows:

1. *Hemoccult slides (Smith-Kline Diagnostics)*
   A stool sample is placed on one side of guaiac paper. Two drops of Hemoccult developer are placed on the other side. Bluish discoloration indicates the presence of occult blood in the stool.
2. *Hematest tablets (Ames)*
   A stool sample is placed on the developer paper. A tablet is placed on top of the stool specimen. Two to three drops of tap water are placed on the tablet and allowed to flow onto the paper. Again, a bluish discoloration indicates occult blood in the stool.

Contraindications. None.

Nursing considerations

Nursing Diagnoses/Collaborative Problems

See Fecal studies, p. 4.

Nursing Implications with Rationale

- If any special dietary restrictions are applicable, instruct the client as indicated.
- Tell the patient how many stool specimens are required and supply specimen containers. Give the patient tongue blades to transfer the specimens from the bedpan to the specimen container.
- Instruct the patient not to mix in urine or toilet paper with the stool specimen. Both can contaminate the specimen and alter the test results.
- Check the stool for occult blood on the unit, following the directions explicitly, or send the specimen to the laboratory for analysis.
- If the stool is obtained by digital examination, explain the procedures to the patient. It is important to be gentle during the rectal exam. The slightest mucosal trauma can cause a positive test result.

Carcinoembryonic antigen test

Normal value: <2 ng/ml.

Rationale. Carcinoembryonic antigen (CEA) is a protein that normally occurs in fetal gut tissue. By birth, detectable levels disappear. In the early 1960s, CEA was found to exist in the bloodstream of adults who had colorectal tumors. The antigen was originally thought to be specific for indicating colorectal cancer. More recently, it has been found to exist in patients with a variety of other carcinomas, sarcomas, and even many benign diseases, such as ulcerative colitis and cirrhosis.

Because of this lack of specificity, a CEA test cannot be used as an initial or screening test in the detection of colorectal cancer. It is usually used to monitor the patient's response to therapy. Preoperatively elevated CEA levels will return to normal after complete excision of a tumor. Also, a steadily rising CEA level occasionally is the first sign of tumor recurrence. Knowledge of this fact makes CEA tests very valuable in the follow-up of patients who have had potentially curative resections.

Procedure. A peripheral blood specimen is taken. The collecting tube varies according to the commercial laboratory measuring the levels.

Contraindications. None.

Nursing considerations

Nursing Diagnoses/Collaborative Problems

See Blood studies, p. 2.

Nursing Implications with Rationale

- After venipuncture apply pressure or a pressure dressing to the site. Observe the site for bleeding.

Sigmoidoscopy

(lower GI endoscopy)

Normal values: normal anus, rectum, and sigmoid colon.

Rationale. Endoscopy of the lower GI tract allows one to visualize and, if desired, take biopsy specimens of tumors, polyps, or ulcerations of the anus, rectum, and sigmoid colon. *Anoscopy* refers to examination of the anus; *proctoscopy* to examination of the anus and rectum, and *sigmoidoscopy* (the procedure done most often) to examination of the anus, rectum, and the distal sigmoid colon. Because the lower GI tract is difficult to visualize radiographically, the direct visualization afforded through sigmoidoscopy is required. Microscopic review of biopsy specimens obtained using this procedure can provide the diagnosis of many lower bowel disorders.

Procedure. The patient is usually given a Fleet's enema on the night before and the morning of the procedure. A light breakfast is usually allowed. The patient is usually not sedated.

Although sigmoidoscopy is usually performed in a specialized room containing all the necessary equipment, it can be performed at the bedside. Examination is carried out with the patient in the knee-chest position. If the patient cannot tolerate this position, the lateral, or Sim's, position is used, with the buttocks positioned 10 to 12 cm over the edge of the bed to facilitate complete rotation of the sigmoidoscope. Maximum convenience and comfort are afforded by using a "proctoscopic" table, which tilts the patient into the required position.

The procedure begins with digital examination of the rectum, which slowly dilates the anal sphincter. The well-lubricated instrument is gently passed into the rectum and then into the sigmoid colon. The sigmoidoscope reaches about 25 cm (10 inches) into the lower bowel. Air is insufflated to distend the bowel, allowing better visualization. Small amounts of stool and mucus can be removed during the procedure with cotton swabs or by suctioning. The procedure usually takes 15 minutes.

Contraindications. The procedure is not performed on the following:

1. Patients who are uncooperative.
2. Patients with painful anorectal conditions, such as fissures, fistulae, or hemorrhoids.
3. Patients with severe rectal bleeding.
4. Patients who are suspected to have a perforated rectum or colon.

Nursing considerations

Nursing Diagnoses/Collaborative Problems

See Endoscopic procedures, pp. 6-7.

Nursing Implications with Rationale

- Explain the procedure to the patient. Warn the patient that he or she will feel discomfort and the urge to defecate as the sigmoidoscope is passed. Encourage verbalization of the patient's fears. Provide emotional support.
- Obtain the patient's written consent for sigmoidoscopy and possible biopsy.
- Allow the patient to have a light breakfast on the morning of the examination.
- Assist the patient with enemas ordered on the morning of and on the evening before the test to ensure optimum visualization of the lower GI tract.
- Assure the patient that he or she will be properly draped to avoid additional unnecessary exposure and embarrassment.
- Tell the patient that because air is insufflated into the bowel during the procedure, he or she may have "gas pains."
- After the study observe the patient for fever, bleeding, abdominal distention, and unusual complaints of pain. Slight rectal bleeding may occur if biopsy specimens are taken.

Barium enema study

(lower GI series)

Normal values: normal filling, contour, patency, positioning, and transit time of barium.

Rationale. The barium enema (BE) study consists of a series of x-ray films of the colon used to demonstrate the presence and location of polyps, tumors (Figure 3-6), and diverticula (Figure 3-7). Positional abnormalities (such as malrotation) and external compression of the bowel from paracolonic tumors can also be detected. Therapeutically, the BE study may be used for attempted reduction of nonstrangulated ileocolic intussusception (infolding of a proximal segment of intestine within a distal segment of intestine) in children.

Procedure. The specific preparation of a BE study varies according to the protocol of the radiologist performing the test. Two sample preparations are shown below:

Sample #1
Two days prior to the examination
  Clear liquid diet
Evening before
  10 ounces of magnesium citrate or X-prep
Day of examination
  NPO after midnight
  Enema in the morning

Sample #2
Day before the examination
  Drink one gallon of Colyte
  Clear liquid diet
Day of examination
  NPO after midnight
Enema in the morning if the patient was unable to drink all of the Colyte

The test begins with the rectal instillation of approximately 500 to 1500 ml of barium. Because the patient often has difficulty retaining the barium, a rectal tube with an inflatable balloon is used. The patient is placed in supine, prone, and lateral positions. The progress of the barium flow is followed on a fluoroscope. Small polyps and early changes in ulcerative colitis are more easily detected with an *air-contrast barium enema* study. In this study, after the bowel mucosa is outlined with a thin coat of barium, air is insufflated to enhance the contrast and outline of small lesions. After the x-ray films are taken, the patient is allowed to expel the barium. This may take as long as 30 minutes. After the barium is expelled, another film is taken for retention of the barium. The colon is examined again for pathologic conditions in the postevacuation film. The entire study is little more uncomfortable than a routine saline enema. It takes about 45 minutes.

The standard procedure for administering a barium enema through a colostomy or ileostomy has been to remove the pouch and instill the contrast medium using a standard enema bag. However, many problems occurred with this procedure. Because these patients have no sphincter control and cannot retain contrast medium, the barium would flow freely from the stoma. This obstructed visualization and caused

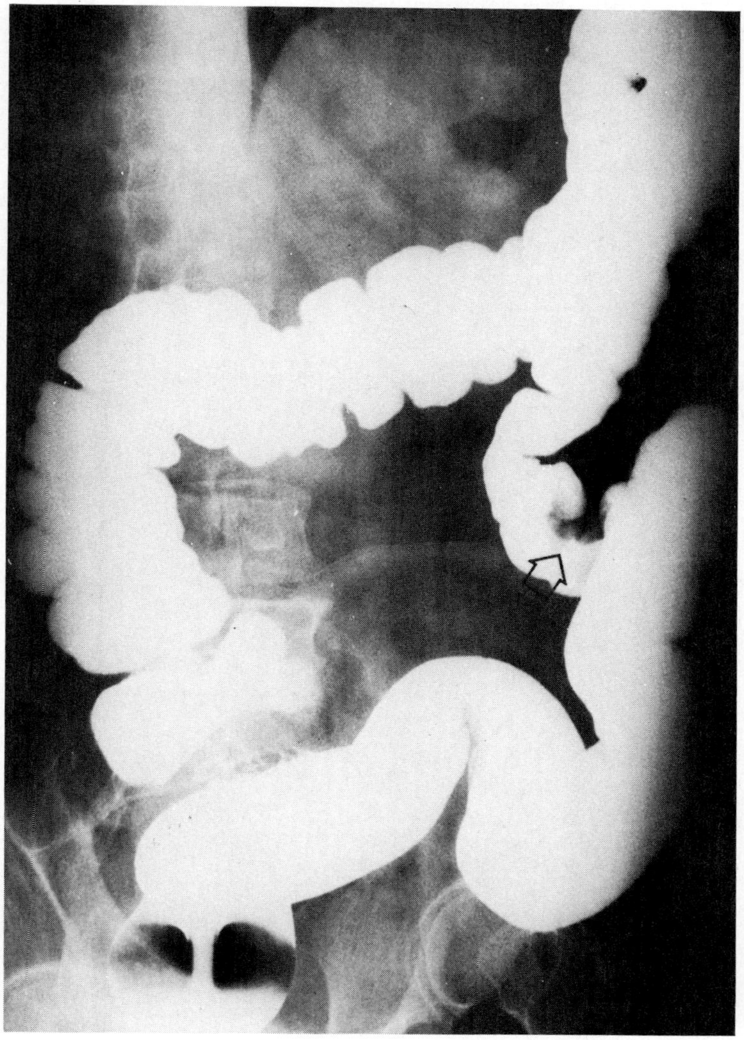

FIGURE 3-6. Barium enema demonstrating a cancer *(arrow)* in the descending colon.

embarrassment. The procedure has now been modified to eliminate some of these problems. The newer method of administering a barium enema is to cover the stoma with a colostomy or bongart pouch to catch any backflow of barium. A cone from a colostomy irrigation kit is inserted into the stoma. This cone is then attached to irrigation tubing with a straight catheter. A clamp is turned on, and the contrast medium is instilled. A collection device (such as a bedpan) can be placed at the patient's side to collect any overflow of contrast medium from the stoma. The end of the pouch can be brought down to rest in the collecting device. When the x-ray studies are completed, a clamp is placed at the bottom of the pouch. This method is very effective because the barium does not get on the patient's skin and obscure the diagnostic x-ray films. Also, the patient is spared the embarrassment of having barium leak from the stoma.

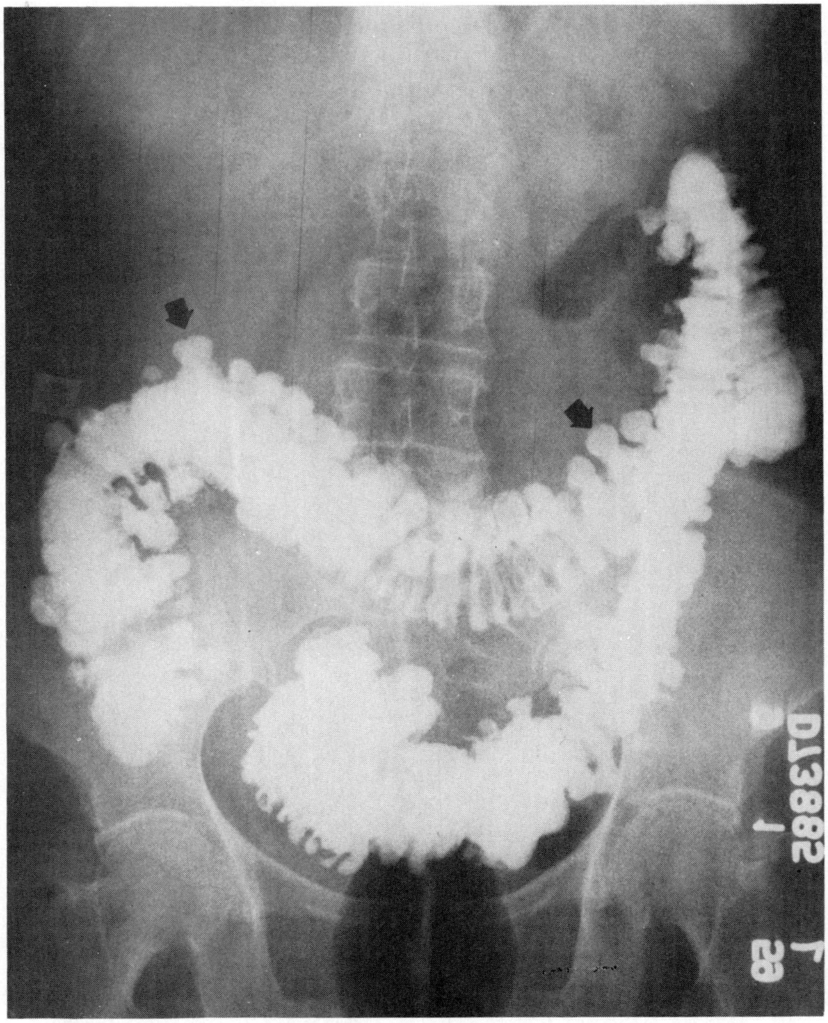

FIGURE 3-7. Barium enema demonstrating multiple diverticula *(arrows)* in the colon.

Contraindications. The use of barium as a contrast medium is contraindicated in cases where a perforated viscus is suspected. (See discussion of Gastrografin in barium swallow, pp. 69-70.)

Nursing considerations

Nursing Diagnoses/Collaborative Problems

See X-ray studies, p. 5.

- Possible alteration in elimination related to barium retention.
- Potential complication: bowel obstruction or fecal impaction.

Nursing Implications with Rationale

- Explain the procedure to the patient. Tell the patient that it is not painful, but that the preparation and procedure may be exhausting. Give written instructions. Encourage verbalization of the patient's questions and fears. Provide needed emotional support.

- Explain the preparations required. Tell the patient that his or her bowel must be free of fecal debris for the barium to outline the lumen of the bowel accurately.
- Assist the patient with the required preparation and chart the effects of the cathartics and suppository.
- Keep the patient NPO after midnight to provide optimum visualization of the bowel.
- Suggest that the patient take reading material to the x-ray department so that he or she may read while expelling the barium.
- The patient may resume a regular diet after the procedure is completed. Force oral fluids to avoid dehydration caused by cathartics.
- After the BE study, assess the patient for complete evacuation of the barium. (Retained barium may cause a hardened impaction.) Stool will be light in color until all of the barium has been expelled. A cathartic such as magnesium citrate or an oil-retention enema may be given.
- A local anesthetic ointment (such as Nupercainal) may be ordered to relieve anal discomfort.
- If a patient is not too tired, a warm bath may be soothing.
- Allow the patient time to rest after the test. The cleansing regimen and the BE procedure may be exhausting.

Colonoscopy

Normal value: normal colon.

Rationale. Before 1960 it was thought that nearly all of the primary colorectal tumors occurred in the sigmoid colon and rectum. Researchers have now recognized that a significant number of tumors occur more proximally and are therefore beyond the visualization ability of the rigid sigmoidoscope. With the development of the fiber-optic colonoscope, the entire colon from anus to cecum can be examined in a high percentage of patients. Therefore, with colonoscopy the detection of lesions in the proximal colon, which would otherwise be missed by sigmoidoscopy, is possible. As with sigmoidoscopy, benign and malignant neoplasms, mucosal inflammation or ulceration, and sites of active hemorrhage can be visualized. Also, biopsy specimens can be obtained and small tumors removed through the scope with the use of cable-activated instruments. Actively bleeding vessels can be coagulated.

Patients who have had previous cancer of the colon are at high risk for developing another colon cancer. For this patient population colonoscopy allows early detection of any secondary tumors. Complications of the procedure include bowel perforation, persistent bleeding from biopsy sites, and oversedation resulting in respiratory depression.

Procedure. The patient's large intestine must be completely free of fecal material. Bowel preparations vary, yet one such successful preparation is as follows:

Day before examination

Clear liquid diet is followed from morning until midnight.

Patient should drink 8 oz. of Colyte every 15-20 minutes over a 2- to 4-hour period beginning about 4 PM until 1 gallon of Colyte is consumed.

Day of examination

The patient is kept NPO after midnight.

One Fleet enema is administered at 6 PM

If patient was unable to drink all the colonic lavage (Colyte), two saline enemas are given.

The patient is premedicated with atropine 0.4 mg and meperidine (Demerol) 50 mg intramuscularly. The study is performed in a room specially equipped for this procedure. An intravenous infusion is begun and the patient is given midazolam (Versed) 1 mg and meperidine 25 to 50 mg intravenously. With the patient in the Sim's position, the scope is inserted into the anus (or colostomy) and slowly advanced to the cecum. For complete colonic examination all the way to the cecum, a significant amount of manipulation of the scope is required. This can be uncomfortable, yet with appropriate sedation, is rarely distressing.

As in all endoscopy, air is insufflated to distend the bowel for better visualization. Endoscopic biopsy-specimen or polyp removal is performed and then the scope is removed. The examination is usually performed in about 1 to 1½ hours.

Contraindications. The test should not be performed on the following patients:

1. Uncooperative patients.
2. Patients whose vital signs are unstable.
3. Patients who are bleeding profusely from the rectum (see Gastroscopy).

The procedure should be delayed if the bowel preparation is not successful in completely removing all fecal material.

Nursing considerations

Potential Nursing Diagnoses/Collaborative Problems

See Endoscopic procedure, pp. 6-7.

- **Potential for injury related to sedation.**
- **Potential complication: respiratory arrest from overdose of sedatives.**

Nursing Implications with Rationale

- Explain the procedure to the patient. Tell the patient that the examination is uncomfortable but that sedation will be given by injection and intravenous infusion. Provide emotional support.
- Obtain the patient's written consent for colonoscopy.
- Assist the patient with the preparation. Record the results from the cathartics and enemas.
- Tell the patient that he or she will be draped to avoid unnecessary embarrassment.
- Tell the patient that because air is insufflated into the bowel during the procedure, he or she may have "gas pains."
- After the test, check for evidence of bowel perforation (abdominal pain, tenderness, and bleeding). Examine the stools for gross blood.
- Unless further studies are needed or bowel perforation is suspected, the patient may resume a normal diet after the procedure. Force fluids to avoid cathartic-induced dehydration.
- If the patient is not too tired, a warm bath may be soothing.
- Allow the patient time to rest after the test. The cleansing regimen and fasting may tire and weaken the patient.
- Take safety precautions until the effect of the medications has worn off.

SUPPLEMENTAL INFORMATION

Stool culture

(stool for culture and sensitivity, C & S; stool for ova and parasites, O & P)

Normal values: normal intestinal flora.

Rationale. The feces (stool) can be examined for the presence of bacteria, ova and parasites, and occult blood (p. 74). Many normal bacteria (such as *Escherichia coli*) are indigenous to the flora in the bowel. Bacterial cultures are usually done to detect enteropathogens (such as *Staphylococcus aureus, Salmonella, and Shigella*).

When a patient is suspected to have a parasitic infection, the stool is examined for ova and parasites (O & P). Usually at least three stool specimens are collected on different days. The major intestinal parasites of clinical significance in the United States include *Ascaris* (hookworms), *Strongyloides* (tapeworms), and *Giardia lamblia* (protozoans). An estimated 3% to 7% of adults in the United States have giardiasis caused by *Giardia lamblia,* which is the most frequent parasite in the United States. This organism is usually transmitted via fecal (sewage) contamination of drinking water. Symptoms of acute infection include foul-smelling watery diarrhea, intestinal gas, and epigastric pain.

Parasitic studies should be done before x-ray studies using barium sulfate because of the excess crystalline material that will be deposited in the stool specimen. This could obscure the detection of parasites. Also, certain medications such as mineral oil, tetracyclines, insoluble diarrheal preparations, and bismuth may inhibit the detection of protozoans.

Procedure. Stools for bacteria or parasites are collected in a clean, wide-mouth plastic or waxed container with a tight-fitting lid. The patient usually defecates into a clean bedpan and transfers either a walnut-size piece of the feces or the entire specimen (as directed by the laboratory) into the specimen container. Urine and toilet paper should not be mixed with the specimen. Since parasites or bacteria are often found in mucus or blood streaks, some of this material, if present, should be included with the sample.

The "tape test" can be done by placing cellophane tape over the perianal area to detect pinworms, which are fairly common in children. Because the female worm lays her eggs at night around the perianal area, the tape is applied before bed and removed in the morning before the patient gets out of bed. The sticky surface is then applied directly to a glass slide and examined microscopically for pinworm ova.

If a rectal swab is to be used, the nurse (wearing gloves) inserts a sterile cotton-tipped swab approximately 1 inch into the anal canal. The swab is gently moved from side to side and left in place for 30 seconds to absorb organisms. This is sometimes done for detection of *Shigella* and gonorrhea (p. 350).

Contraindications. None.

Nursing considerations

Nursing Diagnoses/Collaborative Problems

See Fecal studies, p. 4.

Nursing Implications with Rationale

- Explain the method of stool collection to the patient. Be matter-of-fact to avoid any embarrassment to the patient.
- Instruct the patient not to mix urine or toilet paper with the specimen. Both can contaminate the specimen and alter test results.
- Handle the specimen carefully, as though it is capable of causing infection. If the nurse is assisting with the specimen collection, gloves should be worn.
- Indicate on the lab slip if the patient is taking any medications (such as antibiotics), which can alter the flora of the intestines.
- Generally, barium, oil, or laxatives containing heavy metals are not given 7 days before the stool collection because they interfere with the detection of ova and parasites.
- If the patient received a purgative medication, the complete stool specimen is usually collected.
- If an enema must be administered to collect specimens, only normal saline or tap water should be administered. Soapsuds or any other substance could affect the viability of the organisms collected.
- Send the stool specimen to the laboratory as soon as possible after the stool collection.

Clostridial toxin assay

(Clostridium difficile, antibiotic-associated colitis, pseudomembranous colitis toxic assay)

Normal value: negative (presence of toxin is indicative of disease).

Rationale. It has been shown that there may be an overgrowth of *Clostridium difficile* bacteria in the colon of patients who develop pseudomembranous colitis while taking antibiotics (such as clindamycin, ampicillin, and various combinations of these and other antibiotics). The clostridia bacteria releases a toxin that causes necrosis of the colonic epithelium. This toxin can be detected in the stools of patients afflicted with this superinfection. The detection of this toxin and the presence of this organism in the stool is diagnostic. Management of this antibiotic-associated colitis includes immediate cessation of the antibiotic and IV replacement of fluid and electrolyte losses. Antibiotics such as metronidazole or vancomycin, to which *Clostridium difficile* is sensitive, are administered.

Procedure. Stools are collected in a clean wide-mouth container with a tight-fitting lid as described in the previous study. A rectal swab cannot be used because an adequate amount of stool cannot be obtained by this method. A stool specimen can also be obtained during proctoscopy.

The specimen should be transported immediately to the laboratory in order to prevent deterioration of the toxin. If the specimen cannot be processed immediately, it should then be refrigerated.

Contraindications. None.

Nursing considerations

Nursing Diagnoses/Collaborative Problems

See Fecal studies, p. 4.

Nursing Implications with Rationale

See Stool culture (previous study).

Gastrointestinal bleeding scan

(abdominal scintigraphy, GI scintigraphy)

Normal value: no collection of radionuclide in the gastrointestinal tract.

Rationale. The gastrointestinal bleeding scan is a nuclear medicine test used to localize the site of bleeding in patients who are experiencing a persistent, slow gastrointestinal hemorrhage. Oftentimes localizing the source of bleeding in these patients is quite difficult. If surgery is required for such a patient in whom the exact site of bleeding is not known, the surgery is difficult, cumbersome, and prolonged. Endoscopy has been useful in determining the source of bleeding. However, often the endoscopist does not see the bleeding site, especially if the bleeding is intermittent. Arteriography has been effective in determining the site of bleeding. Unfortunately, the rate of bleeding must exceed 0.5 ml/min to be detected by arteriography. Furthermore, if the gastrointestinal bleeding is intermittent, the arteriogram may be falsely negative.

A gastrointestinal scintigram is much more sensitive for localizing the site of bleeding. It is performed by injecting technetium-99m–labeled sulfur colloid or technetium-99m–labeled red blood cells into the patient. If the patient is bleeding at even a rate as low as 0.1 ml/min, pooling of the radionuclide will be detected in the abnormal segment of intestine. Few false-positive results occur. The test only locates the bleeding and does not indicate the exact pathologic condition causing it. If surgery is required, the operation can easily be directed toward that area, minimizing operating and anesthesia times. No complications are associated with this test.

Procedure. Ten millicuries of freshly prepared technetium-99m–labeled sulfur colloid is administered intravenously to the patient. If red blood cells are used, 3 ml of the patient's own whole blood is combined with technetium and reinjected into the patient. Immediately after the administration of the radionuclide, the patient is placed under a scintillation camera similar to that used in bone or liver scans. Multiple images of the abdomen are obtained at short intervals. The scintigrams are recorded on Polaroid or x-ray film. Detection of the radionuclide in the abdomen indicates the site of bleeding.

Areas of the bowel hidden by the liver or spleen may not be adequately evaluated by this procedure. Also, the rectum cannot be easily evaluated because other pelvic structures (the bladder, for example) obstruct the view. If the initial study is negative and subsequent films give clinical evidence of active bleeding, a repeat scan may be performed with the administration of another dose of technetium-99m.

The test takes about 10 to 20 minutes to perform and is usually done in the nuclear medicine department. No pretest preparation is required. The only discomfort associated with this study is that of injecting the radioisotope.

Contraindications. Pregnant and lactating women.

Nursing considerations

Nursing Diagnoses/Collaborative Problems

See Nuclear scanning, p. 5.

Nursing Implications with Rationale

- Explain the study to the patient. Encourage the patient to verbalize his or her fear of internal hemorrhage.

- Make sure the patient understands that only a small dose of nuclear material is administered.
- Instruct the patient to notify the technician if he or she has a bowel movement during the test. The technician may want to examine the stool for the presence of nuclear material. If nuclear material is present, this highly suggests that the source of the bleeding is in the distal colon or rectum.
- If the patient is having major gastrointestinal bleeding, closely monitor the vital signs during the test.

Schilling test

(vitamin B_{12} absorption test)

Normal values: excretion of 8% to 40% of radioactive vitamin B_{12} within 24 hours

Rationale. The Schilling test is performed to detect vitamin B_{12} absorption. Ingested vitamin B_{12} combines with intrinsic factor produced by the gastric mucosa and is absorbed in the distal part of the ileum. Pernicious anemia (a type of macrocytic anemia) results when the body is unable to absorb vitamin B_{12} because of a lack of intrinsic factor.

The Schilling test can detect whether a defect in vitamin B_{12} absorption or a deficiency in the intrinsic factor exists. With normal absorption of vitamin B_{12}, the ileum absorbs more than the body needs and excretes the excess into the urine. With impaired vitamin B_{12} absorption, no vitamin B_{12} is excreted in the urine. The Schilling test measures the urinary excretion of vitamin B_{12} after the administration of radioactive and nonradioactive doses of vitamin B_{12}.

Decreased levels of vitamin B_{12} are seen in patients with pernicious anemia, malabsorption syndrome, liver diseases, hypothyroidism, and sprue.

Procedure. The Schilling test can be performed in one or two stages. Patients who excrete a normal amount of radioactive vitamin B_{12} in the first stage require no further testing. The second stage is performed if the first stage shows a decreased percentage of radioactive vitamin B_{12} in the urine. The second stage of the test is needed to confirm the diagnosis of pernicious anemia.

First stage (without intrinsic factor). After the patient is kept NPO for 8 to 12 hours before the test, a urine specimen is collected and discarded. The patient then receives an oral dose of radioactive vitamin B_{12} and begins a 24- to 48-hour urine collection. After 1 to 2 hours, the patient receives an intramuscular injection of nonradioactive vitamin B_{12} to saturate tissue-binding sites and to permit some excretion of radioactive vitamin B_{12} in the urine. The patient may resume eating after the injection of vitamin B_{12}.

Second stage (with intrinsic factor). After being kept NPO for 8 to 12 hours before the test, the patient voids and discards the urine. The patient then receives an oral dose of radioactive vitamin B_{12} and human intrinsic factor. A 24-hour urine collection is then begun. After 2 hours the patient receives an intramuscular dose of nonradioactive vitamin B_{12}. The patient may resume eating after the injection. After administration of intrinsic factor and vitamin B_{12} in the second stage, patients who have B_{12} deficiency secondary to lack of intrinsic factor (e.g., chronic gastritis) excrete normal amounts of radioactive B_{12}. Patients who have B_{12} deficiency from primary bowel disease, however, do not have normal B_{12} urinary levels. The second stage is usually performed within 1 week after the first stage.

A combined assay can also be performed to incorporate stages one and two into one procedure. In this method the fasting patient receives a capsule of cobalt-57–labeled vitamin B_{12} plus intrinsic factor and a second capsule of cobalt-58. One hour later, an intramuscular injection of nonradioactive vitamin B_{12} is given. All urine is then collected for 24 hours and the percentages of cobalt-57 and cobalt-58 are calculated.

Contraindications. The test should not be performed within 10 days after a recent radionuclide scan because it could alter the test results.

This study is contraindicated for pregnant and lactating women.

Nursing considerations

Nursing Diagnoses/Collaborative Problems

See Urine studies, p. 3.

Nursing Implications with Rationale

- Explain the purpose and the procedure of the Schilling test to the patient. Also provide written instructions.
- Ensure that laxatives are not given to the patient the evening before the test because they could decrease the rate of vitamin B_{12} absorption.
- Keep the patient NPO for 8 to 12 hours before the test. Food should not be given until after the patient receives the injection. The dietary department should hold the diet tray until the injection is given.
- Be certain that the patient receives the injection of the nonradioactive vitamin B_{12} at the exact time specified. Otherwise, the radioactive vitamin B_{12} will be absorbed by the liver and not excreted in the urine.
- Explain the procedure for collection of the 24-hour urine specimen. (See the creatinine clearance test, p. 231, all but the first and last nursing implications.) Follow the laboratory guidelines in regard to refrigerating the specimen. Patients with elevated BUN levels may be required to collect the urine specimens for longer periods of time, since impaired renal function may slow excretion of vitamin B_{12}.
- Assure the patient that the tracer dose of radioactive vitamin B_{12} is not harmful to them or others because the radioactive dose is extremely small.
- If the patient had a decreased excretion of vitamin B_{12} in the first stage of the test, explain that the second stage of the test is usually performed within 1 week.

Obstruction series

Normal value: no evidence of any bowel obstruction.

Rationale. The obstruction series is a group of x-ray studies performed on the abdomen of patients who have suspected bowel obstruction, paralytic ileus, perforated viscus, or abdominal abscess. This series usually consists of at least two x-ray studies. The first is an erect abdominal x-ray study that should include visualization of both diaphragms. It is examined for evidence of free air under either diaphragm, which is pathognomonic of a perforated viscus. This x-ray study is also used to detect air fluid levels within the intestine. The presence of an air fluid level is compatible with bowel obstruction or paralytic ileus. Occasionally, patients are too ill to stand erect for the erect portion of this series. In these instances, an x-ray film can be taken with the patient in the left lateral decubitus position. If free air is present, it will be seen above the liver on the right side of the abdomen.

The second x-ray film in the obstruction series usually is a supine abdominal x-ray study. An abdominal abscess may be seen as a cluster of small, tiny bubbles within one localized area of the supine abdominal x-ray film. A gas-filled, distended bowel is compatible with a bowel obstruction, the location of which can be determined with this test. Gas-filled large and small bowel detected on this x-ray is compatible with the large bowel obstruction. The presence of only a gas-filled small bowel indicates that the bowel obstruction exists more proximal to the large intestine. In this situation, a small bowel obstruction is probably present.

The obstruction series can be used to monitor the clinical course of patients with gastrointestinal disease. Repeated obstruction series on patients who have partial small bowel obstruction can demonstrate a resolution of the problem or a worsening of the partial bowel obstruction (requiring surgery). Likewise, resolution of the paralytic ileus can be detected by serial use of the obstruction series.

Frequently, a close cross-table lateral view of the abdomen is included in an obstruction series to detect abdominal aorta calcification, which is quite common in older patients. This calcification is easily visualized on the plain radiograph of the cross-table view of the abdomen. This calcification, therefore, demonstrates the outline of the abdominal aorta. If an abdominal aortic aneurysm is present, bulging of the calcified aortic wall will be seen.

Finally, the obstruction series provides the same information as provided by the plain x-ray study of the kidneys, ureters, and bladder (KUB) (see p. 257).

Procedure. Although the procedure varies from hospital to hospital, usually supine abdominal x-ray, erect abdominal x-ray, and perhaps low erect chest x-ray studies are taken. Oftentimes, a cross-table lateral x-ray study is also taken. An obstruction series is performed in the radiology department by an x-ray technician. A radiologist interprets the film. No discomfort is associated with this study. It takes only minutes to perform.

Contraindications. This study is contraindicated in the pregnant patient.

Nursing considerations

Nursing Diagnoses/Collaborative Problems

See X-ray studies, p. 5.

Nursing Implications with Rationale

- Explain the procedure to the patient.
- For adequate visualization, ensure that this study is scheduled before any barium studies.

CASE STUDY 4: ANOREXIA NERVOSA

Becky J., a 14-year-old white girl, was taken to her family nurse practitioner by her mother because of cessation of menses. Once an overweight child, Becky recently had a severe weight loss and was described by her mother as anxious, irritable, and depressed. Despite her weight of 85 pounds (and height of 64 inches), Becky was jogging long distances daily. The physical examination was compatible with signs of starvation (such as sparse, dry hair; dry, flaky skin; muscle wasting; and red, swollen lips).

Studies	Results
Triceps skin-fold thickness (TSF) (Figure 3-8)	65% standard
Midarm circumference (MAC) (Figure 3-8)	65% standard
Midarm muscle circumference (MAMC) (Figure 3-8)	65% standard
Hemoglobin (p. 388)	10 g/dl (normal: 12 g/dl)
Hematocrit (p. 388)	31% (normal: 36%)
Total iron-binding capacity (TIBC) (p. 393)	210 μg/dl (normal: 250-420 μg/dl)
Serum albumin (p. 99)	2.8 g/dl (normal: 3.2-4.5 g/dl)
Total protein (p. 99)	4 g/dl (normal: 6-8 g/dl)
Total lymphocyte count (p. 389)	1200/mm^3 (normal: 1500-3000/mm^3)
Blood urea nitrogen (BUN) (p. 229)	30 mg/dl (normal: 5-20 mg/dl)
24-hour urine for creatinine (p. 330)	Decreased when compared to expected creatinine clearance based on height and sex
Serum triglycerides (p. 34)	200 mg/dl (normal: 40-150 mg/dl)
Skin testing with common antigens	Delayed sensitivity to mumps, purified protein derivative (PPD), and *Candida*

The triceps skin-fold thickness (TSF), which estimates the amount of subcutaneous fat, reflected the depleted caloric stores in the body. The midarm muscle circumference (MAMC), which is calculated using the midarm circumference (MAC) and the TSF (Figure 3-8), reflected moderate to severe muscle protein depletion as a result of catabolism. The decreased hemoglobin and hematocrit levels reflected anemia because of iron and folic acid deficiency. The TIBC level reflected transferrin concentration (p. 393), which is a sensitive and early indicator of protein deficiency. The decreased plasma albumin and protein levels correlated with protein depletion, fatty liver, and edema. The elevated BUN level was the result of catabolism. The decreased lymphocyte count is further evidence of protein malnutrition. Because the 24-hour urinary excretion of creatinine is approximately proportional to lean body mass, its decrease re-

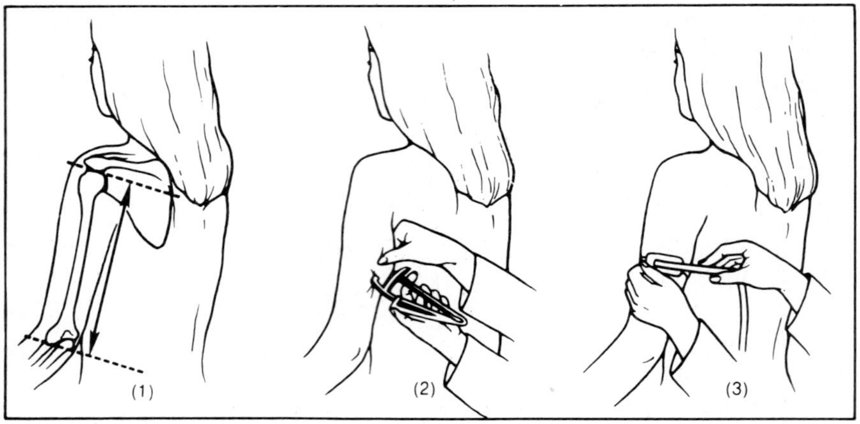

FIGURE 3-8. Techniques for obtaining and evaluating anthropomorphic measurements.
From Jones DA and Jirovec MM: Medical-surgical nursing: a conceptual approach, ed 2, New York, 1982, McGraw-Hill, Inc.

flected a severe degree of muscle protein depletion and decreased muscle mass. The antigen skin test showed decreased immunocompetence, which is seen in nutritional starvation. This also reflects the impaired ability of the white blood cells to fight infection.

Based on the results of these tests and a detailed family history, Becky was placed in the hospital in an adolescent unit for anorectics. After several weeks of nutritional counseling and behavior modification, Becky was discharged to home. Individual and family counseling were continued over the next year.

QUESTIONS AND ANSWERS

1. **QUESTION:** Why is barium, a contrast medium, needed to visualize the GI tract radiographically?
   ANSWER: Diagnostic radiology is based entirely on contrasting densities. If no contrast medium were used, an x-ray film of the abdomen would show only general shadows, fluid levels, and gas. With barium, the inside of the gut can be evaluated for the presence of pathology.
2. **QUESTION:** What is the composition of barium?
   ANSWER: Barium sulfate is a tasteless, odorless, inert, nongranular, and completely insoluble powder that is made into an aqueous suspension. It cannot be absorbed by the GI tract.
3. **QUESTION:** What effect would the administration of narcotics or sedatives have on the results of the UGI?
   ANSWER: Narcotics and sedatives often prolong gastric emptying time. If these drugs are administered before a UGI, the radiologist should be informed to prevent false attribution of the prolonged emptying time of the stomach to a pathologic cause.
4. **QUESTION:** Often the patient admitted for evaluation of the GI tract needs various diagnostic procedures performed in the shortest amount of time possible. If your patient requires a gastric analysis, a UGI, and a BE study, in what order should these procedures be performed and why?
   ANSWER: The gastric analysis should be performed first, since the stomach must not contain any food, fluid, or barium. The BE study should precede the UGI because the ingested barium, descending through the intestine, would obstruct the visualization of the lower GI tract.
5. **QUESTION:** Your patient is receiving antacids and cimetidine (Tagamet) for peptic ulcers. Should these drugs be discontinued before a gastric analysis is performed?
   ANSWER: Yes. Cimetidine is a histamine antagonist. It inhibits gastric acid secretion caused by histamine stimulation. If it is given within 4 hours of gastric analysis, the acid measurements will be artificially low. Administering antacids to the pa-

tient within 2 hours of the study neutralizes the acid produced during the test and, like histamine antagonists, causes artificially low acid measurement.

6. **QUESTION:** The BAO and MAO measurements on your female patient are 5 and 14 mEq/hr, respectively. Are these results alone diagnostic of duodenal peptic ulcers?

   ANSWER: No. Although these values are in the range of most patients with duodenal ulcers, many normal patients have elevated acid levels in the absence of ulcer disease. The diagnosis of ulcers cannot be made on history, physical examination, or gastric analysis alone. These tests only serve to corroborate the findings of the definitive studies—a UGI and gastroscopy.

7. **QUESTION:** Your patient is very anxious before having esophageal function studies. Since admission, the patient has had an order for diazepam (Valium), as needed, for anxiety. Should this drug be given the morning of the test?

   ANSWER: No. Sedation of any kind may reduce the LES pressure and cause greater acid reflux than what might have been present if the patient were not sedated.

8. **QUESTION:** Is colonoscopy more accurate than barium enema studies in diagnosing pathologic colorectal conditions?

   ANSWER: Yes. Several well-controlled studies have indicated the marked superiority of colonoscopy to barium enema studies. The accuracy of BE studies varies from 50% to 75%. Colonoscopy is accurate about 95% of the time.

9. **QUESTION:** Your patient returns to the unit after having a colonoscopy and polypectomy. A regular diet is ordered. He tolerates his lunch well. Before eating supper, he begins to complain of severe abdominal pain and he vomits. What nursing interventions are appropriate in this situation?

   ANSWER: Assessment of the symptomatology present and knowledge of the potential complications of colonoscopy should lead you to suspect perforated colon. The following interventions should be performed:

   a. Hold the supper meal and keep him NPO.
   b. Maintain the patency of the intravenous line, if one is running.
   c. Assess the patient's abdomen for distention.
   d. Record the vital signs.
   e. Contact the physician immediately.

BIBLIOGRAPHY

Bentley DW: *Clostridium difficile*–associated disease in long-term care facilities, Infect Control Hosp Epidemiol 11(8):434-438, 1990.

Bottrill P: Gastrointestinal endoscopy—guidelines for safe clinical practice: a British perspective, Gastroenterol Nurs 13(4):234-238, 1991.

Caffery L and Claussen DS: Inpatient education for fiberoptic/videoptic diagnostic and therapeutic procedures for gastroenterology, Gastroenterol Nurs 14(2):106-109, 1991.

Christie JP and others: Flexible sigmoidoscopy screening, Patient Care 24(12):133-145, 1990.

Cohen S: Disease of the esophagus. In Wyngaarden JB and others, editors: Cecil textbook of medicine, ed 19, Philadelphia, 1992, WB Saunders.

Goyal RK: Diseases of the esophagus. In Wilson J and others, editors: Harrison's principles of internal medicine, ed 12, New York, 1991, McGraw-Hill.

Isselbacher KJ and Podolsky DK: Approach to the patient with gastrointestinal disease. In Wilson J and others, editors: Harrison's principles of internal medicine, ed 12, New York, 1991, McGraw-Hill.

Kelly MT and others: Commercial latex agglutination test for detection of *Clostridium difficile*–associated diarrhea, J Clin Microbiol 25:1244-1247, 1987.

Kidwell JA: Nursing care for the patient receiving conscious sedation during gastrointestinal endoscopic procedures, Gastroenterol Nurs 13(3):134-139, 1991.

Kimmey MB and Silverstein FE: Gastrointestinal endoscopy. In Wilson J and others, editors: Harrison's principles of internal medicine, ed 12, New York, 1991, McGraw-Hill.

Lamont JT and Isselbacher KJ: Disease of the small and large intestine. In Wilson J and others, editors: Harrison's principles of internal medicine, ed 12, New York, 1991, McGraw-Hill.

Lanza FL: Tumors of the stomach. In Rakel RE, editor: Conn's current therapy, Philadelphia, 1991, WB Saunders.

Kerr RB and others: Control of *Clostridium difficile* colitis outbreak by treating asymptomatic carriers with metronidazole, Am J Infect Control 18(5):332-335, 1990.

Martino SM: Gastrointestinal endoscopy education for nursing units within the hospital, Gastrointerol Nurs 12(4):270-273, 1990.

Roberts IM: Malabsorption syndromes. In Rakel RE, editor: Conn's current therapy, Philadelphia, 1991, WB Saunders.

Schiller LR: Peptic ulcer: epidemiology, clinical manifestations, and diagnosis. In Wyngaarden JB and others, editors: Cecil textbook of medicine, ed 19, Philadelphia, 1992, WB Saunders.

Smith LE: Tumors of the colon and rectum. In Rakel RE, editor: Conn's current therapy, Philadelphia, 1991, WB Saunders.

Thibault A and others: Risk factors for the development of *Clostridium difficile*–associated diarrhea during a hospital outbreak, Infect Control Hosp Epidemiol 12(6):345-348, 1991.

Vennes JA: Gastrointestinal endoscopy. In Wyngaarden JB and others, editors: Cecil textbook of medicine, ed 19, Philadelphia, 1992, WB Saunders.

Wall SD: Diagnostic imaging procedures in gastroenterology. In Wyngaarden JB and others, editors: Cecil textbook of medicine, ed 19, Philadelphia, 1992, WB Saunders.

Zeman PK and others: Gallbladder imaging. The state of the art, Gastroenterol Clin North Am 20(1):127-156, 1991.

Chapter 4

DIAGNOSTIC STUDIES USED IN THE ASSESSMENT OF THE

HEPATOBILIARY AND PANCREATIC SYSTEM

ANATOMY AND PHYSIOLOGY

The liver, the biliary tract, and the pancreas (Figure 4-1) are being considered together because of their anatomic proximity, their closely related functions, and the similarity of the symptom complexes caused by many of their closely related functions. The *liver* is the largest gland in the body, occupying most of the right upper quadrant of the abdomen and lying directly beneath the diaphragm. In brief, the main functions of the liver are the following:

1. Formation and secretion of bile. Bile is a collective term that includes bile salts, bilirubin, phospholipids, cholesterol, bicarbonate, and water. Bile salts mix with ingested lipids to provide fat absorption from the gastrointestinal (GI) tract. The bilirubin, cholesterol, and phospholipids are excretory products of metabolism. The bicarbonate and water are secreted into the alimentary tract and neutralize the stomach acid, because digestion and absorption require an alkaline environment.

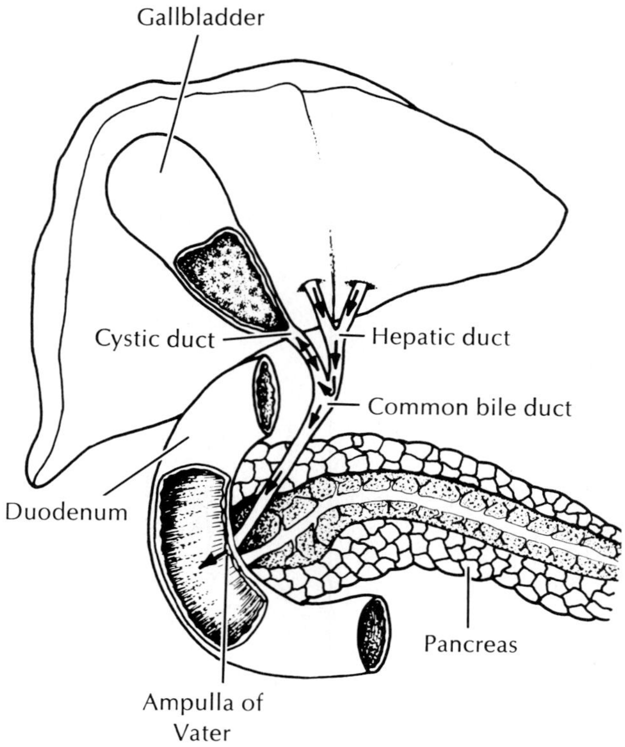

FIGURE 4-1. Normal anatomy of the biliary system.
From Given BA and Simmons SJ: Gastroenterology in clinical nursing, ed 4, St Louis, 1983, The CV Mosby Co.

2. Metabolism and storage of ingested carbohydrates, protein, and fats.
3. Catabolism of many endogenous substances, including insulin, steroids, and gastrin.
4. Detoxification of a variety of drugs.
5. Formation of clotting factors II, VII, IX, and X.
6. Filtration of portal venous blood.

The *biliary system* consists of the gallbladder and the hepatic, cystic, and common bile ducts. The gallbladder is located directly beneath the right lobe of the liver. The principal function of the gallbladder is the storage and concentration of bile. Bile, formed within the liver, flows through an enlarging intrahepatic canalicular system that leads into the *hepatic duct*. The hepatic duct merges with the *cystic duct* of the gallbladder to form the *common bile duct*, which then enters the duodenum at the ampulla of Vater (Figure 4-1). The sphincter of Oddi surrounds the ampulla of Vater and is hormonally controlled to regulate bile flow into the gut. When the food in the alimentary canal flows into the duodenum, cholecystokinin is released from the duodenal mucosa and stimulates contraction of the gallbladder and common bile duct and also relaxation of the sphincter of Oddi.

The *pancreas* lies directly adjacent to the stomach and duodenum and, like the liver, is a complex and multifunctional organ. The primary functions of the pancreas include:

1. Endocrine function: The islets of Langerhans produce and secrete into the bloodstream glucagon, insulin, and also many unnamed, hormonally active peptides.

2. Exocrine function: Pancreatic glandular cells (acini) produce and secrete digestive enzymes such as lipase, amylase, trypsin, and chymotrypsin into the GI tract by way of the pancreatic duct.
3. Neutralizing function: Bicarbonate and water are secreted by the pancreatic glandular cells by way of the main pancreatic duct; they neutralize the stomach acid to provide an alkaline environment for digestion.

The main pancreatic duct enters the ampulla of Vater beside the distal common bile duct (Figure 4-1).

Bilirubin metabolism and excretion

To understand the diagnostic studies used in evaluating the patient with jaundice, one must first be familiar with normal bilirubin metabolism and the pathologic mechanisms of jaundice formation. In the spleen and other organs of the reticuloendothelial system, red blood cells are lysed. Hemoglobin is then released and is broken down to heme and globin molecules. Heme is then catabolized to form biliverdin and then bilirubin. This form of bilirubin is called unconjugated ("indirect") bilirubin. In the liver this substance is conjugated with a glucuronide, resulting in conjugated ("direct") bilirubin. The conjugated bilirubin is then excreted from the liver cell and into intrahepatic canaliculi that eventually lead to the major extrahepatic bile duct system and then into the gut. Once in the GI tract, the conjugated bilirubin is acted on by bacteria to form urobilinogen. Most of this urobilinogen is excreted with the stool. Some, however, is reabsorbed through the enterohepatic pathway and is either excreted in the urine or reexcreted through the bile (enterohepatic circulation of bile salts) (Figure 4-2).

Jaundice is the discoloration of body tissues caused by abnormally high blood levels of bilirubin. Jaundice can usually be recognized when the total serum bilirubin exceeds 2 to 2.5 mg/100 ml. Defects in bilirubin metabolism can occur in any stage of the catabolism of heme. Unconjugated hyperbilirubinemia occurs if the defect exists before glucuronide conjugation (Table 4-1). Unconjugated bilirubin is not water soluble and therefore cannot enter the urine and be excreted.

Physiologic jaundice of the newborn is a result of an immature liver's not having conjugating enzymes. This results in high circulating blood levels of unconjugated bilirubin, which passes through the blood-brain barrier and is deposited in the brain cells of newborns, causing encephalopathy or *kernicterus*.

If the defect occurs after glucuronide addition, conjugated hyperbilirubinemia results (Table 4-1). Conjugated bilirubin is water soluble and can be excreted in the urine by the kidney. It causes the urine to be very dark. Because bilirubin gives the stool its greenish brown color, when obstruction to bilirubin flow occurs, one can expect light yellow or clay-colored stools. In certain situations, as in hepatitis, bilirubin metabolism is interrupted in more than one site, causing a combined conjugated and unconjugated hyperbilirubinemia. When obstructive jaundice is of sufficient duration, hepatocellular dysfunction occurs and may also cause combined conjugated and unconjugated hyperbilirubinemia.

Once the jaundice is recognized clinically or chemically, it is important in terms of therapy to differentiate whether it is predominately caused by unconjugated or conjugated hyperbilirubinemia. This determination helps differentiate prehepatic and intrahepatic jaundice (requiring only medical treatment) from extrahepatic jaundice (usually requiring surgery or therapeutic endoscopy).

CASE STUDY 1: GALLBLADDER AND COMMON DUCT STONES

Mrs. R., a 44-year-old mother of seven children, was an obese woman. Two weeks before she was admitted to the hospital, she began to complain of right upper quadrant abdominal pain associated with nausea and vomiting. Two days before admission she noticed that her urine

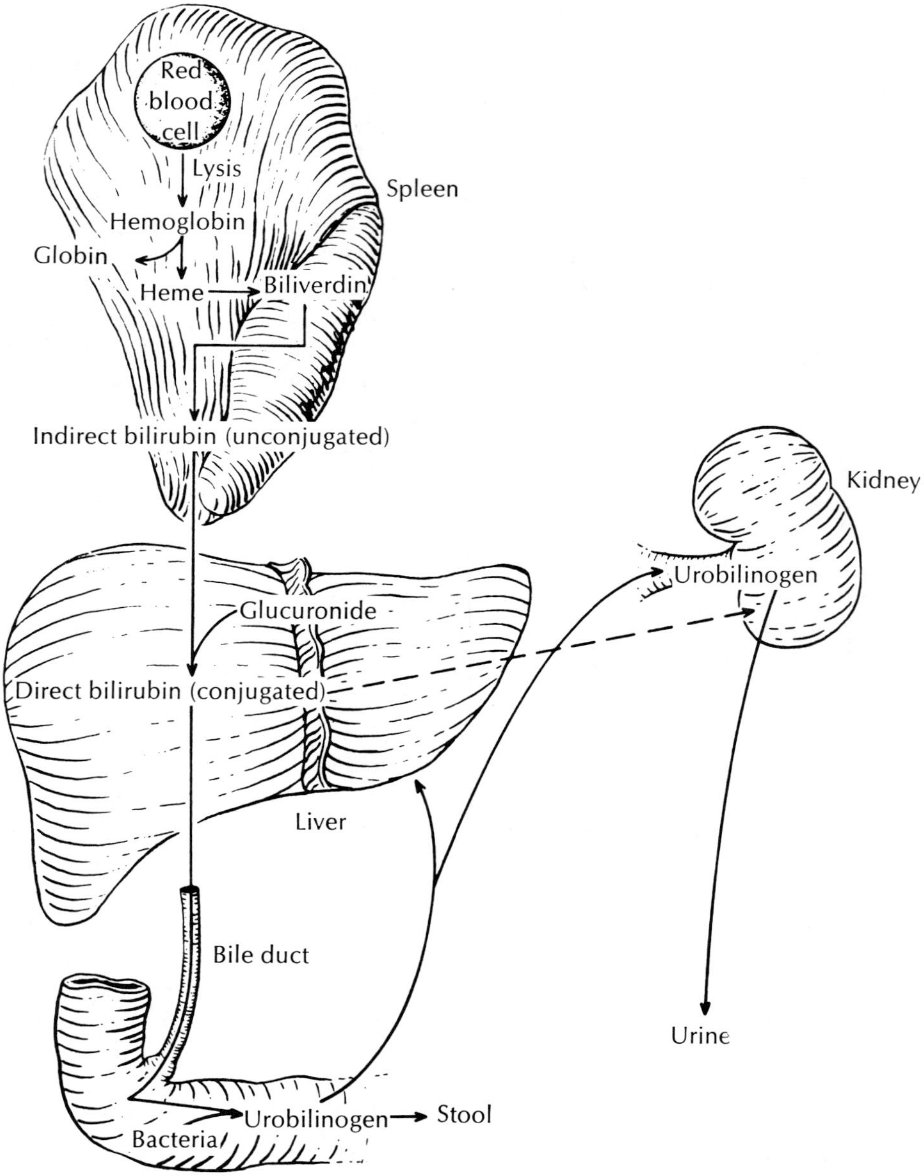

FIGURE 4-2. Bilirubin metabolism and excretion.

TABLE 4-1. Causes and Classification of Jaundice

Condition		Cause	Pathophysiology
Prehepatic cholestasis	Unconjugated (indirect) hyperbilirubinemia	Physiologic jaundice of newborn	Production of bilirubin greater than the liver can accept
		Hemolytic anemia	Overproduction of bilirubin
		Gilbert's disease	Inability to transport bilirubin into the cells
		Crigler Najjar syndrome	Inability to conjugate bilirubin
Intrahepatic (medical) cholestasis	Combined conjugated and unconjugated hyperbilirubinemia	Hepatocellular disease (such as hepatitis)	Inability to transport bilirubin into the cells and to excrete it
		Dubin-Johnson syndrome	Inability to excrete bilirubin from hepatocyte
		Biliary cirrhosis	Obstruction of bilirubin at small intrahepatic bile canaliculi
		Drugs and viruses	
Extrahepatic (surgical) cholestasis	Conjugated (direct) hyperbilirubinemia	Gallstones in common duct Bile duct carcinoma Choledochal cyst Biliary atresia Benign fibrous stricture Periampullary (distal bile duct, pancreas, duodenum, ampulla) carcinoma	Obstruction of bilirubin at extrahepatic ducts

was very dark and her stools were becoming lighter in color. The results of her physical examination revealed she was mildly icteric. Her abdominal examination results indicated mild upper abdominal tenderness and muscle guarding. No other abnormalities were noted during her physical examination.

Studies	Results
Complete blood count (CBC), electrolyte, glucose, and BUN determinations	Normal
Total serum bilirubin determination	3.8 mg/dl (normal: 0.1-1.0 mg/dl)
Indirect fraction	1.0 mg/dl (normal: 0.2-0.8 mg/dl)
Direct fraction	2.8 mg/dl (normal: 0.1-0.3 mg/dl)
Urine bilirubin test	+3 (normal: negative)
Liver enzymes test	
Serum aspartate aminotransferase (AST)	46 IU/L (normal: 5-40 IU/L)
Serum alanine aminotransferase (ALT)	40 IU/L (normal: 5-35 IU/L)
Lactic dehydrogenase (LDH)	228 ImU/ml (normal: 90-200 ImU/ml)
Alkaline phosphatase (ALP)	885 ImU/ml (normal: 30-85 ImU/ml)
5'-Nucleotidase	2.4 units (normal: 0-1.6 units)
Leucine aminopeptidase (LAP)	250 units/ml (normal: 75-185 units/ml)
Serum gamma glutamyl transpeptidase (GGTP)	250 U/l (normal: 5-27 U/l)

Studies	Results
Total serum protein test	7.2 g/dl (normal: 6-8 g/dl)
Serum albumin test	4.2 g/dl (normal: 3.2-4.5 g/dl)
Prothrombin time (PT) test (see Chapter 10)	14.2 sec (patient) 12.0 sec (control)
Oral cholecystography	Nonvisualization of gallbladder
Intravenous cholangiography (IVC)	Faint visualization of common bile duct
Ultrasound examination of the liver and gallbladder	Dilated intrahepatic and extrahepatic bile ducts; presence of stones within the gallbladder (see Figure 4-6)
Endoscopic retrograde cholangiopancreatography (ERCP)	Dilated common bile duct containing a gallstone (see Figure 4-7)
Percutaneous transhepatic cholangiography (PTHC)	Dilated bile duct containing gallstone

Because of the combination of the increased levels of direct bilirubin, alkaline phosphatase, 5′-nucleotidase, GGTP, and LAP, along with the minimally elevated levels of AST and LDH, *obstructive* jaundice was suspected as the cause of this patient's complaints. The bilirubin in the urine (which caused the urine's dark color) further corroborated the clinical finding of a "direct" type of hyperbilirubinemia. The prolonged PT resulted from impaired intestinal absorption of vitamin K and impaired hepatic synthesis of prothrombin and factors VII, IX, and X.

Although oral cholecystography was performed, it probably should not have been, because nonvisualization of the gallbladder could have been predicted on the basis of the high serum bilirubin level. There was a better chance of visualization with IVC, but this also was not helpful since IVCs are usually not visualized when total bilirubin ≥3.0.

Ultrasound examination of the gallbladder permitted the diagnosis of gallstones to be made. However, it had to be made certain that gallstones alone were causing an obstruction in the common bile duct, because patients with gallstones may also have a tumor obstructing this duct. The results of ERCP and PTHC indicated, however, that it was a gallstone alone causing a common bile duct obstruction.

The patient underwent a cholecystectomy and common duct exploration. Several large stones were extracted from the common bile duct. The patient's postoperative course was uneventful. Her serum bilirubin level returned to normal. If her condition precluded laparotomy, she could have undergone ERCP, papillotomy, and endoscopic stone extraction.

DISCUSSION OF TESTS

Serum bilirubin test

Adult/elderly/child:
- Total bilirubin: 0.1 to 1.0 mg/dl or 5.1-17.0 μmol/L (SI units)
- Indirect bilirubin: 0.2-0.8 mg/dl or 3.4-12.0 μmol/L (SI units)
- Direct bilirubin: 0.1-0.3 mg/dl or 1.7-5.1 μmol/L (SI units)

Newborn total bilirubin: 1-12 mg/dl or 17.1-20.5 μmol/L (SI units)

Rationale. (See also discussion of bilirubin metabolism and excretion, pp. 90-91.) The total serum bilirubin determination measures both direct (conjugated) and indirect (unconjugated) bilirubin. The total serum bilirubin level is the sum of the direct and indirect bilirubin levels. In predominantly *unconjugated* hyperbilirubinemia, less than 15% to 20% of the total bilirubin is conjugated. The patient is considered to have predominantly *conjugated* bilirubinemia when more than 50% of the total bilirubin is conjugated. Conjugated hyperbilirubinemia is caused by obstruction of the biliary ducts (as in gallstones) or by hepatocellular disease (such as hepatitis). Unconjugated hyperbilirubinemia is caused by accelerated erythrocyte hemolysis (as in erythroblastosis fetalis), absence of glucuronyl transferase, or hepatocellular disease.

Elevated serum bilirubin test results may be caused by the effects of many different drugs, such as antibiotics, sulfonamides, allopurinol, diuretics, barbiturates, steroids, phenothiazines, or oral contraceptives. Levels of serum bilirubin may be decreased in patients with iron deficiency anemia and in those taking penicillin or large amounts of salicylates.

Procedure. Peripheral venipuncture is performed, and one red-top tube of blood is collected. A heel puncture is used for blood collection in infants, and two blood microtubes are filled. No fasting is required.

Contraindications. None.

Nursing considerations

Nursing Diagnoses/Collaborative Problems

See Blood studies, p. 2.

Nursing Implications with Rationale

- Explain the purpose of the test to the patient and follow specific hospital guidelines for blood collection.
- The blood specimen should not be exposed to sunlight or artificial light because this may reduce the bilirubin content.
- Medications that affect the serum bilirubin level may be held as ordered for at least 24 hours before the test. If these medications are given, they should be listed on the lab slip.
- After the venipuncture, assess the site for bleeding because patients with liver dysfunction often have prolonged clotting times (see p. 406).

Urine bilirubin test

Normal amount: none.

Rationale. (See also discussion of bilirubin metabolism and excretion, pp. 90-91.) Bilirubin is present in normal urine only in minute amounts that cannot be detected by routine test methods. Because unconjugated bilirubin is not water soluble, it cannot be excreted in the urine when the level is elevated. Conjugated bilirubin, however, is water soluble and can be excreted in the urine when serum levels are abnormally high. Therefore, the presence or absence of urinary bilirubin provides important information for determining whether jaundice is predominantly caused by unconjugated or conjugated hyperbilirubinemia. If bilirubin is present in the urine, conjugated hyperbilirubinemia is suggested; if bilirubin is not present in the urine, unconjugated hyperbilirubinemia is suspected.

One of the main values of this test is that it can be performed at the bedside. However, the importance of this test is now diminished because serum fractionation of bilirubin is so easily performed.

Procedure. No food or drink restrictions are necessary in the urine bilirubin test. This test is easily performed with Multistix reagent strips for urinalysis or with Icotest tablets (Ames). Multistix is a firm plastic strip with seven separate areas for testing pH, protein, glucose, ketones, bilirubin, blood, and urobilinogen. For testing bilirubin a fresh urine specimen is obtained and tested as soon as possible. The dipstick is immersed in the well-mixed urine and removed immediately to avoid dissolving the other reagents. After removing the dipstick, the nurse should tap it against the rim of the urine container to remove the excess urine. The strip is held in the horizontal position and compared with the color chart on the label of the bottle at 20 seconds. Results are given in the range of 0 to +3.

Icotest tablets are considered more sensitive for the detection of bilirubin in the urine. For the Icotest, five drops of urine are placed on a special test mat. The tablet is then placed on top of the moistened area of the mat, and two drops of water are added. The bilirubin test is positive if the mat turns blue or purple within 30 seconds. The intensity and the rapidity of the color formation are proportionate to the amount of bilirubin in the urine.

Many drugs interfere with the bilirubin test results. For example, phenazopyridine (Pyridium), ethoxazene (Serenium), and chlorpromazine may give false positive results. Indomethacin (Indocin) can give either a false negative or a false-positive result. High concentrations of ascorbic acid (vitamin C) are associated with false negative results.

Contraindications. None.

Nursing considerations

Nursing Diagnoses/Collaborative Problems

See Urine studies, p. 3.

Nursing Implications with Rationale

- Explain the method of urine collection to the patient, and be sure the patient has the proper urine container.
- Collect a fresh urine sample from the patient and test it as soon as possible (within 1 hour). Bilirubin is not stable in urine, especially when exposed to light.
- Read the directions on the bottle and note the exact time that the test is to be read. Chart the results.
- Immediately after removing the reagent strip or Icotest tablets, replace the cap on the bottle tightly to avoid destruction by moisture in the air.
- Do not use reagent strips or Icotest tablets with test mats after the expiration date.
- List any medications that affect the test results on the lab slip.

Liver enzymes test

Aspartate aminotransferase (AST; formerly called serum glutamic-oxaloacetic transaminase [SGOT])

Normal values:

Adult: 8-20 U/L, 5-40 IU/L, or 8-20 U/L (SI units); women tend to have slightly lower values than men.

Elderly: values slightly higher than adult

Child: values similar to adult

Newborn/infant: 15-60 U/L

Alanine aminotransferase (ALT, formerly called serum glutamic-pyruvic transaminase [SGPT])

Normal values:

Adult/child: 5-35 IU/L

Elderly: may be slightly higher than adult

Infant: may be twice as high as adult

Lactic dehydrogenase (LDH)

Normal values:

Adult/elderly: 45-90 U/L (30° C), 115-225 IU/L, or 0.4-1.7 μmol/L (SI units)

Isoenzymes in adult/elderly values

LDH-1: 17%-27%

LDH-2: 27%-37%

LDH-3: 18%-25%

LDH-4: 3%-8%

LDH-5: 0%-5%

Child: 60-170 U/L (30° C)

Infant: 100-250 U/L

Newborn: 160-450 U/L

Alkaline phosphatase (ALP)

Normal values:

Adults: 30-85 ImU/mL

Elderly: slightly higher than adults

Children and adolescents:

<2 yr: 85-235 ImU/ml

2 to 8 yr: 65-210 ImU/ml

9 to 15 yr: 60-300 ImU/ml (active bone growth)

16 to 21 yr: 30-200 ImU/ml

5′-Nucleotidase

Normal value: 0-1.6 units or 27-233 nmol/s/L (SI units)

Leucine aminopeptidase (LAP)

Normal values:

Blood—male: 80-200 U/ml

female: 75-185 U/ml

Urine—2-18 U/24 hours

Gamma-glutamyl transpeptidase (GGTP), Gamma-glutamyltransferase (GGT)

Normal values:

Male and female >45: 8-38 U/L

Female <45: 5-27 U/L

Elderly: slightly higher than adult

Child: similar to adult

Newborn: five times higher than adult

Rationale. The liver is a storehouse of many enzymes. Injury or disease affecting the liver causes release of these intracellular enzymes into the bloodstream, and their levels become elevated. Some of these enzymes are also produced in other organs, and injury or disease affecting these other organs also cause an elevated serum level. Therefore, although elevation of these serum enzymes is found in pathologic liver conditions, the test is not specific for liver diseases alone.

Serum aspartate aminotransferase (AST) or serum glutamic oxaloacetic transaminase

(SGOT). The enzyme AST is found in very high concentrations in the heart (Chapter 2) and liver and in moderately high amounts in the skeletal muscle, kidneys, and pancreas. High levels are found in the blood after a myocardial infarction (Chapter 2) and with diseases affecting the hepatocyte, e.g., hepatitis.

AST levels are also increased in patients with acute pancreatitis, acute hemolytic anemia, severe burns, acute renal disease, musculoskeletal disease, and trauma. Because intramuscular (IM) injections may also cause increases, IM injections should not be administered before this test. Drugs such as isoniazid (INH), oral contraceptives, opiates, and aspirin can cause increased levels of AST. Levels of this enzyme may be decreased in patients with beriberi or diabetic ketoacidosis and in pregnant patients.

Serum levels of this enzyme are often compared with alanine aminotransferase (ALT). The AST/ALT ratio is usually >1 in alcoholic cirrhosis, liver congestion, and metastatic tumor of the liver. Ratios <1 may be seen in patients with acute hepatitis, viral hepatitis, and infectious mononucleosis.

Serum alanine aminotransferase (ALT) or serum glutamic pyruvic transaminase (SGPT) ALT is found predominantly in the liver, with lesser quantities found in the kidneys, heart, and skeletal muscle. Generally, most ALT elevations are because of liver dysfunction. This enzyme is both sensitive and specific for hepatocellular disease. This test is used primarily to help confirm the liver origin of an AST increase. The AST/ALT ratio is often used in the differential diagnosis of liver disease. This enzyme can be factitiously elevated by the use of isoniazid (INH), some antibiotics, phenothiazines, aminosalicylic acid (PAS), and allopurinol.

Lactic dehydrogenase (LDH). LDH is found in highest concentration in the heart (Chapter 2, page 13), skeletal muscle, and red blood cells (RBCs). Lesser quantities are found in the lung, lymphoid tissue, liver, and kidneys. The LDH level is increased in a wide variety of patient situations, such as acute MI, congestive heart failure, cardiovascular surgery, hepatitis, untreated pernicious anemia, renal disease, muscle disease, pulmonary embolus, hemolysis, or malignant tumors. Because of the wide variety of conditions causing an elevation of LDH, this test is not very helpful as a liver function study.

LDH can be fractionated into five isoenzymes (LDH-1 through LDH-5). The fraction LDH-5 is found predominantly in the liver and skeletal muscle. The LDH-5 fraction is much more sensitive to acute hepatocellular damage than is the total LDH. This fraction may also be elevated with other causes of liver damage even when the total LDH is normal.

Alkaline phosphatase (ALP). Although ALP is found in many tissues, highest concentrations are found in the liver and biliary tract epithelium, bone, intestinal mucosa, and placenta. This enzyme is called *alkaline* because it functions best in an alkaline pH of 9. Detection of this enzyme is important for determining liver and bone disorders. Because ALP exists in the bile duct epithelial cells, the serum enzyme level of ALP is greatly increased in obstructive (both extrahepatic and intrahepatic) biliary disease. The ALP is also increased in patients with metastatic carcinoma to the liver, infarcted bowel, hyperphosphatasia, hepatoma, liver abscess, liver granulomas, hyperparathyroidism, Paget's disease, healing fractures, and rheumatoid arthritis.

Bone is the most frequent extrahepatic source of ALP. For this reason reference values of this enzyme are much higher in children than in adults. When doubt exists about the cause of the elevated ALP, other liver enzymes are tested to obtain a differential diagnosis. Leucine aminopeptidase (LAP), 5′-nucleotidase, and serum gamma glutamyl transpeptidase (GGTP) are elevated in liver disease, but are normal in bone disorders and normal bone growth.

Isoenzymes of ALP are also used to distinguish between liver and bone disease. These isoenzymes are most easily differentiated by the heat stability test. The isoenzyme of liver origin (ALP_1) is heat stable, but the isoenzyme of bone origin (ALP_2) is inactivated by heat.

Elevated levels of ALP may also be seen in

patients receiving intravenous albumin, since many drug manufacturing companies use placental tissue as the source of albumin. Drugs such as antibiotics, colchicine, methyldopa, allopurinol, phenothiazine tranquilizers, indomethacin, some oral contraceptives, isoniazid (INH), and tolbutamide may also cause fictitious elevation of ALP. Because ALP of placental origin is increased during the third trimester of pregnancy, values may increase three times their normal level. Elevated levels can persist until the fourth week postpartum.

Reduced levels of ALP may be seen in patients with the following: hypothyroidism, hypophosphatemia, excess vitamin B ingestion, scurvy, malnutrition, milk-alkali syndrome, celiac disease, and pernicious anemia.

5′-Nucleotidase. 5′-Nucleotidase is thought to be more specific than ALP for the detection of hepatobiliary disease. Its elevation may be an early indication of metastasis in cancer patients, especially if jaundice is absent. It can be used in a differential diagnosis of liver disease from bone disease. In hepatocellular disease, ALP and 5′-nucleotidase are both elevated, whereas in primary bone disease ALP is elevated and 5′-nucleotidase is normal. Because 5′-nucleotidase is normal in pregnancy and the postpartum period, this test may aid in the differential diagnosis of hepatobiliary disease occurring during pregnancy. Elevated enzyme levels are more compatible with obstructive hepatic diseases rather than hepatocellular diseases.

Serum leucine aminopeptidase (LAP). LAP, produced exclusively by the liver, is used in diagnosing liver disorders and in the differential diagnosis of increased ALP levels. LAP levels tend to parallel ALP levels in hepatic disease. LAP is a more sensitive indicator of biliary obstruction. However, unlike ALP, LAP remains normal in bone disease.

LAP can be detected in both blood and urine. Patients with elevated serum LAP levels always show urine elevations. However, when the urine LAP level is elevated, the blood level may have already returned to normal.

Values may be increased during pregnancy and in patients taking estrogens, progesterones, or oral contraceptives.

Gamma glutamyl transferase (GGT) or gamma-glutamyl transpeptidase (GGTP). The enzyme GGT participates in the transfer of amino acids and peptides across the cellular membranes and also possibly participates in glutathione metabolism. Highest concentrations of this enzyme are found in the liver, kidney, spleen, and prostate gland. This test is used to detect liver cell dysfunction and alcohol ingestion.

The rise of GGT generally parallels change in serum ALP, LAP, and 5′-nucleotidase levels in liver disease. However, GGT is more sensitive. Because GGT is not increased in bone disease or growth, it can help distinguish hepatic disease from skeletal disease when serum ALP level is elevated. In this situation a normal GGT level would imply that the elevation was a result of skeletal disease. Levels are normal in pregnancy and in children over 3 months of age. Therefore, this may aid in the differential diagnosis of hepatocellular disease during pregnancy and in children.

An important feature of GGT is that it can detect alcohol ingestion. This enzyme rises rapidly after even a small intake of alcohol and even without evidence of hepatocellular disease. This enzyme, therefore, is very useful in the evaluation of alcoholic patients. The serum level is high in about 75% of those having chronic alcoholism.

GGT may also be increased 4 to 10 days after an acute MI (either because of tissue granulation or as a result of the effect of cardiac insufficiency on the liver). Certain medications (such as phenytoin [Dilantin] and phenobarbital) may also cause elevations of serum GGT levels. Clofibrate and oral contraceptives may decrease the serum levels of this enzyme.

Procedure. Usually no special preparation is necessary for these liver enzyme studies. Some laboratories may require a 12-hour fast. Abstinence from alcohol may be recommended before the GGT test. Approximately 7 to 10 ml of blood is collected in a red-top tube and sent to the laboratory for analysis.

Contraindications. None.

Nursing considerations

Nursing Diagnoses/Collaborative Problems

See Blood studies, p. 2.

Nursing Implications with Rationale

- Many of these liver enzyme tests are affected by medications. Indicate on the lab slip any medications that the patient may be taking to aid in interpretation of test results.
- Some of the enzymes (for example, AST) are affected by IM injections. Try to avoid IM injections for clients scheduled for this particular study to prevent obscuring the test results. If injections are administered, indicate the time given on the lab slip.
- After the venipuncture, assess the site for bleeding because patients with liver dysfunction often have prolonged clotting times (see p. 406).

Serum protein test

(protein, globulin, albumin, total protein)

Normal values:
- Adult/elderly
  - Total protein: 6-8 g/dl
  - Albumin: 3.2-4.5 g/dl
  - Globulin: 2.3-3.4 g/dl
- Total protein
  - Premature infant: 4.2-7.6 g/dl
  - Newborn: 4.6-7.4 g/dl
  - Infant: 6.0-6.7 g/dl
  - Child: 6.2-8.0 g/dl
- Albumin
  - Premature infant: 3.0-4.2 g/dl
  - Newborn: 3.5-5.4 g/dl
  - Infant: 4.4-5.4 g/dl
  - Child: 4.0-5.9 g/dl

Rationale. One way to assess the functional status of the liver is to measure the products that are synthesized there. One of these products is protein, especially albumin, which acts as the main solute in maintaining osmotic pressure of the blood. Furthermore, albumin transports important blood chemicals such as enzymes, hormones, and drugs. When disease affects the liver cell, the hepatocyte loses its ability to synthesize albumin, and the serum albumin level is markedly decreased. However, because the half-life of albumin is 12 to 18 days, severe impairment of hepatic albumin synthesis will not be recognizable until after that period.

Because the total serum protein level is a measure of albumin (made in the liver) and globulin (made in many other organs) by itself, it is a rather inadequate indication of liver function. Although the albumin level may be low because of severe liver dysfunction, the globulin production may be increased, resulting in a normal total serum protein level. This causes a reversal of the normal albumin/globulin ratio (A/G ratio) in chronic liver disease, which results in a decrease in albumin and an increase in globulin. Therefore, if one looked only at the total protein level as a reflection of liver function, one could incorrectly assess liver function as normal when, in fact, it is abnormal. Because of this, one must look specifically at the serum albumin to gain an accurate assessment of liver function. Low serum albumin levels may also result from excessive loss of albumin into urine (as in nephrotic syndrome), or into third-space volumes (as in ascites), or from protein-caloric malnutrition.

Procedure. Peripheral venipuncture is performed, and one red-top tube of blood is collected. Generally, no specific patient preparation is necessary. Some laboratories require the patient be kept NPO for 8 hours except for water.

Contraindications. None.

Nursing considerations

Nursing Diagnoses/Collaborative Problems

See Blood studies, p. 2.

Nursing Implications with Rationale

- Assess the venipuncture site for bleeding.

Oral cholecystography

(gallbladder series, GB series, cholecystogram)

Normal values: visualization of gallbladder; no filling defects; no stones.

Rationale. The oral cholecystogram provides x-ray visualization of the gallbladder after the oral ingestion of a radiopaque, iodinated dye. Adequate visualization of the gallbladder requires concentration of the dye within the gallbladder. The following factors are necessary for adequate dye concentration:

1. The patient must take the correct number of dye tablets. Often the patient's gallbladder is not visualized in the study; later it is found that the patient did not take all of the dye tablets.
2. Adequate absorption of the dye from the GI tract. Vomiting or diarrhea will preclude absorption of the dye.
3. Abstinence from a meal (especially a fatty meal) on the morning of the test. A fatty meal induces emptying of the gallbladder and eliminates the dye from the biliary system before x-ray films are taken. The patient must be kept NPO after midnight.
4. Uptake from the portal system and excretion of the dye by the liver. In hepatocellular dysfunction, the uptake and excretion of the dye are deficient. If the bilirubin level is >1.8, visualization is unlikely.
5. Patency of the cystic duct. The dye is secreted by the liver through the hepatic duct and enters the gallbladder through the cystic duct. A gallstone obstructing the cystic duct (as found in acute cholecystitis) can prevent the dye from entering the gallbladder.
6. Concentration of the dye within the gallbladder. The mucosa of a chronically inflamed gallbladder is unable to absorb the bile waters to concentrate the dye enough for visualization.

On an x-ray film the dye-filled gallbladder is seen as a vesicle filled with radiographic (white) material (Figure 4-3). Calculi are visualized as radiolucent (dark) shadows in a dye-filled gallbladder (Figure 4-4). Gallbladder polyps or tumors occasionally can be seen as filling defects in an otherwise dye-filled gallbladder.

To rule out insufficient dye intake as a cause of nonvisualization, the test is always repeated using a double dose of the contrast dye. Nonvisualization after the double dose is reliable evidence of a chronically inflamed gallbladder that harbors stones. When properly performed, oral cholecystography is considered an accurate and reliable test for pathologic gallbladder conditions. However, occasionally small gallstones may be missed. Oral cholecystography is seldom effective if the serum bilirubin level is >1.8 mg/dl.

Procedure. On the evening before the test Telepaque (iopanoic acid) tablets or some other absorbable iodine dye with a specified amount of water is prescribed. Usually this is given 1 to 2 hours after a low-fat supper. The patient is then allowed only water until bedtime. Thereafter, the patient is kept NPO until the test is completed.

On the morning of the test, the patient goes to the radiology department. The radiologist takes x-ray films of the right upper quadrant of the abdomen as the patient is placed in several positions. The positional changes are necessary to differentiate gallstones from air bubbles. Because gallstones are more dense than bile and air bubbles are less dense than bile, positional change causes the gallstones to descend to the bottom and the air bubbles to ascend to the top of the bile solution contained within the gallbladder. After initial x-ray examination, the patient may be given a fatty meal consisting of eggs, butter, or cream or take a synthetic fat-containing substance (Bilevac) to test the contractibility of the gallbladder (Figure 4-3). (Sincalide can be injected intravenously to cause contraction of the gallbladder within 15 minutes.) X-ray films are then repeated at intervals until the gallbladder has expelled the dye. No

A

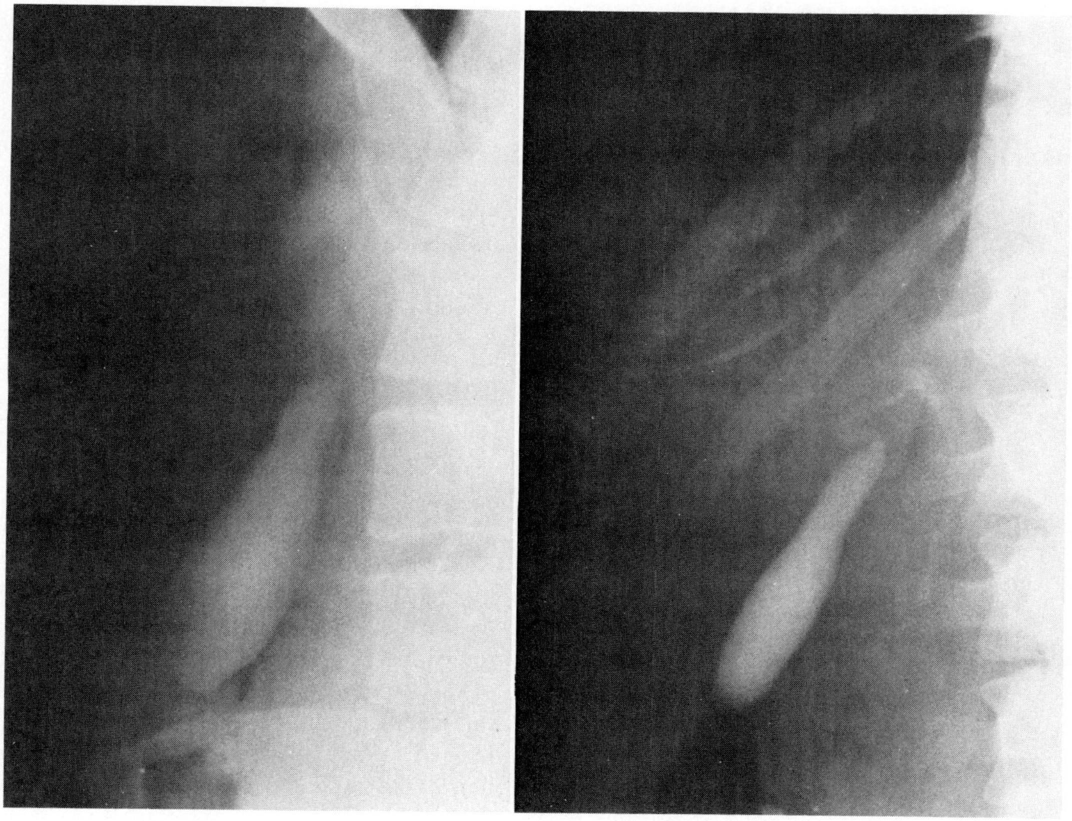

B

FIGURE 4-3. **A,** Normal oral cholecystogram before fatty meal. **B,** Normal oral cholecystogram after fatty meal.

discomfort is associated with a gallbladder series. Examining time is approximately 1 hour. Post–fatty-meal tests require another 1 to 2 hours.

Contraindications. The test is contraindicated in the following:

1. Patients who are allergic to iodine dye
2. Patients in early pregnancy, because x-ray exposure may be teratogenic (causing congenital abnormalities) to an early fetus

Nursing considerations

Nursing Diagnoses/Collaborative Problems

See X-ray studies, p. 2.

- Potential complication: adverse reaction/allergy to dye

Nursing Implications with Rationale

- Explain the procedure to the patient. Assure the patient that no pain or discomfort is associated with the test.
- Be sure that the serum bilirubin level is <1.8 mg/dl so that visualization will be possible. If the level is >1.8 mg/dl, inform the physician; the study will probably be canceled.
- On the evening before the test, give the patient a low-fat or fat-free meal to avoid contraction of the gallbladder. Foods such as milk, butter, cream, and sauces should be avoided.
- Before the administration of the dye, make sure the patient is not allergic to iodine to prevent anaphylaxis.

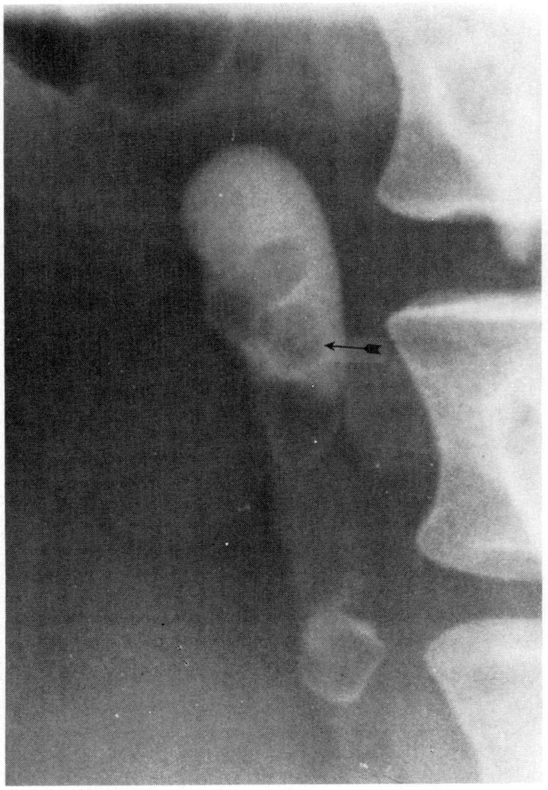

FIGURE 4-4. Oral cholecystogram showing gallbladder filled with stones *(arrow)*.

- Approximately 12 hours before the test, give the patient six 0.5 g iopanoic acid tablets by mouth. The tablets are taken one at a time at 5-minute intervals with specified amounts of water. If the patient vomits after taking the dye, notify the physician. The physician will either prescribe the dye again or postpone the test.
- After the patient takes the dye, assess the patient for side effects, such as abdominal cramps, nausea, vomiting, and diarrhea, which can alter the absorption of the dye. Side effects should be reported to the attending physician and to the radiologist.
- Explain to the patient that after taking the contrast dye, no other food may be eaten. Food will stimulate the gallbladder to contract and therefore eliminate the dye from the gallbladder.
- Explain to the patient that the dye is eventually excreted in the urine. Some patients report slight dysuria following cholecystography.
- If the patient will receive a fatty meal to stimulate emptying of the gallbladder, he or she cannot have any other food or fluid until all follow-up x-ray films are completed. Food may induce emptying of the gallbladder.

Intravenous cholangiography

(intravenous cholangiogram, IVC)

Normal value: patent biliary ducts.

Rationale. In this study intravenously administered radiographic dye is concentrated by the liver and secreted into the bile duct. In contrast to oral cholecystography, in which usually only the gallbladder is filled, IVC allows visualization of the hepatic and common bile ducts and also the gallbladder if the cystic duct is patent. IVC is used to demonstrate stones, stricture, or tumor of the hepatic duct, common bile duct, and the gallbladder. There are four indications for this test:

1. Visualization of the biliary ductal system does not require dye concentration in the gallbladder, as is the case in oral cholecystography. Therefore, this test is helpful in studying the biliary tree for retained gallstones in cholecystectomized patients who have postoperative symptoms suggestive of gallstones.
2. Frequently in patients who have an acute abdominal inflammatory process unrelated to the biliary system (such as pancreatitis), the oral cholecystogram does not visualize the gallbladder. The reason for this is unknown. However, an intravenously administered dye frequently fills the normal gallbladder in these patients and thus rules out the biliary system as a cause of the acute abdominal inflammation.

3. Patients who have proven gallstones in their gallbladders may require IVC to demonstrate passage of the stones into the common bile duct.
4. IVC is used in patients who cannot tolerate the oral administration of the iopanoic acid tablets that are used in oral cholecystography.

On the oral cholecystogram, the gallbladder is rarely visualized when the patient's bilirubin level is over 1.8 mg/dl. An IVC rarely demonstrates the gallbladder when the patient's bilirubin level is over 3.5 mg/dl. Therefore, in patients whose bilirubin is between 1.8 mg and 3.5 mg, the chances of gallbladder visualization are greater when IVC is used. Today, IVC is being replaced by endoscopic retrograde cholangiopancreatography (ERCP) and percutaneous transhepatic cholangiography (PTHC) in most institutions. These newer tests are more sensitive and specific for biliary disease. Further, these tests are not dependent on hepatobiliary function and can therefore be useful in the jaundiced patient.

Procedure. The patient is usually given a laxative (such as two bisacodyl [Dulcolax] tablets) in the morning on the day before the examination. A normal diet is maintained. The patient is then kept NPO after midnight. A cleansing enema may be given on the morning of the test. For this study the patient goes to the radiology department. While in the supine position, the patient is given an IV infusion of iodine dye (cholangiograph). X-ray films of the right upper quadrant of the abdomen are taken intermittently for a period of up to 8 hours, thus allowing the gallbladder and hepatic and common bile ducts to fill. Finally the dye should be seen entering the duodenum. Duct obstruction caused by stones, stricture, or tumor interrupts the sequence of events. Frequently tomography (see p. 139) is used to allow better visualization of the ductal system (Figure 4-5).

IVC is not uncomfortable except for the initial intravenous dye injection. Rarely the patient feels a transient cutaneous flush immediately following infusion of the dye. The duration of this study varies from 1 to 8 hours. This study is performed by a radiologist.

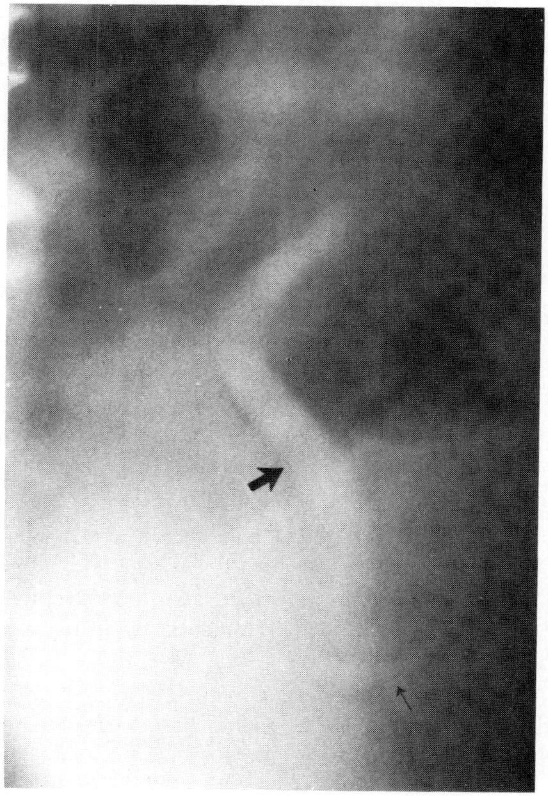

FIGURE 4-5. Intravenous cholangiogram showing a normal common bile duct, with tomography to better delineate the ductal structures. Note the pancreatic duct *(small arrow)*.

Contraindications. IVC is contraindicated in the following:

1. Patients with an allergy to iodine dye
2. Patients with a bilirubin level >3.5 mg/dl.

Nursing considerations

Nursing Diagnoses/Collaborative Problems

See X-ray studies, p. 5.

- Potential complication: adverse reaction or allergy to dye

Nursing Implications with Rationale

- Explain the procedure to the patient. Tell the patient that the dye may cause a burning sensation when injected. Give the patient the opportunity to verbalize his or her feelings.
- Give the patient two bisacodyl tablets on the morning of the day preceding the study. The bisacodyl tablets clear the bowel of hardened feces. Keep the patient NPO after midnight until the test is completed.
- Be sure that the bilirubin level is <3.5 mg/dl so that visualization is possible. If the level is elevated, call the physician; the study may be canceled.
- Before the administration of the dye, make sure that the patient is not allergic to iodine.
- After the dye is administered, observe the patient for allergic reactions, such as dyspnea, tachycardia, sweating, nausea, vomiting, and chills.
- Explain to the patient that the dye is eventually excreted in the urine. Some patients report slight dysuria following IVC.

Ultrasound examination of the liver and biliary system

(echogram of the liver and biliary system)

Normal values: normal gallbladder and biliary ducts.

Rationale. With ultrasound, a harmless high-frequency sound wave is emitted and penetrates the organ being studied. These sound waves are bounced back to a sensor (transducer) and are arranged into a pictorial image of that organ by electronic conversion. A realistic Polaroid picture of the organ studied is obtained.

Diagnostic ultrasound is now the method of choice for detecting gallstones within the gallbladder and biliary tree. It is also useful in detecting cystic structures of the liver (such as benign cysts, hepatic abscesses, or dilated intrahepatic ducts) and solid intrahepatic tumors (primary and metastatic). The gallbladder and extrahepatic ducts can be seen and examined as to their contents, such as gallstones (Figure 4-6) and tumors. If the extrahepatic ducts appear to be normal size in a patient with jaundice, one can safely assume that the cause of jaundice is intrahepatic or prehepatic. If, on the other hand, the ducts are dilated, it is assumed that jaundice is caused by extrahepatic anatomic obstruction of the bile duct.

Diagnostic ultrasound has been beneficial in the study of almost all organs of the body and is discussed, when appropriate, under each system. Because this study requires no contrast material and is not associated with radiation, it is valuable in evaluating pregnant patients.

Procedure. For examination of the gallbladder, it is best to keep the patient NPO after midnight on the day of the study to ensure that the gallbladder is at maximum size for this test. If the patient were to eat, the gallbladder would contract, empty its bile, and become smaller. A smaller gallbladder is more difficult to detect with ultrasound. Fasting is not required for ultrasonography of other organs.

The patient is taken to the ultrasound room (usually in the radiology department) and is placed on an examining table in the supine position. The ultrasonographer, usually a radiologist, applies a greasy paste to the skin overlying the organ. This paste is used to enhance sound transmission and reception. The transducer is moved along the skin in a vertical and then horizontal line. The combination of horizontal (coronal section) and vertical (sagittal section) views printed on Polaroid film allows a three-dimensional look at the organ. This test is noninvasive, has no side effects, and can safely be performed on pregnant patients. It is not associated with any discomfort. The duration of this study is approximately 20 minutes.

Contraindications. None.

Nursing considerations

Nursing Diagnoses/Collaborative Problems

See Ultrasound studies, p. 6.

Nursing Implications with Rationale

- Explain the procedure to the patient. Assure the patient that no discomfort is associated with this study.

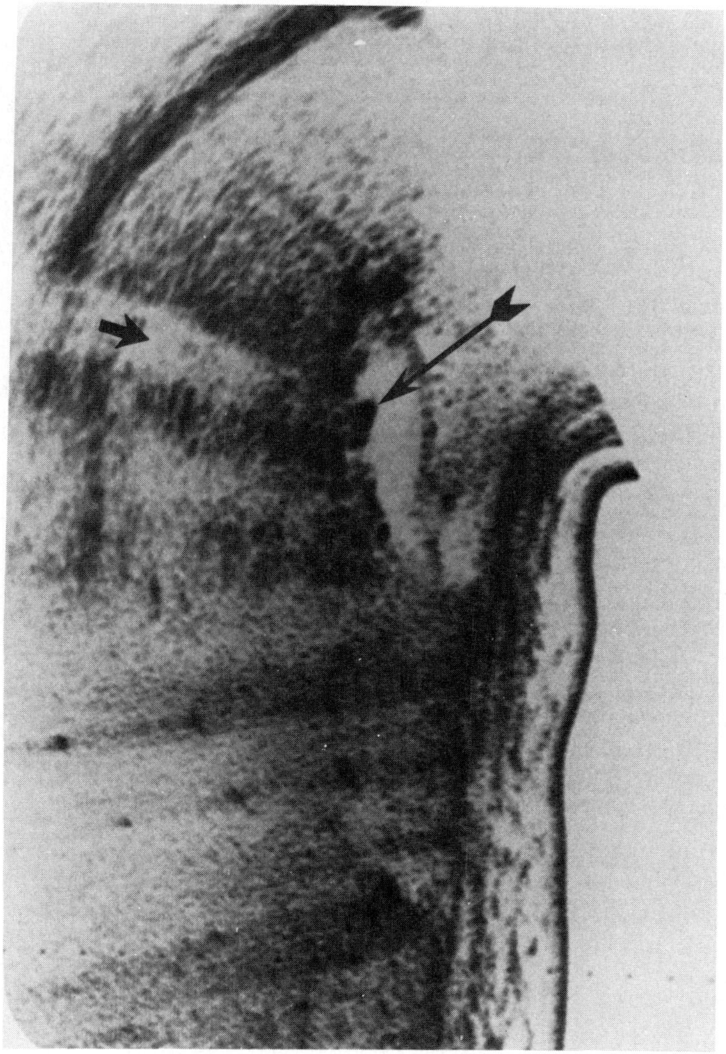

FIGURE 4-6. Ultrasound image of the gallbladder. Long arrow points to stone in the gallbladder. Short arrow indicates areas (posterior to the gallbladder) not penetrated by ultrasound because of the gallstones.

- If the gallbladder is being studied with ultrasound, keep the patient NPO after midnight on the day of the study to prevent contraction of the gallbladder.
- If the patient has had prior barium contrast studies, request an order for cathartics. Ultrasound cannot penetrate barium, and the study will not be adequate.
- Explain to the patient that a liberal amount of gel or lubricant will be applied to the skin over the liver to enhance transmission and reception of the sound waves.
- When the patient returns to the floor after the study, help remove the lubricant from his or her abdomen.

Endoscopic retrograde cholangiopancreatography of the biliary ducts

(ERCP of the biliary ducts)

Normal value: normal biliary ducts.

Rationale. Endoscopic retrograde cholangiopancreatography (ERCP), with the use of a fiberoptic endoscope, is used to visualize the bile and pancreatic ducts (see p. 124). If partial or total obstruction exists, the characteristics of the obstructing lesion will be demonstrated. Stones (Figure 4-7), benign strictures, cysts, and malignant tumors can be identified.

In patients with direct-reaching hyperbilirubinemia caused by obstructive jaundice, the cause and site of obstruction must be identified. If the cause is *intrahepatic* cholestasis, medical therapy alone is used. However, if the jaundice is shown to be caused by an *extrahepatic* ductal pathologic condition, surgery is indicated to relieve the jaundice. To determine whether the pathologic condition is intrahepatic or extrahepatic, the biliary ducts must be visualized radiographically. Only ERCP and PTHC can provide such visualization. Oral cholecystography and IVC do not visualize the biliary tree when the bilirubin level is >3.5 mg/dl. PTHC (discussed later) is an invasive procedure with significant morbidity. ERCP, on the other hand, is associated with much less morbidity but must be performed by an endoscopist with expertise and experience.

As in gastroscopy, the possibility of perforation of the esophagus, stomach, and duodenum exists in ERCP, although it occurs very rarely. Another complication is gram-negative sepsis. An obstructed bile duct frequently contains infected bile. The pressure of dye injection during ERCP can push bacteria into the bloodstream and thus cause bacteremia that may progress to gram-negative sepsis and shock. A broad-spectrum antibiotic (such as cephalothin) is sometimes added to the dye before injection to attempt reduction of this complication. Acute pancreatitis can result from the pressure of dye injection or from transient edema of the ampullary papilla caused by the ERCP catheter.

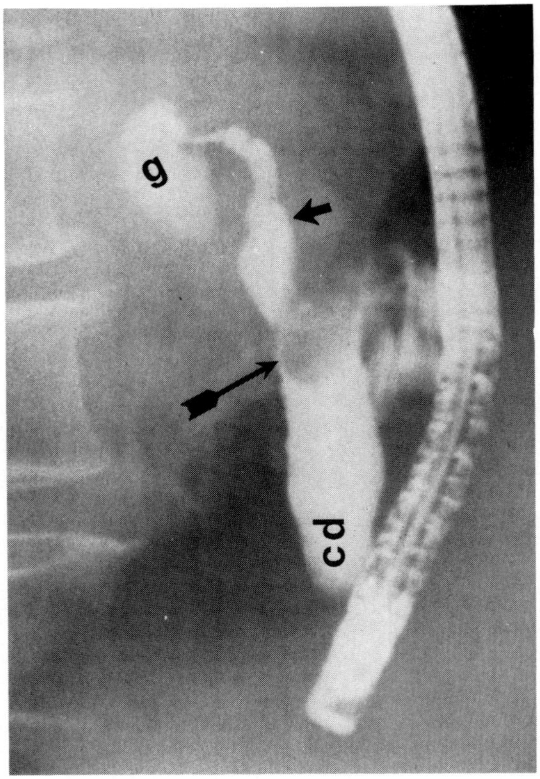

FIGURE 4-7. Endoscopic retrograde cholangiopancreatogram. Endoscope within the duodenum is seen at the right. *Cd,* Common bile duct; *g,* gallbladder. Short arrow indicates cystic duct. Long arrow indicates shadow caused by large gallstone in the common bile duct. The hepatic duct is not visualized because of the obstructing stone.

Procedure. (See also discussion of gastroscopy on pp. 64-65.) The patient is kept NPO after midnight on the day of the test. The patient is placed in the supine or left lateral decubitus position. A flat plate of the abdomen (kidney, ureter, and bladder) may be done before this study to ensure that any barium from previous studies is not obscuring visualization. The patient is usually premedicated with diazepam (Valium) or midazolam (Versed) and meperidine (Demerol) or butorphanol (Stadol) IV. For ERCP, a side-viewing fiberoptic duodenoscope is inserted through the oral pharynx and passed through the esophagus, stomach, and into the

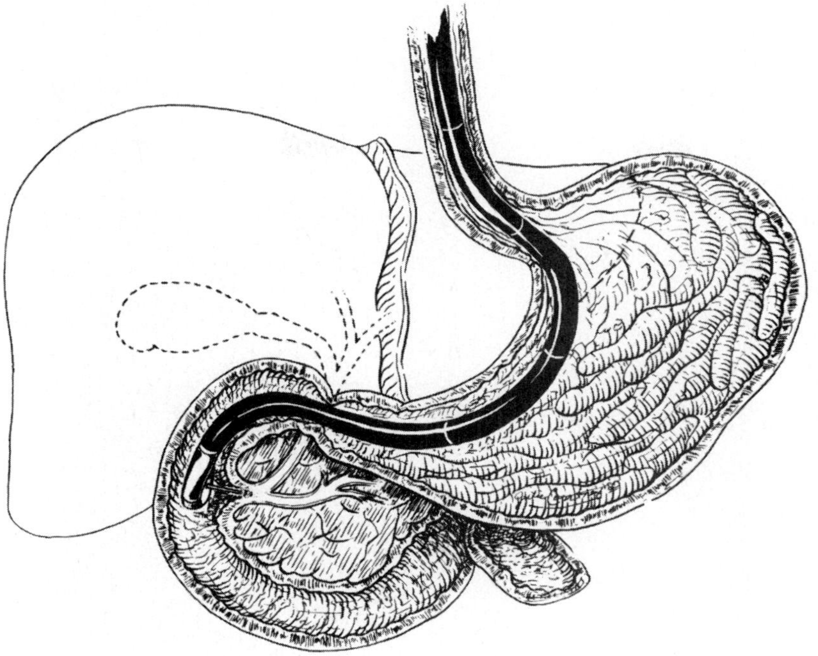

FIGURE 4-8. Endoscopic retrograde cholangiopancreatogram. The fiberoptic scope is passed into the duodenum. Note a small catheter being advanced into the pancreatic biliary ducts.

duodenum (Figure 4-8). At this time, the patient is given 0.4 mg glucagon intravenously to paralyze the duodenum so that the ampulla of Vater can be found more easily. Through an accessory lumen within the scope, a small catheter is passed through the ampulla of Vater and enters into either the common bile or pancreatic ducts (Figures 4-9 and 4-10). Radiographic dye is injected, and x-ray films are taken. The patient does not feel any discomfort with the dye injection. The duration of this test is about 1 hour.

Contraindications. (See also discussion of gastroscopy on pp. 64-65.) ERCP cannot be performed in an uncooperative patient, because cannulation of the ampulla of Vater requires minimum motion on the part of the patient. Like all endoscopy, suspicion of a perforated viscus is an absolute contraindication. Because pancreatitis can be aggravated by pancreatic duct injection, active pancreatitis is a relative contraindication.

Nursing considerations

Nursing Diagnoses/Collaborative Problems

See Endoscopic procedures, pp. 6-7.

- Potential complication: perforation
- Potential complication: sepsis

Nursing Implications with Rationale

- Review the nursing implications for gastroscopy (pp. 65-66).
- Make sure the physician has obtained written and informed consent for this procedure before premedicating the patient.
- Tell the patient that the test takes approximately 1 hour, during which time he or she must lie completely motionless on a hard x-ray table. Remaining still for this period of time may be uncomfortable for the patient.
- Assure the patient that during the test no discomfort occurs, other than the initial gag when the duodenoscope is passed. Encourage the patient to verbalize his or her feelings. Provide emotional support.

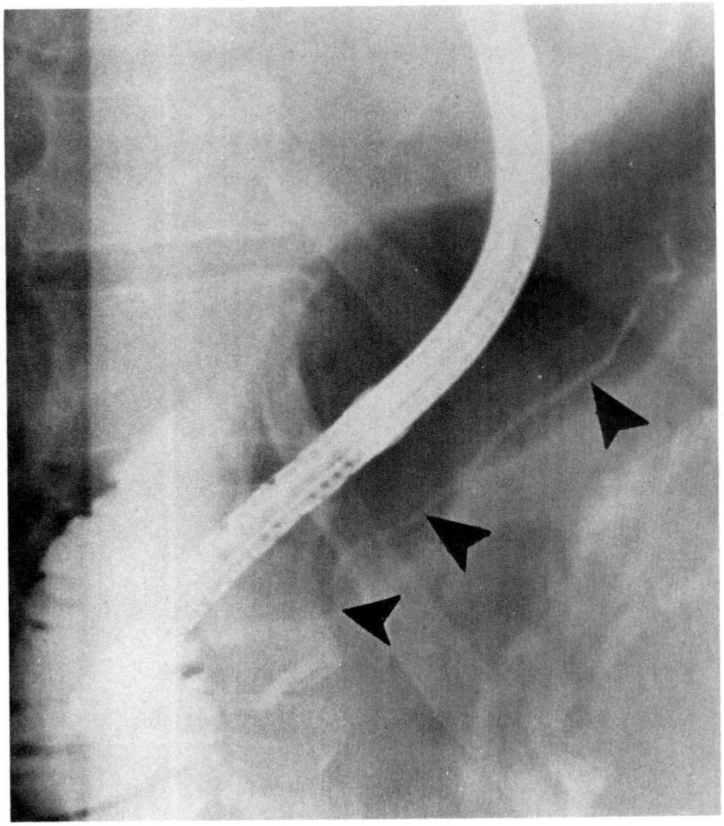

FIGURE 4-9. Endoscopic retrograde cholangiopancreatogram showing a normal pancreatic duct. Scope is within the dye-filled duodenum. Arrows indicate normal pancreatic duct.

- Occasionally the pressure of the injection into the main pancreatic duct causes an acute bout of pancreatitis. This is best diagnosed by obtaining a serum amylase determination the day following the procedure.
- Monitor the patient's temperature, heart rate, and blood pressure as ordered. Assess the patient for signs of bacteremia or septicemia.

Percutaneous transhepatic cholangiography

(PTHC)

Normal values: normal gallbladder and biliary ducts.

Rationale. By the passing of a needle through the skin, the liver and into a dilated intrahepatic bile duct, the biliary system can be directly injected with iodinated dye. The intrahepatic and extrahepatic biliary ducts and occasionally the gallbladder can be visualized and studied for partial or total obstruction caused by gallstones, benign strictures and cysts, and malignant tumor (Figure 4-11). If no obstruction is seen and jaundice is present, intrahepatic cholestasis exists.

Because the bilirubin level of patients with jaundice is elevated, oral cholecystography and intravenous cholangiography cannot visualize the biliary structures. Therefore, PTHC or ERCP are the only methods available to visualize the biliary tree in these patients.

Localized or generalized peritonitis is a potential complication of PTHC. This is caused by

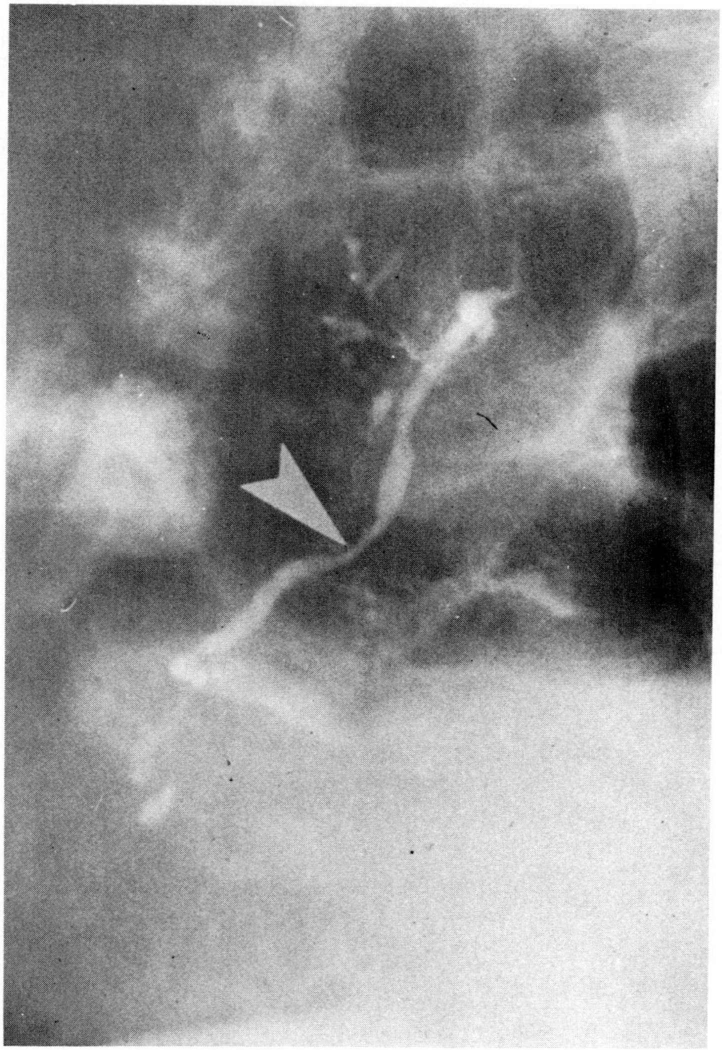

FIGURE 4-10. Endoscopic retrograde cholangiopancreatogram with arrow showing pancreatic ductal narrowing secondary to a cancer. The fiberoptic scope was removed before the x-ray film was taken.

bile extravasation from the liver after the needle is removed. Occasionally surgical repair of the bile leak is necessary. Another potential complication is bleeding caused by inadvertent puncture of a large hepatic blood vessel. This, too, may require surgical repair. These complications can be markedly reduced with the use of the "Chiba Skinny Needle." As described in the discussion of ERCP, bacteremia and sepsis are also potential complications, resulting from injection of the dye into an obstructed bile duct containing infected bile. The pressure of injection pushes the bacteria into the bloodstream. By routinely adding a broad-spectrum antibiotic to the injection, the incidence of bacteremia and sepsis can be almost completely avoided.

Procedure. Usually a bile duct ultrasound is performed. If the bile ducts are found to be di-

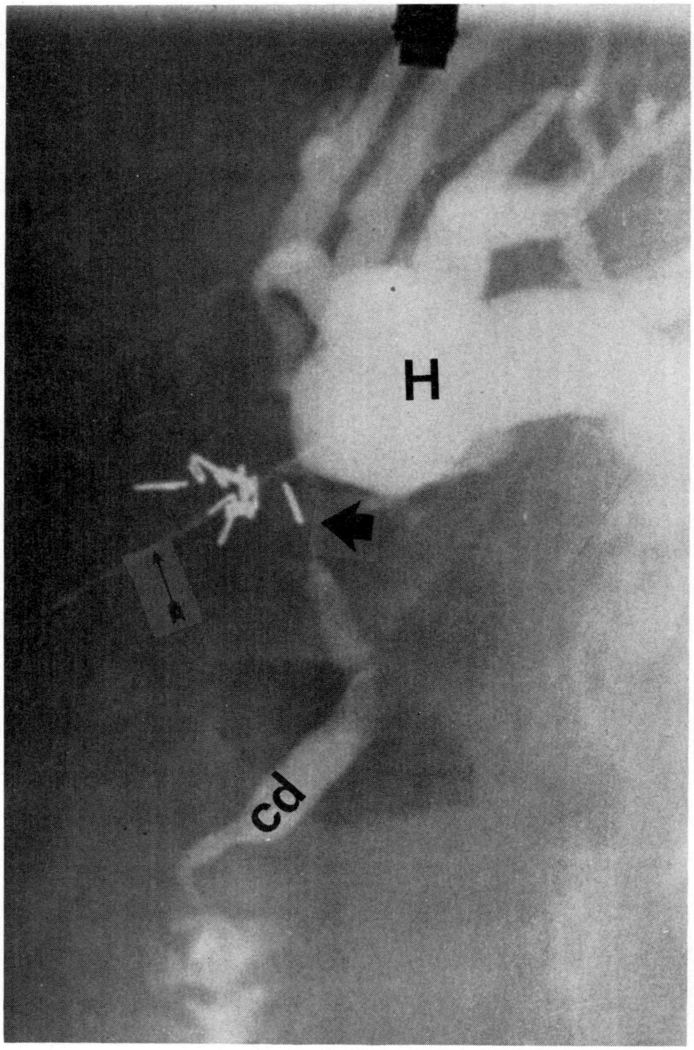

FIGURE 4-11. Percutaneous transhepatic cholangiogram. *H*, Dilated hepatic duct and its branches; *cd*, nondilated common bile duct. Broad arrow indicates a malignant stricture. Thin arrow indicates the cholangiocatheter. Metal hemostatic clips placed during a previous operation are present at left of the stricture.

lated, the patient proceeds to PTC. However, if the bile ducts are not dilated, the chance of gaining bile duct access is small, and the PTC is not attempted. If the PTC is to be carried out, the patient is kept NPO after midnight on the day of the study. A laxative may be given the evening before this study. Sometimes a cleansing enema is given on the morning of the test. Before the patient reports to the radiology department, an IV infusion is started for venous access and the injection of sedatives. Usually the patient is premedicated with atropine, 0.4 mg, and meperidine, 50 mg, IM. In the radiology department the patient is placed in a supine

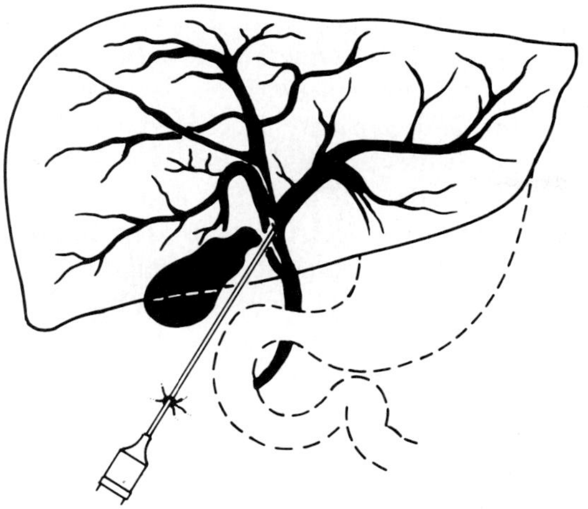

FIGURE 4-12. Percutaneous transhepatic cholangiogram.
From Given BA and Simmons SJ: Gastroenterology in clinical nursing, ed 4, St Louis, 1983, The CV Mosby Co.

position on an x-ray table. The abdominal wall (over the liver) is anesthetized with lidocaine (Xylocaine). With the use of televised fluoroscopic monitoring, the needle is advanced through the skin and into the liver (Figure 4-12) as the physician is aspirating. When bile flows freely into the syringe, a catheter is advanced through the needle and well into the biliary system. Dye containing an antibiotic is injected, and x-ray films are taken immediately. If complete obstruction is found, the catheter may be temporarily left in place to establish drainage and decompression of the biliary tract.

PTHC takes about 1 hour, during which time the patient must lie completely still. If repeated needle sticks must be made to obtain biliary access, the patient may become uncomfortable.

If hemorrhage or bile extravasation occurs, the patient may have severe right upper quadrant abdominal pain. Shoulder-top pain, referred from the right upper quadrant, may be present.

After returning to the floor, the patient is kept on bed rest and NPO in the event that surgery may become necessary to control hemorrhage or significant bile extravasation.

Contraindications. PTHC in contraindicated in:

1. Patients with iodine allergy
2. Patients with evidence of mild cholangitis; dye injections increase biliary pressure and cause bacteremia, which may lead to septicemia and shock
3. Patients who are poor surgical candidates; surgical repair of complications may be necessary
4. Uncooperative patients
5. Patients with prolonged clotting times
6. Patients who recently have had a GI contrast study; residual barium may obscure radiographic visualization of the bile ducts.

Nursing considerations

Nursing Diagnoses/Collaborative Problems

- Possible knowledge deficit related to test purpose, preparation, and procedure
- High risk for alteration in comfort related to test procedure
- Potential complication: bleeding
- Potential complication: peritonitis
- Potential complication: sepsis

Nursing Implications with Rationale

- Explain the procedure to the patient. Encourage verbalization of the patient's feelings, since the patient may be anxious regarding this study.
- Tell the patient that he or she will feel slight discomfort when the abdomen is anesthetized locally. Pressure may be felt when the needle is placed into the liver.
- Be sure the patient is not allergic to iodine.
- Ensure that the patient's written and informed consent for PTHC is obtained before premedicating the patient.
- If GI contrast studies were recently performed, obtain a physician's order for a cathartic to remove any residual barium.
- Prepare the patient as if for surgery because

emergency surgical intervention may become necessary to control hemorrhage or bile leakage. Type and crossmatch the patient's blood before this test. The patient's platelet count and the prothrombin time should be normal.

- On the patient's return to the floor, keep him or her at bed rest and NPO. Place a sandbag over the site of needle insertion, if ordered. Observe the site for bile leakage or hemorrhage. A small amount of bleeding is usually present.
- Take the patient's vital signs frequently (every 15 minutes for four times, then every 30 minutes for four times, then every hour for four times, and then every 4 hours). Assess the vital signs for a decrease in blood pressure or an increase in pulse, either of which would indicate hemorrhage. A hemoglobin and hematocrit determination may be ordered 6 hours after PTHC.
- If the catheter is left in the biliary tract, establish a sterile closed system of drainage.
- Withhold pain medications to avoid blunting the abdominal signs associated with hemorrhage or bile extravasation. Observe the patient for increasing abdominal pain.

SUPPLEMENTAL INFORMATION

Gallbladder scanning

(hepatobiliary scintigraphy, hepatobiliary imaging, biliary tract radionuclide scan, cholescintigraphy, DISIDA scanning, HIDA scanning, IDA scanning)

Normal values: gallbladder, common bile duct, and duodenum visualization within 60 minutes after radionuclide injection. (This confirms cystic and common bile duct patency.)

Rationale. Through the use of iminodiacetic acid (IDA) analogues labeled with technetium-99m (^{99m}Tc), the biliary tract (Figure 4-13) can be evaluated in a safe, accurate, and noninvasive manner. These radionuclide compounds injected into the blood stream are extracted by the liver and excreted in the bile. Cholescintigraphy is a valuable tool in evaluating patients with suspected biliary tract disease. The primary use of this study is in the diagnosis of acute cholecystitis. Early surgical intervention for the patient with acute cholecystitis decreases the morbidity and mortality associated with this condition. If the gallbladder cannot be seen after administration of ^{99m}Tc-IDA, cystic duct obstruction and acute cholecystitis is indicated. This procedure is superior to oral cholecystography, intravenous cholangiography, ultrasonography, and CT scanning of the abdomen for the detection of acute cholecystitis.

Biliary scintigraphy has also been used successfully to evaluate patients with jaundice, ampullary stenosis, duodenal diverticula, biliary-enteric anastomosis, and biliary leaks. This scanning procedure is also useful in acute extrahepatic obstruction because the common bile duct can be visualized even when the serum bilirubin level is elevated. In fact, Diisopropyl IDA (DISIDA) permits visualization in the biliary tract for bilirubin levels up to 30 mg/dl.

Chronic cholecystitis can also be detected by cholescintigraphy. By measuring the contractility of the gallbladder, the ejection fraction of the bile from the gallbladder can be calculated. A reduced fraction <30% is associated with chronic cholecystitis.

Procedure. After a 4-hour fast the patient reports to the radiography department and is placed in the supine position on an x-ray table. After an IV injection of ^{99m}Tc-IDA derivative (for example, DISIDA, PIPIDA, HIDA), the right upper quadrant of the abdomen is scanned. The HIDA or PIPIDA scans are most useful in assessing the patency of the biliary tree since these radionuclides are secreted by the hepatocytes into the bile canaliculi. Serial images are obtained over 1 hour. Subsequent images can be obtained at 10- to 15-minute intervals. A right lateral view is taken to document the anterior position of the gallbladder. If the gallbladder, common bile duct, and duodenum are not seen within 60 minutes after the injection, delayed images up to 4 hours may be obtained. Films are recorded on Polaroid film. Some patients are given a fatty meal or chole-

A 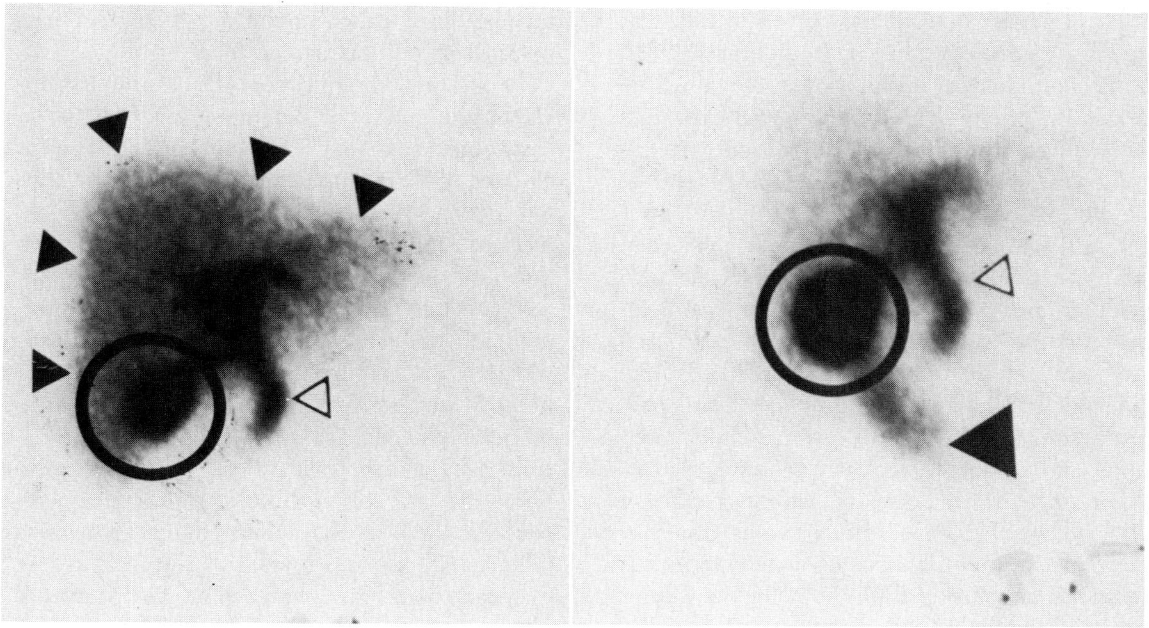 B

FIGURE 4-13. **A,** Normal cholescintigrams. Solid pointers indicate outline of the liver. Gallbladder is circled. Pointer outlines indicate normal common bile duct. **B,** Normal cholescintigram—later in time. Liver is now less well defined because most of the radionuclide is in the biliary tree (as marked in **A**). Duodenum *(solid black arrow)* now visibly contains radionuclide.

cytokinin to evaluate the emptying of the gallbladder and the ejection fraction.

The only discomfort associated with this procedure is that of the IV injection of radionuclide. However, many patients complain about lying on the hard, x-ray table. A radiologist or nuclear medicine physician performs this study in approximately 1 to 4 hours.

Contraindications. Pregnancy.

Nursing considerations

Nursing Diagnoses/Collaborative Problems

See Nuclear scanning, p. 5.

Nursing Implications with Rationale

- Explain the procedure to the patient. Ensure that the patient has fasted the 4 hours before the procedure. The majority of patients without any cystic duct obstruction fail to demonstrate the gallbladder if they are not in the fasting state.
- After the procedure be sure to obtain a meal for the patient.
- Assure the patient that exposure is not to large amounts of radioactivity because only tracer doses of the radioisotopes are used.

Operative cholangiography

In operative cholangiography, the common bile duct is directly injected with the radiopaque dye. As in ERCP and IVC, stones appear as radiolucent shadows, and tumors cause partial or total obstruction of the flow of dye into the duodenum. By visualization of the biliary duct structures, the surgeon is provided with a "road map" of an oftentimes difficult anatomic area. This reduces the possibility of inadvertent common duct injury.

If common duct stones are suspected, not only must a cholecystectomy be performed, but also a common duct exploration (CDE) must be carried out. Before the routine use of operative cholangiography, about 50% of patients undergoing cholecystectomy required CDE, based on the clinical suspicion that common duct stones were present. Stones were found in less than half of the CDEs. Therefore, the CDE was performed unnecessarily on many patients and significantly increased the morbidity associated with cholecystectomy. When intraoperative cholangiography is used routinely, CDE is performed only on those with positive cholangiography and not on those with negative results. This reduces the number of patients requiring CDE to about 25% of the previous number. Therefore, intraoperative cholangiography is useful not only for its ability to recognize stones and other pathologic conditions, but also because it reduces the number of unnecessary CDEs.

T-tube cholangiography

(postoperative cholangiography)

Normal values: no stones.

Rationale. T-tube cholangiography is performed to diagnose retained ductal stones postoperatively in the patient who has had a cholecystectomy and a common bile duct exploration. The test is performed through the use of a T-shaped rubber tube that the surgeon places in the bile duct during the previously performed common bile duct exploration. Dye is injected through the external end of the T tube and x-ray films are taken. Usually T-tube cholangiography is performed 1 week postoperatively. If no stones are evident, the T tube is removed. If the presence of stones is questionable, the T tube is left in place and the study is repeated in 3 weeks. When stones are present, the T tube is left in place until a well-defined tract is established (approximately 3 weeks). At this time the T tube is removed and a basket catheter is inserted into the common duct through the T-tube tract for the purpose of nonoperative stone extraction.

A potential complication of this study is sepsis caused by increased ductal pressure with the dye infusion (as in PTHC and ERCP). The incidence of this complication is reduced by adding a broad-spectrum antibiotic to the dye injection. Another complication is inadvertent removal of the T tube during the study.

Procedure. The patient is kept NPO after midnight on the day of the test. No cathartics or sedatives are required. In the radiology department, a sterile dye solution containing an antibiotic is placed in a sterile container and attached by a catheter to the T tube. The solution drips into the T tube by minimal gravity pressure. When the biliary ductal system is filled, x-ray films are taken of the right upper quadrant of the abdomen while the patient is placed in the supine, prone, and oblique positions. No discomfort is associated with this study. A radiologist usually performs this procedure in approximately 15 minutes.

Contraindications. This test is contraindicated in the uncooperative patient or in patients with dye allergy.

Nursing considerations

Nursing Diagnoses/Collaborative Problems

- Possible knowledge deficit related to test purpose, preparation, and procedure
- Potential complication: sepsis
- Potential complication: adverse reaction/allergy to dye

Nursing Implications with Rationale

- Explain the procedure to the patient. Assure the patient that he or she should not have any discomfort when the dye is injected through the T tube.
- Observe the patient for signs of sepsis. Take the vital signs frequently, as ordered, and assess the patient for increased temperature, tachycardia, chills, hypertension, and disorientation.

- If the T tube is left in place, connect it to a sterile closed drainage system to avoid bacteria entering the ductal system through the catheter.
- If the T tube is removed, keep the T tube tract site covered with a sterile dressing to prevent bacteria from entering the ductal system. Assess the site for drainage and record the amount of drainage. This is important because the bile duct can be torn open during the removal of the T tube, causing a significant bile leak. This bile loss can cause steatorrhea (large amounts of fat in the feces), fluid and electrolyte imbalance, and skin excoriation at the drain site.

Liver biopsy

Normal value: normal liver histology.

Rationale. Liver biopsy is a safe, simple, and valuable method of diagnosing pathologic liver conditions. For this study, a specially designed needle is inserted through the skin and abdominal wall and then into the liver. A piece of liver tissue is removed for microscopic examination. Percutaneous liver biopsy is used in the diagnosis of various liver disorders such as cirrhosis, hepatitis, drug reactions, granuloma, and tumor.

Percutaneous liver biopsy is indicated in

1. Patients with unexplained hepatomegaly (enlargement of the liver)
2. Patients with persistently elevated liver enzyme levels
3. Patients in whom primary or metastatic tumor is suspected
4. Patients with unexplained jaundice
5. Patients in whom hepatitis is suspected
6. Patients in whom infiltrative disease, such as sarcoidosis, amyloidosis, Wilson's disease, or miliary tuberculosis, is suspected.

Although liver biopsy is generally considered a safe procedure, complications do exist. These include:

1. Hemorrhage caused by inadvertent puncture of a blood vessel within or surrounding the liver
2. Peritonitis caused by inadvertent laceration of a bile duct with leakage of bile into the abdominal cavity
3. Pneumothorax (collapse of the lung) caused by improper placement of the biopsy needle upward into the adjacent chest cavity.

Complications are markedly diminished when this study is performed by an experienced and skillful physician.

Procedure. Before the study a coagulation profile (prothrombin time, partial thromboplastin time, and platelet count) is performed to ensure adequate hemostasis if a small intrahepatic blood vessel is punctured. The patient's blood may be typed and crossmatched so that blood can be made available for transfusion if necessary.

The patient is kept NPO from midnight on the day of the examination. Meperidine and atropine are often administered 30 to 60 minutes before the study. The patient is placed in the supine or left lateral position. The skin overlying the area of the liver from which the biopsy specimen is desired is aseptically cleansed and anesthetized. A small incision (<1 cm) is made in the skin. The patient is instructed to exhale and "hold it" because during exhalation the diaphragm ascends, thus reducing the possibility of pneumothorax. It is best to practice the sustained exhalation two or three times before the insertion of the needle. During a sustained exhalation the physician rapidly introduces the biopsy needle into the liver, obtains the liver tissue, and then immediately withdraws the needle.

Several different needles are available for a liver biopsy. The one with which the physician feels most comfortable is used. A long, thin needle attached to a syringe is usually used for an aspiration biopsy. Also, one may use Vim-Silverman or Tru-cut needles, which have cutting edges to allow excision of a small piece of liver tissue. The use of these latter needles provides more tissue for examination, but a slightly higher complication rate is associated with them.

The tissue sample is placed into a specimen bottle containing formalin (or saline solution if a frozen section is requested) and sent to the pathology laboratory. A small dressing is placed over the needle insertion site, and the patient is placed on his or her right side to provide pressure on the biopsy site as the liver lays against the upper abdominal wall. The entire procedure is usually performed at the bedside in about 20 minutes. Minor discomfort may be experienced during the injection of the local anesthetic. Some patients complain of right shoulder pain as the biopsy needle passes the diaphragm.

Contraindications. Liver biopsies are contraindicated in:

1. Uncooperative patients who will not hold their breath during sustained exhalation
2. Patients with impaired hemostasis, because inadvertent puncture of a blood vessel may cause exsanguination
3. Patients with profound anemia, who cannot afford a major blood loss
4. Patients with infection of the right pleural space and those with septic cholangitis, because the needle biopsy may spread the infection
5. Patients with obstructive jaundice who have large dilated intrahepatic bile ducts; the chance of laceration of these ducts, with subsequent continued bile leakage, is too great.

Nursing considerations

Nursing Diagnoses/Collaborative Problems

- Possible knowledge deficit related to test purpose, preparation, and procedure
- High risk for alteration in comfort related to test procedure
- Possible anxiety related to unknown sensations of the procedure
- Potential complication: hemorrhage
- Potential complication: pneumothorax
- Potential complication: bile leakage and peritonitis

Nursing Implications with Rationale

- Explain the procedure to the patient. Most patients are very apprehensive about this biopsy. Encourage verbalization of the patient's fears.
- Make sure the physician obtains the written and informed consent for this procedure before the study.
- Check the results of the patient's hemostasis studies to make certain that the patient has no coagulation disorders. As discussed earlier, many patients with liver disease have coagulation problems that make them prone to hemorrhage. Inform the physician of any abnormal test results.
- Keep the patient NPO after midnight on the day of test in case emergency surgery is needed to control hemorrhage or biliary leakage.
- Inform the patient that it is vital to lie very still during this procedure and to hold his or her breath during exhalation when instructed. Any movement of the chest may cause the needle to slip and lacerate the liver or diaphragm.
- Administer sedatives, if ordered, before the study.
- Support the patient during the procedure. Assist the physician as needed. Place the tissue obtained into the appropriate specimen container and have it sent to the pathology department.
- After the procedure, place the patient on the right side for 1 to 2 hours. In this position the liver capsule is compressed against the chest wall, thereby tamponading any hemorrhage or bile leak. The patient should remain at bed rest for 12 to 24 hours.
- Assess the patient's vital signs frequently (usually every 15 minutes for four times, then every hour for four times, and then every 4

hours) for evidence of hemorrhage (increased pulse, decreased blood pressure) and peritonitis (increased temperature). Evaluate the patient for increasing abdominal pain. Be aware that some pain in the right upper quadrant of the abdomen and the right shouldertop area is common. This pain is caused by the inevitable leakage of blood or bile or both from the biopsy site in the liver. This fluid causes a localized and mild peritonitis. When the leak involves a large quantity of blood or bile, the peritoneal reaction is great, and the resulting pain is severe. Report this immediately to the physician.

Liver scanning

(radioisotope liver scanning)

Normal values: normal size, shape, and position of the liver.

Rationale. This radionucleotide procedure is used to outline and detect structural changes of the liver. A radionucleotide (usually a ^{99m}Tc sulfur–labeled albumin colloid) is given intravenously. Later, a gamma ray detecting device (Geiger counter) is passed over the patient's abdomen. This records the distribution of the radioactive particles in the liver. The spleen can also be visualized by the detector when ^{99m}Tc sulfur is used. Because the scan can only demonstrate filling deficits greater than 2 cm in diameter, false negative results can occur in patients who have space-occupying lesions (such as tumors, cysts, and granulomas) smaller than 2 cm. The scan may be incorrectly interpreted as positive in patients who have cirrhosis, because of the distortion of the patient's liver parenchyma.

Rose bengal radioactive iodine (^{131}I) scanning is useful in differentiating intrahepatic cholestasis from extrahepatic obstruction. This isotope is normally taken up and excreted by the hepatocytes. With complete biliary ductal obstruction, the dye will not be detected in the duodenum by the gamma ray detector. However, with intrahepatic cholestasis, some isotope may be visualized within the duodenum and small bowel.

Procedure. No special preparation is required for colloidal technetium (^{99m}Tc) and rose bengal (^{131}I) scanning. Thirty minutes after a peripheral IV injection of the radiosotope, a gamma ray detecting device is slowly passed over the patient while he or she is moved from the supine to the lateral, and prone positions to visualize all surfaces of the liver. The radionucleotide uptake is recorded on either x-ray or Polaroid film.

This procedure is performed in the nuclear medicine department by a trained technician in approximately 1 hour. A physician trained in nuclear medicine interprets the reports. The only discomfort is associated with the IV injection of the radioisotope. Because only tracer doses of radioisotopes are used, no precautions need to be taken against radioactive exposure.

Contraindications. Liver scanning is contraindicated in the pregnant patient and in the uncooperative patient.

Nursing considerations

Nursing Diagnoses/Collaborative Problems

See Nuclear scanning, p. 5.

Nursing Implications with Rationale

- Explain the procedure to the patient. Encourage verbalization of the patient's fears. Provide emotional support.
- Assure the patient that he or she will not be exposed to large amounts of radioactivity because only tracer doses of isotopes are used.

Blood ammonia

Normal values:
Adults: 15-110 μg/dl or 47-65 μmol/L (SI)
Children: 40-80 μg/dl
Newborns: 90-150 μg/dl

Rationale. Ammonia, a by-product of protein metabolism, is normally converted by the liver into urea and then secreted by the kidneys (see BUN, p. 229). With severe liver dysfunction or when the blood flow is diverted from the liver (e.g. from portal hypertension), the blood ammonia level rises and the BUN level decreases. The blood ammonia level is primarily used as an aid in diagnosing hepatic encephalopathy or coma. Elevated blood ammonia levels suggest liver dysfunction as the cause of these symptoms. Elevated levels may also be seen in patients with hepatic failure, erythroblastosis fetalis, cor pulmonale, pulmonary emphysema, and congestive heart failure. Exercise may also cause an increase in ammonia levels. Decreased blood ammonia levels may be seen in patients with renal failure, essential hypertension, and malignant hypertension. It is important to note that certain antibiotics (such as neomycin and tetracycline) can decrease ammonia levels.

Procedure. Fasting is not usually required. Venous blood (5 to 7 ml) is collected in a green-top tube and sent to the laboratory for analysis.

Contraindications. None.

Nursing considerations

Nursing Diagnosis/Collaborative Problems

See Blood studies, p. 2.

Nursing Implications with Rationale

- Assess the venipuncture site for bleeding. Many patients with liver disease have prolonged clotting times.
- List any antibiotics the patient is currently taking on the lab slip. Certain antibiotics can cause a decreased ammonia level, thus giving inaccurate test results.

Hepatitis virus studies

(hepatitis-associated antigen, HAA, Australian antigen)

Normal value: negative.

Rationale. Hepatitis is an inflammation of the liver caused by a virus. Three common viruses are now recognized that can cause this disease—hepatitis A virus, hepatitis B virus, and hepatitis C virus (also called hepatitis non-A, non-B virus).

Hepatitis A virus (HAV), which causes what was originally called "infectious hepatitis," has a short incubation period of 2 to 6 weeks. The virus is usually excreted in the stool and transmitted via the fecal-oral route. Usually there is complete recovery from this relatively benign form of hepatitis. Although tests are not yet available to detect HAV, tests are available to detect the two types of antibody the body makes to HAV.

The first type of antibody is IgM (HAV-Ab/IgM), which appears around 3 to 4 weeks after exposure or just before the AST rise. The IgM level returns to normal in about 8 weeks. The second type of antibody is IgG (HAV-Ab/IgG), which appears around 2 weeks after the beginning of the IgM increase and slowly returns to lower levels, although remaining detectable for more than 10 years. If the IgM antibody is elevated in the absence of the IgG antibody, acute infection is indicated. If the IgG is elevated in the absence of the IgM, the convalescent stage of a recent infection or residual elevation from a previous HAV infection may be indicated.

Hepatitis B (HBV), which causes what was originally called "serum hepatitis," has a long incubation period of 5 weeks to 6 months. Although hepatitis B is most frequently transmitted by blood transfusions, it can also be contracted via the blood, saliva, or semen. Although less infectious than HAV, HBV may cause a severe, unrelenting form of hepatitis ending in liver failure and death. Increased incidence of this virus is seen in the following: blood transfusion recipients, male homosexuals, patients undergoing renal dialysis, renal transplant patients, patients with drug dependencies, and patients with leukemia or lymphoma.

The HBV, also called the Dane particle, is made up of an inner core surrounded by an outer capsule. The outer capsule contains the hepatitis B surface antigen (HBsAG), formerly called Australian antigen. The inner core contains HBV core antigen (HBcAg) and, within the core, the hepatitis B e-antigen (HBeAg) is found. The antibodies made by the body in response to these antigens are called the HBsAb, HBcAb, and HBeAb. The tests used to detect these antigens and antibodies are as follows:

1. *Hepatitis B surface antigen (HBsAg).* Detection of this surface antigen is the most commonly and easily performed test for hepatitis B. The test for surface antigen is the first indicator to become abnormal. Surface antigen level rises before the onset of clinical symptoms, peaks during the first week of symptoms, and returns to normal by the time jaundice subsides. Therefore, detection of HBsAg generally means active infection by HBV. If the levels of this antigen persist in the blood, the patient is considered to be a carrier.
2. *Hepatitis B surface antibody (HBsAb).* This antibody appears about 4 weeks after the disappearance of HBsAg and signifies the end of acute infection and immunity to further infection. Concentrated forms of this agent constitute the hyperimmunoglobulin given to patients who have come in contact with hepatitis B–infected patients (for example, an inadvertent needle prick from a needle previously used on a patient with HBV infection).
3. *Hepatitis B core antigen (HBcAg).* No tests are currently available to detect this antigen.
4. *Hepatitis B core antibody (HBcAb).* This antibody's level rises about 1 month after the appearance of HBsAg, peaks in 1 month, and declines (although remains elevated) for several years. The core antibody is usually present in chronic hepatitis. The core antibody level is elevated during the time lag between the disappearance of HBsAG and the appearance of HBsAb. This time interval is called the *core window.* During the core window the core antibody is the only detectable marker of recent infection.
5. *Hepatitis B e-antigen (HBeAg).* The e-antigen is generally not employed for diagnostic purposes but is instead used as an index of infectivity. Its presence correlates with early and active disease as well as high infectivity in acute HBV infection. The persistent presence of this antigen in the blood predicts the development of chronic HBV infection.
6. *Hepatitis B e-antibody (HBeAb).* Detection of this antibody means that the acute phase of HBV infection is over or nearly over and that infectivity is much less. HBeAb titers reach their peak during the core window time interval.

Hepatitis C virus (HCV), also called hepatitis non-A, non-B, is transmitted in a manner similar to hepatitis B. The incubation period ranges from 2 to 12 weeks after exposure. The clinical illness is similar to hepatitis B, but much less severe. The majority of blood transfusion hepatitis cases are now because of hepatitis C. HCV antibody testing is available and, when positive, indicates that infection has occurred. However, the chronology and transmissibility of the disease when HCV antibodies are detected have yet to be determined. Donor blood screening with alanine aminotransferase (ALT) to eliminate some cases of hepatitis C has been suggested. The ALT enzyme is very sensitive to acute liver cell injury.

Procedure. No special preparation is necessary for these antigen-antibody studies. A peripheral venipuncture is performed, and generally one red-top tube of blood is obtained. Most of the testing is done by radioimmunoassay techniques.

Contraindications. None.

Nursing considerations

Nursing Diagnoses/Collaborative Problems

See Blood studies, p. 2.

- Possible knowledge deficit related to spread of disease

Nursing Implications with Rationale

- Explain the procedure to the patient.

- Handle the serum specimen as if it were capable of transmitting viral hepatitis. Wash your hands very carefully after handling all equipment. Gloves should always be worn during venipuncture.
- Apply pressure or a pressure dressing to the venipuncture site after the blood is drawn.
- Observe the site for bleeding.
- Enteric precautions should be taken in caring for patients suspected of hepatitis A infection.

CASE STUDY 2: PANCREATITIS

Mr. D., 52 years old, was admitted to the hospital complaining of severe epigastric pain with radiation to his back. The pain started on the day before admission and was associated with nausea and vomiting. On examination he was found to be dehydrated and to have only mild epigastric midline tenderness and guarding. He denied a recent alcohol debauch. Because of previous symptoms, Mr. D. had undergone oral cholecystography, the results of which were normal.

Studies	Results
Routine laboratory studies	Within normal limits (WNL) except for WBC, which was 15,000/mm^3 (normal WBC: 5000-10,000/mm^3)
Serum amylase test	640 IU/L (normal: 56-190 IU/L)
Urine amylase test	1240 IU/hr (normal: 3-35 IU/hr)
Serum lipase test	240 units/L (normal: 0-110 units/L)
Ultrasound examination of pancreas	Edematous and enlarged head of the pancreas
CT scanning of abdomen	Diffusely edematous and enlarged gland
ERCP	Normal pancreatic duct

The diagnosis of pancreatitis was quite certain in light of the elevation of both the serum and the urine amylase levels and also of the serum lipase level. Alcohol and gallstones are the two most common causes of pancreatitis. However, the patient denied drinking alcohol and previous oral cholecystography excluded gallstones. Because cancer of the pancreas can also cause distal pancreatic inflammation, tumor had to be ruled out as a cause of this pancreatitic episode. Ultrasound, which is occasionally inaccurate for pathologic pancreatic conditions, indicated an enlarged head of the pancreas that could be compatible with a tumor. However, CT scanning and ERCP results eliminated the possibility of cancer.

The patient was treated with nasogastric (NG) suction and IV infusions until his gastrointestinal function returned to normal. His pancreatitis was subsequently found to be drug-induced (by hydrochlorothiazide). The drug was stopped, and he had no further problems.

DISCUSSION OF TESTS

Serum amylase test

Normal values: 56-190 IU/L or 80-150 Somogyi units/dl (values may be slightly increased during pregnancy and in the elderly).

Rationale. The serum amylase test is an easily and rapidly performed test for pancreatitis. Amylase is normally secreted from the pancreatic acinar cell into the pancreatic duct and then into the duodenum. Once in the intestine, it aids in the catabolism of carbohydrates to their component sugars. Damage to these acinar cells (as in pancreatitis) or obstruction to the pancreatic ductal flow (as in pancreatic carcinoma) causes an outpouring of this enzyme into the intrapancreatic lymph system and also into the free peritoneum. Blood vessels draining the free peritoneum and absorbing the lymph pick up this excess amylase. An abnormal rise in the serum level of amylase is the result, which occurs within 12 hours of the onset of pancreatic disease. Because amylase is rapidly cleared by the kidney, serum levels may return to normal within 48 to 72 hours. Ongoing inflammation (as in severe hemorrhagic pancreatitis), duct obstruction (as in cancer), or pancreatic ductal leakage (as in pseudocysts) causes persistently elevated serum amylase levels. Although serum amylase is a sensitive test for pancreatic disorders, it is far from specific. This is because it is found in many other organs, such as salivary glands, liver, intestines, kidneys, and the female genital tract. Disorders affecting these organs (such as parotitis, cholecystitis, renal infarction, or ectopic pregnancy) also cause a high serum amylase level. Serum levels are also increased in patients with perforated ulcer or bowel. The amylase secreted by the pancreas into the bowel leaks out of the perforation and is absorbed by the blood vessels of the peritoneum. A patient receiving an intravenous dextrose solution may have decreased serum amylase levels, causing a false-negative result. Many drugs (such as narcotic analgesics, aspirin, and loop diuretics) can cause a false-positive result.

Procedure. Blood is withdrawn from a peripheral vein and placed in a red-top tube. No fasting is required of the patient.

Contraindications. None.

Nursing considerations

Nursing Diagnoses/Collaborative Problems

See Blood studies, p. 2.

Nursing Implications with Rationale

- Apply a pressure dressing to the site after the venipuncture is completed. Observe the site for bleeding.
- Note on the lab slip if the patient is receiving IV dextrose because dextrose can cause a false-negative result.
- Note on the lab slip if the patient is taking any medication which can cause a false-positive result.

Urine amylase test

Normal values: 3-35 IU/hr, or 6-30 Wohlgemuth units/ml, or up to 5000 Somogyi units/24 hours.

Rationale. Because the kidney rapidly clears amylase, disorders affecting the pancreas cause elevated amylase levels in the urine. The serum amylase level may rise only transiently in acute (uncomplicated) pancreatitis. The serum levels frequently return to normal 1 to 2 days after the onset of disease. Levels of amylase in the urine, however, remain elevated for 7 to 10 days after the onset of disease. This fact is important if one is to make the diagnosis of pancreatitis in patients who have had symptoms for 3 days or longer. Like the serum levels, amylase levels in the urine can be elevated in many other nonpancreatic disorders (see the discussion of the previous test), but the urine levels are highest with pancreatitis. A comparison of the renal clearance of amylase to creatinine provides more diagnostic information for pancreatitis than does either the urine amylase level or the serum amylase level. When the renal amylase/creatinine clearance ratio is 5% or more, the diagnosis of pancreatitis can be made with certainty. With ratios less than 5% in a patient with elevated serum and urine amylase levels, pathologic conditions other than pancreatitis should be sought.

Procedure. Generally a timed 2-hour or 24-hour urine collection is required. A standard specimen container is used, and the specimen is refrigerated or kept on ice during the collection period. No patient fasting is required.

Contraindications. None.

Nursing considerations

Nursing Diagnoses/Collaborative Problems

See Urine studies, p. 3.

Nursing Implications with Rationale

- Explain the procedure to the patient. Give the patient the necessary urine containers.
- Record the exact times of the beginning and end of the collection period. The collection begins *after* the patient empties his or her bladder and discards that specimen. All subsequent urine is collected, including the one at the end of the collection period.
- Encourage the patient to drink fluids during the collection period unless fluids are restricted for medical reasons.
- Keep the specimen on ice or refrigerated until it is sent to the laboratory.

Serum lipase test

Normal values: 0-110 units/L or 0-417 U/L (SI).

Rationale. The most common cause of an elevated serum lipase level is acute pancreatitis. Lipase is an enzyme secreted by the pancreas into the duodenum to break triglycerides down to fatty acids. Like amylase (see previous test), lipase appears in the bloodstream following damage to the pancreas. Since lipase is produced only in the pancreas, elevated serum levels are specific to pathologic pancreatic conditions.

In acute pancreatitis elevated lipase levels usually parallel serum amylase levels. However, the lipase level rises 24 to 48 hours after the onset of pancreatitis and remains elevated for 5 to 7 days. Because it peaks later and remains elevated longer than the serum amylase level, serum lipase levels are useful in the late diagnosis of acute pancreatitis. Lipase levels are less useful in patients with chronic alcoholic pancreatitis, pancreatitis secondary to biliary tract disease, or pancreatic carcinoma.

Procedure. Blood is withdrawn from a peripheral vein and placed in a red-top tube. The blood is drawn after an overnight fast. No water restrictions are necessary.

Contraindications. None.

Nursing considerations

Nursing Diagnoses/Collaborative Problems

See Blood studies, p. 2.

Nursing Implications with Rationale

- Apply a pressure dressing to the venipuncture site. Observe the site for bleeding.
- Order the patient's breakfast after the blood sample is obtained.
- Many narcotics (such as morphine, codeine, meperidine) may interfere with test results if given within the 24 hours preceding the test. Note the time of their administration on the lab slip if they were given during this time period.

Ultrasound examination of the pancreas

(pancreas echogram)

Normal values: normal size and position of the pancreas.

Rationale. Through the use of reflected sound waves, ultrasonography of the pancreas provides diagnostic information of this rather inaccessible abdominal organ. In diagnostic ultrasound, a harmless high-frequency sound wave is emitted from a transducer and penetrates the organ being studied. These sound waves are bounced back to the transducer and electronically converted into a pictorial image of that organ. A realistic Polaroid picture of the pancreas is obtained.

Ultrasound examination of the pancreas is mainly used to establish the diagnosis of carcinoma, pseudocysts, pancreatitis, and pancreatic abscess. Because ultrasound abnormalities persist from several days to weeks, the diagnosis of pancreatitis can be supported by this study even after the serum amylase and lipase levels have returned to normal. Furthermore, follow-up ultrasound study can be used to monitor the resolution of pancreatic inflammation and the response of a tumor to therapy.

Procedure. Fasting is usually not required although preferred. The study is performed in the radiology department, with the patient supine on an examining table. The ultrasonographer, usually a radiologist or technician, applies mineral oil or glycerin to the skin of the abdomen over the organ. This paste is used to enhance transmission and reception. The transducer is moved along the skin in a horizontal (cross-sectional) and a vertical (sagittal) line. The depth and intensity recordings of these echoes produce a realistic anatomic photograph of the section being examined. Review of these prints allows a three-dimensional look at the pancreas. Ultrasound is noninvasive, has no side effects, and can be safely performed on pregnant patients. Because the ultrasonic beam is almost totally reflected by air-filled organs, this study cannot be used diagnostically if the patient's intestine is filled with gas. Since barium also reflects the sound wave, ultrasound examination should be performed before barium studies. This test is not associated with any patient discomfort. The duration of the study is about ½ hour. The accuracy of this test depends on the ability of the technician to obtain good films and of the radiologist to read them.

Contraindications. This test is contraindicated in the uncooperative patient.

Nursing considerations

Nursing Diagnoses/Collaborative Problems

See Ultrasound studies, p. 6.

Nursing Implications with Rationale

- Explain the procedure to the patient. Assure the patient that no discomfort is associated with this test.
- Explain to the patient that a liberal amount of gel or lubricant will be applied to the skin over the pancreas to enhance the transmission and reception of sound waves.
- If the patient's abdomen appears to be distended with gas or if the patient has had a recent barium study, this study should be canceled, because gas and barium interfere with sound-wave transmission.
- When the patient returns to the floor, help him or her remove the gel or lubricant from the abdomen.

Computed tomography of the abdomen

(CT of the abdomen)

Normal values: no evidence of tumor or pathologic condition.

Rationale. Computed tomography (CT) of the abdomen is a noninvasive yet very accurate x-ray procedure used to diagnose pathologic conditions of the abdominal organs such as inflammation, tumor, cysts, ascites, aneurysms, abscesses, lymphadenopathy, and infiltrative processes of the liver and spleen. The recognizable cross-sectional image produced by a CT scan is especially important for studying the pancreas because this organ is retroperitoneal and well hidden by the overlying peritoneal organs.

The image results from passing x-rays through the patient's abdomen at many angles. The variation in density of each tissue allows for variable penetration of the x-rays. Each density is given a numeral value called a coefficient, which is digitally computed into shades of gray. This is then displayed on a television screen as thousands of dots in various shades of gray. The final display appears as an actual photograph of the anatomic area sectioned by the x-rays (Figure 4-14). The study is only two-dimensional (that is, anterior to posterior and right to left). However, if one looks at a series of cross-sectional views from the foot to the head, a three-dimensional appearance is created and allows the abdominal organs to be examined in detail. For example, in acute pancreatitis, the pancreas is seen as a diffusely enlarged edematous organ. In chronic pancreatitis, pancreatic calcification can be seen. Pancreatic cancer is shown as a localized mass with a density coefficient different and distinct from that of the surrounding normal pancreatic tissue. Peripancreatic cysts (such as pseudocysts and abscesses) are easily seen as masses with a density coefficient indicating fluid. The radiation exposure that the patient incurs with this procedure is minimal.

Procedure. The patient is kept fasting for 4 hours before the test. Sedation is rarely required and is given only to the patient who cannot remain still during the length of the procedure. The patient is taken to the radiology department and is asked to remain motionless in the supine position, because any motion causes blurring and streaking of the final picture. An encircling x-ray camera (body scanner) takes pictures at varying levels (usually 1 to 2 cm apart) of the abdomen from the pubis to the xiphoid process. A monitor allows for immediate display, and the images are recorded on x-ray type film. The procedure takes about 30 minutes and is painless.

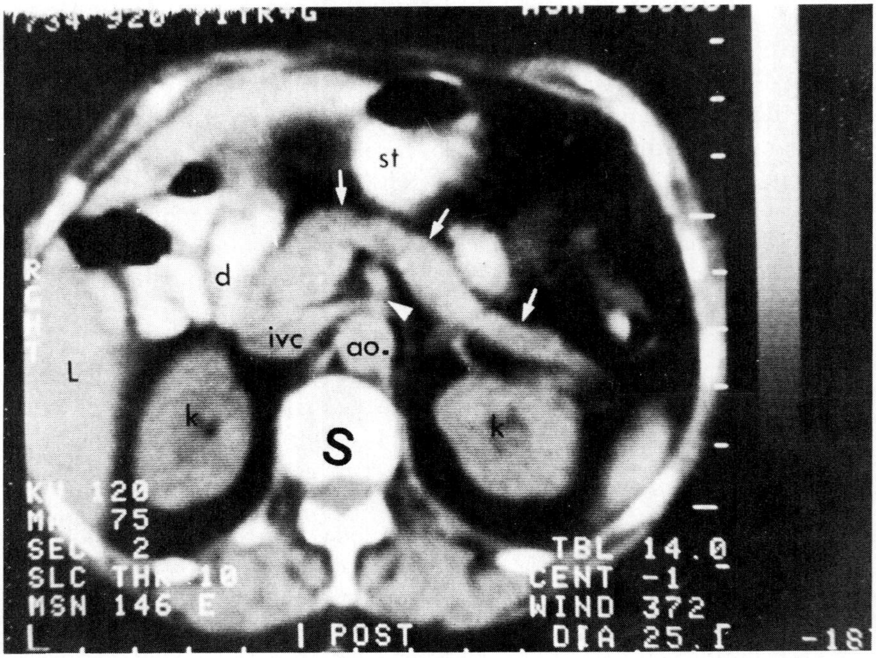

FIGURE 4-14. Computed tomogram of the abdomen showing a cross-sectional view of the abdomen at the level of the pancreas. *St,* Stomach; *d,* duodenum (both the stomach and the duodenum contain gastrografin); *L,* liver; *k,* kidneys; *ivc,* inferior vena cava; *ao.*, aorta; *S,* spine. Arrows indicate pancreas; pointer indicates superior mesenteric vessels.

The patient is given radiographic water-soluble dye by mouth, by IV, and occasionally via the rectum depending on the type of scan being performed. This contrast agent helps delineate the margins of the abdominal structure to afford better visualization.

Contraindications. This test is contraindicated in the uncooperative patient and during pregnancy. Patients with iodine allergies should not receive IV contrast.

Nursing considerations

Nursing Diagnoses/Collaborative Problems

See X-ray studies, p. 5.

- High risk for anxiety related to placement within large body scanner

Nursing Implications with Rationale

- Explain procedure to the patient. The patient's cooperation is necessary, since he or she must lie still during the procedure.
- If possible, show the patient a picture of the machine and encourage the patient to verbalize his or her fears, since some patients may suffer claustrophobia when their bodies are enclosed in the machine.
- Keep the patient NPO for 4 hours before the test. Food in the stomach or duodenum may confuse the final picture.
- Not all hospitals have CT equipment. You may have to make arrangements to transport the patient to another facility.

Endoscopic retrograde cholangiopancreatography of the pancreatic duct

(ERCP of the pancreatic duct)

Normal values: patent pancreatic duct.

Rationale. Not only can the biliary system be visualized by ERCP (see p. 106) but also the pancreatic duct (Figure 4-9). ERCP of the pancreas is a sensitive and reliable procedure for detecting clinically significant degrees of pancreatic dysfunction. Localized pancreatic duct narrowing indicates tumor (Figure 4-10). Chronic pancreatitis is demonstrated by multiple areas of ductal narrowing, alternating with duct dilatation.

Pathologic leakage of the pancreatic duct (secondary to tumor or inflammation) will be contained by pseudocyst formation or will leak freely into the peritoneal cavity. ERCP visualization of the pancreatic duct will demonstrate the site of the leakage. This is very helpful to the surgeon in deciding on the appropriate therapy.

Procedure. See previous section on ERCP, pp. 106-107.

Contraindications. See p. 107.

Nursing considerations

Nursing Diagnoses/Collaborative Problems

See Endoscopic procedures, pp. 6-7.

- Potential complication: perforation
- Potential complication: sepsis

Nursing Implications with Rationale

See pp. 107-108.

SUPPLEMENTAL INFORMATION

Provocative morphine-prostigmine (Nardi) test

Normal value: negative.

Rationale. A considerable number of patients have intermittent epigastric discomfort as a presenting symptom. These patients usually have been thoroughly evaluated for gallstones or recurrent pancreatitis. When the results are negative, the cause of the pain is often labeled as "psychogenic." Unfortunately, the patient's pain persists, frustrating the surgeon, internist, and psychiatrist. The provocative morphine-prostigmine test for pancreatitis and pappilitis is described by George Nardi. In this test, morphine and prostigmine are given intramuscularly causing marked contractions of the pancreatobiliary tract. If obstruction to outflow of the pancreatobiliary tract exists (e.g., by stenosis or inflammatory edema of the ampulla of Vater papillae), the patient will have recurrence of pain and elevation of at least one serum pancreatic enzyme (amylase or lipase), liver enzymes, or bile acids. When this happens, the test is considered positive, suggesting that the patient has an outflow obstruction of the pancreatobiliary tree. Many of these patients will improve after surgical sphincterotomy or endoscopic papillotomy. (See p. 89 for further discussion of pancreatic biliary anatomy.) Complications to the test may include such severe pain as to require admission to the hospital.

The accuracy of the Nardi test is not great. Normal patients and those with other diseases (such as irritable bowel syndrome) may have a positive morphine-prostigmine provocative test. Furthermore, the same patient may have a positive test one day and not on another. When biliary duct manometric pressures are measured in addition to symptomatic experience of pain and the measuring serum pancreatic enzyme levels, the accuracy of the Nardi provocative test is increased.

Procedure. Patients are given an IM injection of 10 mg of morphine sulfate and 1 mg of prostigmine. Baseline blood samples for serum amylase, bile acids, AST, ALT, and lipase are drawn initially and subsequently every 30 minutes for 4 hours. The patient is observed for clinical signs of abdominal pain, nausea, or vomiting. The patient is assessed to determine whether the provoked symptoms were similar to the previous abdominal pain episodes. A test is considered positive when enzyme levels are increased four-fold over baseline values. The reproduction or recurrence of symptoms are confirmatory and suggestive of a positive test. The patient is usually asked not to eat anything for at least 8 hours before testing and not to eat any fatty foods for the subsequent 12 hours. The study takes about 4 to 5 hours and is often done in the GI endoscopy suite, although it can also be done in the laboratory or in the same-day surgery department. No anesthesia or sedation is required and is, in fact, contraindicated. Results may be affected by sedation.

Contraindications. This test is contraindicated

in patients with jaundice, gallstones, and pancreatobiliary obstructions.

Nursing considerations

Nursing Diagnoses/Collaborative Problems

See Blood studies, p. 2.

Nursing Implications with Rationale

- Make sure the baseline blood samples are drawn before the study and at the designated 30-minute intervals.
- Carefully assess the patients for provoked symptoms of pain similar to those experienced in previous painful episodes.
- Institute safety measures to protect the patient because of the sedative effect of the medications.

CASE STUDY 3: CHILD WITH CYSTIC FIBROSIS

R.T., 9 months old, was brought to his pediatrician by his mother for evaluation of recurrent respiratory tract infections. During the examination the doctor noted the infant's thin extremities and distended abdomen. No weight gain was evident since the child's checkup at the age of 6 months. When questioned about the baby's stools, his mother said they had gotten large and foul smelling since she had started him on solid foods.

Studies	Results
Chest x-ray study	Patchy atelectasis, segmental hyperaeration, and air trapping
Sweat electrolytes test (by iontophoresis)	
Sodium	95 mEq/L (normal: <70 mEq/L)
Chloride	65 mEq/L (normal: <50 mEq/L)
Secretin-pancreozymin test (duodenal aspirate)	Absence of trypsin
Fecal fat (fat absorption) test	
72-hour collection	Fat retention coefficient: 80% (normal: ≥95%)

The findings of the chest x-ray study indicated a significant degree of bronchiolar obstruction causing atelectasis distally. Compensatory hyperaeration was also seen. With the history compatible with fat malabsorption and the bronchiolar obstruction (most probably caused by thickened mucus), the diagnosis of cystic fibrosis was considered. The sweat electrolytes test confirmed the diagnosis, as did the secretin-pancreozymin and fat absorption tests.

The parents were instructed in appropriate pulmonary therapy. A high-protein, low-fat diet (with medium-chain triglycerides) and pancreatic enzyme replacement were prescribed. Water-soluble vitamins were started. The patient gradually gained weight and returned to a near-normal growth pattern.

DISCUSSION OF TESTS

Sweat electrolytes test

(iontophoretic sweat test)

Sodium

Values in children
Normal: <70 mEq/L
Equivocal: 70-90 mEq/L
Abnormal: >90 mEq/L

Chloride

Values in children
Normal: <50 mEq/L
Equivocal: 50-60 mEq/L
Abnormal: >60 mEq/L

Rationale. Patients with cystic fibrosis have increased sodium and chloride content in their sweat. This fact forms the basis of this test, which is both sensitive and specific for this disease. Cystic fibrosis is an inherited disorder characterized by abnormal secretion of exocrine glands within the bronchi, small intestines, pancreatic and bile ducts, and skin (sweat glands). Sweat, induced by electrical current (pilocarpine iontophoresis), is collected, and its sodium and chloride contents are measured. The degree of abnormality is no indication of the severity of cystic fibrosis; it merely indicates that the patient has the disease.

This test is indicated to rule out cystic fibrosis in children with recurrent respiratory tract infection, malabsorption syndrome, or failure to thrive. The test is not reliable during the first few weeks of life. When the test results are positive in a patient with the clinical features suggestive of cystic fibrosis, the diagnosis is certain. Almost all patients with cystic fibrosis have sweat sodium and chloride contents two to five times greater than the normal values.

High serum concentrations of immunoreactive trypsin may prove to be diagnostic during the first 4 to 6 weeks of life when it is difficult to obtain sufficient sweat for testing. This can be used for routine newborn screening.

Procedure. No fluid or food restrictions are necessary. The test is usually performed in a lab by an experienced technician. For iontophoresis, a low level of electric current is applied to the test area (the thigh in infants, the forearm in older children). The iontophoresis unit contains two electrodes. The positive electrode is covered by gauze saturated with pilocarpine hydrochloride, a stimulating drug that induces sweating. The negative electrode is covered by gauze saturated with a bicarbonate solution. The electrodes are strapped onto the test area, and the iontophoresis unit is turned on for 5 to 12 minutes. The electrodes are then removed, the arm is washed with distilled water, and paper disks are placed over the test site by the use of dry, clean forceps. The disks are then covered with paraffin to obtain an airtight seal to prevent evaporation. After 1 hour, the paraffin is removed and the paper disks are transferred immediately by forceps to a weighing jar and sent for sodium and chloride analysis.

The sweat test takes about 1 to 1½ hours to perform. The electrical current is small, and no discomfort or pain is generally associated with the test. However, some patients report a slight stinging sensation. Inadvertent contact of the electrodes with the skin may cause a low-voltage shock or burn.

A screening test can now be done to detect sweat chloride levels. For this procedure a test paper containing silver nitrate is pressed against the child's hand for several seconds. The test is positive when the excess chloride combines with the silver nitrate to form white silver chloride on the paper. The child with cystic fibrosis will leave a heavy handprint on the paper. A positive screening test is usually validated by iontophoresis.

Contraindications. None.

Nursing considerations

Nursing Diagnoses/Collaborative Problems

- Possible knowledge deficit related to test purpose, preparation, and procedure
- Possible anxiety related to unknown sensations of procedure
- Possible alteration in comfort related to procedure
- Possible anxiety related to possible test results

Nursing Implications with Rationale

- Explain the procedure to the parent and the child (depending on the child's age). Role-playing with a doll may be helpful.
- Assure the parents and the child that the child will not be shocked by the electrical current.
- Completely saturate the gauze with the appropriate solution and cover the metal electrodes to avoid discomfort, pain, or skin burns.

Secretin-pancreozymin test

(pancreatic enzymes test)

Volume
Normal values: 2-4 cc/kg of body weight
HCO_3^- (bicarbonate)
Normal values: 90-130 mEq/L
Amylase
Normal values: 6.6-35.2 units/kg of body weight

Rationale. Measurement of the pancreatic enzymes (amylase, lipase, trypsin, and chymotrypsin) may be used to confirm the diagnosis of cystic fibrosis and other exocrine pancreatic diseases. Children with cystic fibrosis have mucous plugs that obstruct their pancreatic ducts. The pancreatic enzymes cannot be expelled into the duodenum and are therefore either completely absent or present only in diminished quantities in a duodenal aspirate. Secretin and pancreozymin are hormones used to stimulate pancreatic secretion of these enzymes. The duodenal contents are aspirated through a Dreiling tube and the pH, bicarbonate level, and enzyme content of the aspirate are determined. Variations in the enzyme levels usually parallel one another so that ordinarily only one enzyme determination is necessary. Amylase is most commonly measured.

Procedure. After a 12-hour fast, the patient goes to the radiology department. With the use of fluoroscopy (an x-ray picture displayed immediately on a television screen) a Dreiling tube is passed through the nose. The distal lumen is to be placed within the duodenum; the proximal lumen lies within the stomach. Both lumens are aspirated separately. This avoids gastric contents mixing with duodenal contents and altering the test results. The duodenum is aspirated until the contents are clear and the pH is basic. This ensures that no gastric (acid) contents are within the duodenum. A control specimen is collected for 20 minutes. The patient is then tested intradermally for sensitivity to secretin and pancreozymin. If no sensitivity is present, these hormones are administered intravenously. Secretin stimulates pancreatic water and bicarbonate secretions. Pancreozymin stimulates pancreatic enzyme secretion. Four duodenal aspirates are collected at 20-minute intervals and placed in specimen containers. These are placed on ice and sent to the laboratory for analysis of volume, bicarbonate content, pH level, and enzyme determination. A pH reading of less than 7 indicates contamination by gastric contents and thus invalidates the test results.

This test takes approximately 2 hours. It can be performed in the laboratory or on the ward. The patient may have discomfort and gagging during placement of the NG tube.

Contraindications. This test is contraindicated in the uncooperative patient.

Nursing considerations

Nursing Diagnoses/Collaborative Problems

- Possible knowledge deficit related to test purpose, preparation, and procedure
- Possible anxiety related to unknown sensations of procedure
- High risk for alteration in comfort related to procedure

Nursing Implications with Rationale

- Explain the procedure to the patient (and to parents if appropriate).
- Keep the adult patient NPO for 12 hours before the study to avoid the presence in the duodenum of food, which may block the aspirating lumen. The NPO time for children varies according to age.
- Tell the patient (and the parents) that he or she will receive an intradermal injection to identify sensitivities to the drugs before they are administered intravenously.
- After the test is completed, clamp and withdraw the NG tube. Give mouth and nose care. Allow the patient to resume a normal diet.

Fecal fat test

(fat absorption test, quantitative stool fat determination)

Normal values: 5 g/24 hours or fat retention coefficient ≥95%.

Rationale. This test measures the fat content in feces. The total output of fecal fat per 24 hours in a 3-day stool collection provides the most reliable measurement.

Obstructed pancreatic ducts caused by mucous plugs (as in cystic fibrosis) or tumors (as in pancreatic cancer) prevent the pancreatic enzymes from entering the gut. Some of these enzymes are lipolytic, and without them fat is not catabolized for absorption. This results in impaired fat absorption (malabsorption). The patient's stools are large, greasy, and foul-smelling. This passage of large amounts of fat into feces is called *steatorrhea.* Steatorrhea can also occur in malabsorption syndromes.

Analysis of fecal fat, although reliable, is not specific to cystic fibrosis. Any condition affected by malabsorption or maldigestion is associated with increased fecal fat. Also, when the gastrointestinal absorption surface area or the time of absorption is markedly decreased, fecal fat is increased (as in bowel hypermobility, massive bowel resection, and antiobesity surgical procedures).

Procedure. For quantitative stool analysis, a timed stool collection and a standard amount of fat content in the diet are essential. Generally, a 3- to 5-day stool collection is required to eliminate daily variations in the amount of fecal fat. The standard fat-content diet should begin 2 to 3 days before the stool collection and continue throughout the collection period. Usually 100 g of fat per day is suggested for adults. In children and infants who cannot eat a 100 g fat per day, a fat retention coefficient is determined by measuring the difference between ingested fat and fecal fat and then expressing that difference (the amount of fat retained) as a percentage of the ingested fat.

$$\frac{\text{Ingested fat} - \text{Fecal fat}}{\text{Ingested fat}} \times 100\%$$

The fat retention coefficient in normal children and adults is 95% or higher. A lower value is indicative of steatorrhea. Each stool specimen is collected and labeled with the name of the patient, the time of collection, and the date and is sent immediately to the laboratory.

Contraindications. None.

Nursing considerations

Nursing Diagnoses/Collaborative Problems

See Fecal studies, p. 4.

Nursing Implications with Rationale

- Explain the purpose of this test and the procedure of stool collection to the patient (and to the parents).
- Tell the patient to defecate into a dry, clean bedpan or container. Give the patient tongue blades to transfer the stool if needed. For an infant the diapers must be examined for stools and the stools transferred to the stool container.
- Tell the patient not to urinate into the stool container or bedpan.
- Tell the patient that diarrheal stools should also be collected.
- Explain to the patient that toilet paper should not be placed into the stool container because it interferes with stool analysis.
- Do not administer laxatives (especially mineral oil) or enemas to the patient, because they interfere with intestinal motility and alter the results.
- Label all specimens appropriately and send them to the laboratory as soon as they are collected.

QUESTIONS AND ANSWERS

1. **QUESTION:** Why is the biliary tract rarely visualized by oral cholecystography or IVC in patients with jaundice?

   ANSWER: The dye used in these studies must be processed by the liver. In patients who have jaundice, hepatocyte function is usually decreased. Therefore, the liver is unable to process the dye adequately for excretion within the biliary tract. The excretion of the dye into the biliary ducts allows for radiographic visualization.
2. **QUESTION:** In a nonjaundiced patient who is suspected of having cholecystitis, which should be performed initially, oral cholecystography or IVC?

   ANSWER: Oral cholecystography should be performed first because:
   a. Oral cholecystography is less invasive than IVC.
   b. Oral cholecystography allows for better and more frequent visualization of the gallbladder than IVC.
3. **QUESTION:** Your patient is scheduled to have oral cholecystography, an upper GI series, and ultrasound examination of the gallbladder. Which should be done first and why?

ANSWER: Because ultrasound cannot penetrate the radiopaque contrast medium used in oral cholecystography or in an upper GI series, the ultrasonography should be done first. Next, the oral cholecystography should be done. If the upper GI series were to precede the oral cholecystography, residual barium could obstruct the radiographic visualization of the gallbladder. The upper GI series is done last.

4. **QUESTION:** Your patient is having nothing by mouth and has an NG tube in place. Oral cholecystography has been ordered. When you come to administer the iopanoic acid tablets, the patient tells you he will vomit them if he tries to swallow. What is the appropriate intervention?
   ANSWER: Crush the tablets and inject them through the NG tube. Flush the NG tube to make sure all of the tablet material is out of the tube. Clamp the tube for 2 hours. If the patient vomits before that time, notify the physician. Either the oral cholecystography will have to be rescheduled or IVC will have to be performed.
5. **QUESTION:** Your patient is 2 months pregnant and is being evaluated for pancreatitis. An ultrasound examination of her gallbladder and pancreas has been ordered. The patient is concerned that the test may harm her unborn child. What is the appropriate intervention?
   ANSWER: Reassure the patient that ultrasound has been proven to be harmless to pregnant women and unborn children. Explain that ultrasonography is based on sound-wave transmission and that no x-ray films are taken.
6. **QUESTION:** Is ERCP necessary in all patients who have acute pancreatitis?
   ANSWER: No. On the contrary, ERCP is rarely performed on patients with acute pancreatitis because the cause of the inflammation is usually obvious (gallstones, alcohol, or penetrating peptic ulcer). However, when the cause of pancreatitis is not obvious, tumor must be ruled out. ERCP is the most reliable method to rule out pancreatic tumor.
7. **QUESTION:** A patient with jaundice is scheduled for ERCP. He has been complaining of vague right upper quadrant abdominal pain. He tells you that he needs a shot for pain before he goes for ERCP. (Morphine has been ordered for him every 4 hours.) What is the appropriate intervention?
   ANSWER: Explain that morphine sulfate cannot be given because it causes severe spasm of the sphincter of Oddi. With the patient having that spasm, the endoscopist will not be able to catheterize the sphincter and perform the ERCP. Inform the patient that he will receive meperidine before the test and that this will alleviate his pain.
8. **QUESTION:** Before sending your jaundiced patient for PTHC his prothrombin time (PT) test results come to the floor. The PT is 50% of normal. What should you do?
   ANSWER: Notify the physician. He most probably will want to cancel the study, because inadvertent puncture of a large blood vessel in a patient with a coagulation disorder could be disastrous. The physician most probably will recommend vitamin K be given for 2 to 3 days. Then the PT test should be repeated. If the PT test results are normal, the PTHC can be performed.
9. **QUESTION:** On returning from having PTHC, your patient becomes hypotensive. What is the appropriate nursing intervention?
   ANSWER:
   a. Notify the physician.
   b. Increase the IV rate and place the patient in the Trendelenburg position.
   c. Assess the patient for signs of gram-negative septic shock: fever, chills, warm and flushed skin, disorientation.
   d. Assess the patient for signs of hemorrhagic shock secondary to inadvertent puncture of a large blood vessel: coldness, clamminess, pallor, air hunger, tachycardia.
   e. Draw a complete blood count and a hemoglobin/hematocrit count. If the count of white cells is elevated, consider sepsis. If the hemoglobin/hematocrit count is decreased, consider hemorrhage.
   f. If septic shock exists, the physician will order appropriate antibiotics.
   g. If hemorrhagic shock exists, blood and volume replacement should be given. Surgery may be necessary for repair of the ruptured blood vessel.
10. **QUESTION:** Your patient has an increase in urine amylase level and a normal serum amylase level. Could this patient have pancreatitis?
    ANSWER: Yes. The early transient rise in the serum level amylase may have been missed. The

urine level stays elevated for a longer period of time.

11. **QUESTION:** Your patient returns from T-tube cholangiography. The study was normal, and the physician removed the tube in the radiology department. After arriving on the floor, you notice a large quantity of bile draining from the former T-tube site. What is appropriate intervention?
ANSWER:
a. Notify the physician.
b. Culture the bile; the results may be important if the bile causes a subsequent peritonitis.
c. Establish a sterile drainage system that will protect the skin from autodigestion from the bile.
d. Accurately measure and collect the quantity of bile drainage daily.
e. If the bile leak persists, bile salt depletion may ensue. Check with the physician about refeeding the bile drainage to the patient either by a feeding tube or orally, mixed in orange juice.

BIBLIOGRAPHY

Aldrete JS: Acute pancreatitis. In Rakel RE, editor: Conn's current therapy, Philadelphia, 1991, WB Saunders.

Bone R: Cystic fibrosis. In Wyngaarden JB and others, editors: Cecil textbook of medicine, ed 19, Philadelphia, 1992, WB Saunders.

Beeler MF, Kao YS, and Scheer WD: Malabsorption, diarrhea, and examination of feces. In Henry JB, editor: Todd-Sanford-Davidsohn clinical diagnosis and management of laboratory methods, ed 16, vol 1, Philadelphia, 1979, WB Saunders.

Boat TF: Cystic fibrosis. In Behrman RE, editor: Nelson textbook of pediatrics, ed 14, Philadelphia, 1992, WB Saunders.

Conn M: Preoperative evaluation of patients with liver disease, Mt Sinai J Med 58 (1):75-80, 1991.

Dienstag JL, Wands JR, and Isselbacher KJ: Acute hepatitis. In Wilson J and others, editors: Harrison's principles of internal medicine, ed 12, New York, 1991, McGraw-Hill.

Greenberger NJ and Toskes PP: Approach to the patient with pancreatic disease. In Wilson J and others, editors: Harrison's principles of internal medicine, ed 12, New York, 1991, McGraw-Hill.

Iber FL: Cirrhosis. In Rakel RF, editor: Conn's current therapy, Philadelphia, 1991, WB Saunders.

Linn HH and others: Is preoperative ultrasound cancer screening necessary in patients with normal liver function tests? J Clin Gastroenterol 13(1):108-110, 1991.

Malet PF and Soloway RD: Diseases of the gallbladder and bile duct. In Wyngaarden JB and others, editors: Cecil textbook of medicine, ed 19, Philadelphia, 1992, WB Saunders.

Podolsky DK and Isselbacher KJ: Diagnostic procedures in liver disease. In Wilson J and others, editors: Harrison's principles of internal medicine, ed 12, New York, 1991, McGraw-Hill.

Saltzstein EC and Mercer LC: Cholecystitis and cholelithiasis. In Rakel RF, editor: Conn's current therapy, Philadelphia, 1991, WB Saunders.

Sarr MG and others: Chronic pancreatitis. In Rakel RE, editor: Conn's current therapy, Philadelphia, 1991, WB Saunders.

Scharschmidt BF: Hepatic tumors. In Wyngaarden JB and others, editors: Cecil textbook of medicine, ed 19, Philadelphia, 1992, WB Saunders.

Tanaka S and others: Effectiveness of periodic checkup by ultrasonography for early diagnosis of hepatocellular carcinomas, Cancer 66(10):2210-2214, 1991.

Thibodeau GA: Anatomy and physiology, St Louis, 1987, CV Mosby.

Thoeni RF: Clinical application of magnetic resonance imaging of the liver, Invest Radiol 26(3):266-273, 1991.

Thoeni RF: Imaging of the liver, Curr Opin Radiol 3(3):427-439, 1991.

Weisinger RA: Laboratory tests in liver disease. In Wyngaarden JB and others, editors: Cecil textbook of medicine, ed 19, Philadelphia, 1992, WB Saunders.

Chapter 5

DIAGNOSTIC STUDIES USED IN THE ASSESSMENT OF THE
PULMONARY SYSTEM

ANATOMY AND PHYSIOLOGY

The lungs are elastic sponge-like structures located within the thoracic cavity, one on either side of the chest. Their outer surface is enveloped by a two-layered membrane (pleura) that covers each lung and lines the thoracic cavity. The pleura is termed *visceral* where it covers the lungs and *parietal* where it lines the thorax. Between the two layers is a potential space called the pleural space. A small amount of fluid lubricates the pleural surfaces and prevents any friction between the lungs and the thorax during respiration.

Each lung is divided into subsections called lobes. The right lung has three lobes (upper, middle, lower); the left lung has two lobes (upper and lower). Each lobe is further divided into segments. Each pulmonary segment is ventilated by its own bronchiole, perfused by its own pulmonary arteriole, and drained by its own pulmonary venule. These structures are branches of the bronchus, pulmonary artery, and pulmonary vein respectively. These structures enter the lung at its root (hilus) (Figure 5-1).

Air travels through the nose, trachea, bronchus and bronchiole to end up in the alveoli (tiny air sacs). Each alveolus is in close association with a pulmonary arteriole and venule. Together the alveoli and their blood supply form the basic unit of the pulmonary system, where the exchange of oxygen and carbon dioxide ultimately takes place. The human lung contains approximately 300 million of these microscopic units (alveoli). Cells contained within the alveolar walls secrete a lipoprotein called *surfactant*. This substance prevents complete alveo-

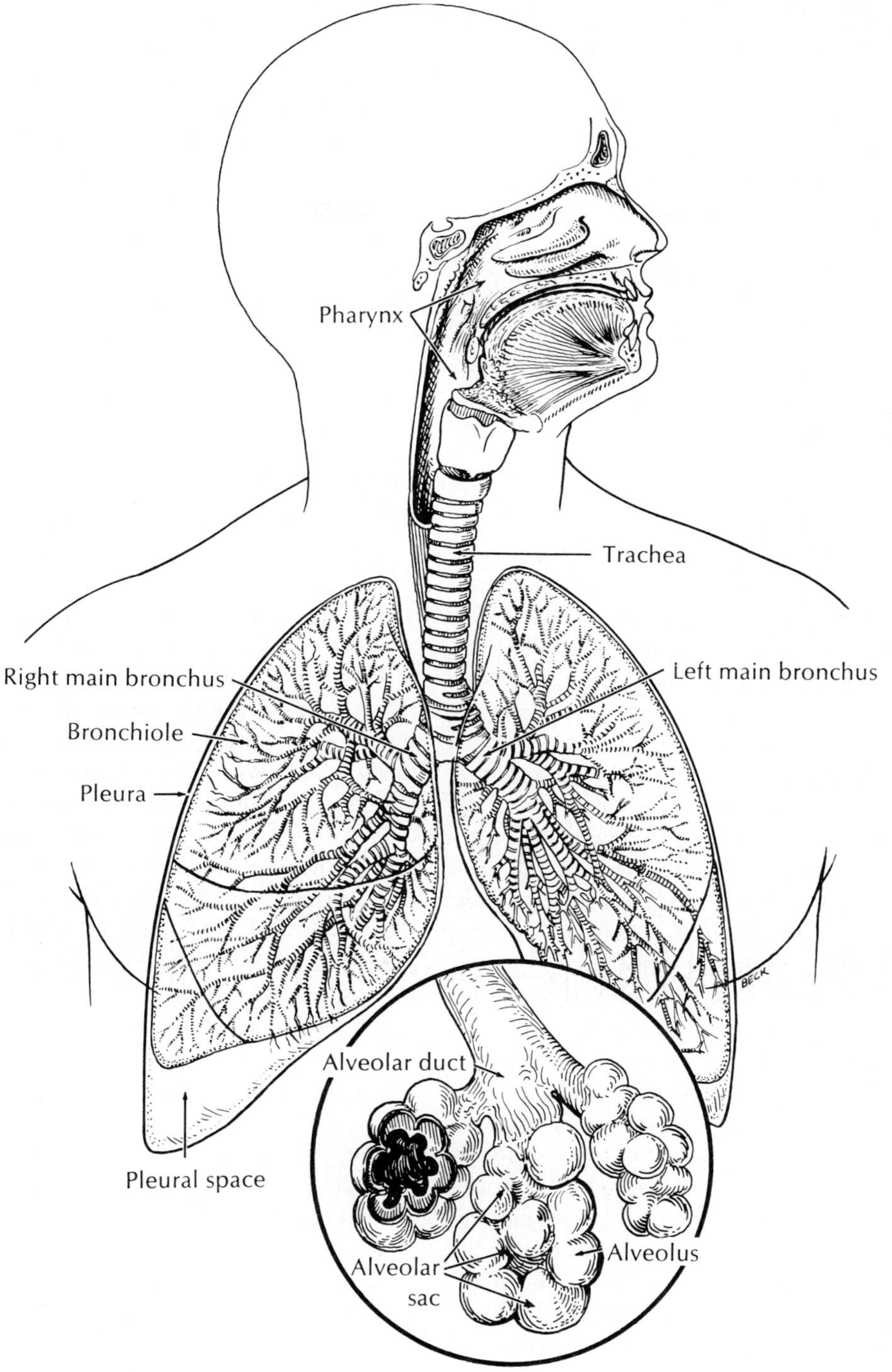

FIGURE 5-1. Normal anatomy of the pulmonary system: pharynx, trachea, and lungs. The inset shows the grapelike alveolar sacs, where air and blood exchange oxygen and carbon dioxide through the thin walls of the alveoli. Capillaries (not shown) surround the alveoli. From Anthony CP and Kolthoff NJ: Textbook of anatomy and physiology, ed 9, St Louis, 1975, The CV Mosby Co.

lar collapse at the end of expiration. If this collapse were to occur, high inflating pressures would be required for reexpansion. This would increase the work of respiration.

Ventilation

The process of ventilation includes two phases: inspiration and expiration. During inspiration, contraction of the diaphragm and intercostal muscles causes the thoracic cavity to enlarge and thus to decrease intrathoracic pressure below atmospheric pressure. Air is then drawn into the lungs.

During expiration the muscles of respiration relax, causing the thoracic cavity to decrease in size. The intrathoracic pressure then becomes greater than atmospheric pressure, causing air to flow from the lungs into the atmosphere.

The stimulus for respiration is controlled by the respiratory center in the medulla of the brain. Chemoreceptors located in the aortic arch and the carotid bifurcation assess the level of CO_2 and O_2 in the blood. CO_2 is most important in respiratory control. When the CO_2 level of the blood increases (hypercapnia), the chemoreceptors relay that message to the medulla. The medulla then stimulates the person to breathe. Central (brain) chemoreceptors sensitive to CO_2 and O_2 are also in the cerebrospinal fluid. O_2 is a much less forceful stimulant to the chemoreceptors in normal people. Yet in patients with chronic obstructive pulmonary disease (COPD), these chemoreceptors get used to chronically high blood-CO_2 levels and become insensitive to CO_2. O_2 then assumes the role of respiratory stimulant. This is important, because when the O_2 level in a patient with COPD is artificially raised (for example, by use of an oxygen mask) to high levels, the stimulus for breathing (that is, a low O_2 level or, hypoxemia) is lost and the patient may stop breathing.

In addition to the effect of pressure gradients existing between the thoracic cavity and the atmosphere, inspiration and expiration are also affected by lung and thoracic cavity compliance. The term *compliance* refers to the ease with which lung tissue may be stretched. Compliance is expressed as the volume inhaled per unit of pressure required to expand the lung during that inhalation (volume in cubic centimeters and pressure in centimeters of water). A compliant lung (high compliance) expands easily when pressure is applied. A noncompliant or stiff lung (low compliance) requires greater than normal amounts of pressure for reexpansion; therefore the patient must expand greater energy to achieve normal ventilation.

Pulmonary circulation

Almost the entire cardiac output of the right ventricle passes through the capillaries of the lung and comes into close contact with the alveoli. Here the O_2 moves from the alveoli to the blood, and CO_2 moves in reverse. A small percentage of the right ventricle's output does not participate in gas exchange and bypasses the alveoli. This unoxygenated blood returns to the left atrium, where it mixes with the oxygenated blood. The movement of this blood, which bypasses the pulmonary circulation, is referred to as a "right-to-left shunt." The end result of this shunt, although it is physiologically normal, is to lower the O_2 in the arterial blood. If the amount of shunted blood were to increase, severe hypoxia could be the result. Examples of this include pneumonia, where some of the alveoli are filled with pus, and adult respiratory distress syndrome (as in shock lung and pulmonary edema), where alveoli are filled with fluid. When the alveoli are filled, no air can ventilate them; therefore the blood supplying those alveoli must return to the left atrium without the opportunity for gas exchange and oxygenation. This causes an increase in the amount of blood shunted from the right to the left side of the heart, and profound hypoxemia results.

CASE STUDY 1: LUNG CANCER

Mr. N. was a 63-year-old man who had a long history of cigarette smoking. He had a chronic cough but more recently had noticed blood-

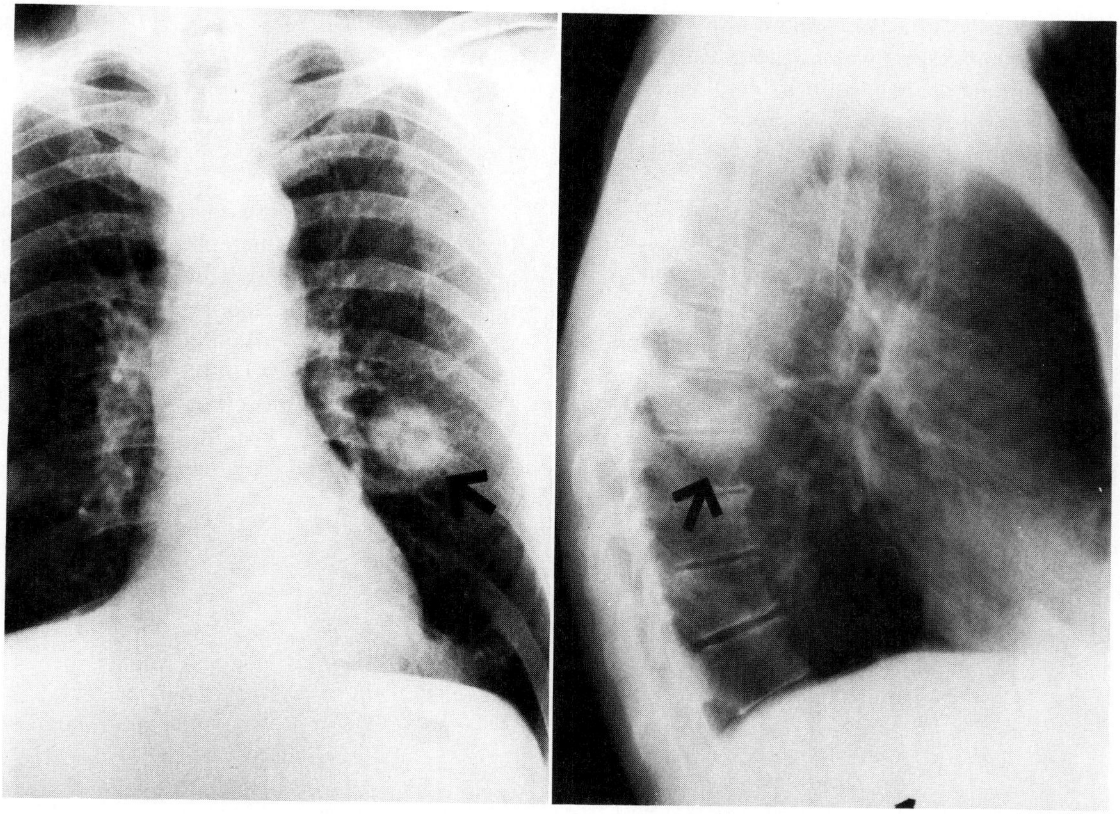

FIGURE 5-2. Chest x-ray film showing tumor in the left lung. **A,** Posterior-anterior view. **B,** Lateral view.

streaked sputum. The results of his physical examination were normal.

Studies	Results
Routine laboratory work	Normal
Chest x-ray film	Mass in left lower lobe (Figure 5-2)
Tomograms of chest	Solid mass in left lower lobe (see Figure 5-6)
Sputum study for cytology, acid-fast bacilli (AFB), and culture and sensitivity	Positive for malignant cells; no AFB; normal throat flora
Bronchoscopy	Partially obstructing tumor in basal segment of left lower lobe
Lung biopsy	Squamous cell carcinoma
Mediastinoscopy	No lymph nodes affected by tumor

Studies	Results
Pulmonary function studies	
Forced vital capacity	3400 cc (predicted: 3800 cc)
Forced expiratory volume	2600 cc (predicted: 3000 cc)
Maximal midexpiratory flow	340 L/min (predicted: 360 L/min)
Maximal volume ventilation	120 L/min (predicted: 130 L/min)
Aterial blood gases study	pH: 7.41 (normal: 7.35-7.45)
	Po_2: 70 mm Hg (normal: 80-100 mm Hg)
	Pco_2: 33 mm Hg (normal: 35-45 mm Hg)
	(HCO_3^-: 24 mEq/L (normal: 22-26 mEq/L)

The mass seen in the lung on x-ray examination and tomography was considered to be malignant based on the sputum cytology study, bronchoscopy, and the lung biopsy results, indicating squamous cell carcinoma. Mediastinoscopy showed no involved mediastinal lymph nodes. If positive for metastasis, the tumor would have been considered to be inoperable. Preoperative pulmonary functions indicated that the patient could tolerate an aggressive surgical approach to this tumor, and a left lower-lobe lung resection, by means of a thoracotomy, was performed. Postoperatively Mr. N. had no problems. He died of unrelated problems 6 years later.

DISCUSSION OF TESTS

Chest x-ray study

(chest roentgenogram)

Normal values: normal lungs and surrounding structures.

Rationale. The chest x-ray study is important in the complete evaluation of the pulmonary and cardiac system. This procedure is often part of the general admission workup in adult patients (Figure 5-3). Much information can be provided by the x-ray study. One can identify or follow (by repeated chest x-ray studies) the following:

1. *Tumors* of the lung (primary, Fig 5-2, and

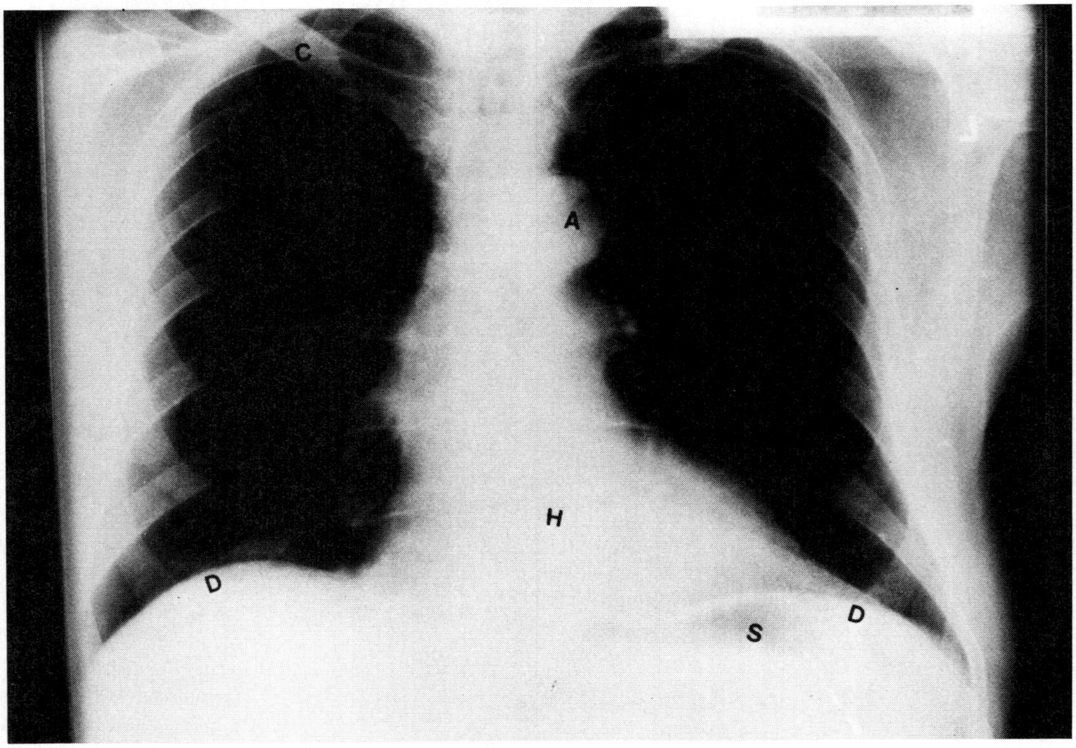

FIGURE 5-3. Normal chest x-ray film. *H,* heart; *D,* diaphragm; *A,* aortic arch; *S,* stomach bubble; *C,* clavicle.

metastatic, Fig 5-4), heart (myxoma), chest wall (soft-tissue sarcomas), and bony thorax (osteogenic or metastatic sarcoma)

2. *Inflammation* of the lung (pneumonia, Figure 5-5), pleura (pleuritis), and pericardium (pericarditis)
3. *Fluid accumulation* in the pleural cavity (pleural effusion), pericardium (pericardial effusion), and lung (pulmonary edema)
4. *Excess air accumulation* in the lung (COPD) and pleura (pneumothorax)
5. *Fractures* of the bones of the thorax
6. *Diaphragmatic hernia* (hiatal, Bochdalek, and Morgagni)

Procedure. Chest x-ray studies are best performed in the radiology department. Studies using a portable chest x-ray camera may be done at the bedside and are commonly performed on critically ill patients who cannot leave the nursing unit. The patient's clothing is removed down to the waist, and a gown or drape is put on the patient. Metal objects (such as necklaces, watches, and pins) must be removed; otherwise, they will show up on the x-ray film and obscure visualization of part of the chest.

A

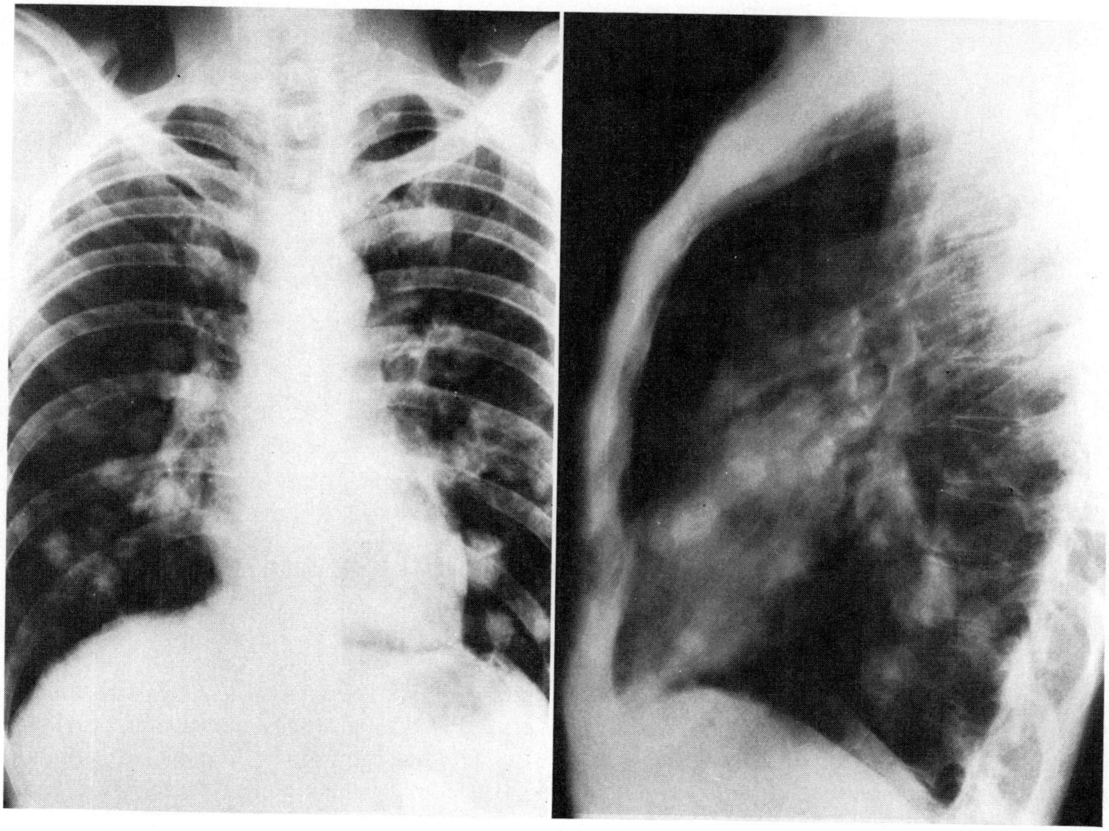

B

FIGURE 5-4. Chest x-ray film showing multiple metastatic nodules within the lung field. **A,** Posterior-anterior view. **B,** Lateral view.

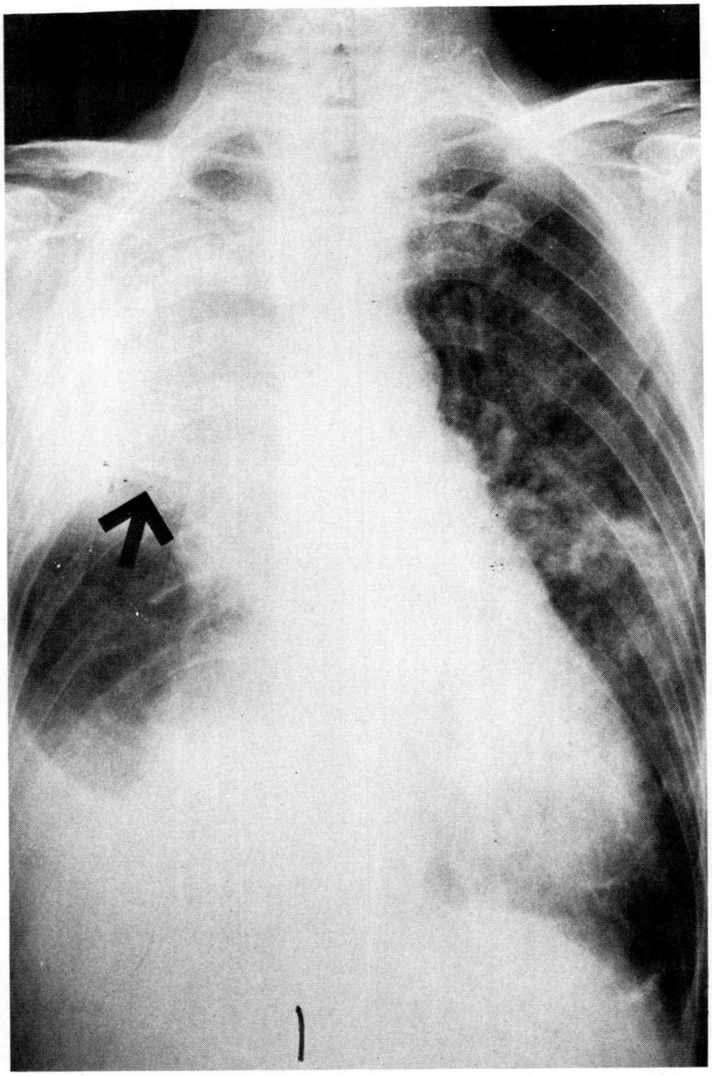

FIGURE 5-5. Chest x-ray film showing pneumonia consolidation *(arrow)*.

Most chest x-ray films are taken at a distance of 6 feet, with the patient standing. The sitting or supine position can also be used, but x-ray films taken with the patient in the supine position do not demonstrate fluid levels, if fluid is present. A *posteroanterior* (PA) view, with the x-rays passing through the back of the body (posterior) to the front of the body (anterior), is taken first. Then a *lateral* view, with the x-rays passing through the patient's side, is taken.

Oblique views may be taken with the x-rays slanted at specific angles as they pass through the body. *Lordotic* views provide visualization of the apices (rounded upper portions) of the lungs and are commonly used for tuberculosis detection. *Decubitus* films are taken with the patient in the recumbent lateral position to localize fluid in the pleural space (pleural effusion).

After the patient is correctly positioned, he or she is told to take a deep breath and hold it until the x-ray film is taken. X-ray films are taken by a radiologic technician in several minutes. The patient feels no discomfort.

Contraindications. X-ray studies are contraindicated in pregnancy. However, if such a study is needed, a lead shield should be placed over the uterus.

Nursing considerations

Nursing Diagnoses/Collaborative Problems

See X-ray studies, p. 5.

Nursing Implications with Rationale

- Explain the procedure to the patient.
- Tell the patient that clothing above the waist needs to be removed and that a gown will be supplied. If the patient will be going from a ward to the radiology department having the patient put on a gown before leaving the nursing unit is a good idea. This eliminates the need for dressing and undressing in the radiology department.
- Inform the patient that any metal objects (such as necklaces) need to be removed. Metal objects block the body structures that they cover and appear on the x-ray film.
- Tell the patient that he or she will be asked to take a deep breath and hold it while the x-ray film is being taken. This ensures that a maximum amount of air fills the lungs and allows a clear view of the pulmonary system. Any movement will blur the film.
- Premenopausal women who are not presently in their menstrual cycle should wear a metal apron over their abdominal organs. This is to prevent x-ray exposure to a fetus in the event that the woman is in early pregnancy.
- Men should cover their testes and women should cover their ovaries with a lead shield to prevent radiation-induced abnormalities that may result in congenital abnormalities in future children.

Tomography of the lung

(laminography, planigraphy)

Normal values: normal lungs and surrounding structures.

Rationale. Tomography is a radiographic technique by which a sequence of x-ray films, each representing a "slice" of the lung at different depths, is taken. Usually, the slices are made at 0.5 to 1.0 cm apart throughout the organ being studied. Tomography permits examination of a single layer or plane of tissue that would otherwise be obscured by the surrounding structures on an ordinary film.

For tomography, the x-ray tube and the film cassette are rapidly moved in opposite directions while the x-ray film is taken. This technique effectively blurs all tissue planes except that plane, or slice, being studied.

Tomography is often a helpful adjunct to a routine chest x-ray study for several reasons:

1. It may reveal properties of a lung lesion, such as cavitation and tumor margins, that normally are not seen on chest x-ray films. This is important because if, for example, a coin lesion found on a chest x-ray film were subsequently found on tomograms to be a well-defined cavity, tumor would be unlikely. If the lesion were found to be solid with ill-defined margins, malignancy would be suggested (Figure 5-6).
2. Many structures (such as the hilus, trachea, and mediastinum) are not seen clearly on routine chest x-ray films. Tomography provides better visualization of these structures.
3. Occasionally, many small lesions (as in metastasis) are not seen on routine chest x-ray films and can only be seen on certain tomographic cuts of the lung.

Indications for chest tomography have markedly diminished since the advent of CT of the

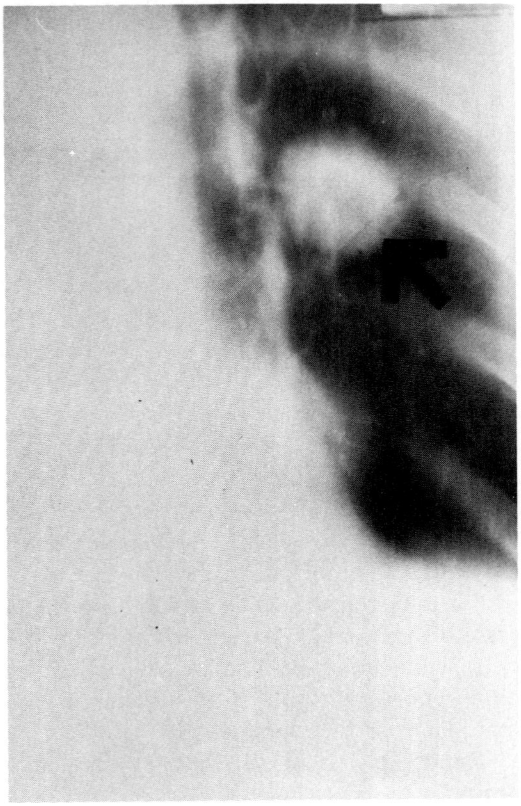

FIGURE 5-6. Tomogram of left lung. Arrow indicates a "solid" tumor.

chest (see p. 161) and magnetic resonance imaging (see p. 201). Tomography is mainly used in facilities where more advanced technology is not available.

Procedure. The nonfasting patient goes to the radiology department as for a routine chest x-ray study (see preceding discussion). With the patient remaining completely still, an x-ray tube is rapidly moved back and forth in one direction while the film is rapidly moved in the opposite direction. The excursion of this movement regulates the plane of tissue photographed. Prone, supine, and lateral positions may be required. The patient is unable to recognize these fine, synchronized movements of the tube and the x-ray film. The test is no more uncomfortable than a routine chest x-ray study, and it takes about 15 minutes. A radiologist usually performs tomography.

Contraindications. This procedure is contraindicated in the pregnant patient.

Nursing considerations

Nursing Diagnoses/Collaborative Problems

See X-ray studies, p. 5.

Nursing Implications with Rationale

- Explain to the patient the purpose and procedure for tomography.
- See the preceding discussion on the chest x-ray study.

Sputum studies

Culture and sensitivity (C & S)
Normal value: normal throat flora.
Acid-fast bacilli (AFB)
Normal value: no bacilli seen.
Cytology
Normal value: normal epithelial cells.

Rationale. Study of the patient's sputum can provide valuable information in the diagnostic workup of a patient with pathologic pulmonary conditions.

Culture and sensitivity (C & S). Sputum cultures are obtained to determine the presence of pathogenic bacteria in patients with respiratory infections, such as pneumonia. *Gram staining* is the first step in the microbiologic analysis of sputum. After staining the sputum, bacteria are classified as gram-positive or gram-negative. This may be used to guide drug therapy until determination of bacterial sensitivity to various antibiotics is done to identify the appropriate antimicrobial drug therapy. It is preferable that sputum for C & S be collected before antimicrobial therapy is initiated. Antibiotics can limit the growth of pathogenic bacteria in culture and thereby create a false-negative result.

Acid-fast bacilli (AFB). This sputum collection and analysis is usually ordered when tuberculosis is suspected. *Mycobacterium tuberculo-*

sis, after taking up a dye such as basic fuchsin, is not decolorized by acid-alcohol (that is, it is acid-fast) and is seen under the microscope as a red, rod-shaped organism. If this bacillus is seen, the patient has active tuberculosis. A special medium is required to culture this bacterium.

Cytology. Tumors within the pulmonary system frequently slough malignant cells into the sputum. When the sputum is gathered, the cells are examined. If the test is positive, malignant cells can be seen, indicating tumor. If only normal epithelial cells and no malignant cells are seen, either no malignancy exists or the tumor is not shedding cells. Therefore, a positive test indicates malignancy and a negative test cannot rule out cancer.

Procedure. Sputum specimens are best collected when the patient awakes and before the patient eats or drinks. Only sputum that has come from deep within the lungs should be collected. At least one teaspoon of sputum must be collected in a sterile, wide-mouth sputum container. Sputum is usually obtained by having the patient cough after taking several deep breaths. If the patient is unable to produce a sputum specimen, coughing can be stimulated by lowering the head of the patient's bed or by giving the patient an aerosol administration of a warm hypertonic solution. Other methods used to collect sputum include endotracheal aspiration, fiberoptic bronchoscopy (direct visualization and aspiration of bronchial secretion), and transtracheal aspiration (needle puncture into the trachea and aspiration through a catheter). These methods exclude oropharyngeal contamination of the specimen. For cytology or AFB determinations, sputum is usually collected on three separate occasions.

Contraindications. None.

Nursing considerations

Nursing Diagnoses/Collaborative Problems

- Possible knowledge deficit related to test purpose, preparation, and procedure

Nursing Implications with Rationale

- Explain the procedure for sputum collection to the patient. Remind the patient that the sputum must be coughed up from the lungs and that saliva is not sputum. The laboratory technician will evaluate the specimen according to specified criteria (such as the number of epithelial cells) to determine whether the specimen is sputum or saliva before studying it. Sputum contains columnar (bronchial) cells; saliva is identified by squamous (mouth) cells.
- Hold antibiotics until after the sputum has been collected. If the patient has been taking these drugs, they should be listed on the lab slip.
- Give the patient a sterile sputum container on the night before the sputum is to be collected, so that the morning specimen may be obtained on the patient's arising. Obtaining an early morning specimen is best because secretions pool and collect in the lungs during sleep. The early morning specimen is likely to be the most productive.
- Instruct the patient to rinse out his or her mouth with water before the sputum collection to decrease contamination of the sputum specimen by particles in the oropharynx. The patient should not use toothpaste or mouthwash because they can affect the viability of microorganisms in the sputum specimen.
- If an aerosol treatment is necessary, explain the procedure to the patient and point out that it will stimulate coughing and sputum expectoration.
- Inform the patient to notify the nurse as soon as the specimen is collected so it can be labeled appropriately and sent to the laboratory as soon as possible. For aesthetic reasons the sputum container should be wrapped in paper towels so that the contents cannot be seen.
- Provide the patient with an ample supply of tissues with which to wipe his or her mouth after expectorating.

Bronchoscopy

Normal values: normal larynx, trachea, bronchi, and alveoli.

Rationale. Bronchoscopy permits endoscopic visualization of the larynx, trachea, and bronchi by a flexible fiberoptic bronchoscope. Diagnostic uses of the bronchoscope include:

1. Direct visualization of the tracheobronchial tree for abnormalities such as tumors, inflammation, and strictures
2. Removal of biopsy specimens from observed lesions
3. Aspiration of "deep" sputum for C & S and cytology determinations

Therapeutic uses of the bronchoscope include:

1. Aspiration of retained secretions in patients with airway obstruction or postoperative atelectasis
2. Control of bleeding in areas within the bronchus
3. Removal of small, aspirated foreign bodies
4. Brachytherapy, which is endobronchial radiation therapy using iridium placed via the bronchoscope
5. Laser therapy for vaporization of bronchial obstructions

The rigid bronchoscope is a wide-bore metal tube that permits visualization of only the larger airways. Presently, it is mainly used for the removal of large foreign bodies. Its use has radically diminished since the advent of the newer flexible fiberoptic bronchoscope.

Because of its smaller size and its flexibility, the flexible fiberoptic scope has increased the diagnostic reach of bronchoscopy to the smaller bronchi. This newer scope has an accessory lumen through which cable-activated instruments can be used for removing biopsy specimens of pathologic lesions. Also, the collection of bronchial washings (obtained by flushing the airways with saline solution), pulmonary toilet, and the instillation of anesthetic agents can be carried out through this extra lumen. Double-sheathed, plugged-protected brushes can be passed through this accessory lumen. This allows more accurate determination of causative pulmonary infective agents and better cytology specimens. Laser vaporization can now be done through the bronchoscope to burn out endotracheal tumors. Complications of bronchoscopy include fever, hypoxemia, laryngospasm, bronchospasm, pneumothorax, or hemorrhage if a biopsy was performed. Complications are rare when this procedure is performed by an experienced endoscopist.

Procedure. The patient is kept NPO after midnight on the day of the bronchoscopy. *Fiberoptic bronchoscopy* is performed by a surgeon or pulmonary specialist at the bedside or preferably in an endoscopy room. Preoperative medications, such as atropine, 0.6 to 1.0 mg, and meperidine (Demerol), 50 mg, intramuscularly (IM) may be administered approximately 1 hour before the study.

The patient's nasopharynx and oropharynx are anesthetized topically with lidocaine (Xylocaine) spray before the insertion of the bronchoscope. Often this topical spray is preceded by an aerosol treatment with lidocaine. The patient is then placed in the sitting or supine position, and the tube is inserted through the nose or mouth and into the pharynx. After the tube passes into the larynx and through the glottis, more lidocaine is sprayed into the trachea to prevent the cough reflex. The tube is passed farther, well into the trachea, bronchi (Figure 5-7), and the first- and second-generation bronchioles for systematic examination of the bronchial tree. Biopsy specimens and washings are taken if a pathologic condition is seen or strongly suspected. If bronchoscopy is performed for pulmonary toilet (removal of mucus), each bronchus is aspirated until clear. This procedure takes less than 30 minutes and is somewhat uncomfortable for most patients.

Rigid bronchoscopy is usually performed in the operating room under general anesthesia. The patient is placed in the supine position with

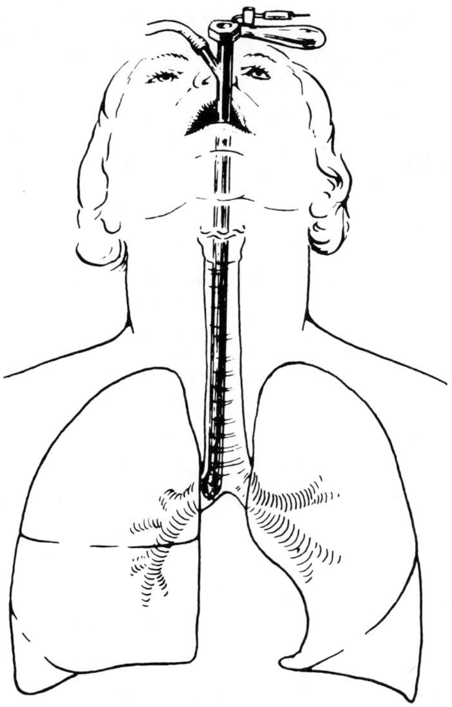

FIGURE 5-7. Bronchoscope inserted through trachea and into bronchus.
From DeWeese DD and Saunders WH: Textbook of otolaryngology, ed 6, St Louis, 1982, The CV Mosby Co.

the neck hyperextended. The tube is inserted through the mouth and larynx and then into the trachea.

Contraindications. Patients with hypercapnia and with severe shortness of breath who cannot tolerate interruption of high-flow O_2 should not have bronchoscopy studies.

Nursing considerations

Nursing Diagnoses/Collaborative Problems

See Endoscopic procedure, pp. 6-7.

- Potential complication: fever
- Potential complication: hypoxemia
- Potential complication: laryngospasm
- Potential complication: bronchospasm
- Potential complication: aspiration

Nursing Implications with Rationale

- Explain the procedure to the patient to reduce anxiety so that the patient can cooperate more fully. Encourage verbalization of the patient's feelings and fears.
- Ensure that the informed consent for this procedure is obtained before the patient is premedicated.
- Keep the patient NPO after midnight on the day of the study to prevent possible aspiration of gastric contents induced by gagging.
- Administer the preoperative medications as ordered. Atropine is used to prevent vagally induced bradycardia and to minimize secretion. (The patient may complain of having a dry mouth.) Meperidine or morphine is used to sedate the patient and relieve anxiety.
- Remove and safely store the patient's dentures, glasses, or contact lenses before administering the preprocedure medication.
- Reassure the patient that he or she will be able to breathe during this procedure.
- Instruct the patient not to swallow the local anesthetic sprayed into the throat. An emesis basin should be provided for expectoration of the lidocaine.
- After the procedure do not allow the patient to eat or drink anything until the tracheobronchial anesthesia has worn off and the gag reflex has returned, usually about 2 hours. A patient who eats or drinks anything before that time could unknowingly aspirate the food or drink and develop pneumonia.
- Observe the patient's sputum for hemorrhage if biopsy specimens were removed. A small amount of blood streaking is to be expected for several hours after bronchoscopy. Large amounts of bleeding (several ounces within 30 minutes) are disconcerting, because this blood may be drawn into the pulmonary alveoli and create a chemical pneumonitis.
- Monitor vital signs frequently, as ordered. Fever may be seen for 2 to 6 hours after the procedure because of chemical pneumonitis. Observe the patient closely for evidence of

impaired respiration or laryngospasm. Transient hoarseness is a complication. The vocal cords may go into spasms after intubation. Emergency resuscitation equipment (including tracheal tube, laryngoscope, and medications such as steroids and epinephrine) should be readily available.

- Observe postanesthesia precautions for the patient until the effect of the sedative medications no longer exist.
- Be aware that fever after bronchoscopy is very common within the first 24 hours.
- If tumor is suspected, collect postbronchoscopy sputum for a cytology determination. Frequently the deep secretions loosened by bronchoscopy may contain malignant cells diagnostic of lung tumor.
- Warm saline gargles and lozenges may be helpful if the patient complains of a sore throat.

Lung biopsy

Normal values: no evidence of pathology.

Rationale. This invasive procedure is used to obtain a specimen of pulmonary tissue for a histologic examination by either an open or closed technique. The open method involves a limited thoracotomy. The closed technique includes methods such as transbronchial lung biopsy, transbronchial needle aspiration biopsy, and transcatheter bronchial brushing, which are done through a bronchoscope.

Lung biopsy is indicated to identify the cause of a parenchymal pulmonary disease or a pulmonary tumor. Carcinomas, granulomas, and sarcoidosis can be diagnosed with this procedure. This procedure is also useful in detecting environmental risks, infections, or familial disease, which may lead to better patient prevention and treatment. Complications of lung biopsy are dictated by the procedure used to obtain them. However, the most common complications are pneumothorax, pulmonary hemorrhage, and empyema.

Procedure. The general procedure for a patient having a lung biopsy is keeping the patient NPO after midnight on the day of the biopsy. The patient is usually sedated ½ to 1 hour before the procedure. The position of the patient depends on the method used. The histologic specimen may be obtained by several different methods.

A *transbronchial lung biopsy* is performed via a flexible fiberoptic bronchoscopy using cutting forceps. Fluoroscopy is used to assure the proper opening and positioning of the forceps on the lesion. Fluoroscopy also permits visualization of the "tug" of the lung as the specimen is removed. For this procedure the patient is usually premedicated with atropine to reduce bronchial secretions and sedated with either meperidine or morphine.

Another technique of obtaining a lung specimen is by *transbronchial needle aspiration biopsy,* where the specimen is obtained via a fiberoptic bronchoscope using a needle. Before this procedure the patient is usually premedicated with atropine to reduce bronchial secretions. The bronchoscope is inserted. After the target site has been identified by fluoroscopy, the needle is inserted into the tumor, and aspiration is performed with the attached syringe and catheter. The needle is then retracted within its sheath, and the entire catheter is withdrawn from the fiberoptic bronchoscope. The bronchoscope is then removed.

A *transcatheter bronchial brushing* is also performed via a fiberoptic bronchoscope. During bronchoscopy a small brush is moved back and forth over the suspicious area. The cells adhere to the brush, which is then removed and wiped on microscopic slides. The bronchoscope is then removed.

Another method of obtaining a lung specimen is by *percutaneous needle biopsy.* This biopsy is obtained after using x-ray determination of the desired site. The procedure is carried out by using a cutting needle or by aspiration with a spinal-type needle to obtain a specimen. The main problem with this procedure is potential damage to major blood vessels and pneumothorax.

A final method of obtaining a lung specimen is by an *open-lung biopsy.* For this procedure the patient is taken to the operating room and general anesthesia is used. The patient is placed in the supine position, and a small thoracic incision is made in the chest wall. After a piece of lung tissue is removed, the lung is closed. Chest tube drainage is used for about 24 hours after an open-lung biopsy.

Contraindications. Lung biopsies are contraindicated in patients with bullae or cysts, suspected vascular anomalies, bleeding abnormalities, pulmonary hypertension, and respiratory insufficiency that is so severe that a small pneumothorax would present a distinct risk. This test is also contraindicated in the uncooperative patient. All these contraindications are relative; the risk must be weighed against the importance of securing a diagnosis by performing lung biopsy.

Nursing considerations

Nursing Diagnoses/Collaborative Problems

- Possible knowledge deficit related to test purpose, preparation, and procedure
- Possible alteration in comfort related to procedure
- Possible injury related to effects of sedatives
- Possible anxiety related to unknown sensations or procedure
- Potential complication: bleeding
- Potential complication: pneumothorax
- Potential complication: empyema

Nursing Implications with Rationale

- Explain the procedure to the patient and describe the method of obtaining a specimen. Ensure that the informed and signed consent is obtained.
- Ensure that the patient fasts as ordered. Usually the patient is kept NPO after midnight on the day of the test to prevent aspiration during the procedure.
- Administer the preprocedure medications as ordered 30 to 60 minutes before the test. Atropine is usually given before bronchoscopic examinations to decrease the bronchial secretions. Meperidine (Demerol) may be given to sedate anxious patients.
- During the lung biopsy instruct the patient to remain still. Any movement or coughing could cause perforation of the lung by the biopsy needle.
- During the procedure observe the patient carefully for signs of respiratory distress (such as shortness of breath, rapid pulse, or cyanosis). If these symptoms are observed, report them immediately to the physician.
- After the specimens are obtained, place them in the appropriate jars for histologic and microbiologic examinations to ensure appropriate test results.
- After the lung biopsy procedure, vital signs are taken frequently (usually every 15 minutes for four times, then every 30 minutes for four times, and then every hour for four times, and then every 4 hours). They should be evaluated for signs of bleeding (increased pulse and decreased blood pressure) and for shortness of breath. The patient's breath sounds should be evaluated, and any decrease noted on the biopsy site should be reported immediately.
- After the lung biopsy a chest x-ray examination is usually ordered to check for complications, such as pneumothorax. Observe the patient for signs of pneumothorax (such as dyspnea, tachypnea, decrease in breath sounds, anxiety, and restlessness).

Mediastinoscopy

Normal value: no abnormal mediastinal lymph node tissue.

Rationale. Mediastinoscopy is a procedure in which a mediastinoscope (a lighted instrument with a viewing lens) is inserted through a small incision made at the suprasternal notch. The scope is passed into the superior mediastinum for the purposes of inspecting the mediastinal lymph nodes and removing biopsy specimens from them. Because these lymph nodes receive lymphatic drainage from the lungs, their assessment can provide information diagnostic of intrathoracic diseases such as carcinoma, lymphoma, granulomatous infections, and sarcoidosis. Therefore, mediastinoscopy is used in establishing the diagnosis of a variety of intrathoracic diseases. It is also employed to "stage" patients with lung cancer and to assess their condition's operability. Approximately 35% of all patients with lung cancer who are examined are found to have metastases by mediastinal lymph node biopsy. Metastasis is a contraindication to thoracotomy because the tumor is inoperable.

The possibility of inadvertent puncture of the esophagus, trachea, or central vessels exists. If a puncture were to occur, immediate thoracotomy may be necessary.

Procedure. Mediastinoscopy is a surgical procedure performed in the operating room. The patient is kept NPO after midnight on the day of the study.

With the patient under general anesthesia, an incision is made in the suprasternal notch and the mediastinoscope is passed through this neck incision into the superior mediastinum. After the lymph nodes are examined and biopsy specimens are removed, the scope is withdrawn and the incision is sutured closed.

This procedure is performed by a surgeon in approximately 1 hour. The patient is asleep during the procedure.

A chest x-ray is usually performed after the procedure to ensure that a pneumothorax or hemorrhage has not occurred.

Contraindications. This procedure is contraindicated in any patient in whom the risk involved in anesthesia is high.

Nursing considerations

Nursing Diagnoses/Collaborative Problems

See Endoscopic procedures, pp. 6-7.

Nursing Implications with Rationale

- Explain the procedure to the patient. The physician performing mediastinoscopy should inform the patient of the potential complications.
- Ensure that the physician has obtained the informed consent for the procedure before premedicating the patient.
- Encourage verbalization of the patient's feelings, fears, and anxieties regarding mediastinoscopy.
- Provide the same preoperative and postoperative care as for any other surgical procedure.
- Keep the patient NPO after midnight on the day of the test.
- Be sure that the patient's blood has been typed and cross matched, that several units of blood are available, and that the patient is ready for thoracotomy if necessary.
- A chest x-ray is usually performed after the procedure to ensure that pneumothorax or hemorrhage has not occurred.

Pulmonary function studies

Normal values: vary with the age, sex, height, and weight of the patient.

Rationale. Pulmonary function tests are performed to detect abnormalities in respiratory function and to determine the extent of any pulmonary abnormality. The main reasons for pulmonary function studies include the following:

1. *Preoperative evaluation.* When planned thoracic surgery will result in loss of functional pulmonary tissue, as in lobectomy (removal of part of a lung) or pneumonectomy (removal of an entire lung), a significant risk of pulmonary failure exists if preoperative pulmonary function is already severely compromised by other diseases, such as COPD.

2. *Evaluation of response to bronchodilator therapy.* Some patients with COPD have a spastic component to their obstructive disease that may respond to long-term use of bronchodilators. Pulmonary function studies performed before and after the use of bronchodilators will identify that group of patients.
3. *Differentiation between restrictive forms of chronic pulmonary disease and obstructive forms.* Restrictive defects (such as pulmonary fibrosis, tumors, and chest wall trauma) occur when ventilation is disturbed by a limitation in chest expansion. Inspiration is primarily affected. Obstructive defects (such as emphysema, bronchitis, and asthma) occur when ventilation is disturbed by an increase in airway resistance. Expiration is primarily affected.
4. *Determination of the diffusing capacity of the lungs.* Rates are based on the difference in concentration of gases in inspired and expired air.
5. *Performance of inhalation tests in patients with inhalant allergies.* Results may establish a cause-and-effect relationship in some patients.
6. *Preoperative nonthoracic surgery evaluation.* Abdominal surgery can inhibit lung function. Preoperative evaluation of lung function is an important part of assessing operative risks.

Pulmonary function studies routinely include determinations of:

1. Forced vital capacity (FVC)
2. Forced expiratory volume in 1 second (FEV_1)
3. Maximal midexpiratory flow (MMEF)
4. Maximal voluntary ventilation (MVV)
5. Arterial blood gases (ABG) (discussed as a separate test; see the next section)

One must be aware that there are no absolute normal values for these functions. Values vary according to factors such as the patient's height, weight, sex, and age. Predicted or "expected" normal values may be obtained from tables correlated for such factors. The patient's values, then, are recorded as a percentage of expected values. When the volumes or flow rates are 100% of the predicted value, this represents good pulmonary function. Values less than 50% of that predicted norm indicate poor pulmonary function; high mortality exists for patients in this group who require surgery. The normal values given below are for a healthy, young, 70 kg, 6-foot-tall man.

FVC
Normal values: 4800 cc
FEV_1
Normal value: 3980 cc
MMEF
Normal value: 400 L/min
MVV
Normal values: 125-170 L/min

Forced vital capacity. FVC is the amount of air that can be forcefully expelled from a maximally inflated lung position. This volume is decreased below the expected value in obstructive and restrictive pulmonary disease. One needs a FVC of at least 750 cc to mount an effective cough to keep the bronchial tree clear.

Forced expiratory volume in 1 second. FEV_1 is the volume of air expelled during the first second of the FVC. In patients with obstructive disease, airways are narrowed and resistance to flow is high. Therefore, not as much air can flow out in 1 second, and FEV_1 is reduced below the predicted value. In restrictive lung disease, FEV_1 is decreased not because of airway resistance but because the amount of air originally inhaled is less (that is, decreased FVC). One should therefore measure FEV_1/FVC. A normal value of 80% is found in patients with restrictive lung disease. In obstructive disease this ratio is well below 80%. The FEV_1 measurement will reliably improve with bronchodilator therapy if a spastic component to obstructive disease exists.

Maximal midexpiratory flow. MMEF is the maximum rate of air flow through the pulmonary tree during forced expiration. This is also called forced midexpiratory flow ($FEF_{25\%-75\%}$). This test is independent of the patient's effort or cooperation. MMEF is reduced below expected value in obstructive diseases and normal in restrictive disease. If it is below 60 L/min, surgery carries a prohibitive mortality risk.

Maximal volume ventilation. MVV, which was formerly called maximal breathing capacity (MBC), is the maximal volume of air that the patient can breathe in and out during 1 minute. It is decreased below the expected value in both restrictive and obstructive pulmonary diseases.

▪ ▪ ▪

A comprehensive pulmonary function study may also include evaluation of the following lung volumes and lung capacities, many of which are illustrated in Figure 5-8.

Tidal volume. TV, or V_T, is the volume of air inspired and expired with each normal respiration.

Inspiratory reserve volume. IRV is the maximum volume of air that can be inspired from the end of a normal inspiration. It represents forced inspiration over and beyond the tidal volume.

Expiratory reserve volume. ERV is the maximum volume of air that can be exhaled after a normal expiration.

Residual volume. RV is the volume of air remaining in the lungs following forced expiration.

Inspiratory capacity. IC is the maximal amount of air that can be inspired after a normal expiration (IC = TV + IRV).

Functional residual volume. FRV is the amount of air left in the lungs after a normal expiration (FRV = ERV + RV).

Vital capacity. VC is the maximal amount of air that can be expired after a maximal inspiration (VC = TV + IRV + ERV).

Total lung capacity. TLC is the volume to which the lungs can be expanded with the greatest inspiratory effort (TLC = TV + IRV + ERV + RV).

Minute volume. MV (sometimes called minute ventilation) is the volume of air inhaled and exhaled per minute.

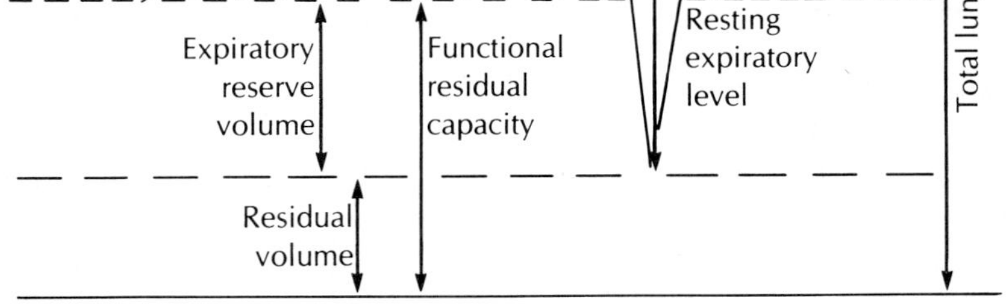

FIGURE 5-8. Lung volumes and capacities illustrated by spirography tracing.
From Phipps WJ, Long BC, and Woods NF: Medical-surgical nursing: concepts and clinical practice, ed 2, St Louis, 1983, The CV Mosby Co.

Dead space. Dead space is the part of the tidal volume that does not participate in alveolar gas exchange.

Procedure. The unsedated patient is taken to the pulmonary function laboratory. The patient breathes into a sterile cylinder, which is connected to a computerized machine able to measure and record the desired values.

The patient is asked to inhale as deeply as possible and then to exhale as much air as possible. From this the machine computes FVC, FEV_1, FEV_1/FVC, and MMEF. Next the patient is asked to breathe in and out as deeply and frequently as possible for 15 seconds. The total volume breathed is recorded and multiplied by 4 to obtain the MVV. This test takes approximately 10 minutes and is painless. It is usually performed by an inhalation therapist or a technician.

The *diffusing capacity* of the lung (DL) for any gas can be measured as part of pulmonary function study. The DL measures the diffusion of gases per minute across the alveolar-capillary membrane. Most laboratories employ carbon monoxide (CO) for measuring DL because CO has a great affinity for hemoglobin, and therefore, only a small concentration of CO is needed in clinical tests. Because of this, the major limiting factor to the transfer of the gas is its rate of diffusion across the alveolar-capillary membrane and not pulmonary blood flow. The DL of carbon monoxide (DLCO) is usually measured by having the patient inhale a CO mixture. DLCO is then calculated by analysis of the amount of CO exhaled compared with the amount inhaled. The normal value for DLCO is calculated from a nomogram and varies according to body size, age, body position, and exercise. DLCO may be altered in diseases of the alveolar-capillary membrane (such as interstitial fibrosis); in conditions that decrease the surface area for gas exchange (such as emphysema and pneumonectomy); and in other disorders such as severe anemia where the DLCO may be decreased because of the decreased number of RBCs and lower levels of hemoglobin. Determination of DL is a sensitive, noninvasive method for detecting pulmonary interstitial parenchymal disease, determining the severity of the disease, and following the disease process and the effect of therapy. The DL of oxygen (DLO_2) may be obtained by multiplying DLCO by 1.23.

Inhalation tests may also be performed during pulmonary function studies to establish a cause-and-effect relationship in some patients with inhalant allergies. The *methacholine* or *histamine challenge test* is commonly used to detect the presence of hyperactive airway diseases. This test would not be indicated for a patient known to have asthma. A positive methacholine challenge is a greater than 20% reduction in the patient's FEV_1 after the administration of that drug. Care is taken during this challenge test to reverse any severe bronchospasm with prompt administration of an inhalant bronchodilator (such as isoproterenol).

Contraindications. Pulmonary function studies are contraindicated in:

1. Patients who are in pain because they cannot cooperate by deep inspiration and expiration
2. Patients who because of age or mental incapability are unable to cooperate.

Nursing considerations

Nursing Diagnoses/Collaborative Problems

- Possible knowledge deficit related to test purpose, preparation, and procedure
- Possible anxiety related to fear of breathing tests
- Possible activity intolerance and fatigue related to procedure

Nursing Implications with Rationale

- Explain the test completely. The patient's cooperation is necessary to obtain accurate results. Assure the patient that his or her air supply will be adequate during this procedure. Many people with respiratory disorders are anxious about undergoing breathing tests.

- Instruct the patient not to use any bronchodilators or to smoke for 6 hours before this study.
- Withhold the use of small-dose meter inhalers and aerosol therapy before this study.
- Measure and record the patient's height and weight before this study to determine the predicted values.
- Occasionally patients with severe respiratory problems are exhausted after the testing; plan needed periods of rest.

Arterial blood gases study

Normal values:

pH
- Adult/child: 7.35-7.45
- Newborn: 7.32-7.49
- 2 months-2 years: 7.34-7.46

Pco_2
- Adult/child: 35-45 mm Hg
- Child <2 years: 26-41 mm Hg

HCO_3^-
- Adult/child: 21-28 mEq/L
- Newborn/infant: 16-24 mEq/L

Po_2
- Adult/child: 80-100 mm Hg
- Newborn: 60-70 mm Hg

O_2 saturation
- Adult/child: 95%-100%
- Elderly: 95%
- Newborn: 40%-90%

Possible critical values:
- pH: <7.25, >7.55
- Pco_2: <20, >60
- HCO_3^-: <15, >40
- Po_2: <40
- O_2 saturation: 75% or lower

Rationale. Measurement of the arterial pH, Po_2, Pco_2, and bicarbonate ion (HCO_3^-) concentrations provides valuable information in assessing and managing a patient's respiratory and metabolic (renal) disturbances.

pH. The pH is the hydrogen ion (H^+) concentration expressed as a negative logarithm (p). Because it is a negative logarithm, pH is *inversely proportional* to the actual hydrogen ion concentration. Therefore, as pH increases, the hydrogen ion concentration decreases; and as pH decreases, the hydrogen ion concentration increases. The pH is a measurement of alkalinity (pH >7.45) and acidity (pH <7.35). In respiratory or metabolic alkalosis pH is elevated. In respiratory or metabolic acidosis pH is decreased (Table 5-1).

Pco_2. Pco_2 is a measurement of the partial pressure of CO_2 in the blood. Pco_2 is referred to as the *respiratory* component in acid-base determination because this value is primarily controlled by the lung. The equation below demonstrates the relationship between CO_2 and H^- concentration, or pH.

$$H_2O + CO_2 \leftrightarrows \underset{\textit{Carbonic acid}}{H_2CO_3} \leftrightarrows H^+ + HCO_3^-$$

As the CO_2 level increases, the equation is shifted to the right and hydrogen ion is formed, which causes a decrease in pH. Therefore, one can see that the CO_2 level and the pH are inversely proportional.

The Pco_2 level is elevated in primary respiratory acidosis and decreased in primary respiratory alkalosis (Table 5-1). Because the lungs are used to compensate for primary metabolic acid-base derangements, Pco_2 levels are affected by metabolic disturbances as well. In metabolic acidosis, the lungs attempt to compensate by "blowing off" CO_2 to raise pH. In metabolic alkalosis, the lungs attempt to compensate by retaining CO_2 to lower pH (Table 5-2).

HCO_3^-. The bicarbonate ion is a measure of the *metabolic* (renal) component of the acid-base equilibrium. This ion can be measured directly by the bicarbonate value or indirectly as CO_2 content, or total CO_2. Again the equation demonstrates the relationship between HCO_3^- and pH.

$$H_2O + CO_2 \leftrightarrows H_2CO_3 \leftrightarrows H^+ + HCO_3^-$$

As the HCO_3^- level increases, the equation is shifted to the left. Because less H^+ is present, the pH increases. Therefore, one can see that the relationship of HCO_3^- to pH is a directly

TABLE 5-1. Normal Values for Arterial Blood Gases and Abnormal Values in Uncompensated Acid-Base Disturbances

Acid-base disturbance	pH	Pco_2 (mm Hg)	HCO_3^- (mEq/L)	Common cause
None (normal values)	7.35-7.45	35-45	22-26	
Respiratory acidosis	↓	↑	Normal	Respiratory depression (drugs, central nervous system trauma) Pulmonary disease (pneumonia, COPD, respirator underventilation)
Respiratory alkalosis	↑	↓	Normal	Hyperventilation (emotions, pain, respirator overventilation)
Metabolic acidosis	↓	Normal	↓	Diabetes, shock, renal failure, intestinal fistula
Metabolic alkalosis	↑	Normal	↑	Sodium bicarbonate overdose, prolonged vomiting, or nasogastric drainage

TABLE 5-2. Acid-Base Disturbance and the Compensatory Mechanism

Acid-base disturbance	Mode of compensation
Respiratory acidosis	Kidneys will retain increased amounts of HCO_3^- to increase pH.
Respiratory alkalosis	Kidneys will excrete increased amounts of HCO_3^- to lower pH.
Metabolic acidosis	Lungs "blow off" CO_2 to raise pH.
Metabolic alkalosis	Lungs retain CO_2 to lower pH.

proportional one. HCO_3^- is elevated in metabolic alkalosis and decreased in metabolic acidosis (Table 5-1). The kidneys are also used to compensate for primary respiratory acid-base derangements. For example, in respiratory acidosis, the kidneys attempt to compensate by reabsorbing increased amounts of HCO_3^-. In respiratory alkalosis, the kidneys excrete HCO_3^- in increased amounts in an attempt to lower pH through compensation (Table 5-2).

Po_2. The Po_2 level is an indirect measurement of the O_2 content of arterial blood. It is a measure of the tension (pressure) of O_2 dissolved in the plasma. The Po_2 level is decreased in the following patients:

1. Patients who are unable to oxygenate the arterial blood because of O_2 diffusion difficulties (such as pneumonia and shock lung)
2. Patients who have premature mixing of venous blood with arterial blood (such as in congenital heart disease)
3. Patients who have underventilated and overperfused pulmonary alveoli (pickwickian syndrome), that is, obese patients who cannot ventilate properly when in the supine position.

Oxygen saturation. O_2 saturation is an indication of the percentage of hemoglobin saturated with O_2. When 95% to 100% of the hemoglobin carries O_2, the tissues are easily provided with O_2. As the Po_2 level decreases, the percentage of hemoglobin saturation also decreases. This decrease (see an oxyhemoglobin dissociation curve) is linear to a point. However, when the Po_2 level drops below 60 mm Hg, small drops in the Po_2 level cause large drops in the percentage of hemoglobin saturated with O_2. At O_2 saturation levels of 70% or below, the tissues are unable to extract enough O_2 to carry out their vital functions.

With an understanding of the foregoing material, the ABG report can be interpreted easily in several steps. A more detailed and comprehensive discussion of ABG is beyond the scope of this book.

Step 1: Look at the pH and determine whether acidosis (pH <7.35) or alkalosis (pH >7.45) exists.

Step 2: Next look at the Pco_2 level. If it is shifted in a way to cause the previously noted pH, the primary problem is a respiratory one. For example, a shift in the Pco_2 level to >45 with an acidotic pH indicates respiratory acidosis. A shift in the Pco_2 level to <35 with an alkalotic pH indicates respiratory alkalosis. However, if the Pco_2 level is shifted in a way opposite to what one would expect to cause the pH value, *compensation* is present and the problem is primarily a metabolic one. (For example, a pH of 7.3 and a Pco_2 level of 28 indicates metabolic acidosis with compensation.)

Step 3: Now look at the HCO_3^- level. If it is shifted in such a way as to cause the previously noted pH, the problem is primarily metabolic. For example, a shift in the HCO_3^- to <22 with an acidotic pH indicates metabolic acidosis. However, if the HCO_3^- level is shifted in a way opposite to what one would expect to cause the pH value, *compensation* is present and the problem is primarily a respiratory one. (For example, a pH of 7.3 and HCO_3^- level of 32 indicates respiratory acidosis with compensation.)

Procedure. The arterial blood can be obtained from any area of the body where good pulses are palpable (usually the radial, brachial, or femoral artery). The arterial site is cleaned with povidone-iodine (Betadine) or alcohol. A 20-gauge needle is attached to a syringe containing about 0.2 ml of heparin (to ensure adequate heparinization of the syringe) and inserted into the artery. After 3 to 5 ml of blood is drawn, the needle is removed and pressure is applied to the arterial site for 3 to 5 minutes. The syringe is capped and gently rotated to mix the blood and heparin. The arterial blood sample is placed in an iced container and immediately taken to the chemistry laboratory for analysis.

This arterial puncture is performed by laboratory technicians, respiratory inhalation therapists, nurses, or physicians. The patient is placed in a sitting or supine position. The arterial puncture takes 5 to 10 minutes, depending on the skill of the person drawing the blood. An arterial blood gas test is more painful than a venous puncture. For ongoing respiratory monitoring an arterial line can be inserted to avoid multiple punctures.

Contraindications. None.

Nursing considerations

Nursing Diagnosis/Collaborative Problems

See Blood studies, p. 2.

- Potential complication: thrombosis and distal ischemia

Nursing Implications with Rationale

- Explain the procedure to the patient and tell him or her that it will cause slightly more discomfort than a venous puncture.
- If you are drawing the blood, know the anatomy of the arterial sites to avoid nerve damage.
- If you plan to use the radial artery, perform an *Allen test* to evaluate the presence of the ulnar artery. The Allen test is done by causing the hand to blanch by obliterating both the radial and ulnar pulses. The pressure is then released over the ulnar artery only. If flow through the ulnar artery is good, flushing will be seen immediately. The Allen test is then positive, and the radial artery can be used for puncture. If the Allen test is negative (no flushing), repeat the Allen test on the other arm. If both arms give a negative result, choose another artery for puncture. The Allen test ensures collateral circulation to the hand

if thrombosis of the radial artery should follow the puncture.

- Notify the laboratory before drawing the arterial blood gases so that the necessary equipment can be calibrated before the blood sample arrives.
- If bubbles are present in the blood sample, expel them immediately. Air bubbles affect the oxygen level of the blood gases measurement.
- Place the blood sample in an iced container, because the lower temperature reduces blood cell metabolism, which may alter the pH, Pco_2, and HCO_3^- values.
- Maintain pressure to the arterial site for 3 to 5 minutes to avoid hematoma formation. If the patient has an abnormal clotting time or is taking anticoagulants, apply pressure longer.
- Be sure that no active subcutaneous bleeding exists before leaving the patient.

SUPPLEMENTAL INFORMATION

Oximetry

(pulse oximetry, ear oximetry)

Normal values: 95% or higher.
Possible critical values: <90%

Rationale. Oximetry is a noninvasive method of monitoring arterial oxygen saturation (SaO_2). The SaO_2 is the ratio of oxygenated hemoglobin to the total amount of hemoglobin. The SaO_2 is expressed as a percentage; for example, a saturation of 95% indicates that 95% of the total hemoglobin attachments for oxygen have oxygen attached to them. The SaO_2 is an accurate approximation of O_2 saturation obtained from arterial blood gases (see previous study). By correlating the SaO_2 and the patient's physiologic status, a close estimate of the Po_2 can be obtained.

Oximetry is commonly used in many clinical situations, such as pulmonary rehabilitation programs, stress testing, and sleep laboratories. It can be used to assess the body's response to various drugs such as theophylline, which causes bronchodilation, and methacholine, which evokes bronchospasm in people having asthma. Oximetry can also be used for monitoring the oxygen status during the perioperative period and in patients on mechanical ventilation.

Procedure. The earlobe, pinna (upper portion of the ear), or the fingertip is rubbed to increase blood flow. The monitoring probe or sensor is then clipped to the ear or finger. The sensor warms and increases blood flow to the tissue. A beam of light passes through the tissue and the sensor measures the amount of light the tissue absorbs. SaO_2 values are recorded. The study is usually performed by a respiratory therapist or nurse at the bedside, and takes only a few minutes to carry out.

Contraindications. None.

Nursing considerations

Nursing Diagnoses/Collaborative Problems

- Possible knowledge deficit related to test purpose, preparation, and procedure

Nursing Implications with Rationale

- Explain the procedure to the patient, assuring him or her that this is a noninvasive test.

CASE STUDY 2: TUBERCULOSIS

Ms. N., a 32-year-old nurse, worked in an inner city hospital. She had a 3-month history of weight loss, cough, hemoptysis, low-grade fever, and drenching night sweats over the upper half of her body several times per week.

Studies	Results
Routine laboratory work	Within normal limits (WNL) except for hemoglobin (10.5 g/dl) and hematocrit (32%) (Normal hemoglobin: 12-16 g/dl) (Normal hematocrit: 37-47%)
Erythrocyte sedimentation rate (sed rate) (see Chapter 12, p. 444)	30 mm/hour (Normal: up to 20 mg/hour)

Studies	Results
Chest x-ray (see p. 136)	Multinodular infiltration in the apical posterior segments of the upper lobes and superior segments of the lower lobes (Normal: No pathology)
Sputum culture (see p. 140)	*Mycobacterium tuberculosis* (Normal: None)
Tuberculin skin test	17 mm tranverse diameter of induration (Normal: <5 mm)

The diagnosis of tuberculosis was confirmed in light of the sputum culture, tuberculin test, and chest x-ray. An elevated sedimentation rate and modest anemia are common components of the clinical pathology.

The treatment of tuberculosis is based on the administration of effective drugs. Two effective drugs are required to prevent the emergence of drug-resistant mutants. The patient was placed on a 9- to 12-month regimen of isoniazid, 300 mg, and rifampin, 600 mg, daily.

DISCUSSION OF TESTS

Tuberculin skin test

(tuberculin skin test with purified protein derivative, PPD)

Normal value: negative; reaction <5 mm

Rationale. Although this test is used to detect tuberculosis infection, it is unable to indicate whether the infection is active or dormant. For the tuberculin skin test a purified protein derivative (PPD) of the tubercle bacillus is injected intradermally. Usually an intermediate strength (0.1 ml or 5 tuberculin units) of PPD is used. If the patient is infected with tuberculosis (whether active or dormant) lymphocytes recognize the PPD antigen and cause a local reaction. If the patient has not been exposed to tuberculosis, no reaction occurs. If the test is negative and the physician strongly suspects tuberculosis, a "second strength" PPD (100 or 250 tuberculin units) can be used. If this test is then negative, the patient most certainly does not have active or dormant tuberculosis.

A word of caution should be mentioned concerning positive PPD reactions. If a patient with a particular complaint has a positive PPD reaction, it does not necessarily mean that active tuberculosis is the cause of the complaint. It may only mean that the patient has had tuberculosis in the past and that is now dormant and not causing any problems.

The PPD test can also be used as part of a series of skin tests done to assess the immune system. Because many older patients have been exposed to TB, it is fairly common to have a positive PPD. If the immune system is nonfunctioning because of poor nutrition or chronic illness (such as neoplasia or infection), the PPD test will be negative despite the fact that the patient has had an active or dormant tuberculosis infection. It has been well established that surgery is associated with greater mortality in these patients (with immunoincompetence) than in patients whose immune systems are intact.

Laboratory testing for tuberculosis is usually performed as part of the routine prenatal evaluation in pregnant women. Oftentimes this may be the mother's first contact with the health care system in a number of years.

When a patient known to have active tuberculosis receives a PPD test, the local reaction may be so severe as to cause a complete skin slough requiring surgical care. When these patients are eliminated from PPD testing, the test has no complications. One cannot get active tuberculosis from a PPD test because there are no live organisms in the test solution.

Other selected skin tests are described in Table 5-3. All skin tests must be read at the designated time, and all results must be based on established criteria as seen in Table 5-3.

Procedure. A nurse prepares the volar (inner) aspect of the forearm with alcohol and intradermally injects 0.1 ml of PPD with a tuberculin syringe. A skin wheal should result. The test site should be marked with indelible ink. A

TABLE 5-3. Selected Skin Tests

Disease	Test	Antigen	Time to read	Positive reaction
Diphtheria susceptibility	Schick	Diphtheria toxin	3-6 days	>10 mm
Echinococcosis	Casoni	Fluid from hydatid cyst	15-20 min	Immediate erythema and swelling
Lymphogranuloma venereum	Frei	Killed virus	48-72 hours	6 × 6 mm raised papule
Sarcoidosis	Kveim-Siltzback	Sarcoid tissue	6 weeks	Palpable nodule
Scarlet fever	Schultz-Charlton	Antitoxin	24 hours	Blanched area
Scarlet fever susceptibility	Dick	Erythrogenic toxin	24 hours	>10 mm
Systemic fungal infection	Histoplasmin-latex	Killed fungi	48 hours	>5 mm
Toxoplasmosis	Toxoplasma	Antigen	24-48 hours	>10 mm
Trichinosis	*Trichinella*	Killed larvae	15-20 min	Blanched wheal surrounded by erythema
Tuberculosis	PPD	Tuberculin antigen	48-72 hours	>10 mm
Tularemia	Foshay	Killed bacteria	48 hours	Erythema and induration

nurse or physician reads the test 48 to 72 hours later. The test site is examined for induration (hardening), and the hardened area (*not* the reddened area) is marked and measured. If the thickened, swollen area measures more than 10 mm, the test is considered positive. Induration measurements between 5 and 10 mm are considered doubtful, and results <5 mm are labeled negative.

Contraindications. PPD testing is contraindicated in the following:

1. Patients with known active tuberculosis infections
2. Patients who have received bacille Calmette-Guérin (BCG) immunization against PPD because they will demonstrate a positive reaction to the PPD vaccination even though they have never had tuberculous infection

Nursing considerations

Nursing Diagnoses/Collaborative Problems

- Possible knowledge deficit related to test purpose, preparation, and procedure
- Possible anxiety related to unknown sensations or procedure
- Possible anxiety related to possible test results

Nursing Implications with Rationale

- Explain the procedure to the patient. Assure the patient that he or she will not get tuberculosis from this test.
- Assess the patient for previous tuberculosis. Report significant findings to the physician.
- Obtain from the patient a history of previous PPD results and BCG immunization.
- Prepare the forearm with alcohol and allow it to dry. Intradermally inject the PPD and then

circle the area with indelible ink. Record the time at which the PPD was injected.

- Read the results in 48 to 72 hours and record the results. Some hospitals require readings at both 48- and 72-hour intervals.
- If the test is positive, be sure that the physician is notified and that the patient is treated appropriately.
- If the test is positive, check the arm 4 to 5 days after the test to be certain that a severe skin reaction has not occurred that requires surgical debridement.
- If the patient is an outpatient, do not give the PPD test when the reading time (48 to 72 hours later) falls on a weekend. Frequently, no one is available at such a time to read the results.

CASE STUDY 3: PULMONARY EMBOLISM

Mrs. K., a 68-year-old woman, fell on the ice while shopping. She was taken to the local hospital, where a fracture of her hip was diagnosed and repaired. She had been doing well until the sixth postoperative day, when she complained of an acute onset of right-sided chest pain, shortness of breath, and palpitations. Physical examination revealed her to be tachypneic and anxious. The pulse rate was 140 per minute. Her chest was clear, with minimal wheezing noted on the right side. Her heart was normal except for the tachycardia and an accentuated pulmonic sound.

Studies	Results
Routine laboratory work	Normal
Chest x-ray study (see case study 1)	Positive lucent area on the right side of her chest
LDH determination (see Chapter 4)	600 ImU/ml (normal: 90-200 ImU/ml)
Total bilirubin determination (see Chapter 4)	1.9 mg/dl (normal: 0.1-1.0 mg/dl)
AST determination (see Chapter 4)	33 IU/L (normal: 5-40 IU/L)
EKG (see Chapter 2)	Severe right-sided heart strain
Aterial blood gases test (see case study 1)	
pH	7.44 (normal: 7.35-7.45)
P_{CO_2}	22 mm Hg (normal: 35-45 mm HG)
P_{O_2}	48 mm Hg (normal: 80-100 mm Hg)
HCO_3^-	23 mEq/L (normal: 22-26 mEq/L)
Lung scanning	Multiple filling defects: right side worse than left side (Figure 5-9)
Pulmonary angiography	Complete obstruction of right pulmonary artery and upper branch of left pulmonary artery (Figure 5-10)

In light of the clinical findings, pulmonary embolism was highly suspected. Lucency on the chest x-ray film was compatible with pulmonary embolism, as were the features shown on the lung scan and the pulmonary angiogram. The trend of elevated LDH and bilirubin levels in the presence of normal AST level is considered classic for pulmonary embolism. The arterial blood gas levels indicate severe hypoxemia compatible with a significant pulmonary embolism. Heparin was prescribed. One day later the patient's partial thromboplastin time (PTT) was 72 seconds (control value: 32 seconds; normal value: 30-40 seconds). Warfarin (Coumadin) was started 5 days after the heparin was begun. Four days after starting warfain therapy, the patient's prothrombin time (PT) was 15 seconds (control value: 12 seconds; normal value: 11.0-12.5 seconds). The heparin was stopped, and the patient was discharged on warfarin therapy. She had no further problems, and warfarin was discontinued after 6 months. (See Chapter 10 for PTT and PT monitoring of heparin and warfarin therapy.)

DISCUSSION OF TESTS

Lung scanning

(pulmonary scintiphotography, ventilation/perfusion scanning, V/Q scan)

Normal value: diffuse and homogeneous uptake of nuclear material by the lungs.

Rationale. This nuclear medicine procedure is

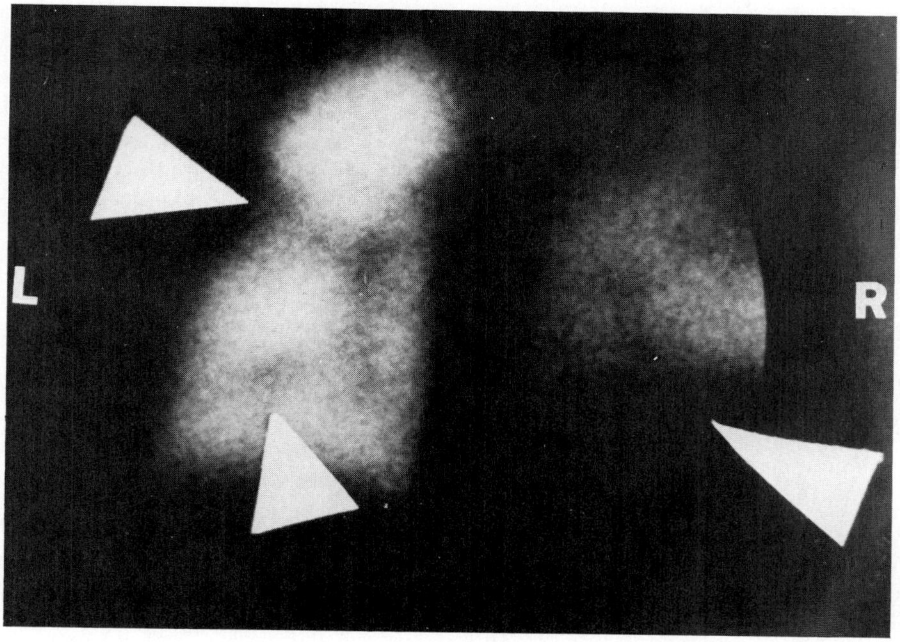

FIGURE 5-9. Lung scan (posterior view). Pointers indicate areas of decreased blood perfusion. The right side is worse than the left.

used to identify defects in blood *perfusion* of the lung in patients with suspected pulmonary embolism (Figure 5-9). Blood flow to the lungs is evaluated using a macroaggregated albumin (MAA) tagged with technetium, which is injected into the patient's peripheral vein. Because the diameter of the radionucleotide aggregates is larger than that of the pulmonary capillaries, the aggregates become temporarily lodged in the pulmonary vasculature. A gamma ray detecting device passed over the patient records the distribution of the particles within the lung.

A homogeneous uptake of particles that fills the entire pulmonary vasculature conclusively rules out pulmonary embolism. If a defect in an otherwise smooth and diffusely homogeneous pattern is seen, a perfusion abnormality exists, which may indicate pulmonary embolism. Unfortunately, other serious pulmonary lesions (such as atelectasis, pleural effusion, and emphysema), which decrease the ventilation of a part of the lung, also cause a defect in pulmonary blood perfusion. One can see, then, that although the scan is sensitive (easily recognizes pathologic conditions), it is not specific because many different pathologic conditions can cause the same abnormal results.

The chest x-ray study may aid in assessing the perfusion scan, since a perfusion defect that occurs in the same area as a defect on x-ray film does not indicate pulmonary embolus. It may represent pneumonia, atelectasis, or pleural effusion. However, when a perfusion defect occurs in an area of the lung that is normal on a chest x-ray study, pulmonary embolus probably exists. Lung scan specificity can be enhanced by performance of a *ventilation scan*, which detects abnormalities in ventilation. The ventilation lung scan reflects the patency of the pulmonary airways using krypton gas or Tc-DTPA as an aerosol. When vascular obstruction (for example, embolism) is present, ventilation lung scans demonstrate a normal wash-in and a normal wash-out of radioactivity from the embolized lung area. However, if parenchymal disease is responsible for the perfusion abnormality, wash-in or wash-out is abnormal. Therefore, the "mismatch" of perfusion and ventilation is characteristic of vascular embolic disorders, while the "match" is indicative of parenchymal disease.

Procedure. The unsedated, nonfasting patient who is suspected of having a pulmonary embolism is taken to the nuclear medicine department. A peripheral intravenous injection of radionucleotide-tagged albumin aggregate is given for the *perfusion* portion of the scan. While the patient lies in the appropriate position, a gamma ray detecting device is passed over the patient and records nucleotide uptake on either x-ray film or Polaroid film. This is done with the patient in the supine, prone, and various lateral positions, which allows for anterior, posterior, and lateral views, respectively. The results are interpreted by a physician trained in diagnostic nuclear medicine. The procedure is painless except for the initial injection.

For the *ventilation* scan, the patient breathes the tracer through a face mask with a mouthpiece. Less patient cooperation is needed with krypton. Ventilation scans can even be performed on comatose patients using krypton. Krypton images can be obtained before, during, or after perfusion images. In contrast, Tc-DTPA images are usually done before perfusion images and require patient cooperation with deep breathing and appropriate use of breathing equipment to prevent contamination.

The amount of radiation that the patient receives is minimal. The test takes about 30 minutes. If an iodine-tagged agent (^{131}I) is used, the patient's thyroid gland should be blocked by administration of Lugol's solution (10 drops) several hours before the administration of the iodine.

Contraindications. Lung scanning is contraindicated in the following patients:

1. Patients with hypotension and instability. Quite naturally no patient can be considered stable when pulmonary embolism is suspected, yet one must recognize the patient who cannot safely tolerate the lack of intensive nursing care that exists when the study is being performed.
2. Patients with pulmonary parenchymal problems, such as pneumonia, emphysema, pleural effusion, or tumors. These problems definitely give the picture of a perfusion defect (false-positive result) and simulate pulmonary embolism.
3. The pregnant patient. One tries to avoid unnecessary radiation during pregnancy.

Nursing considerations

Nursing Diagnoses/Collaborative Problems

See Nuclear scanning, p. 5.

Nursing Implications with Rationale

- Explain the procedure to the patient. Encourage verbalization of patient's fears and provide emotional support
- Monitor the patient's vital signs during the test if the patient is unstable.
- If ^{131}I is used, obtain the physician's order and administer 10 drops of Lugol's solution several hours before the test. This will block thyroid uptake of the iodine.

Pulmonary angiography

Normal value: normal pulmonary vasculature.

Rationale. Through an injection of a radiographic contrast material into the pulmonary arteries, pulmonary angiography permits visualization of the pulmonary vasculature. Angiography is used to detect pulmonary embolism (Figure 5-10) and a variety of congenital and acquired lesions of the pulmonary vessels.

When pulmonary embolism is suspected, lung scanning should be performed first. If the lung scan is normal, pulmonary embolism is ruled out. However, if the scan is suggestive but not definitive of pulmonary embolism, diagnosis can only be made with certainty with pulmonary angiography. Definitive diagnosis for pulmonary embolism requires pulmonary angiography. Obtaining this proof of pulmonary

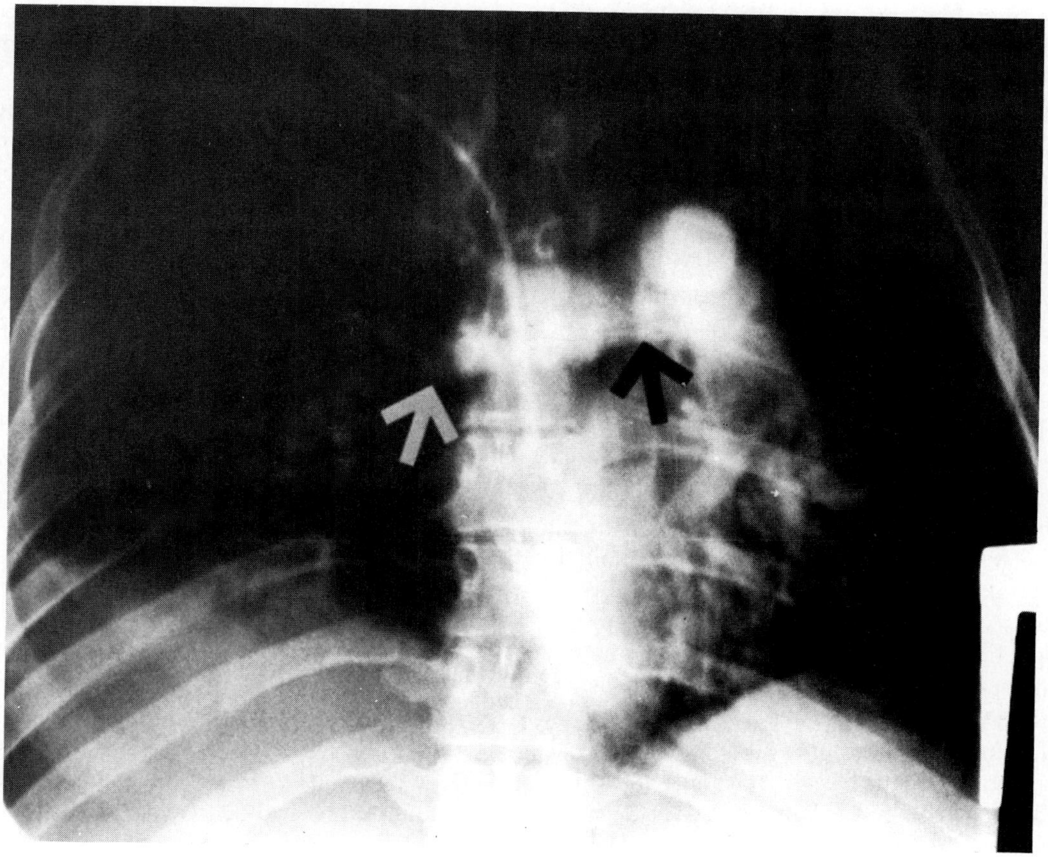

FIGURE 5-10. Pulmonary angiogram. White arrow indicates absence of dye in right pulmonary artery (caused by large obstructing embolism). Black arrow indicates normal left pulmonary artery.

embolism is especially important in elderly patients and in patients with diseases for which anticoagulation therapy is risky, e.g., peptic ulcers. Also, in rare instances, pulmonary embolectomy (removal of an embolus), rather than anticoagulation, is considered crucial for patient survival. In these cases the angiographic location of the clot is important.

The complications associated with pulmonary angiography are the following:

1. *Cardiac arrhythmia.* Premature ventricular contractions (PVCs) during right-sided heart catheterization may lead to ventricular tachycardia and ventricular fibrillation.
2. *Anaphylaxis.* The dye used in this test can produce anaphylaxis in patients with dye allergies.
3. *Risk of death.* Without the close monitoring of the intensive care unit, unstable patients may develop severe medical problems that can go unrecognized in the x-ray department and lead to death.

Bronchial angiography is now being done in some hospitals to identify bleeding sites in the lungs. For this procedure catheters are placed transarterially into the orifice of bronchial arteries. Radiopaque material is then injected and the arteries are visualized. If a bleeding site is identified, the site can be injected to prevent further bleeding.

Procedure. The patient is kept NPO after midnight on the day of the examination. He or she is sedated, usually with atropine and meperidine. In the angiography room, usually located in the radiology department, the patient is placed on an x-ray table. The groin is prepared and draped in a sterile manner. A catheter is placed into the femoral vein and passed into the inferior vena cava. With fluoroscopic visualization (motion picture x-ray images displayed on a television monitor), the catheter is advanced to the right atrium and right ventricle. With expertise, the angiographer (a physician) can manipulate the catheter into the main pulmonary artery, where the dye is injected through the catheter. X-ray films of the chest are immediately taken in timed sequence. This allows all vessels visualized by the injection to be photographed. If filling defects are seen in the contrast-filled vessels, a pulmonary embolism is present.

During the actual injection of dye material, the patient may feel a burning and flush throughout the body. This is transient, usually passing within seconds. The test takes about 1 hour. Lying on the hard table for that time is uncomfortable for the patient.

Contraindications. This study is contraindicated in:

1. Patients with dye allergies
2. Unstable patients
3. Uncooperative patients

Nursing considerations

Nursing Diagnoses/Collaborative Problems

See X-ray studies, p. 5.

- Potential complication: cardiac arrhythmias
- Potential complication: anaphylaxis

Nursing Implications with Rationale

- Explain the procedure to the patient. Tell the patient where the catheter will be inserted (usually the femoral vein). Inform the patient that a warm flush may be felt when the dye is injected. Provide emotional support.
- Ensure that the written and informed consent for this procedure is obtained before premedicating the patient.
- Assess the patient for allergies to the iodine dye.
- Keep the patient NPO after midnight on the day of the study.
- Administer the preprocedure medications as ordered. Atropine may be ordered to decrease secretions, and meperidine is used to sedate the patient and relieve anxiety.
- After the procedure observe the catheter insertion site for inflammation, hemorrhage, hematoma, or absence of peripheral pulse.
- Assess the vital signs for evidence of bleeding (decreased blood pressure and increased pulse). Vital signs are usually ordered to be taken every 15 minutes for four times, then every 30 minutes for four times, and then every 4 hours.

CASE STUDY 4: PLEURAL EFFUSION

Mr. D.L., 54 years old, developed shortness of breath. He was in otherwise good health. He had no chest pain. His physical examination indicated that he had decreased breath sounds in the left lung and also dullness to percussion in this area.

Studies	Results
Routine laboratory work	Within normal limits (WNL)
Chest x-ray study (see p. 136)	Possible pleural effusion (noted on decubitus views)
CT scan of the chest	No intraparenchymal lung tumor; there is, however, free fluid in the pleural cavity and a thickened parietal pleura especially in the lower chest cavity
Thoracentesis and pleural fluid analysis	
Gross appearance	Bloody
Cell count	WBC >1000 mm^3; 70% of WBC are small lymphocytes RBC >100,000/mm^3 (all suggestive of exudate)

Studies	Results
Specific gravity	1.016 (suggestive of exudate)
Protein content	3.9 g/dl (characteristic of exudate)
LDH	Pleural fluid to serum LDH ratio 0.7 (typical of exudate)
Glucose	80 mg/dl (serum: 90 mg/dl)
C & S	No growth
Mycobacterium and fungus	Negative
Cytology	Malignant-appearing mesothelial cells
Pleural biopsy	Undifferentiated mesothelium

The pleural effusion suspected on the chest x-ray study and documented on the CT scan could have been caused by infection, tumor, or other forms of inflammation. The thickening of the parietal pleura on the CT scan did, however, strongly point to a tumor affecting the parietal mesothelial pleural surface. The thoracentesis analysis indicated that it was an exudative type of fluid consistent with either an infection or tumor. Since the pleural fluid glucose was not markedly diminished, infection was unlikely as a possibility. The negative cultures for bacteria, tuberculosis, and fungus ruled out the possibility for these infections. Cytology strongly pointed toward a mesothelial type of tumor. Pleural biopsy, however, made the definitive diagnosis of mesothelioma.

The patient was treated with chemotherapy, which unfortunately did not help. He attempted, ineffectually, several unconventional forms of anticancerous therapy outside the country. He died 3 months after the diagnosis of his neoplastic disease.

DISCUSSION OF TESTS

Computed tomography of the chest

(CT of the chest or lung)

Normal values: no evidence of tumor or pathology.

Rationale. Computed tomography (CT) scanning of the chest is a noninvasive yet very accurate x-ray procedure used to diagnose and evaluate pathologic conditions such as tumors, nodules, coin lesions, cysts, pleural effusion, and enlarged lymph nodes. When an intravenous contrast material is given, vascular structures can be identified and a diagnosis of aortic aneurysm can be made. This procedure provides a cross-sectional view of the chest and is especially useful in detecting small differences in tissue densities, thus demonstrating lesions that cannot be seen on conventional radiology and tomography. At this time, magnetic resonance imaging (MRI) (see Chapter 6) has limited application in parenchymal lung problems.

The CT x-ray image results from using a body scanner machine to pass x-rays through the patient's chest at many different angles. The variation in density of each tissue allows for variable penetration of the x-rays. Each density is given a numerical value called a coefficient, which is digitally computed into shades of gray. This is then displayed on a television screen as thousands of dots in various shades of gray. The final display appears as an actual photograph of the anatomic area sectioned by the x-rays. The study is only two-dimensional (that is, anterior to posterior and right to left). However, if one looks at a series of cross-sectional views, a three-dimensional appearance is created. Because each point within a cross-sectional field is viewed from hundreds of different angles, the density of each point can be precisely determined. The mediastinal structures can be visualized in a manner that cannot be equaled with conventional x-ray and tomography scans.

Procedure. The patient is usually kept fasting for 4 hours before the CT of the lung in case contrast dye is administered. Sedation is rarely required and is given only to the patient who cannot remain still during the length of the procedure. The patient is taken to the radiology department and is asked to remain motionless in the supine position because any motion causes blurring and streaking of the final picture. An encircling x-ray camera (body scanner) takes pictures at varying intervals (usually 1-4 cm apart). Television equipment allows for immediate display, and the image is recorded on x-ray type film. The procedure takes 30 to 45 minutes to perform and is painless. However, many patients are uncomfortable lying on a hard x-ray table for this amount of time.

Often intravenous dye is administered to the patient and the x-ray studies are repeated. This adds an additional 30 to 45 minutes to the procedural time. During the dye injection the patient may feel a warm flush of the face or body. Many patients have momentary nausea with the dye injection.

Contraindications. This test is contraindicated in the pregnant patient and in patients who are allergic to iodine dye.

Nursing considerations

Nursing Diagnoses/Collaborative Problems

See X-ray studies, p. 5.

- Potential for claustrophia (related to x-ray equipment)

Nursing Implications with Rationale

- Explain the procedure to the patient. Assure the patient that CT scanning of the lungs is a safe and painless x-ray method that incurs no more radiation than a series of regular x-ray studies.
- If possible, show the patient a picture of the doughnut-like x-ray scanner. Tell the patient that he or she will be alone in the x-ray room, but will be observed from a control room by a specialized technician. The patient and the technician can communicate through an intercom system. Inform the patient that clicking noises from the scanner will be heard. People often describe the clicking noise as sounding similar to that of a washing machine. The patient will not be able to feel the scanning machine rotate.
- Keep the patient NPO for 4 hours before the test, because the iodine dye may cause nausea. It is usually not known before the test if enhanced visualization by the dye injection is needed.
- Assess the patient for allergies to iodinated dye to prevent dye-induced anaphylaxis. Sometimes the patient is pretested for dye allergies. Observe the patient for signs of anaphylaxis (such as respiratory distress, palpitations, blood pressure drop, itching, urticaria [hives], or diaphoresis). Emergency drugs should always be available to counteract any severe allergic reaction. If iodine allergy is suspected and is not severe, diphenhydramine (Benadryl) and steroids can be administered before scanning.
- Inform the patient that lying motionless is required during the study. Even talking or sighing may cause artifacts on the computer image.
- No special postprocedure care is required. The patient may resume all activities.
- Encourage patients who receive the dye injection to increase their fluid intake, because the dye is excreted by the kidneys and causes diuresis.

Thoracentesis and pleural fluid analysis

(pleural tap)

Normal values: normal pleural fluid.

Rationale. Thoracentesis is an invasive procedure that entails the insertion of a needle into the pleural space for removal of fluid or air (Figure 5-11). Pleural fluid is removed for both diagnostic and therapeutic purposes. Therapeutically, it is done to relieve pain, dyspnea, and other symptoms of pleural pressure. Removal of this fluid also permits better radiographic visualization of the lung. Diagnostically, thoracentesis is performed whenever a pleural effusion (abnormal accumulation of fluid in the pleural space) of unknown etiology is recognized. A decubitus chest x-ray is obtained before thoracentesis to ensure that the pleural fluid is mobile and, therefore, accessible to a needle placed within the pleural space.

The pleural fluid is usually evaluated for gross appearance; cell counts; protein, LDH, glucose, and amylase levels; gram stain and bacteriologic cultures; *Mycobacterium tuberculosis* and fungus cultures; cytology; CEA levels; and

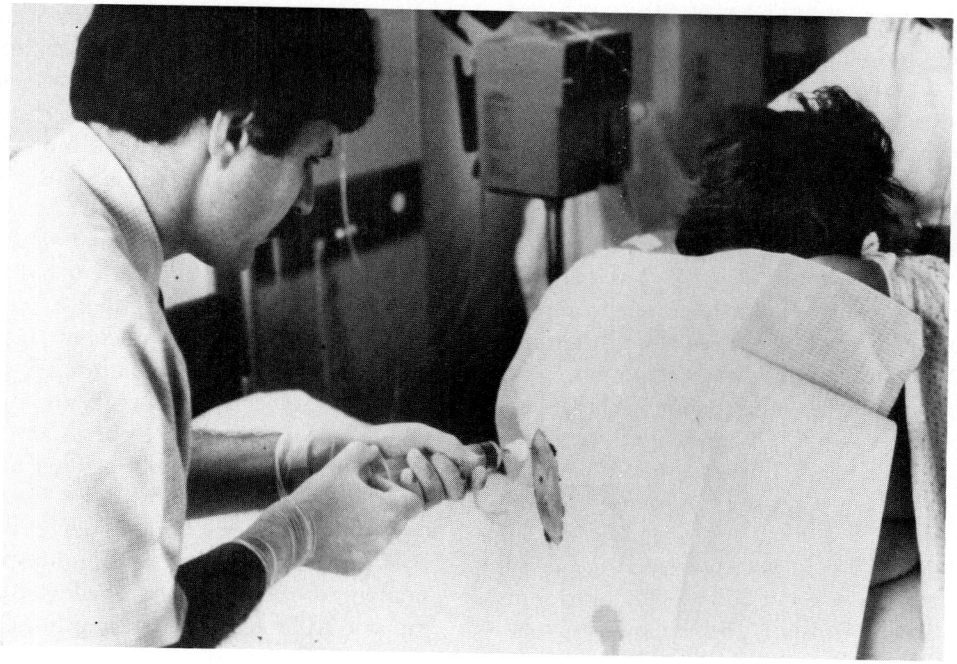

FIGURE 5-11. Performance of thoracentesis.

sometimes for other specific tests. Each is discussed separately here.

Gross appearance. The color, optical density, and viscosity are noted as the pleural fluid appears in the aspirating syringe. Empyema is characterized by the presence of a foul odor and the appearance of thick puslike fluid. An opalescent, pearly fluid is characteristic of chylothorax (chyle in the pleural cavity).

Cell counts. The white blood cell (WBC) and differential counts are determined. A WBC count exceeding 1000 mm^3 is suggestive of an exudate. The predominance of polymorphonuclear leukocytes (PMNs) usually is an indication of an acute inflammatory condition (such as pneumonia, pulmonary infarction, or early tuberculosis effusion). When more than half of the white cells are small lymphocytes, the effusion is usually because of tuberculosis or tumor.

Protein content. Levels >3 g/dl are characteristic of exudates, while transudates usually have a protein content of <3 g/dl. Transudates are most commonly caused by congestive heart failure. Cirrhosis, nephrotic syndrome, myxedema, peritoneal dialysis, and acute glomerulonephritis are other causes. *Exudates* are most commonly found in infectious disease and in neoplastic conditions. However, collagen vascular disease, pulmonary infarction, gastrointestinal diseases, trauma, and drug hypersensitivity are also causes of exudative effusions.

Lactic dehydrogenase (LDH). A pleural fluid to serum LDH ratio of >0.6 is typical of an exudate.

An exudate is identified with a high degree of accuracy if the pleural fluid to serum protein ratio is >0.5 and the pleural fluid to serum LDH ratio is >0.6.

Glucose. Usually pleural glucose levels approximate serum levels. Low values appear to be a combination of glycolysis by the extra cells and impairment of glucose diffusion because of damage of the pleural membrane. Values <60 mg/dl are occasionally seen in tuberculosis or malignancy and are common in rheumatoid arthritis and empyema.

Amylase. In a malignant effusion, the amylase concentration is slightly elevated. Very high amylase levels are seen when the effusion is caused by pancreatitis or rupture of the esophagus with leakage of salivary amylase.

Gram stain and bacteriologic culture. These tests are routinely performed when bacterial pneumonia or empyema is a possible cause of the effusion. If possible, these should be done before the initiation of antibiotic therapy.

Cultures for Mycobacterium tuberculosis *and fungus.* Tuberculosis or fungus may be a cause of pulmonary effusion especially in patients with compromised immunologic defenses.

Cytology. Cytologic study is reported to detect tumor cells in about 50% to 60% of patients with malignant effusions. Breast and lung cancers are the two most frequent tumors; lymphoma is the third.

Carcinoembryonic antigen (CEA). Pleural fluid CEA levels are elevated in various malignancies (e.g., of the colon, breast, or pancreas) and some benign conditions.

Special tests. The pH of pleural fluid is usually 7.4 or greater. The pH is commonly below 7.2 when infection is present. The pH may be between 7.2 and 7.4 in tuberculosis or malignancy. A total lipid and cholesterol count should be done if chylothorax is suspected by the opalescent, pearly appearance of the fluid. In some instances the rheumatoid factor and complement levels are also measured in pleural fluid.

Pleural fluid ANA (see Chapter 12) and pleural fluid–ANA ratios are often used to evaluate pleural effusion secondary to systemic lupus erythematosus.

The most common complication of the thoracentesis procedure is pneumothorax because of puncture of the visceral pleura or entry of air into the pleural space through the aspirating needle. If pneumothorax is suspected, its extent is determined by a chest x-ray study. Other complications of thoracentesis include intrapleural bleeding because of tissue puncture (such as of the lung, liver, or spleen) or a blood vessel; hemoptysis caused by needle puncture of a pulmonary vessel or an area of inflammation; reflex bradycardia and hypertension; pulmonary edema; pain (shouldertop pain on the affected side); and seeding of the needle track with tumor.

Procedure. No fasting or sedation is necessary for thoracentesis. If the patient has a troublesome cough, a suppressant such as codeine may be given before the procedure to prevent coughing during the procedure. For this test the patient is usually placed in an upright position (Figure 5-11) with the arms and shoulders raised and supported on a padded overbed table. This position spreads the ribs and enlarges the intercostal space for insertion of the needle. Patients who cannot sit upright are placed in a sidelying position on the unaffected side with the side to be tapped uppermost.

The thoracentesis is performed under strict sterile technique. The needle insertion site, which is determined by percussion, auscultation, and examination of a chest x-ray film, ultrasound scanning, or fluoroscopy, is aseptically cleansed and anesthetized with a local anesthetic such as lidocaine. The needle is then positioned in the pleural space, the fluid is withdrawn with a syringe and a three-way stopcock. A spring or Kelly clamp may be placed on the needle at the chest wall to stabilize the needle depth during the fluid collection. A short polyethylene catheter (Intracath) may be inserted into the pleural space for fluid aspiration. The advantage of inserting this catheter is that it decreases the risk of puncturing the visceral pleura and inducing a pneumothorax. Also, large volumes of fluid may be collected by connecting the catheter to a gravity-drainage system.

After the fluid is obtained, the needle is removed and a small bandage is placed over the site. The patient is then usually turned on the unaffected side for 1 hour to allow the pleural puncture site to heal.

This procedure can be performed by a physician at the patient's bedside, in a procedure room, or in the physician's office. Although the local anesthetic eliminates pain at the insertion site, some patients complain of feeling pressure when the pleura is entered and the fluid is removed.

Contraindications. Thoracentesis is contraindicated in the uncooperative patient and in the patient with clinically significant thrombocytopenia. The patient who is fully anticoagulated with heparin or warfarin (Coumadin) presents a risk of bleeding. This risk should be evaluated in relation to the importance of the information to be obtained by the thoracentesis procedure.

Nursing considerations

Nursing Diagnoses/Collaborative Problems

- Possible knowledge deficit related to test purpose, preparation, and procedure
- Possible alteration in comfort related to test procedure
- Potential complication: pneumothorax
- Potential complication: bleeding
- Potential complication: pulmonary edema
- Potential complication: reflex bradycardia and hypertension

Nursing Implications with Rationale

- Explain the purpose of the test and the procedure to the patient. Be certain that the patient knows that movement or coughing during the procedure is prohibited to avoid inadvertent needle damage to the lung or pleura. A cough suppressant is usually given before the procedure if the patient has a troublesome cough. If the patient must cough during the procedure, the physician may withdraw the needle slightly to avoid puncture.
- Ensure that an informed consent for this procedure is obtained.
- Before the procedure make certain that a sterile thoracentesis tray has been obtained from the central supply.
- Be sure that the patient's chest x-ray study or ultrasound scan is available at the procedure site before thoracentesis, so the fluid location can be determined and the puncture site decided. Fluoroscopy may also be used. The site is dull on percussion because of the fluid accumulation. The presence of this fluid indicates that the needle should enter the pleural space and not the lung.
- Help position the patient appropriately (usually in a sitting position) to enhance the patient's comfort and to allow the fluid to pool in the base of the pleural space.
- During the procedure monitor the pulse for reflex bradycardia and evaluate the patient for diaphoresis and a feeling of faintness. If these occur, the procedure should be terminated and the patient placed in the recumbent position. A second attempt at thoracentesis may be tried several hours later.
- Label the specimen with the patient's name, date, source of fluid, and diagnosis. Record the exact location of the thoracentesis, the quantity of the fluid obtained, and the gross appearance of the fluid.
- After the test obtain a chest x-ray study as ordered to check for the complication of pneumothorax, which could be induced by the pleural tap.
- After the study monitor the vital signs as ordered. Observe the patient for coughing or for the expectoration of blood (hemoptysis), which might indicate trauma to the lung. Evaluate the patient for signs and symptoms of pneumothorax, tension pneumothorax, subcutaneous emphysema, and pyogenic infection (such as tachypnea, dyspnea, decrease in breath sounds, anxiety, restlessness, or fever). Pulmonary edema or cardiac distress may also be produced because of a sudden shift of mediastinal contents if a large amount of fluid was aspirated.
- After the procedure listen to the patient's lungs for diminished breath sounds, which could be a sign of pneumothorax. Compare these sounds to the baseline breath sounds auscultated before thoracentesis.
- If the patient has no complaints of dyspnea,

normal activity usually can be resumed 1 hour after the procedure.

Pleural biopsy

Normal values: no evidence of pathology.

Rationale. Pleural biopsy is the removal of pleural tissue for histologic examination. It is indicated when the pleural fluid obtained via thoracentesis (see previous study) obtains exudative fluid, which is suggestive of neoplasm or tuberculosis. The pleural biopsy is indicated to distinguish between these two disease processes.

Pleural biopsy is usually performed via needle biopsy of the pleura. It can also be performed via *pleuroscopy*, which is done by inserting a videoscope into the pleural space for inspection and biopsy of the pleura. Pleural tissue may also be obtained by an *open pleural biopsy*, which involves a limited thoracotomy and requires general anesthesia. For this procedure a small intercostal incision is made, and biopsy of the pleura is done under direct observation. The advantage of this procedure is that a larger specimen may be obtained.

Serious complications of pleural biopsy are rare. The major risk of this procedure is bleeding and injury to the lung, which can produce pneumothorax.

Procedure. No fasting or sedation is required before pleural biopsy. This procedure is usually performed with the patient in a sitting position with the shoulders and arms elevated and supported by a padded overbed table. The patient should be instructed to remain very still during the procedure.

Several special needles are available for performing biopsy of the parietal pleura. All have a cutting edge and some device for retaining the biopsy. The most commonly used needle is the Cope instrument, which consists of an 11-gauge outer cannula with a sharp cutting edge and a 13-gauge, blunt-tipped, hooked biopsy trocar. A metal pointer is attached to the hub of the trocar to indicate the direction of the hook.

After the presence of the fluid has been determined by the thoracentesis technique, the skin overlying the biopsy site is anesthetized and pierced with a no. 11 scalpel blade. (The presence of fluid at the insertion site indicates that the needle should enter the pleural space and not the lung. The visceral pleura should not be penetrated because the needle should be placed in the space between these two sheaths.) The 13-gauge needle is then inserted within the cannula until fluid is removed (some fluid is left in the pleural space after the thoracentesis to make the biopsy easier). The inner needle is then removed, and the blunt-tipped, hooked biopsy trocar, attached to a three-way stopcock, is substituted in the cannula. The patient is instructed to expire all air and then to perform the Valsalva maneuver to prevent air from entering the pleural space. The cannula and the biopsy trocar are then withdrawn, while the hook catches the parietal wall and takes a specimen with its cutting edge. Usually three biopsy specimens are taken from different sites at the same session. The specimens are placed in a fixative solution (such as formaldehyde) and sent to the laboratory immediately. After the specimens are taken, additional parietal fluid can be removed. However, postbiopsy bleeding may obscure the true character of the fluid. An adhesive bandage is applied to the site. A chest x-ray test is usually performed after the study to detect the potential complication of pneumothorax.

This procedure is done by a physician at the bedside, in a special procedures room, or at the physician's office in about 30 minutes. Because of the instillation of the local anesthetic, little discomfort is associated with this procedure.

Contraindications. A pleural biopsy is contraindicated in patients with prolonged bleeding or clotting times.

Nursing considerations

Nursing Diagnoses/Collaborative Problems

- Possible knowledge deficit related to test purpose, preparation, and procedure

- Possible alteration in comfort related to test procedure
- Potential complication: bleeding
- Potential complication: pneumothorax

Nursing Implications with Rationale

- Explain the procedure to the patient. Ensure that the signed and informed consent is obtained before the procedure.
- Position patient and instruct him or her to remain still during procedure. Any movement can cause inadvertent needle damage.
- After the test check the vital signs frequently (usually every 15 minutes for four times, then every 30 minutes for four times, then every hour for four times, and then every 4 hours).
- After the test, observe the patient for signs of respiratory distress (such as shortness of breath and diminished breath sounds on the side of the biopsy site). Make sure the chest x-ray study is repeated if ordered to check for pneumothorax.
- Ensure that the biopsy specimen is placed in the proper fixative solution and immediately sent to the laboratory after the study. Failure to do so may interfere with accurate test result interpretation.

SUPPLEMENTAL INFORMATION

Bronchography

(bronchogram, laryngography)

Normal values: normal tracheobronchial tree.

Rationale. A bronchogram is an x-ray examination of the tracheobronchial tree produced after the instillation of iodine dye into the bronchi via a catheter or bronchoscopy. Positioning of the patient and the catheter allows the radiopaque material to coat all portions of the tracheobronchial tree so that their outline can be recorded on a chest x-ray film (Figure 5-12). X-ray films are then taken to demonstrate the outline and structure of the trachea, bronchi, and the entire tracheobronchial tree.

Bronchography is indicated to diagnose bronchiectasis, to identify obstruction in the distal bronchi, and to detect congenital or acquired forms of tracheobronchial malformation. Bron-

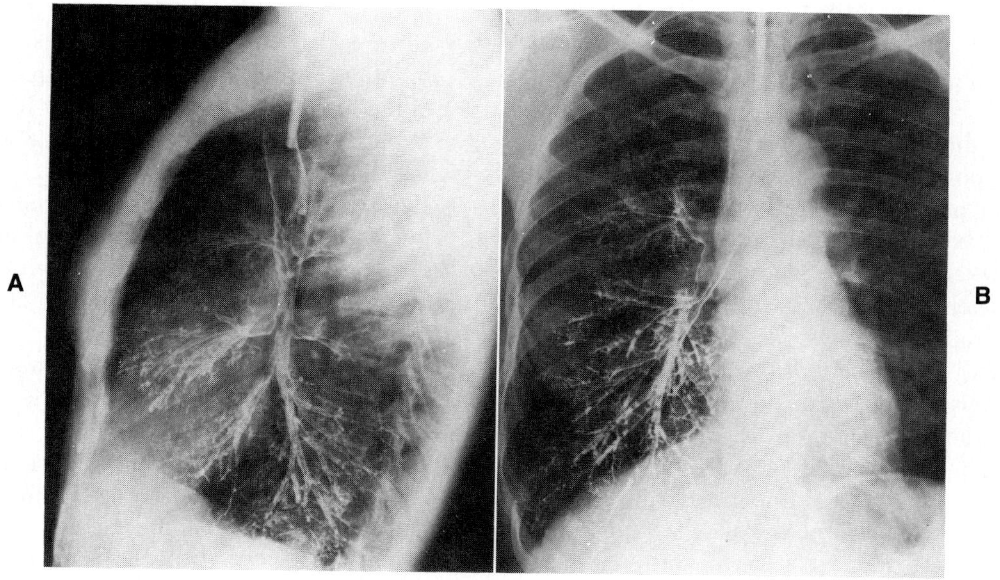

FIGURE 5-12. Normal bronchogram of right lung; lateral (**A**) and anteroposterior (**B**) views. From DeWeese DD and Saunders WH: Textbook of otolaryngology, ed 6, St Louis, 1982, The CV Mosby Co.

chography is used in the evaluation of patients for possible surgery (resection of a bronchopulmonary segment) and in those patients with recurrent, localized pneumonia or severe hemoptysis. When indicated, bronchography should not be performed when patients have an exacerbation of cough or sputum production. The test should be performed after the symptoms are treated and when the secretions of mucus are minimal. Because of the alterations in pulmonary function and occasional inflammatory reactions induced by this procedure, studying one lung at a time is safer than studying both. The indications for bronchography have diminished since the development of a flexible fiberoptic bronchoscope (see p. 142). Bronchospasm is a potential complication of bronchography.

Procedure. Before this procedure the patient should be NPO for at least 8 to 12 hours. The patient should perform thorough oral hygiene the night before and the morning of bronchography. Preprocedure medications may include atropine to decrease secretions and diazepam (Valium) for its sedative effect. If the patient has a productive cough, usually an expectorant is administered and postural drainage is performed for 1 to 3 days before the procedure. Postural drainage may be indicated for all patients to remove secretions from the small bronchi.

For this procedure the patient is placed in a sitting position. After spraying a local anesthetic into the patient's nose or mouth to suppress the gag reflex, a catheter or bronchoscope is passed into the trachea. The pharynx, larynx, and major bronchi are anesthetized before introduction of the radiopaque dye. The position of the patient and the placing of the catheter allow the radiologist to fill regions of interest selectively with radiopaque material. The positions that the patient is placed in are usually the reverse of those used in postural drainage. Multiple x-ray views are then obtained. Following this procedure postural drainage is usually indicated to remove the radiopaque dye from the lungs.

Bronchography is performed by a physician in approximately 45 minutes. Most patients would describe the test as being uncomfortable. During the test patients are instructed not to cough. Rapid, shallow breathing helps suppress the urge to cough.

Contraindications. Bronchography is contraindicated in the following: pregnant patients, patients allergic to iodine dye, patients with acute pulmonary infections, and patients with respiratory insufficiency.

Nursing considerations

Nursing Diagnoses/Collaborative Problems

See X-ray studies (p. 5) and Endoscopic procedures (pp. 6-7).

- Potential complication: bronchospasm

Nursing Implications with Rationale

- Explain the procedure to the patient to reduce anxiety and increase cooperation. Encourage verbalization of the patient's feelings and fears. Assure the patient that he or she will be able to breathe during this study.
- Keep the patient NPO after midnight on the day of the study to prevent possible aspiration of gastric contents induced by gagging during passage of the bronchoscope or catheter.
- Ensure that the patient performs thorough mouth care the night before and the morning of the test to decrease the number of bacteria in the mouth, which could be introduced during this procedure.
- Before this procedure postural drainage may be ordered to promote expulsion of mucus or exudate from the lungs. Drainage clears the air passages and allows for more satisfactory x-ray results.
- Ensure that the informed consent for this procedure is obtained before the patient is premedicated.
- Remove and safely store the patient's dentures, glasses, or contact lenses before administering the preprocedure medication.
- Administer the preprocedure medications as ordered. These are usually given 1 hour before the test.

- Instruct the patient not to swallow the local anesthetic sprayed into the throat. An emesis basin should be provided for expectoration of the lidocaine.
- Emphasize to the patient that a great effort should be made to suppress coughing during the procedure. Coughing prevents adequate alveolar filling and also expels the contrast medium before the test is completed. Rapid, shallow breathing helps to suppress the cough reflex.
- After the procedure postural drainage is usually performed to help remove the radiopaque dye from the tracheobronchial tree. However, no permanent damage occurs if some of the dye remains in the lungs.
- After the procedure do not allow the patient to eat or drink anything until the tracheobronchial anesthesia has worn off and the gag reflex returns. Usually this takes about 2 hours. The patient who drinks or eats anything before that time could unknowingly aspirate food or fluid and develop pneumonia.
- Monitor the vital signs as ordered. Observe the patient closely for evidence of impaired respiration or laryngospasm. The vocal cords may go into spasms after intubation. Emergency resuscitation equipment (including tracheal tube, laryngoscope, and medications such as steroids and epinephrine) should be readily available.
- Observe postanesthesia precautions for the patient until the effect of the sedative medications no longer exists.
- After the procedure encourage the patient to cough, which helps clear the tracheobronchial tree.
- Be aware that a slight temperature elevation is common for 2 to 3 days after the test.
- After the procedure a sore throat is often common. This discomfort can usually be relieved by gargling or administration of throat lozenges.
- Follow-up x-ray films may be taken at a later date to ascertain if any dye remains in the tracheobronchial tree.
- Normal activities may usually be resumed 24 hours after completion of this study.

Alpha$_1$-antitrypsin determination

Normal values:
Newborn: 147-200 mg/dl
Adult: >250 mg/dl

Rationale. Serum alpha$_1$-antitrypsin (α_1-antitrypsin) determinations are obtained when an individual has a family history of early onset emphysema because there is a familial tendency to have a deficiency of this antienzyme. Deficient or absent serum levels of this antienzyme can be found in these patients. These people usually develop a severe, disabling emphysema. The exact mechanism by which antitrypsin deficiency is responsible for emphysema is unclear.

Through genetic typing it has been found that most of the normal population have two M genes, designated as MM, and have alpha$_1$-antitrypsin levels >250 mg/dl. Z and S genes are commonly associated with alterations of serum levels of alpha$_1$-antitrypsin. Individuals who are homozygous ZZ or SS always have serum levels <50 mg/dl and often have levels near zero. These people develop severe panacinar emphysema in the third or fourth decade of life. Their major clinical symptoms usually include progressive dyspnea with minimal coughing. However, chronic bronchitis is prominent in those who smoke.

Individuals of the heterozygous state MZ or MS have serum levels of alpha$_1$-antitrypsin between 50 to 200 mg/dl. Approximately 5% to 14% of the adult population are in the heterozygous state, which is considered to be a risk factor for emphysema. Levels can be fictitiously increased with the use of estrogens or tamoxifen.

Procedure. Peripheral venipuncture is performed and one tube of blood is collected as specified by the laboratory.

Contraindications. None.

Nursing considerations

Nursing Diagnoses/Collaborative Problems

See Blood studies, p. 2.

Nursing Implications with Rationale

- Observe the venipuncture site for bleeding and hematoma formation.
- If the test results show that the patient is at risk for developing emphysema, patient teaching should begin and include factors such as avoidance of smoking, avoidance of infections, avoidance of inhaled irritants, proper nutrition, proper environment, adequate hydration, and education about the disease process of emphysema.

Angiotensin-converting enzyme (ACE)

(serum angiotensin converting enzyme, SACE)

Normal values: 23-57 U/ml (over age 20 years)

Rationale. Angiotensin-converting enzyme is found in pulmonary epithelial cells and converts angiotensin I to angiotensin II (a potent vasoconstrictor). For this reason the ACE levels may be used in the evaluation of special cases of hypertension. Elevated levels of ACE are found in a high percentage of patients with sarcoidosis. This test is primarily used to support the diagnosis of sarcoidosis and to evaluate the severity of the disease and the response to therapy. Other diseases associated with elevated serum levels include Gaucher's disease (a rare familial disorder of fat metabolism), leprosy, alcoholic cirrhosis, active histoplasmosis, tuberculosis, hemolysis, Hodgkin's disease, myeloma, scleroderma, pulmonary embolism, and idiopathic pulmonary fibrosis. ACE inhibitors, e.g., captopril, reduce serum levels of ACE.

ACE studies are not done on patients under 20 years of age because these people normally have very high levels.

Procedure. A peripheral venipuncture is performed, and approximately 2 to 5 ml of blood is obtained and sent to the laboratory.

Contraindications. None.

Nursing considerations

Nursing Diagnoses/Collaborative Problems

See Blood studies, p. 2.

Nursing Implications with Rationale

- Assess the venipuncture site for bleeding.
- Note on the laboratory slip if the patient is taking steroid drugs. These drugs usually cause decreased SACE levels.

QUESTIONS AND ANSWERS

1. **QUESTION:** When chest x-ray films are taken in the nursing unit with a portable x-ray camera, what precautions should the staff observe to prevent radiation exposure?
   ANSWER: The nursing staff should, if necessary, assist the radiologic technician in the placement of the x-ray film cassette behind the patient. Then the nursing staff, visitors, and other patients should leave the room before the x-ray films are taken. If constant bedside care is needed, a lead apron should be worn for protection from exposure.
2. **QUESTION:** A 42-year-old patient develops a clinical picture compatible with a pulmonary embolism. Lung scanning is done and is positive. Does this patient need pulmonary angiography?
   ANSWER: Not necessarily. As discussed in this chapter, a positive lung scan is not definitive evidence of pulmonary embolism, because other pathologic pulmonary conditions (pneumonia or pleural effusion) can create the same results. However, angiography is not always necessary. If the chest x-ray study results are normal (that is, no pneumonia or pleural effusion, for example), then one can be confident that the patient has a pulmonary embolism. If the chest x-ray study results are abnormal, pulmonary angiography is needed to establish the diagnosis of pulmonary embolism.
3. **QUESTION:** The physician orders oxygen for your patient, who is short of breath. How long after the start of oxygen would arterial blood gases be drawn to evaluate the patient's Po_2 level?
   ANSWER: Twenty to 30 minutes. It takes this long for any change in inspired oxygen concentration to be reflected in the Po_2 level. Whenever oxygen therapy is initiated or changed, an arterial blood gas study should be done 10 to 40 minutes

later, depending on the patient's underlying lung disease, to evaluate the effect of the new oxygen therapy. Likewise, when a patient is started on a respirator or a respiratory setting is changed, an arterial blood gas study should be performed 30 to 40 minutes later.

4. **QUESTION:** Interpret the following arterial blood gas results on a patient admitted to your unit with uncontrolled diabetes mellitus: pH, 7.25; Pco_2, 36 mm Hg; HCO_3^-, 19 mEq/L; Po_2, 84 mm Hg.
   ANSWER: The patient's arterial blood gases show metabolic acidosis. This is because the pH is acidotic, the Pco_2 level is within the normal range, and the HCO_3^- is altered in a way (decreased) compatible with acidosis.
5. **QUESTION:** One hour later, before therapy is initiated, the above patient's ABG shows the following: pH, 7.32; Pco_2, 28; HCO_3^-, 19. Interpret these results.
   ANSWER: The results indicate persistent metabolic acidosis with partial respiratory compensation. The Pco_2 level is decreased because the lungs are "blowing off" CO_2 in an attempt to compensate for the acid-base derangement.
6. **QUESTION:** Interpret the blood gas results on this patient seen in the emergency room with pneumonia: pH, 7.28; Pco_2, 60 mm Hg; HCO_3^-, 32 mEq/L.
   ANSWER: The results indicate respiratory acidosis with partial metabolic compensation. Respiratory acidosis is present because the increased CO_2 level is compatible with the acidotic pH. The kidneys are retaining bicarbonate to attempt to compensate for the acidotic pH.
7. **QUESTION:** Your patient, who is being evaluated for lung surgery, is scheduled for pulmonary function studies. Shortly before going for this test, the patient complains of severe back pain. The patient has an order for meperidine, 50 mg IM for pain. Should the drug be given?
   ANSWER: Yes. Remember that sedation should not be given to a patient before pulmonary function studies, because many of these tests are effort-related and the sedated patient cannot cooperate completely. However, a patient in severe pain cannot cooperate either. Therefore, the drug should be given to alleviate the pain, and the study should be canceled and rescheduled for another time.

BIBLIOGRAPHY

Birdsall C: How and when do you use pulse oximetry? Am J Nurs 87:158, 1987.

Blue PN and others: The need for oblique or lateral ventilation images in the diagnosis of pulmonary embolism, Clinical Nucl Med 15(12):917-919, 1990.

Braunwald E: Approach to the patient with disease of the respiratory system. In Wilson J and others, editors: Harrison's principles of internal medicine, ed 12, New York, 1991, McGraw-Hill.

Davies SF: Bacterial pneumonia. In Rakel RE, editor: Conn's current therapy, Philadelphia, 1991, WB Saunders.

Deslauriers J: Atelectasis. In Rakel RE, editor: Conn's current therapy, Philadelphia, 1991, WB Saunders.

Hirsh J and Anderson DR: Pulmonary embolism. In Rakel RE, editor: Conn's current therapy, Philadelphia, 1991, WB Saunders.

Ihde DC: Primary lung cancer. In Rakel RF, editor: Conn's current therapy, Philadelphia, 1991, WB Saunders.

Moser KM: Diagnostic procedures in respiratory diseases. In Wilson J and others, editors: Harrison's principles of internal medicine, ed 12, New York, 1991, McGraw-Hill.

Reynolds HY and Root RK: Bronchiectasis and broncholithiasis. In Wilson J and others, editors: Harrison's principles of internal medicine, ed 12, New York, 1991, McGraw-Hill.

Scoggin CH: Pulmonary neoplasms. In Wyngaarden JB and others, editors: Cecil textbook of medicine, ed 19, Philadelphia, 1992, WB Saunders.

Senior RM: Pulmonary embolism. In Wyngaarden JB and others, editors: Cecil textbook of medicine, ed 19, Philadelphia, 1992, WB Saunders.

Stein PD and others: Diagnostic utility of ventilation/perfusion lung scan in acute pulmonary embolism is not diminished by pre-existing cardiac or pulmonary disease, Chest 100(3):604-606, 1991.

Weinberger SE and Drazen JM: Disturbances of respiratory function. In Wilson J and others, editors: Harrison's principles of internal medicine, ed 12, New York, McGraw-Hill.

Chapter 6

DIAGNOSTIC STUDIES USED IN THE ASSESSMENT OF THE NERVOUS SYSTEM

ANATOMY AND PHYSIOLOGY

The nervous system may be divided conveniently into three areas:

1. The central nervous system, consisting of the brain and spinal cord
2. The peripheral nervous system, which includes the cranial and spinal nerves
3. The autonomic nervous system, made up of the sympathetic and parasympathetic nerves

Since the diagnostic procedures discussed in this chapter relate primarily to the brain and the spinal cord, this brief discussion of anatomy and physiology is limited to these areas.

The brain is encased and protected by the bony skull, which is a composite of several bones (frontal, parietal, occipital, and temporal). At the base of the skull is the *foramen magnum,* through which the spinal cord passes. Numerous small openings in the skull permit the passage of cranial nerves and blood vessels.

The brain is divided into the cerebrum, cerebellum, and brainstem (Figure 6-1). The *cerebrum* is the largest part of the brain. It is divided into two hemispheres, each consisting of five lobes. The *frontal* lobe, located anteriorly, contains nerves that primarily affect the emotional responses, attitudes (personality), and thought processes (such as judgment, volition, ethical values, and abstract and creative thinking). The *parietal* lobe, located in the midcentral area, contains nerves associated with somatic sensations such as pain and temperature. The *temporal* lobe is located laterally and inferiorly to the frontal and parietal lobes. It contains the hearing center. The posterior part of each cerebral hemisphere is called the *occipital* lobe, which is primarily concerned with visual perception. A fifth lobe, the *insula* (island of Reil), lies hidden from view in the lateral fissure.

Within the cerebrum are fluid-filled spaces called ventricles. The large lateral ventricles

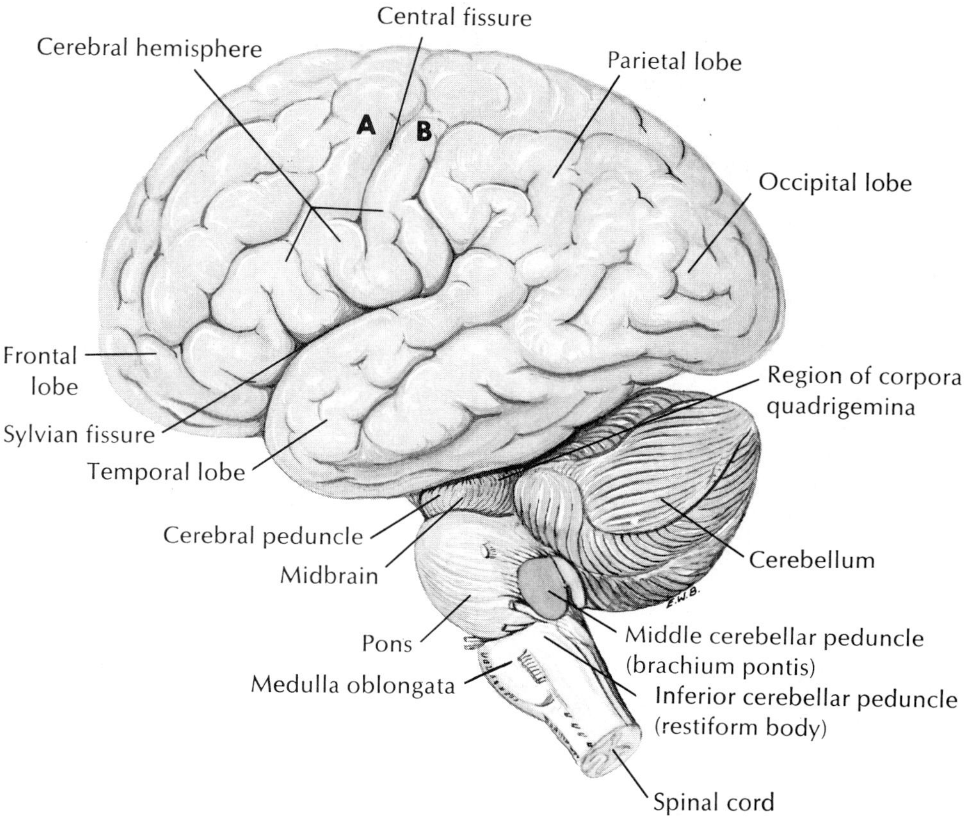

FIGURE 6-1. Human brain as it appears on left side. **A,** Precentral and, **B,** postcentral convolutions.
From Schottelius BA and Schottelius DD: Textbook of physiology, ed 18, St Louis, 1978, The CV Mosby Co.

empty into a smaller central, or third, ventricle. This, in turn, drains to a fourth ventricle located within the brainstem. The fluid within the four ventricles normally flows into the subarachnoid space.

The *cerebellum* is located just below the cerebral occipital lobe (Figure 6-1). It is separated from the cerebrum by the tentorium cerebelli and is responsible for the control and coordination of skeletal function and spatial equilibrium.

The *brainstem* extends from the cerebral hemispheres through the foramen magnum, where it then is called the spinal cord. The brainstem includes the midbrain, pons, and medulla oblongata (Figure 6-1) and neurologically controls breathing, heart rate, blood pressure, and consciousness.

The vertebral column (Figure 6-2) supports the head and protects the spinal cord contained within. The vertebral column consists of cervical, thoracic, lumbar, sacral, and coccygeal vertebrae. Between two vertebrae is an opening called a vertebral foramen, through which spinal nerves leave the spinal cord. The vertebrae are held together by strong ligaments. True joint spaces separate the vertebrae. Within these joints are vertebral discs. Each disc is composed of a central core called the *nucleus pulposus* and an outer rim called the *anulus fibrosus*.

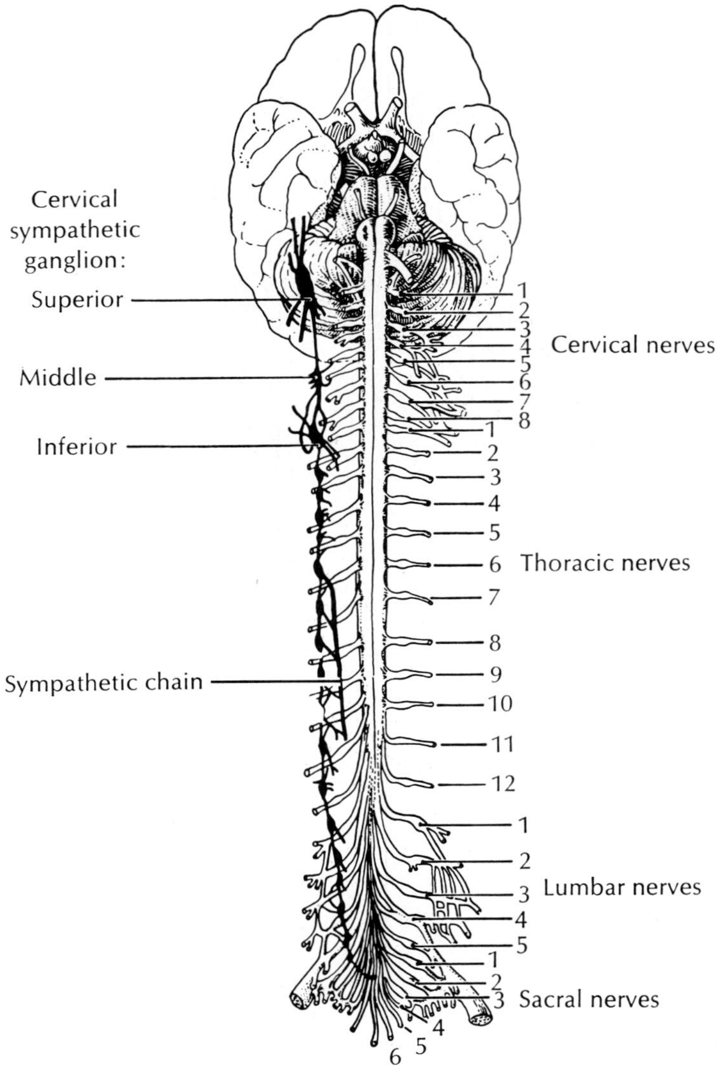

FIGURE 6-2. Ventral view of brain and spinal cord, with spinal nerves. Left side shows sympathetic chain.
From Schottelius BA and Schottelius DD: Textbook of physiology, ed 18, St Louis, 1978, The CV Mosby Co.

The spinal cord, which is contained within the spinal canal, is about 45 cm (18 inches) long and approximately the width of a finger. The spinal cord is a direct continuation of the medulla oblongata. It contains the motor and sensory relay fibers to and from the higher centers within the cord and the brain.

Because the brain and spinal cord are vital yet delicate organs, they are well protected by three membranes called *meninges* (dura mater, arachnoid, and pia mater). The *dura mater* is the dense fibrous outer layer. The *arachnoid* lies next to the dura mater. The *pia mater* is that layer most closely adherent to the brain and spinal cord. The space between the arachnoid mater and the pia mater is called the *subarachnoid* space. Within this space cerebrospinal fluid (CSF) circulates.

The choroid plexuses, found in the lateral and third and fourth ventricles of the brain, are the sites of CSF formation. CSF is secreted from the blood as the blood circulates through the capillaries of the choroid plexuses. The CSF passes through the channels from the lateral ventricles to the third and fourth ventricles, and then into the subarachnoid space surrounding the brain and spinal cord. Subsequently, the CSF is reabsorbed by the venous circulation of the skull.

The function of the CSF is to cushion and support the brain and spinal cord within the skull and vertebral column. This fluid acts as a "shock absorber" and therefore reduces the impact of trauma to the central nervous system. CSF also carries nutrients to various areas of the brain and spinal cord. The average person has approximately 150 ml of CSF in the ventricular and subarchnoid systems.

The brain has a dual blood supply (that is, carotid and vertebral). There are left and right carotid and vertebral arteries. This double blood supply serves to protect the brain from tissue necrosis in the event of occlusion of one of the four vessels. Unique to the brain is the blood-brain barrier. This prevents the movement of large molecules from the blood into the extracellular fluid surrounding the brain cell. This barrier eliminates the need for the brain to compensate rapidly for sudden and transient changes in blood volume and composition.

CASE STUDY 1: SEIZURE DISORDER

Johnny C. was a 12-year-old boy who began to complain of frequent headaches 4 months before his hospital admission. On the day of his admission, he had a major motor seizure, which his parents observed. During the seizure he lost bladder and bowel control. On physical examination he appeared to be in deep "postictal" sleep. He had no focal neurologic signs. On examination of the optic fundi, no evidence of papilledema was found.

Studies	**Results**
Routine laboratory work	Within normal limits (WNL)
Skull x-ray study	No evidence of skull fracture
Lumbar puncture	
Opening pressure	250 cm H_2O (normal: <200 cm H_2O)
Closing pressure	220 cm H_2O (normal: <200 cm H_2O)
Cerebrospinal fluid (CSF) examination	
Blood	Negative
Color	Clear
Cells	
Lymphocytes	0-2/mm^3 (normal: <5/mm^3)
Polymorphonuclear leukocytes	None (normal: none)
Protein	120 mg/dl (normal: 15-45 mg/dl)
Glucose	50 mg/dl (normal: 50-75 mg/dl)
Cytology	Questionably malignant cells
Serologic test for venereal disease	Negative (normal: negative)
Electroencephalography (EEG)	Focal slowing of the wave pattern in the posterior aspect of the cerebrum (normal: regular, rhythmic, electrical waves)
Brain scanning	Increase in radioactivity in the posterior aspect of the brain (normal: homogenous and minimal uptake of radioactive material)
Cerebral angiography	Neovascularity (tumor vessels) in the posterior aspect of the brain, involving the cerebellum and the occipital lobe of the cerebrum (normal: normal carotid vessels and terminal branches)
CT (computed tomography) scanning	A soft-tissue mass arising out of the cerebellum and invading the occipital lobe of the cerebrum

The skull x-ray study ruled out the possibility of a skull fracture as the cause of the boy's problem. Lumbar puncture excluded the possibility of meningitis or subarachnoid hemorrhage. However, the high protein count and questionably positive cytology indicated a possible neoplasm. EEG located an area of nonspecific abnormality in the posterior aspect of the brain. Brain scanning, cerebral angiography, and CT scanning all indicated a posterior fossa tumor.

Because of these findings, the patient underwent a craniotomy. A very invasive medulloblastoma was found to be arising from the patient's cerebellum and involving the occipital lobe of the cerebrum. The tumor was unresectable. Postoperatively, the patient was given phenytoin (Dilantin) and radiation therapy to the involved area. A chemotherapy regimen was administered. The patient's tumor did not respond to the therapy, and he died 4 months after the onset of disease.

DISCUSSION OF TESTS

Skull x-ray study

Normal values: normal skull and surrounding structures

Rationale. An x-ray study of the skull allows the visualization of the bones making up the

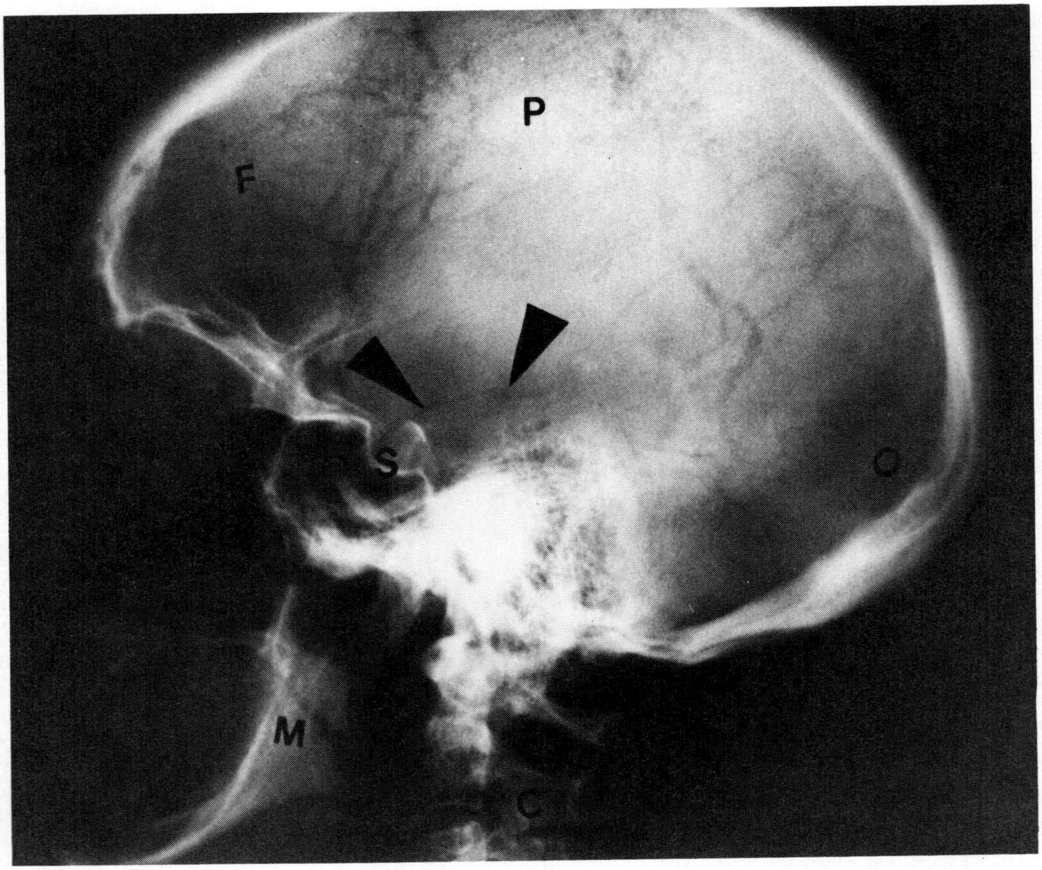

FIGURE 6-3. Lateral view of skull. Pointers indicate fracture line in temporal bone. *F*, Frontal bone; *P*, parietal bone; *O*, occipital bone; *S*, sella turcica; *M*, mandible; *C*, cervical vertebrae.

skull, the nasal sinuses, and any cerebral calcification. The study is indicated in patients in whom a pathologic condition is suspected in any of these structures.

Fractures of the skull are easily seen as abnormal radiolucent lines in an otherwise radiopaque skull bone (Figure 6-3). Metastatic tumors of the skull can easily be seen as radiolucent spots in an otherwise normal skull (Figure 6-4). Opacification of the nasal sinuses may indicate sinusitis, hemorrhage, or tumor.

The pineal gland, located in the midline of the brain, is thought to regulate the biorhythms of mammals. This gland may become calcified anytime after puberty. When calcified, it is a very useful marker and allows the midline of the brain to be easily identified on a skull x-ray film. Conditions such as unilateral hematoma or tumor cause a shift of midline structures (and the calcified pineal gland) to the side opposite the site of the pathologic condition. Simple skull x-ray films, then, allow for the easy detection of these unilateral space-occupying lesions.

The sella turcica is the bony structure surrounding and protecting the pituitary gland (Figure 6-3). Tumors of the pituitary gland may cause an increase in size or an erosion of the sella. These changes can be detected by skull x-ray studies. No complications are associated with this test when it is used appropriately and selectively.

Procedure. The unsedated patient is taken to the radiology department and placed on an x-ray table. Metal objects (such as bobby pins, barrettes, and earrings) and dentures must be removed, because they will obscure visualization

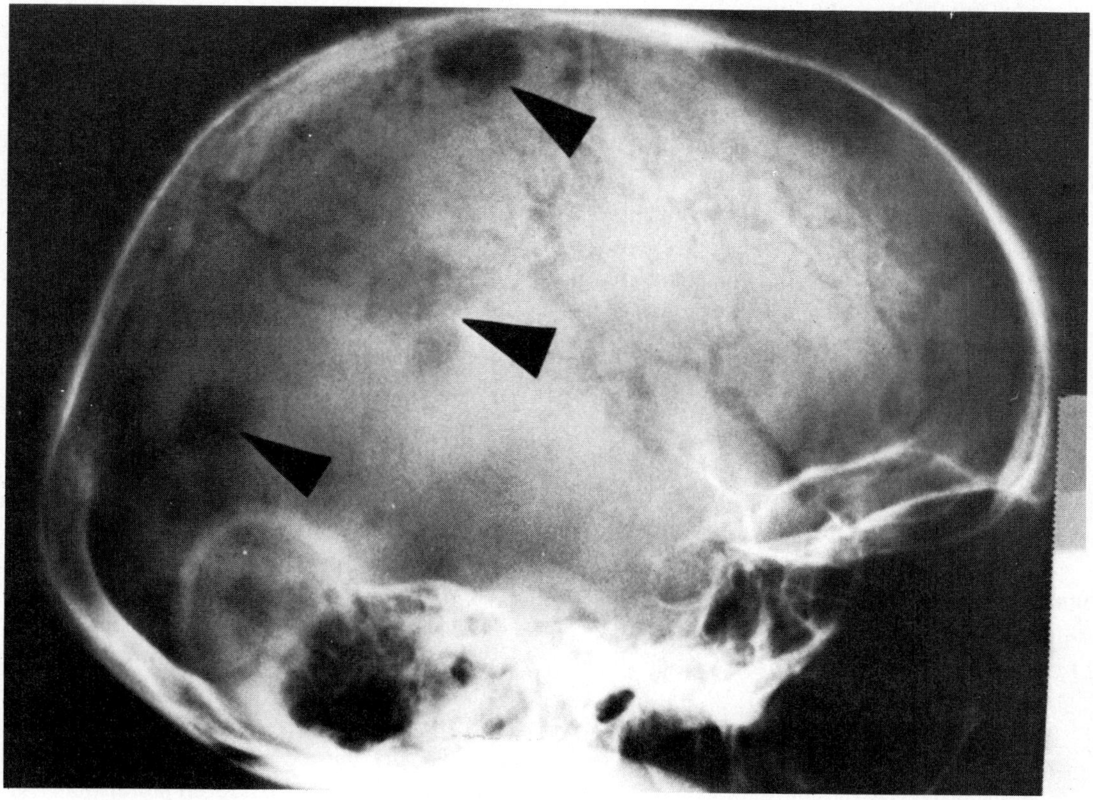

FIGURE 6-4. Lateral view of skull. Pointers indicate osteolytic metastasis to skull. Primary site of tumor was breast.

of part of the skull. If a glass eye is present, it should be noted on the x-ray examination request slip because it can present a confusing shadow. Axial (submentovertical, i.e., chin to top of head), half-axial (Towne), posteroanterior, and lateral views of the skull are usually taken. The test is painless and requires only a few minutes for its completion. Skull x-ray films are taken by a radiologic technician and interpreted by a radiologist.

Contraindications. This procedure is contraindicated in uncooperative patients who cannot remain still.

Nursing considerations

Nursing Diagnoses/Collaborative Problems

See X-ray studies, p. 5.

Nursing Implications with Rationale

- Explain the procedure to the patient.
- Tell the patient that all objects above the neck must be removed. Metal objects and dentures prevent x-ray visualization of the structures they cover.
- If the patient is unstable or unconscious, supervise to and from the radiology department and during the x-ray examination. Hyperextension and manipulation of the head should not be permitted until cervical injuries are ruled out.
- In trauma cases where the scalp has been lacerated, dress the wound in a sterile manner before the x-ray film is taken.
- As in all patients with head trauma, sedation solely for the purpose of completing any test should be avoided.

Lumbar puncture and cerebrospinal fluid examination

(LP, spinal tap, spinal puncture)

Pressure
Normal values: <200 cm H_2O
Color
Normal values: clear and colorless
Blood
Normal value: none
Cells
Normal values: no red blood cells; <5 lymphocytes per mm^3
Culture and sensitivity
Normal value: no organisms present
Protein
Normal values; 15-45 mg/dl CSF
Glucose
Normal values: 50-75 mg/dl CSF or >40% of blood glucose level
Chloride
Normal values: 700-750 mg/dl
Lactic dehydrogenase (LDH)
Normal values: <2.0-7.2 U/ml
Cytology
Normal value: no malignant cells
Serology for syphilis
Normal value: negative
Glutamine
Normal value: 6-15 mg/dl

Rationale. By placing a needle in the subarachnoid space of the spinal column, one can measure the pressure of that space and obtain spinal fluid for examination. The examination may assist in the diagnosis of brain or spinal cord neoplasm, cerebral hemorrhage, meningitis, encephalitis, degenerative brain disease, autoimmune disorders involving the CNS, neurosyphilis, and demyelinating disorders (such as multiple sclerosis or acute demyelinating polyneuropathy). Lumbar puncture may be used therapeutically yet very rarely to relieve intracranial pressure, to inject therapeutic or diagnostic agents, and to administer spinal anesthetics. Examination of the CSF usually includes evaluation for the presence of blood, bacteria, and malignant cells, along with quantitation of the amount of glucose and protein present. Color is noted and tests are performed to detect syphilitic organisms.

Pressure. By attaching a sterile manometer to the needle used in lumbar puncture, the pressure within the subarachnoid space of the spinal canal can be measured. A pressure above 200 cm H_2O is considered abnormal. As discussed earlier, the subarachnoid space surrounding the brain is freely connected to the subarachnoid space of the spinal cord. Therefore, any increase in intracranial pressure (because of tumor, hemorrhage, hematoma, or tissue edema) is directly reflected as an increase at the lumbar site. In cases where this normal connection is suspected to be obstructed above the puncture (as by a tumor, scarring, foreign body, or intervertebral disc), a Queckenstedt-Stookey test is performed (see page 181).

Color. CSF is normally clear and colorless. A cloudy appearance may indicate an increase in the WBC count. Normally, CSF contains no blood. A red tinge to the CSF indicates the probable presence of blood from subarachnoid bleeding or because the needle used in the lumbar puncture has penetrated a blood vessel. These causes of the bleeding must be differentiated. In the traumatic puncture the blood within the spinal fluid clots. No clotting occurs in a patient with a subarachnoid hemorrhage. Also, in a traumatic tap the fluid tends to become clear toward the end of the procedure, as successive CSF samples are obtained. This clearing does not occur with a subarachnoid hemorrhage.

Blood. Blood in the CSF indicates a cerebral hemorrhage into the subarachnoid space or a traumatic tap. (See the previous paragraph.)

Cells. The number of red blood cells is merely an indication of the amount of blood present within the CSF. Except for a few lymphocytes, the presence of white blood cells in the CSF is abnormal. The presence of polymorphonuclear leukocytes (neutrophils) in the CSF is indicative of bacterial meningitis or cerebral abscess. When mononuclear leukocytes are present, viral or tubercular meningitis or encephalitis is suspected.

Culture and sensitivity. The organism that causes meningitis or brain abscess can be cultured from the CSF. Organisms found may include atypical bacteria, fungi, or *Bacterium tuberculosis.* A gram stain of the CSF may give the clinician some early information about the causative infectious agent. This may allow appropriate antibiotic therapy to be initiated before the 24 hours necessary for completion of the culture and sensitivity report.

Protein. Normally, very little protein (15 to 45 mg/dl) is found in CSF from the subarachnoid space. The amount of protein is usually lower in CSF obtained from the cisterna magna and even lower in the ventricle. Small amounts of protein are found in CSF because protein is a large molecule that does not cross the blood-brain barrier. However, disease processes can alter the permeability of this protective membrane.

The protein content within CSF is increased in patients who have infectious or inflammatory processes such as meningitis, encephalitis, or myelitis (inflammation of the spinal cord). Tumors may also cause an increase in the protein content. Normally, less than 12% to 20% of the total protein consists of gamma globulin. The proportion of albumin to globulin is higher in CSF than in blood plasma because albumin is smaller in size than globulin and therefore can pass more easily through the blood-brain barrier. Patients with multiple sclerosis, neurosyphilis, or degenerative cord or brain disease have an elevation of the globulin fraction of total protein. An increase in the CSF level of immunoglobulin G (IgG), an increase in the ratio of IgG to other proteins (such as albumin), and the detection of *oligoclonal gamma globulin bands* are highly suggestive of inflammatory and autoimmune diseases of the CNS, in particular, multiple sclerosis.

Glucose. The glucose level in CSF is decreased when there is an increase in the number of cells within CSF. These cells may be inflammatory cells in response to infection (as in meningitis), shedded tumor cells (as in brain tumors), or bacterial cells. A blood sample for glucose is usually drawn before the spinal tap is performed. A CSF glucose level less than 40% of the blood glucose level may indicate meningitis or neoplasm.

Chloride. The chloride concentration in CSF may be decreased in patients with meningeal infections, tubercular meningitis, and conditions of low blood chloride levels. If the chloride level in CSF is increased, it is not of any neurologic significance. It correlates with the blood levels of chloride. CSF is not routinely evaluated for chloride; this test is done only if specifically requested.

Lactic dehydrogenase (LDH). Quantitation of LDH (specifically fractions 4 and 5) is helpful in diagnosing bacterial meningitis. The source of LDH is the neutrophils that fight the invading bacteria. When the LDH level is elevated, infection or inflammation is suspected.

Cytology. Examination of the cells in the CSF can determine if they are malignant or benign. Primary cortical tumors and metastatic tumors in the central nervous system shed cells from their surface, which float freely in CSF. Their presence incriminates neoplasm as the cause of the neurologic problem.

Serology for syphilis. Latent neurosyphilis is diagnosed by performing one of many presently available serologic tests on CSF. These include: (1) the Wassermann test, (2) the Venereal Disease Research Laboratory (VDRL) test, and (3) the fluorescent treponemal antibody (FTA) test. The FTA test is presently considered to be the most sensitive and specific. When test results are positive, the diagnosis of neurosyphilis is made and appropriate antibiotic therapy is required.

Glutamine. The CSF can also be evaluated for detection of glutamine. This test is useful in the detection and evaluation of hepatic encephalopathy and coma. In many instances, levels of glutamine are increased with Reye's syndrome.

Complications of lumbar puncture include the following:

1. Persistent CSF leak, causing severe headache.
2. Introduction of bacteria into CSF, causing suppurative meningitis.
3. Herniation of the brain through the tentorium cerebelli or herniation of the cerebellum through the foramen magnum. In patients who have increased intracranial pressure, the quick reduction of pressure in the spinal column by the lumbar puncture may induce herniation of the brain, causing compression of the brainstem. The result is deterioration of the patient's neurologic status and death.
4. Inadvertent puncture of the spinal cord, caused by an inappropriately high puncture of the spinal canal.
5. Puncture of the aorta or vena cava, causing serious retroperitoneal hemorrhage. This puncture is the result of a misdirected spinal needle probe.
6. Transient back pain and pain or paresthesia in the legs.

Procedure. No fasting or sedation is required for lumbar puncture. This study is a sterile procedure that can easily be performed at the bedside by a qualified physician. (Cisternal magna puncture [see p. 197], however, requires the expertise of a neurologic specialist.) The patient is usually placed in the lateral decubitus (fetal) position (Figure 6-5). The patient should clasp the hands on the knees to maintain this position. It is important that the lumbar area be flexed as much as possible to assure maximum bowing of the spine and to allow as much space as possible between the vertebrae. A vertebral interspace between L2 and S1 is chosen for the puncture, because the spinal cord ends around L2. This procedure can also be performed with the patient sitting up and leaning over a table if pressure readings are not required.

A local anesthetic (usually 1% lidocaine) is injected into the skin and subcutaneous tissues after the site has been aseptically cleansed. Next, a spinal needle containing an inner obturator is placed through the skin and into the spinal canal. The subarachnoid space is entered. The insert (obturator) is removed, and CSF can be seen slowly dripping from the needle. The needle is then attached to a sterile manometer and the pressure (called the *opening pressure*) is recorded. Before the pressure reading is taken the patient is asked to relax and straighten the legs to reduce the intraabdominal pressure, which causes an increase in CSF pressure. Next, three

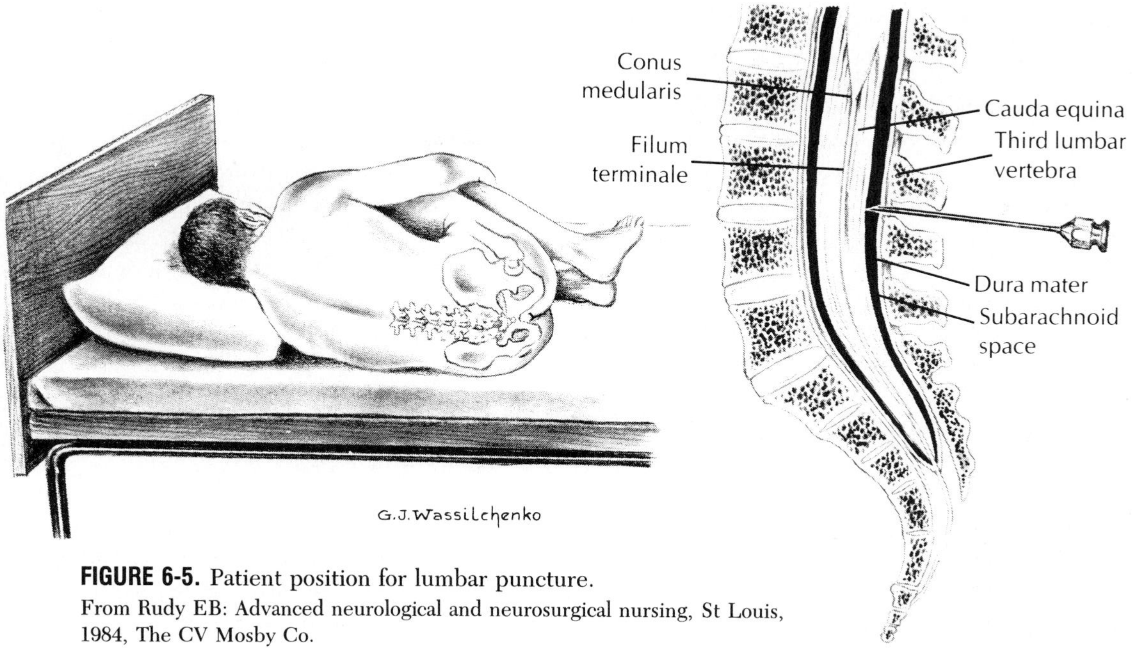

FIGURE 6-5. Patient position for lumbar puncture.
From Rudy EB: Advanced neurological and neurosurgical nursing, St Louis, 1984, The CV Mosby Co.

sterile test tubes are filled with 5 to 10 ml of CSF and sent for appropriate testing. Finally, the pressure (called the *closing pressure*) is measured.

If blockage in CSF circulation in the spinal (subarachnoid) space is suspected, a *Queckenstedt-Stookey test* is performed. For this test the jugular veins are occluded either manually by digital pressure or by a medium-sized blood pressure cuff inflated to approximately 20 mm Hg. Within 10 seconds after jugular vein occlusion, CSF pressure should increase from 15 to 40 cm H_2O and then promptly return to normal within 10 seconds after release of the pressure. A sluggish rise or fall of CSF pressure with venous compression suggests partial blockage of CSF circulation. No rise after 10 seconds suggests complete obstruction within the spinal canal.

After the procedure the spinal needle is removed, and digital pressure is placed over the area of needle insertion. An adhesive bandage can be placed over the puncture site. The patient is then placed in the prone position with a pillow under the abdomen to increase the intraabdominal pressure, which indirectly increases the pressure on the tissues surrounding the spinal canal. This acts to retard continued CSF flow from the spinal canal. The patient is encouraged to drink increased amounts of fluid to replace the CSF removed during the lumbar puncture. The patient is asked to maintain the reclining position usually for 4 to 12 hours to avoid the discomfort of potential postpuncture spinal headache.

This procedure is usually described as painful by the patient. Patients usually complain of a feeling of pressure from the needle. Some patients complain of a shooting pain in their legs. This may be caused by the needle's touching the spinal nerves of the lower extremities. The procedure lasts approximately 20 minutes.

Contraindications. This procedure is contraindicated in:

1. Uncooperative patients
2. Patients with increased intracranial pres-

sure, because the lumbar puncture may induce cerebral or cerebellar herniation
3. Patients who have severe degenerative spinal joint disease because the physician is most always unsuccessful in trying to place the needle through the degenerated interspinal space
4. Patients who are prone to psychosomatic illness because these patients may occasionally associate a lumbar puncture with the potential of paraplegia
5. Patients with an infection near the LP site; meningitis can result from contamination with infected material

Nursing considerations

Nursing Diagnoses/Collaborative Problems

- Possible knowledge deficit related to test purpose, preparation, and procedure
- Possible alteration in comfort related to test procedure
- Possible anxiety related to unknown sensations of procedure
- Possible anxiety related to test results
- Potential complication: headache
- Potential complication: meningitis
- Potential complication: herniation of brain
- Potential complication: perforation of spinal cord, aorta, or vena cava

Nursing Implications with Rationale

- Explain the procedure and the postprocedure routine to the patient. This is necessary to minimize anxiety and ensure the patient's cooperation. Many patients have misconceptions regarding this procedure. Assure the patient that insertion of the needle will not cause paralysis because the needle is inserted into the area below the spinal cord.
- Ensure that the physician has obtained written and informed consent for this procedure.
- Order the necessary lumbar puncture tray from the central supply department of the hospital.
- Have the patient empty the bladder before the procedure, if possible. A misdirected needle may puncture the bladder if distended with urine.
- Explain to the patient that he or she must lie very still throughout this procedure. Movement may cause traumatic injury.
- Assist the patient in assuming the appropriate position. The patient's head and neck are flexed into the chest, and the knees are pulled up into the chest. You may place a pillow between the patient's legs to prevent the upper part of the legs from rolling forward. Stand facing the patient, with one hand on the patient's shoulder and the other hand on the patient's knees.
- You may be required to assist the physician by holding the manometer straight. If you are not wearing sterile gloves, hold the very top of the manometer with your fingertips.
- Label and number the specimen jars appropriately and have them delivered immediately to the appropriate laboratory.
- After the procedure keep the patient on bed rest with his or her head flat because of the high risk of spinal headache. This headache is probably caused by the loss of CSF at the puncture site. The patient may turn from side to side. Encourage the patient to drink fluids through a straw.
- After the procedure assess the patient for movement of the extremities, pain at the injection site, drainage of blood or CSF at the injection site, and the ability to void. Notify the physician of any unusual occurrences.

Electroencephalography

Normal values: normal frequency, amplitude, and characteristics of brain waves

Rationale. The electroencephalogram (EEG) is a graphic recording of the electrical activity the brain generates. Brain waves are detected by electrodes in a manner similar to the EKG's recording of electrical impulses generated by the heart (Chapter 2). EEG electrodes are placed on the scalp over multiple areas of the brain to detect and record electrical impulses produced within the brain. Moving graph paper is used. Considerable sophistication is necessary for interpreting the frequency, amplitude, and characteristics of the brain waves. This study is invaluable in the investigation of epileptic states, where the focus of seizure activity is characterized by rapid, spiking waves seen on the graph (Figure 6-6). Patients with cerebral lesions (such as hemorrhage, abscess, neoplasm, or infarction) have abnormally slow EEG waves, depending on the size and location of the lesion.

Because this study determines the overall activity of the brain, it can be used to evaluate trauma and drug intoxication and to determine cerebral death in comatose patients. The EEG is also valuable in the diagnosis of hysterical blindness. Visual stimulation causes EEG changes if sight is present. Similarly, a response evoked by a noise during light sleep can confirm hearing in a patient who feigns deafness.

The EEG can also be used to monitor cerebral blood flow during surgical procedures. For example, during carotid endarterectomy (re-

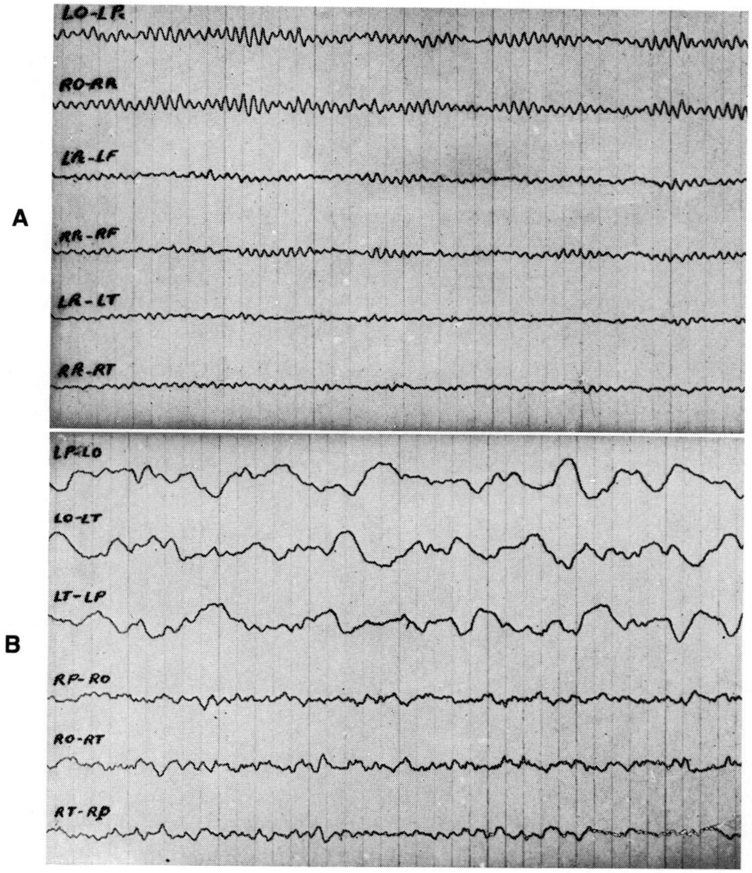

FIGURE 6-6. Electroencephalographic recordings. Placements are indicated by *L*, left; *R*, right; *F*, frontal; *T*, temporal; *O*, occipital; *P*, parietal; *Pc*, precentral. Calibration for time and amplitude is the same for all and can be noted in **E. A,** Normal record with regular, 10-per-second alpha waves dominant throughout. **B,** Irregular, high-amplitude delta waves (1-2 per second) prominent over left side. This patient had an intracranial tumor.

Continued.

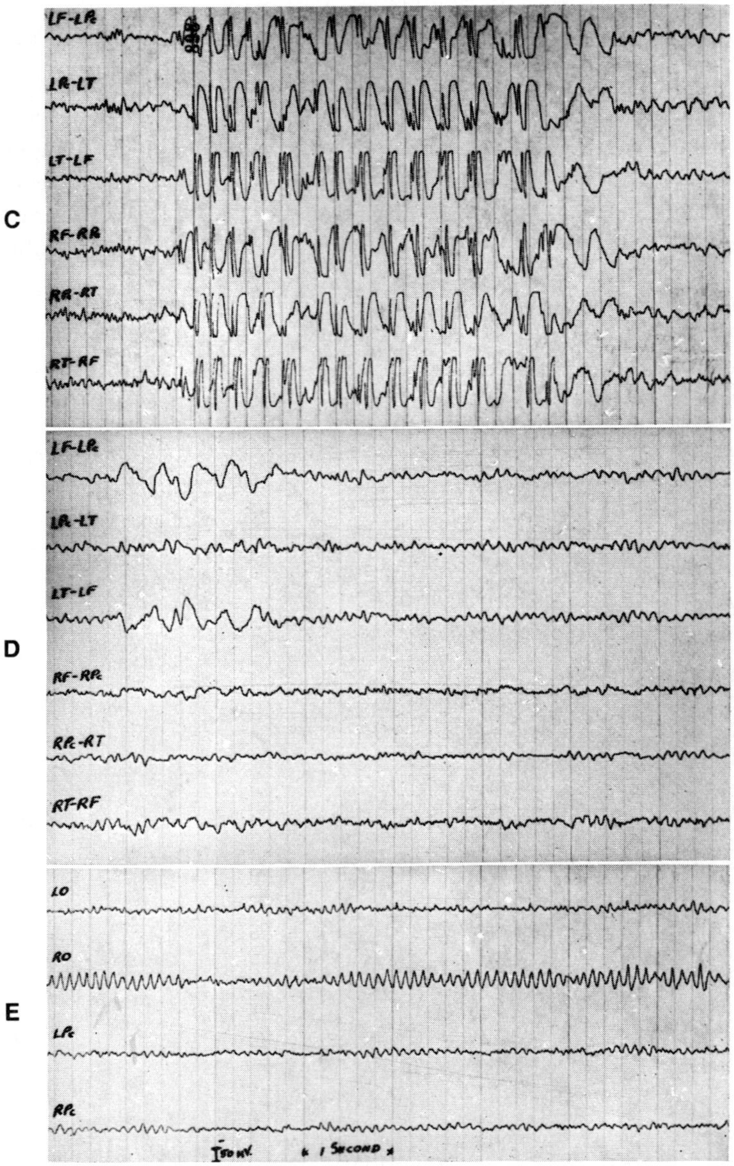

FIGURE 6-6, cont'd. **C,** Three-per-second, synchronous "spike and dome" waves present in all areas, as seen in minor epilepsy. **D,** Irregular, high-amplitude, 2-3-per-second waves out of phase in left frontal area. Patient had jacksonian epilepsy. **E,** Greatly diminished amplitude in occipital area. Patient had head trauma with fracture of left occipital bone.

A to **E** from Conway BL: Carini and Owens' neurological and neurosurgical nursing, ed 8, St Louis, 1982, The CV Mosby Co.

moval of atherosclerotic plaque from the inner lining of the vessel) the carotid vessel must temporarily be occluded. When this surgery is performed with the patient under general anesthesia, the EEG can be used for the early detection of cerebral tissue ischemia, which would indicate that continued carotid occlusion results in a stroke syndrome. Temporary shunting of blood during the surgery is then required. No complications are associated with EEG.

Brain mapping can be performed using EEG data and computer digitalization to show a topographic map of the brain. This technique can also map evoked responses. The information can be used to evaluate patients with migraine headaches, vertigo, generalized seizures, dementia, ischemic abnormalities, psychiatric disorders, dyslexia, hyperactivity, and Alzheimer's disease.

Procedure. The patient is instructed to shampoo his or her hair the night before the study. No oils, sprays, or lotions may be used. The patient should not fast before this study. Coffee, tea, and cola are not permitted on the morning of the procedure. Anticonvulsants are rarely discontinued before the study because of the risk of precipitating seizures. Usually only a limited amount of sleep is allowed the night before the study.

EEG is often performed in a specially constructed room (Figure 6-7) that is shielded from outside disturbances (electrical, auditory, and

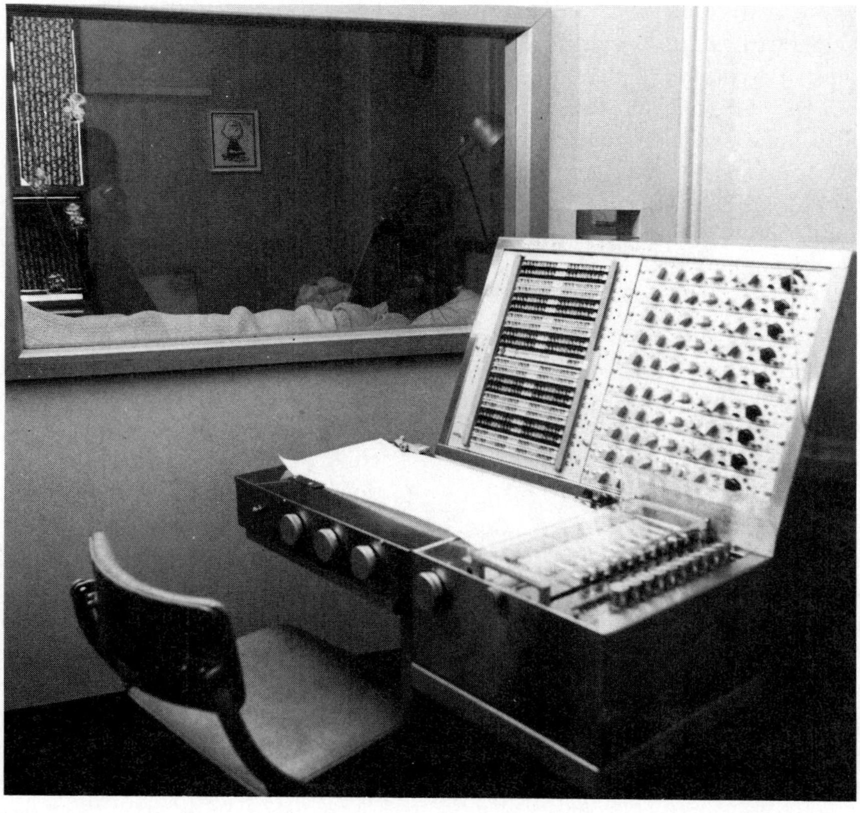

FIGURE 6-7. Electroencephalography suite, showing patient isolated from equipment. Electroencephalography room is specially constructed to shield out noise and other artifacts.

From Conway BL: Carini and Owens' neurological and neurosurgical nursing, ed 8, St Louis, 1982, The CV Mosby Co.

visual). EEG can be done at the bedside if the patient is too ill to be moved.

The patient is placed in a supine position on a bed or reclining on a chair. Sixteen or more electrodes are applied to the scalp with electrode paste in a uniform pattern over both sides of the head, covering the prefrontal, frontal, temporal, parietal, and occipital areas. One electrode may be applied to each earlobe for grounding.

After the electrodes are applied, the patient is instructed to lie still with his or her eyes closed. The technician continuously observes the patient during the EEG recording for any movements that could alter the results. Approximately every 5 minutes the recording is interrupted to permit the client to move, if desired. In addition to the resting EEG, a number of "activating" procedures can be performed:

1. The patient is hyperventilated (asked to breathe deeply 20 times a minute for 3 minutes) to induce alkalosis and cerebral vasoconstriction, which may activate abnormalities.
2. Photostimulation is performed by flashing a light (stroboscope) over the patient's face with the patient's eyes opened or closed. Photostimulated seizure activity may be seen on the EEG.
3. A sleep EEG may be performed to aid in the detection of some abnormal brain waves that are seen only if the patient is sleeping (such as frontal lobe epilepsy). The sleep EEG is performed after orally administering methyprylon (Noludar) and secobarbital (Seconal). (Secobarbital should not be administered to children.) A recording is performed while the patient is falling asleep, while the patient is asleep, and while the patient is waking.

After the study the electrode paste and the electrodes are removed. The patient is either returned to the unit or is released. This study is performed by an EEG technician in approximately 45 minutes to 2 hours. Other than the fatigue caused by missing sleep before and the discomfort of remaining still during the study, no pain is associated with this study.

Contraindications. None.

Nursing considerations

Nursing Diagnoses/Collaborative Problems

- Possible knowledge deficit related to test purpose, preparation, and procedure
- Possible anxiety related to test results

Nursing Implications with Rationale

- Explain the procedure to the patient. Many patients fear that the EEG can "read the mind" or detect senility. Some patients fear that the EEG is a form of electric shock therapy. Reassure the patient that these ideas are false. Encourage verbalization of the patient's fears.
- Assure the patient that the flow of electrical current is *from* the patient. He or she will feel nothing during this study.
- Instruct the patient to wash his or her hair the night before the study. No hair oils, sprays, or lotions should be used, because these can cause movement of the scalp electrodes.
- Check if the physician desires to discontinue any medications before the study.
- Instruct the patient if sleep time should be shortened on the night before the test. Adults should not sleep more than 4 to 5 hours and children not more than 5 to 7 hours. This is done to allow the patient to relax and possibly fall asleep during the study.
- Administer the sedatives or hypnotics before the study, as indicated for the sleep EEG. (These are usually given in the EEG room.) Otherwise, sedatives or hypnotics should not be given because they cause abnormally low-voltage, fast waves to appear on the EEG.
- Do *not* allow the patient to fast before the study. Fasting may cause hypoglycemia, which could modify the EEG pattern. Coffee, tea, and cola are not permitted on the morning of the study because of their stimulating effect.

- Tell the patient that during the recording of the EEG, his or her activity should be minimal, if any. Movement (including opening of the eyes) creates interference and alters the EEG recording.
- After the study help the patient remove the electrode paste. The paste may be removed with acetone or witch hazel, and the hair should be shampooed.
- Ensure safety precautions (side rails up) after the test until the effect of the sedatives has worn off. If the patient is having the study done as an outpatient, an adult should accompany the patient and provide transportation home after the study.

Brain scanning

Normal value: no areas of increased radionuclide uptake within the brain

Rationale. Brain scanning allows for the detection of pathologic cerebral conditions by Geiger counter scanning of the patient's cranial contents after the IV administration of a radioisotope. This study is routinely performed in patients who have frequent and severe headaches, stroke syndrome, seizure disorders, or other major neurologic complaints. Normally, the blood-brain barrier does not allow the blood to come in direct contact with the brain tissue. Commonly used radioisotopes (such as technetium-99m pertechnetate, mercury-201, or radioiodinated albumin) are unable to cross this blood-brain barrier. However, in localized pathologic conditions, such as cerebral neoplasms, brain abscess, acute infarction, cerebral hemorrhage, acute hematoma, and arteriovenous (AV) malformation, the normal barrier is disrupted. The isotopes are then preferentially localized or concentrated in these regions of the brain. A scintillation (Geiger) counter recognizes this relative increase in radioactive material through the intact skull and graphically displays this brain feature (Figure 6-8).

The precise cause of the disruption of the blood-brain barrier can be any of a number of pathologic processes. Unfortunately, the brain scan is not a specific indicator of the exact pathologic process. Study of the location, size, and shape of the abnormality, along with the timing of the scan, may help specify the pathologic process. Tumors appear as discrete, marginated, and spherical lesions, usually within the center of the brain. Subdural hematomas are also discrete

A

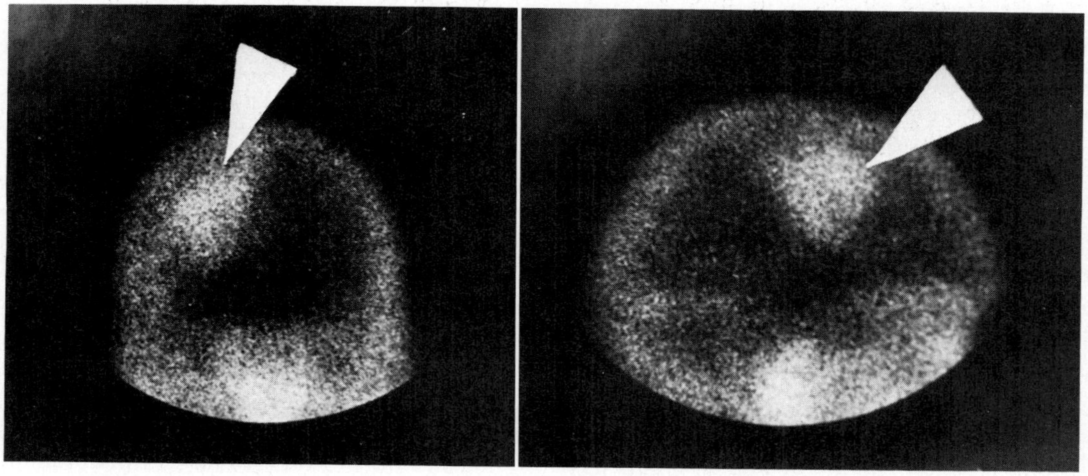

B

FIGURE 6-8. Brain scans. **A,** Anteroposterior view. **B,** Lateral view. White pointers indicate tumor seen in both views.

and spherical, but always appear in the periphery. A brain abscess is characterized as a lesion with an outer rim of increased uptake of isotopes and a core with little uptake.

Timing of brain scanning in relation to the onset of strokelike symptoms is usually significant. For example, in cerebral infarction, scanning performed soon after the onset of symptoms may be normal and then become abnormal 2 weeks later. This combination is virtually pathognomonic of infarction. Scanning in patients with cerebral thrombosis without infarction may never become abnormal. Tumors and abscesses cause abnormalities on the first scan.

The injection of isotopes followed by immediate scanning can be used to detect changes in the dynamics of cerebral blood flow by comparing one side of the brain with the other. For example, cerebral vascular occlusive disease is characterized by a decreased flow rate, in contrast to an AV malformation, which is associated with an increased flow rate.

Cisternal scans may be performed by injecting radioactive material into the subarachnoid space and then taking serial scans of the head. These scans are useful in evaluating ventricular size and patency of the CSF pathways and reabsorption. Normally, because only a small amount of CSF enters the ventricles, their uptake of radioactive material should be minimal. However, blocks in the CSF pathways may prevent this reabsorption, and thus large amounts of isotopes may appear in the ventricles. Cisternal scans may also be used to evaluate CSF leakage in patients with recurrent meningitis and to evaluate hydrocephalus. This noninvasive study is essentially without complications.

Procedure. The nonfasting, unsedated patient is given a potassium chloride capsule 2 hours before the IV injection of technetium-99m pertechnetate. The potassium chloride prevents an inordinate amount of technetium uptake by the choroid plexus, which would simulate a pathologic cerebral condition. Similar solutions may be used to enhance uptake by other available radioisotopes and to block irradiation to other organs. Blocking agents are not necessary with technetium-99m diethylenetriamine pentaacetic acid (DTPA). Shortly after the technetium injection, the patient is placed in the supine, lateral, and prone positions while a counter is passed over the patient's head. The radioisotope counts are anatomically displayed and photographed while the patient remains very still.

When cerebral flow studies are performed, the patient is placed in the supine position and injected with isotopes, and the counter is immediately placed over the head. The counts are anatomically recorded in timed sequence to follow the isotope during its first flow through the brain. Another scan is obtained later for identification of pathologic tissue.

Brain scanning is performed by a technician in the nuclear medicine department. The duration of this study is approximately 35 to 45 minutes. No discomfort is associated with this study other than that of the peripheral IV puncture required for the injection of the radioisotopes.

Contraindications. This study is contraindicated in the uncooperative patient and in the pregnant patient.

Nursing considerations

Nursing Diagnoses/Collaborative Problems

See Nuclear scanning, p. 5.

Nursing Implications with Rationale

- Explain the procedure to the patient. Encourage verbalization of the patient's fears and provide emotional support.
- Administer the potassium chloride as ordered before the scanning.
- Assure the patient that the radioactive material will be excreted from the body within 24 hours. Encourage fluids to aid the excretion of the isotope.
- Monitor confused or unstable patients in the nuclear medicine department throughout the procedure.

Cerebral angiography

(cerebral arteriography)

Normal value: normal cerebral vessels

Rationale. Cerebral angiography provides radiographic visualization of the cerebral vascular system after the intraarterial injection of radiopaque dye into the carotid or vertebral arteries. This procedure is used for the detection of abnormalities of the cerebral circulation, such as aneurysms, occlusion, or AV malformations (Figure 6-9). Vascular tumors are seen as masses containing multiple, small AV fistulas. Nonvascular tumors, abscesses, and hematomas

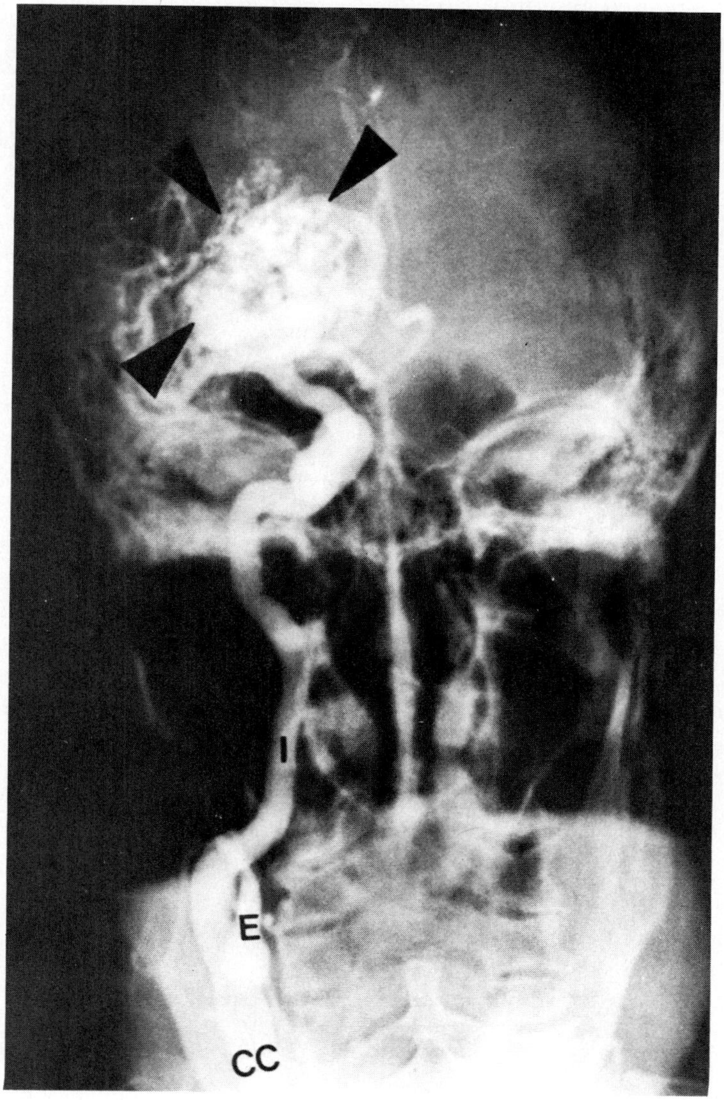

FIGURE 6-9. Cerebral angiogram. Black pointers indicate large arteriovenous malformation. *CC*, Common carotid artery; *E*, external carotid artery; *I*, internal carotid artery.

present an avascular mass, distorting the normal vascular location.

Cerebral angiography is an invasive procedure and is therefore associated with complications. These include:

1. Anaphylaxis caused by an allergic reaction to the iodinated contrast material
2. Hemorrhage or hematoma formation at the puncture site used for arterial access
3. Neurologic deficits caused by the angiocatheter dislodging an atherosclerotic plaque, which can travel to the brain and cause infarction

Procedure. The patient is usually kept NPO for solid foods after midnight on the day of cerebral angiography. Liquids are usually allowed because the patient should be well hydrated. The patient is usually sedated with atropine and meperidine (Demerol) 30 minutes before the study and taken to the angiography room, located in the radiology department. This procedure is usually performed with the patient under local anesthesia. General anesthesia is reserved for the confused or extremely restless patient.

Puncture site selection is determined by the clinical problem under investigation and by the personal preference of the physician performing the test. A needle or cannula may be placed percutaneously into the lumen of the common carotid, vertebral, or subclavian artery. Selective catheterization may also be performed to cannulate any of the major cervical vessels in retrograde fashion by way of the brachial or femoral artery. Fewer complications occur with the retrograde technique. The catheter is followed under fluoroscopy as it passes into the desired artery. Radiopaque contrast material is then injected, and the flow of blood through the cranial cavity is seen. Serial x-ray films are taken in timed sequence to show the arterial and venous phases of the cerebral circulation.

The patient is required to lie quietly in the supine and lateral positions. During the dye injection, the patient will feel a severe, transient burning sensation and flush. The only other discomfort associated with this study is from the arterial puncture needed for dye injection. After the x-ray films are completed, the catheter is removed and a pressure dressing is applied to the puncture site.

A relatively new procedure called *digital subtraction angiography* (DSA) or *digital venous subtraction angiography* (DVSA) is a type of computerized fluoroscopy that uses *venous* or *arterial* catheterization to visualize the arteries of the body (especially the carotid and cerebral arteries). This procedure enables small differences in x-ray absorption between an artery and the surrounding tissues to be converted to digital information and stored. DSA is especially useful when bone blocks visualization of the blood vessels under study. This study is valuable in the preoperative and postoperative evaluation of patients having vascular and tumor surgery. For DSA an image "mask" is made of the area of clinical interest and then stored in the computer. After the IV injection of the contrast material, subsequent images are made. The computer then subtracts the preinjection "mask" image from the postinjection image. This removes all undesired tissue images (such as bone) and leaves an arterial image of high contrast and quality. If venous injection of the dye is used rather than arterial injection, the complications and risk associated with conventional arteriography are avoided. However, DSA is more often performed via an arterial injection of contrast material.

Conventional angiography and DSA are usually performed by an angiographer (radiologist) in approximately 1 hour.

Contraindications. This test is contraindicated in the patient with dye allergies and in the unstable patient.

Nursing considerations

Nursing Diagnoses/Collaborative Problems

- Possible knowledge deficit related to test purpose, preparation, and procedure
- Possible anxiety related to unknown sensations of procedure
- Possible anxiety related to test results

- High risk for alteration in comfort related to test procedure
- Possible injury related to effects of sedatives
- Potential complication: adverse reaction/allergy
- Potential complication: bleeding
- Potential complication: stroke
- Potential complication: peripheral arterial problems
- Potential complication: infection

Nursing Implications with Rationale

- The physician who obtains written permission for this study should thoroughly explain the procedure to the patient. Reinforce the patient's understanding.
- Tell the patient where the catheter will be inserted (usually into the femoral artery). Inform the patient that an uncomfortably warm flush during dye insertion will be felt. Most patients are very frightened about this procedure. Encourage verbalization of the patient's fears and provide emotional support.
- Assess the patient for allergies to iodine dye. A sensitivity test may be performed on the day before the study.
- Assess the patient for anticoagulant therapy because of the potential complication of bleeding. If the procedure is not postponed, it is done with the awareness that severe bleeding can occur.
- Before the study obtain baseline data on which to evaluate patient response after the procedure. Baseline data should include vital signs, level of consciousness, pupil reaction, facial symmetry, strength and motion of the extremities, and distal pulses (if the femoral artery approach is to be used).
- Keep the patient from having solid foods after midnight on the day of the test. If a sedative has been ordered, administer it on the evening before the study to ensure that the patient gets a good night's sleep.
- Administer the preprocedure drugs as ordered before angiography.
- Ensure that emergency drugs and equipment, along with personnel trained to perform cardiopulmonary resuscitation, are available during the study in the event of anaphylaxis. Assess the patient after the study for a delayed reaction to the dye.
- After the procedure, monitor vital signs and perform a neurologic evaluation frequently (every 15 minutes for four times, then every 30 minutes for four times, then every hour for four times, and then every 4 hours) and compare these findings with the preprocedure data base. An increase in pulse rate and a decrease in blood pressure may indicate bleeding. Notify the physician immediately of any signs of hemorrhage or embolism.
- Assess the catheter insertion site for hemorrhage, hematoma, and inflammation each time the vital signs are taken. If the neck arteries were used for arterial access, assess the neck region for swelling or hematoma that could compromise respiration. If the brachial or femoral arteries were cannulated, assess the involved extremity for peripheral pulses, numbness, tingling, pain, color, temperature, and loss of function. Any abnormalities should be immediately reported to the physician.
- Keep the patient on bed rest for 12 hours after the procedure to allow for complete sealing of the arterial puncture. During this time, the involved extremity should be extended and immobilized to prevent kinking of the vessel and clot formation.
- Apply an ice bag to the puncture site to reduce swelling and pain.
- Check if the patient can resume a regular diet after the procedure. Unless proscribed for medical purposes, encourage fluids to promote dye excretion by the kidneys. Renal function can deteriorate in dehydrated patients who receive iodine dye injection.

CT scanning

(computed tomography; CT scan of the brain; computerized axial tomography, CAT scan; CATT, computed axial transverse tomography; EMI scanning)

Normal value: no evidence of a pathologic condition

Rationale. Computed tomography is a remarkable study, which may be performed with or without a dye injection, consisting of a computerized analysis of multiple tomographic x-ray films taken of the brain tissue at successive layers to provide a three-dimensional view of the cranial contents. The CT x-ray image provides a view of the head as if one were looking down through its top. The variation in density of each tissue type allows for variable penetration of the x-ray beam. An attached computer calculates the amount of x-ray penetration of each tissue (coefficient) and displays this as shades of gray. This image is placed on a television screen and photographed. Radiodense tissue appears white, and radiolucent tissue appears darker. The final result is a series of realistic anatomic pictures of coronal sections of the brain.

CT scanning is used in the diagnosis of intracranial neoplasms (Figure 6-10), cerebral infarctions, ventricular displacement or enlargement, cortical atrophy, cerebral aneurysms, intracranial hemorrhage and hematoma, and AV malformation.

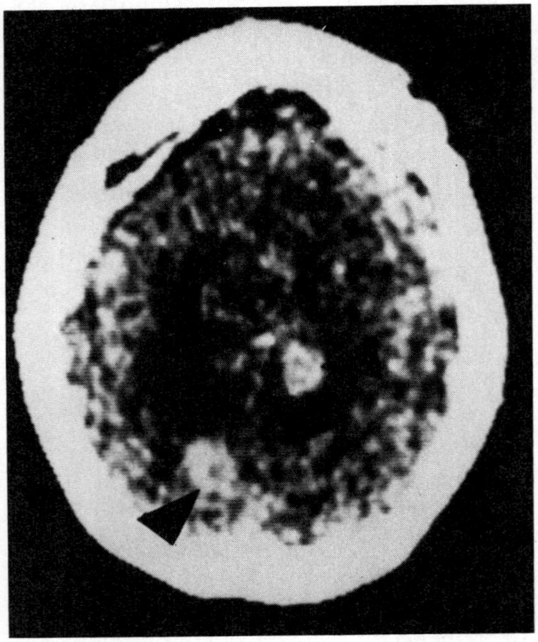

FIGURE 6-10. Computed tomogram (CT scan) of head. Black pointers indicate metastatic tumors within brain. Primary site of tumor was melanoma of lower extremity.

Visualization of neoplasms, old infarctions, or any pathologic process that destroys the blood-brain barrier may be enhanced by the IV injection of iodinated contrast dye. CT scans may be repeated frequently to monitor the progress of the disease or to monitor the healing process.

In many cases, CT scanning has eliminated the need for more invasive procedures such as cerebral arteriography (discussed in this chapter) and pneumoencephalography, rarely done anymore. CT scans of the spinal column are frequently performed to diagnose herniated cervical or lumbar discs.

No complications are associated with CT scanning other than the possibility of an allergic reaction to the dye if a contrast medium is used. The amount of radiation incurred during CT scanning is comparable to that incurred during a routine series of skull x-ray films. Although this form of x-ray scanning is considered revolutionary, magnetic resonance imaging (MRI) (see p. 201) has replaced CT scanning of the CNS, when an MRI unit is available. The accuracy, specificity, and clarity of the MRI is superior to a CT scan.

Procedure. The patient is usually kept fasting for 4 hours before the study. Sedation is required only for young children and other patients who cannot remain still during the procedure. Wigs and hairpins are removed from the patient's head. The patient lies in the supine position on an examining table with his or her head resting in a snug-fitting rubber cap within a water-filled box. The patient's head is enclosed only to the hair line (as in a hair dryer) (Figure 6-11). The face is not covered, and the patient can see out of the machine at all times. Sponges are placed along the side of the head to ensure that the patient's head is cushioned but does not move during this study. Any movement causes computer-generated artifacts on the image produced. The patient is instructed not to talk or sigh during the scanning.

The scanner passes a small x-ray beam through the brain from one side to the other. The machine then rotates 1 degree; the procedure is repeated at each degree through a 180° arc. The machine is then moved down about 0.5 to 2 cm, and the entire procedure is repeated for a total of about 3 to 7 "slices," or planes. This procedure requires about 15 to 30 minutes.

A

B

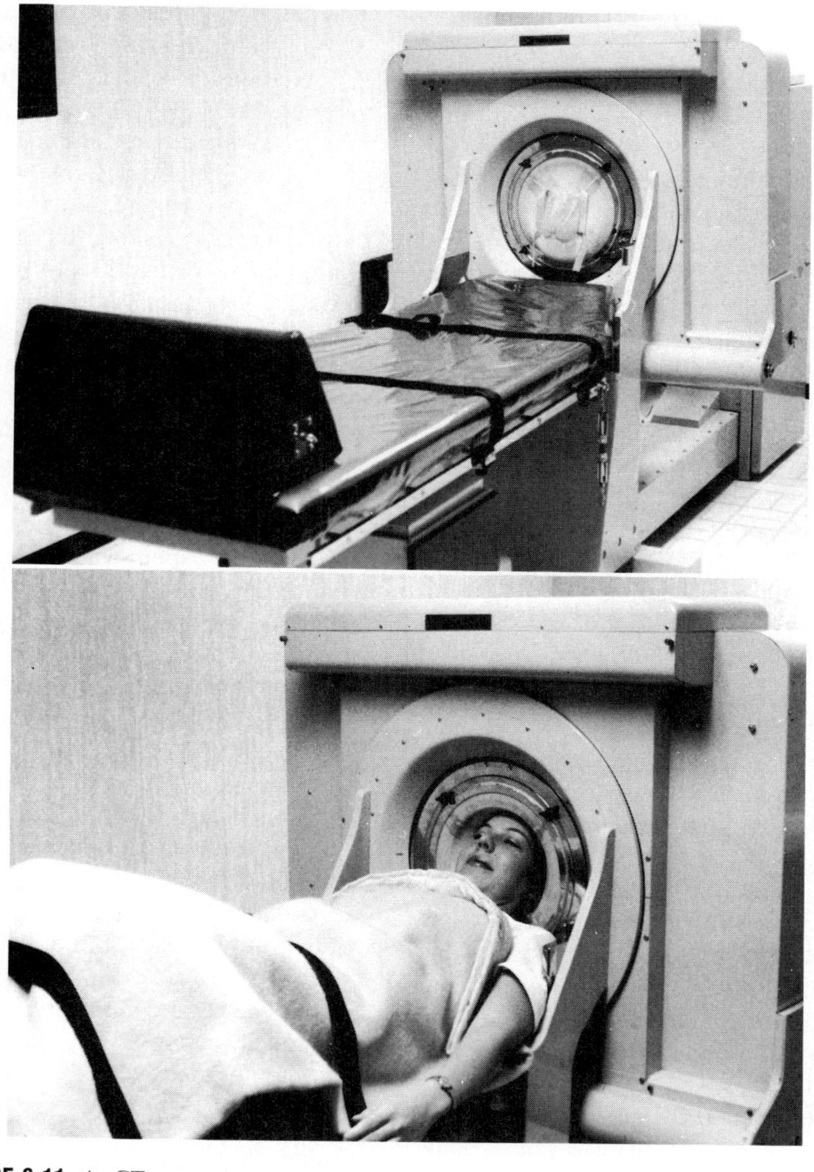

FIGURE 6-11. **A,** CT scanning equipment. **B,** Patient receiving CT scanning.
From Conway BL: Carini and Owens' neurological and neurosurgical nursing, ed 8, St Louis, 1982, The CV Mosby Co.

Usually an iodinated dye is then used. A peripheral IV line is started, and the iodine dye is then administered through it. The entire scanning process is repeated. The patient may feel facial flushing with the dye injection.

The data are immediately available in the form of an x-ray film or as a Polaroid print. CT scanning is performed by a technician in approximately 45 to 60 minutes. This is a painless procedure. The only discomfort associated with this study are those of lying still on a table and of the peripheral venipuncture. Occasionally patients become claustrophobic or uncomfortable during this study. Hospitalization is not required for this procedure. The patient may wear street clothes during the study. The amount of radiation exposure incurred with CT scanning is equal to that of a skull x-ray examination.

Contraindications. CT scanning is contraindicated in uncooperative patients and in patients allergic to iodine dye.

Nursing considerations

Nursing Diagnoses/Collaborative Problems

See X-ray studies, p. 5.

Nursing Implications with Rationale

- Explain the procedure to the patient. Assure the patient that CT scanning is a safe and painless x-ray method of studying the structures of the brain. Encourage verbalization of the patient's fears.
- If possible, show the patient a picture of the scanning machine and encourage verbalization of anxieties.
- Keep the patient NPO for 4 hours before the study, because the iodine dye may cause nausea. It is not usually known before the test if enhanced visualization by dye injection will be indicated.
- Instruct the parents if their child should be sleep-deprived before this study. This is done by keeping the child awake until midnight the night before the study. The child is then awakened every hour beginning at 4 A.M. for a 5- to 10-minute period. The child should not be allowed to fall asleep in the car on the way to the hospital.
- Instruct the patient that wigs, hairpins, or clips cannot be worn during this procedure because they hamper visualization of the brain.
- Assess the patient for allergies to iodinated dye to prevent dye-induced anaphylaxis. Sometimes the patient is pretested for dye allergies. Observe the patient for signs of anaphylaxis (such as respiratory distress, palpitations, or diaphoresis).
- Sedate the patient, if ordered. Sedation is used for children and other patients who cannot lie still during the procedure.
- Inform the patient that he or she must lie motionless during the study. Even talking or sighing may cause artifacts on the computer image.
- Tell the patient that during the procedure he or she will hear a "clicking" noise as the scanner moves around the head. Some describe the sound as being like that of a washing machine. The patient will not be able to feel the scanner rotate.
- No special postprocedure care is required. The patient can resume all activities. If the patient was sedated, observe safety precautions until the effects of the sedative have worn off.
- Encourage patients who received a dye injection to increase their fluid intake, because iodine contrast can cause renal function deterioration especially in the dehydrated patient.
- Some hospitals do not have CT scanning devices. Transportation arrangements may have to be made for patients from smaller facilities unless a mobile CT scanner can be brought to the hospital.

SUPPLEMENTAL INFORMATION

Oculoplethysmography

(OPG)

Normal value: normal and equal blood flow in both carotid arteries

Rationale. Oculoplethysmography (OPG) is a noninvasive study used to indirectly measure the blood flow in the ophthalmic artery. Since the ophthalmic artery is the first major branch of the internal carotid artery, its blood flow reflects the carotid blood flow and the ultimate blood flow to the brain.

For this study, pressure in the eyes is measured by suction cups placed on the eye for the recording of eye pressures (Figure 6-12). OPG is indicated in patients who have symptoms of transient ischemic attacks (TIAs), cardiac bruits, and neurologic symptoms (such as dizziness or fainting). If indicated, this procedure may be followed by cerebral angiography (p. 189). This test is often performed as a follow-up study after carotid endarterectomy, which involves cleaning out the inside of the carotid artery.

Procedure. No fasting or sedation is necessary before OPG. This study is usually performed in a special room designed for neurologic studies. The patient lies on his or her back on a table or a bed. The blood pressure in both arms is taken before the test. EKG electrodes are applied to the patient's extremities to demonstrate any abnormal cardiac rhythms or blinking of the eyes during the study.

Anesthetic eyedrops are then instilled in both eyes to minimize discomfort during OPG. Small detectors are attached to the earlobes to detect blood flow to the ear through the external carotid artery. Tracings for both ears are taken and compared. Eyecups resembling contact lenses (Figure 6-12) are applied directly to the eyeball. Tracing of the pulsations within each eye are then recorded. A vacuum source is then applied to the suction cup. This increased pressure causes the pulse in both eyes to disappear temporarily because all the blood flow to the eye is stopped. When the suction source is stopped, the blood flow returns to the eyes. Both pulses should return simultaneously. Time difference in the pulse rate from one eye to the other, from one ear to the other, and from

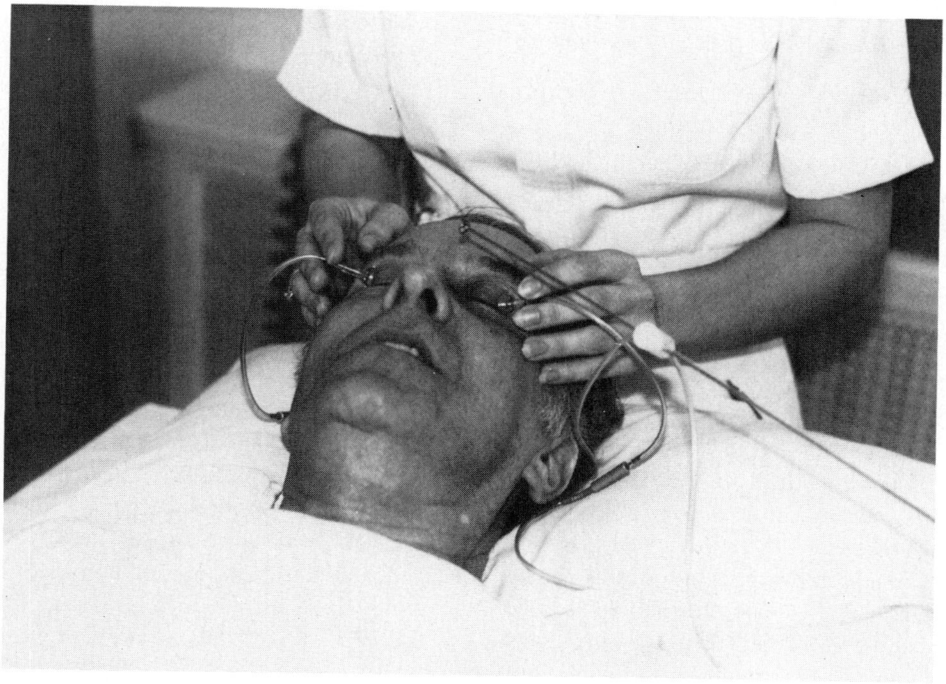

FIGURE 6-12. Suction cups ready to be placed on the eyeballs for oculoplethysmography (OPG).

the ear to the eye on each side is measured in milliseconds. If internal carotid stenosis is present, blood flow to the eye would be delayed. A trained technician performs this test in approximately 20 to 30 minutes. The patient's eyes usually burn slightly when the ophthalmic drops are applied. When suction is applied to the suction cup, the patient may feel a pulling sensation. During the suction application, vision may temporarily be lost; it will immediately return, however. After the study vision should be unaffected.

Complications of OPG include conjunctival hemorrhage and corneal abrasions. If corneal abrasions occur, the eye is patched and a lubricant such as Dacriose solution is applied. Patients may also experience photophobia for a short time after the procedure.

Contraindications. OPG is contraindicated in patients who have had recent eye surgery or had retinal detachment and those with cataracts.

Nursing considerations

Nursing Diagnoses/Collaborative Problems

- Possible knowledge deficit related to test purpose, preparation, and procedure
- Possible anxiety related to unknown sensations of procedure
- Possible anxiety related to test results
- Possible alteration in comfort related to test procedure
- Potential complication: conjunctival hemorrhage
- Potential complication: corneal abrasion

Nursing Implications with Rationale

- Explain the procedure to the patient. If the patient is wearing contact lenses, they should be removed before the study.
- After the study inform the patient that the eye anesthesia usually wears off in about ½ hour.
- Instruct the patient not to rub the eyes for at least 2 hours. If tears appear, the eye should only be blotted dry.
- If the patient wears contact lenses, they should not be reinserted for at least 2 hours after OPG.
- The patient's eyes may appear bloodshot for several hours after the test. Explain this to the patient so he or she knows that this is normal. Artificial tears may be instilled to soothe any irritation in the eyes.

Ventriculography

(ventriculogram)

Normal values: no ventricular abnormalities

Rationale. For ventriculography, serial x-ray examinations are taken of the skull after air or contrast material is injected *directly* into the ventricles through burr holes in the skull or via spinal canal puncture. The size, shape, and filling of the ventricles are observed. Lesions (for example, brain tumors), cerebral anomalies, and the patency of the ventricular system are identified. This procedure should not be performed when less invasive procedures (such as the CT scan) would suffice for diagnosis.

Procedure. For this procedure a specified area (for example, top, back, or side) of the head must be shaved according to the neurosurgeon's orders. The patient is prepared as for brain surgery because if brain displacement occurs, an immediate craniotomy must be performed.

The fasting patient is taken to the operating room for this procedure and placed in a special chair. Using either general or local anesthesia, the neurosurgeon makes trephines (burr holes) through scalp incisions and then punctures the ventricles with a special needle or catheter. After removing some CSF, either air or contrast material is injected into the ventricles. The patient is then repositioned during the x-ray study that follows to ensure adequate visualization of the ventricular structures.

Immediate surgery (craniotomy) may be necessary if an intracranial tumor is detected or if the procedure itself caused dangerous intracranial pressure shifts. For this reason the procedure permission form must include both a ventriculogram and craniotomy.

If the test results reveal no abnormalities, the needle is removed and the skin over the burr holes is sutured closed. The scalp wounds are covered with a sterile dressing. The sutures are usually removed within 4 to 5 days. Headache, nausea, and vomiting may occur.

Contraindications. See lumbar puncture, p. 181.

Nursing considerations

Nursing Diagnoses/Collaborative Problems

See Lumbar puncture, p. 182.

Nursing Implications with Rationale

- Explain the procedure to the patient and follow the usual preoperative routine (for example, remove dentures and have the patient void). Tell the patient that a hole will be drilled into the skull and a special needle will be inserted into the ventricle of the brain.
- Explain the postprocedure routine to the patient. Much anxiety can be allayed if the patient is reassured that measures will be taken to alleviate any discomfort associated with this procedure.
- Ensure that the physician has obtained the written and informed consent forms for ventriculography and craniotomy before premedicating the patient. Craniotomy may be necessary to prevent brainstem compression.
- After the procedure monitor the vital and neurologic signs frequently (every 15 minutes to every hour for the first 12 to 24 hours). The head of the bed is elevated 10 to 15 degrees for the first 24 hours and then elevated as tolerated. The patient is usually allowed out of bed on the second or third day after the procedure. Side rails are used as indicated.
- After the procedure check the scalp dressing for drainage. Reinforce it as necessary to keep the dressing dry and prevent the entrance of microorganisms.
- After the procedure and when the patient is conscious, encourage fluids to replace the CSF lost during the procedure. Most patients have a headache after this procedure, which usually disappears within 24 to 48 hours after the intracranial air is absorbed in the CSF. An ice bag may help relieve the headache.
- Administer analgesics as ordered and as necessary to relieve severe discomfort.

Cisternal puncture

Normal values: see lumbar puncture and CSF examination, pp. 178-182.

Rationale. In certain conditions a spinal needle is inserted into the cisterna magna for a cisternal puncture (Figure 6-13) instead of into the subarachnoid space (see Lumbar puncture, p. 178). A cisternal puncture may be indicated in the following conditions:

1. To obtain CSF for examination when it cannot be obtained at the lumbar level
2. To demonstrate a subarachnoid block by performing a cisternal puncture simultaneously with a lumbar puncture
3. For drainage of CSF when a lumbar puncture is contraindicated
4. To introduce contrast material or air for myelography
5. To perform encephalography

The risk is negligible and the ill effects are minimal when done by an experienced neurologic specialist. This test requires more skill than the lumbar puncture does.

Procedure. The occipital area at the back of the head is shaved and cleansed with an antiseptic. Strict sterile technique must be maintained throughout this procedure to avoid problems such as brain abscess and meningitis. The patient is placed on his or her side with a pillow under the head to keep the head and spine aligned. The chin rests on the chest and is held in place by a nurse or an assistant to prevent rotation. The needle is inserted about 4 to 5 cm between the first cervical vertebrae and the rim of the foramen magnum (Figure 6-13). The rest of this procedure is then the same as that of the lumbar puncture.

After the procedure the patient usually remains in bed for several hours and is observed

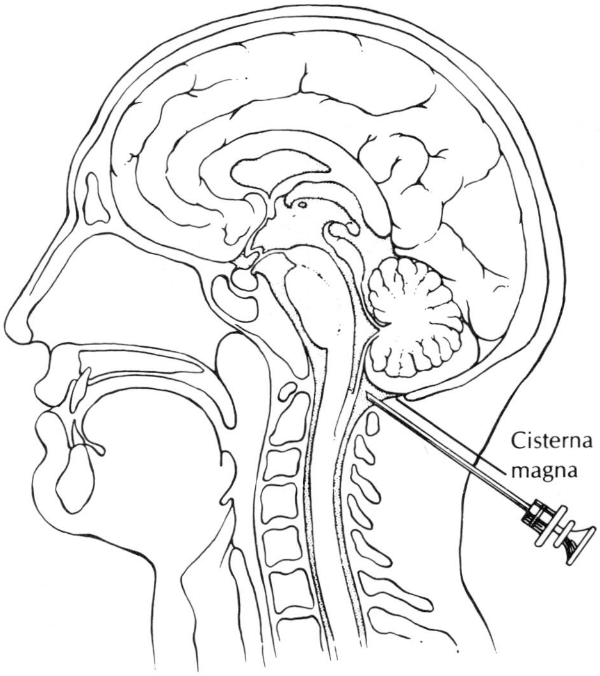

FIGURE 6-13. Position of needle when cisternal puncture is performed. Note needle length and short bevel.
From Phipps WJ, Long BC, and Woods NE: Medical-surgical nursing: concepts and clinical practice, ed 2, St Louis, 1983, The CV Mosby Co.

for respiratory complications (such as cyanosis, dyspnea, and apnea) and irregularities in the heartbeat, which might indicate injury to the medulla. Headaches do not usually occur as a result of this procedure. If no problems occur, the patient is allowed out of bed and may resume normal activities within 2 to 3 hours.

This procedure is usually described as painful by most patients. The duration of this procedure is 20 to 60 minutes. Cisternal puncture is usually performed by an experienced neurologic specialist in a treatment room for outpatients or in the hospital bed for inpatients.

Contraindications. See Lumbar puncture, p. 181. This procedure should also be avoided if a possibility of a lesion in the cisterna magna exists or if a developmental anomaly is suspected at the foramen magnum level.

Nursing considerations

Nursing Diagnoses/Collaborative Problems

See Lumbar puncture, p. 182.

Nursing Implications with Rationale

- Explain the procedure to the patient. A cisternal puncture is often more frightening than a lumbar puncture, since the needle insertion site is closer to the brain.
- Ensure that a written and informed consent form is obtained before this procedure.
- Assist the patient in keeping his or her head still during this procedure. Rotation of the neck could cause needle injury to the medulla.
- After the procedure assess the patient for cyanosis, dyspnea, apnea, and irregularities of the heart rate, which could indicate injury to

the medulla. Headaches do not usually follow this procedure.

Caloric study

(oculovestibular reflex test)

Normal value: nystagmus with irrigation (other observations depend on specific procedure performed)

Rationale. Caloric studies are used to examine the vestibular portion of the eighth cranial nerve by irrigating the external auditory canal with hot or cold water. Normally, stimulation with cold water causes rotary nystagmus (involuntary rapid eye movement) away from the ear being irrigated; hot water induces nystagmus toward the ear being irrigated. If the labyrinth is diseased or, for example, the eighth nerve is compressed by a tumor, no nystagmus is induced. This study aids in the differential diagnosis of lesions in the brainstem and cerebellum because reflex nerve pathways pass through these areas.

Procedure. Solid food is usually held for several hours before this study to reduce the possibility of vomiting. Sedatives are not used because they may alter the patient's response. This procedure usually takes place in a treatment room. The exact procedure for caloric studies varies. Before the test is performed, the patient is examined for the presence of nystagmus, Romberg's sign (postural deviation), and past-pointing (when evaluating coordination and fine motor skills). This examination provides the baseline value for comparison during the study.

The ear on the affected side is irrigated first, since the client's response may be minimal. After an emesis basin is placed under the ear, the irrigation solution is directed into the external auditory canal until the client complains of nausea and dizziness or until nystagmus is seen. Usually this occurs within 20 to 30 seconds. If after 3 minutes no symptoms occur, the irrigation is stopped. The patient is tested for nystagmus, past-pointing, and Romberg's sign. After approximately 5 minutes the procedure is repeated on the other ear. When the test is over, the client is usually taken back to bed via a wheelchair. Bed rest is usually maintained until the subjective symptoms subside.

Contraindications. Caloric study is contraindicated in the following:

1. Patients with a perforated eardrum (however, cold air may be used as a substitute for the fluid).
2. Patients with an acute disease of the labyrinth (such as Ménière's syndrome). The test can be performed when the acute attack subsides.

Nursing considerations

Nursing Diagnoses/Collaborative Problems

- Possible knowledge deficit related to test purpose, preparation, and procedure
- Possible anxiety related to unknown sensations of procedure
- High risk for alteration in comfort (nausea, vomiting, and dizziness) related to test procedure

Nursing Implications with Rationale

- Explain the procedure to the patient. Hold solid foods before the test to reduce the incidence of vomiting.
- After the test bed rest is prescribed until the nausea and vomiting subside, usually 30 to 60 minutes. After that time inform the patient that fluid, food, and normal activities may be resumed.

CASE STUDY 2: MULTIPLE SCLEROSIS

Mrs. W., 35 years old, has been very active in jogging and horseback riding until 1 year ago. During the past year she began to notice severe weakness and paresthesias in her legs. Her gait became unsteady, and she developed loss of vision in one eye. A neurologist suspected multiple sclerosis (MS) and ordered the following studies.

Studies	Results
Routine laboratory work	WNL
Lumbar puncture with CSF examination (see p. 178-182)	
Immunoglobulin G (IgG) index	0.8 (normal: 0.3-0.7)
Immunoglobulin G (IgG) determination	20% (normal: 0-11% of total protein)
Oligoclonal bands	Present (normal: none)
Evoked potentials	
Visual evoked responses	Abnormal latency
Auditory brainstem evoked potentials	Normal
Somatosensory evoked responses	Abnormal latency
Magnetic resonance imaging	Plaques indicative of multiple sclerosis

The wide variety of symptom manifestation often makes MS difficult to diagnose. However, the above studies clearly identified the patient's problem to be that of MS. The CSF study results were classic for the diagnosis of MS. The abnormal latency demonstrated on the evoked potential studies was the result of the demyelination process of MS. One of the amazing qualities of magnetic resonance imaging (MRI) is its ability to detect the plaques of MS.

The patient was given prednisone to decrease the inflammation and associated edema of the myelin sheath. When remission occurred, the patient was instructed about factors that exacerbate, prevent, or ameliorate symptoms.

DISCUSSION OF TESTS

Evoked potential studies

(EP studies, evoked brain potentials)

Normal values: vary according to the laboratory performing the test; values also vary between persons and in the same person over time

Rationale. Evoked potential (EP) studies focus on changes and responses in brain waves that are evoked from stimulation of a sensory pathway. The EP is a sensitive, noninvasive, and objective study that is beginning to play a large part in diagnostic, prognostic, and monitoring techniques.

The study of EPs grew out of early work with the electroencephalogram (EEG) (see p. 182). Though the EEG measures "spontaneous" brain electrical activity, the sensory EP study measures minute voltage changes produced in response to a specific stimulus (such as a light pattern, a click, or a shock). In contrast to the EEG, which records signals that reach amplitudes up to 50 to 100 μV, EP signals are usually less than 5 μV. Because of this, they can only be detected with an averaging computer. The computer averages out (or cancels) unwanted random waves to sum up the evoked response that occurs at a specific time after a given stimulus. Latency refers to the delay between the stimulus and the wave response. Latency depends on factors such as body size, position on the body where the stimulus is applied, conduction velocity of axons in the neural pathways, number of synapses in the system, location of nerve generators of EP components (brainstem or cortex), and presence of CNS pathology. Clinical abnormalities are generally detected by abnormalities (increases) in latency.

EPs are divided by sensory modality into visual, auditory, and somatosensory responses.

Visual evoked responses (VERs) are usually stimulated by a strobe light flash, reversible checkerboard pattern, or retinal stimuli. A visual stimulus to the eye causes an electrical response in the occipital area that can be recorded with electrodes placed along the vertex and the occipital areas of the skull. Ninety percent of patients with multiple sclerosis show abnormal latencies in VERs, a phenomenon attributed to demyelination of nerve fibers. In addition to multiple sclerosis, patients with other neurologic disorders such as Parkinson's disease show an abnormal latency with VERs. The degree of latency seems to correlate with the disease severity. Abnormal results may also be seen in patients with glaucoma and lesions of the optic nerve, optic tract, visual center, or eye. Absence of binocularity, which is a neurologic developmental disorder in infants, can be detected and evaluated with VERs.

Auditory brainstem evoked potentials (or ABEPs or brainstem auditory evoked potentials, or BAEPs) are usually stimulated by clicking sounds to evaluate the central auditory pathways of the brainstem. Either ear can be evoked to detect lesions in the brainstem that involve the auditory pathway without affecting hearing. One of the most successful applications of ABEPs has been screening low birth weight newborns for auditory disorders. This enables infants with poor hearing to be fitted with corrective devices as soon as possible before learning to speak. ABEPs have significant therapeutic implications in the early detection of posterior fossa tumors.

Somatosensory evoked responses (SERs) usually are stimulated by a sensory stimulus (such as electrical) to an area of the body. The time is then measured for the stimulus's current to travel along the nerve to the cortex of the brain. SERs are used to evaluate patients with spinal cord injuries, to monitor spinal cord functioning during surgery or treatment (such as for multiple sclerosis), to evaluate the location and extent of areas of brain dysfunction after head injury, and to pinpoint tumors at an early stage.

One of the main benefits of EPs is their objectivity, since voluntary patient response is not needed. This makes EPs useful with nonverbal (such as young children and infants) and uncooperative patients. This objectivity permits the distinction of organic from psychogenic problems. (This is invaluable in settling law suits concerning workmen's compensation insurance.) In the future EPs may aid in diagnosing and monitoring childhood learning disabilities and mental disorders and in detecting adult mental disorders (such as schizophrenia and alcoholic brain damage).

Procedure. No fasting or sedation is required before administration of EP studies. The position of the electrode depends on the type of EP study to be done.

For VERs, electrodes are placed on the scalp along the vertex and the occipital areas. Stimulation occurs by using a strobe light, checkerboard patterns, or retinal stimuli.

Auditory brainstem evoked potentials are stimulated with clicking noises or tone bursts delivered via earphones. The responses are detected by scalp electrodes placed on the vertex and on each earlobe.

Somatosensory EPs are performed using electrical stimuli applied to nerves at the wrist (medial nerve) or the knee (peroneal). The response is detected by electrodes placed over the sensory cortex of the opposite hemisphere on the scalp.

Contraindications. None.

Nursing considerations

Nursing Diagnoses/Collaborative Problems

- Possible knowledge deficit related to test purpose, preparation, and procedure
- Possible anxiety related to unknown sensations of procedure
- Possible anxiety related to test results

Nursing Implications with Rationale

- Explain the procedure to the patient. Allow plenty of time for verbalization of the patient's fears and questions. Many patients fear the diagnosis that may be substantiated by EP studies.
- Instruct the patient to shampoo his or her hair before the test and to avoid oils and sprays. After the test remove the gel used for adherence of the electrodes.

Magnetic resonance imaging

(MRI, nuclear magnetic resonance or NMR)

Normal values: No evidence of pathology

Rationale. Magnetic resonance imaging (MRI) is a noninvasive diagnostic scanning technique that provides valuable information about the body's anatomy by placing the patient in a magnetic field that is approximately 40,000 times that of the earth's magnetic field. Although the magnet is strong enough to jerk a 2-pound wrench out of the hand, the magnetic field does not harm body tissues. MRI is dependent on how hydrogen atoms behave when placed in a magnetic field and then disturbed by radio-frequency signals. The unique feature of MRI (unlike CT and PET scanning) is that it does not require exposure to ionizing radiation.

Some experts say the images obtained by MRI are clearer than those obtained in PET studies (see Chapter 14). They suggest that MRI will supplant PET scans, since both assay chemicals within the body. However, MRI does this without administration of any chemical contrast agents. MRI will probably replace CT scanning as a primary neurologic diagnostic modality because its advantages over CT scanning include:

1. It provides better contrast between normal tissue and pathologic tissue.
2. Since cortical bone is low in density, it generates little signal on MRI imaging. Therefore obscuring bone artifacts that occur in CT scanning do not occur in MRI scanning.
3. Since rapidly flowing blood appears dark because of its rapid motion, many blood vessels appear as dark lumens. This provides a natural contrast to the blood vessels.
4. Since spatial information is dependent only on how the magnetic fields are varied in space, it is possible to image the transverse, sagittal, and coronal planes directly.

During an MRI scan the patient is placed inside a giant, doughnut-shaped electromagnet to align the magnetic nuclei of hydrogen atoms in the water of the body cells. Hydrogen is used in clinical MRI imaging because it is naturally very abundant in the body. Short bursts of alternating energy are then introduced to knock the nuclei out of alignment. As the nuclei flip back into alignment, tiny radio-frequency signals are emitted, which are then detected by the MRI machine and computer-processed into cross-sectional images of the area under study.

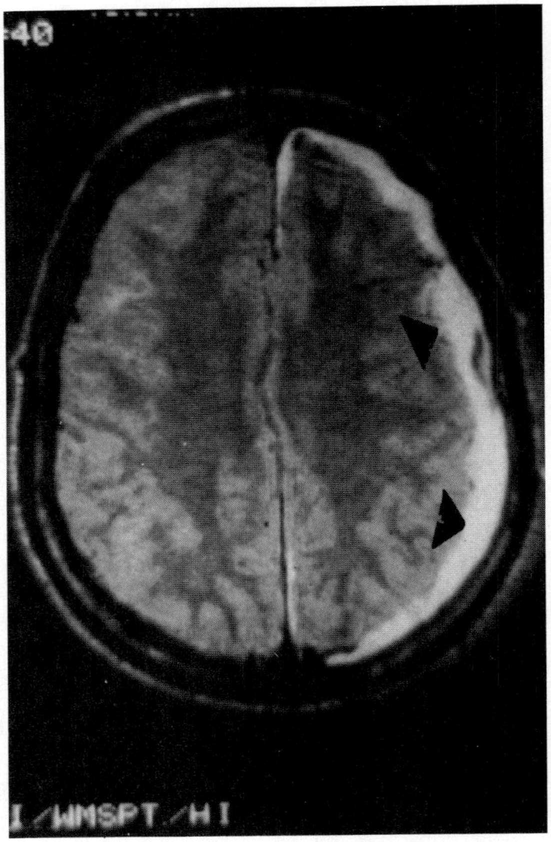

FIGURE 6-14. Magnetic resonance imaging (MRI) of the brain with arrows indicating a subdural hematoma.
Courtesy Central Pennsylvania Magnetic Imaging, Williamsport, Pa.

Although the full usefulness of this technique has yet to be determined, MRI scanning shows promise in the following areas:

1. Visualization of the brain, the base of the skull, and the interior of the spine. (It can detect cerebral lesions not evident on the CT scan, especially posterior fossa lesions.)
2. Detection of cerebral infarctions, arteriovenous (AV) malformation, hemorrhage, and subdural hematoma (see Figure 6-14).

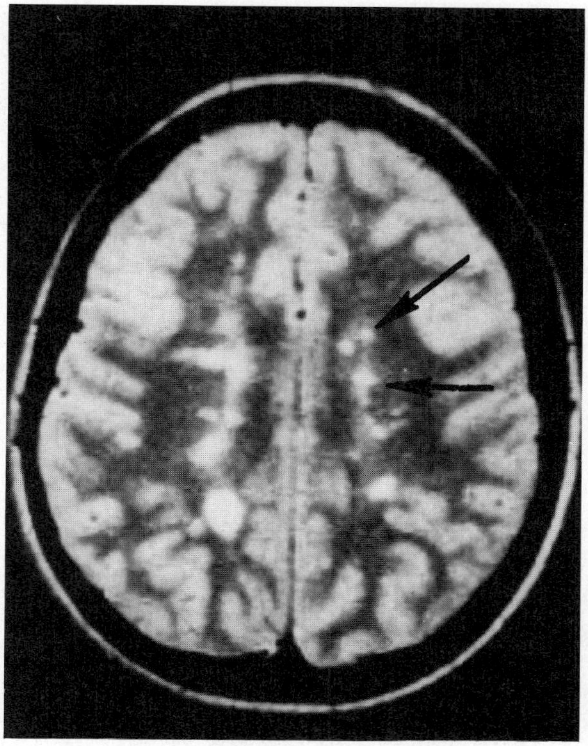

FIGURE 6-15. MRI with arrows demonstrating areas of MS plaques seen in the brain of a patient diagnosed with multiple sclerosis.
Courtesy Central Pennsylvania Magnetic Imaging, Williamsport, Pa.

3. Depiction of lesions in degenerative diseases, such as multiple sclerosis (see Figure 6-15).
4. Determination of the extent of chronic myocardial infarction.
5. Identification of coronary arteries and by-pass grafts.
6. Detection of atherosclerotic plaques in large arteries.
7. Diagnosing diseases of the mediastinum, kidney, liver, pancreas, pelvis, and prostate gland.
8. Detection of tumors. (It is possible to determine if a tumor is progressing or regressing.) (See Figure 6-16.)
9. Evaluation of the trauma patient because the vertebral column, spinal cord, and adjacent soft tissue can be visualized in multiple projections without moving the patient.
10. Differentiation between normal and degenerated discs.
11. Detection of aortic aneurysm, aortic dissection, aortic occlusion and stenosis, and aortic AV malformation.
12. Accurate visualization of bone joint and soft tissue disease or injury.

An important advantage of MRI imaging is that serial studies can be performed in patient without any known risk. This is useful in assessing the response of cancer and lymphoma to radiotherapeutics and chemotherapy. A major disadvantage of MRI is that its patient population is more limited than that of CT scanning. Examination of patients requiring cardiac monitoring or having metal implants, pacemakers, or cerebral aneurysm clips will result in MRI image degradation and may endanger the patient. Claustrophobic patients have difficulty with the procedure.

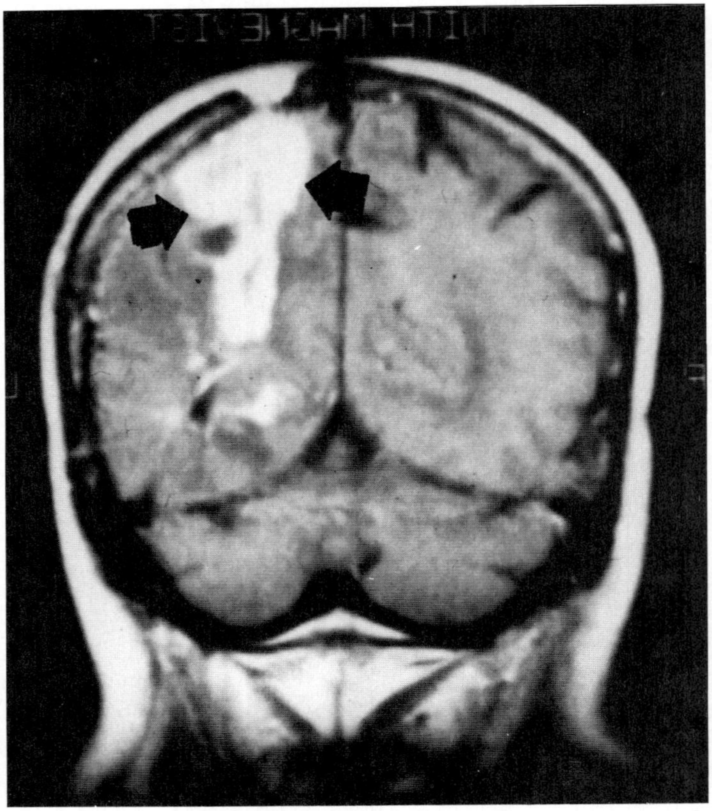

FIGURE 6-16. MRI with arrows indicating a brain tumor accentuated by Magnavist dye. Courtesy Central Pennsylvania Magnetic Imaging, Williamsport, Pa.

Procedure. There are no fluid or food restrictions before MRI for adults. Young children should fast for 4 hours before the test and should also be sleep-deprived so that mild sedation can be used. Because the procedure may last for 1 hour, the patient should empty his or her bladder before the test for comfort reasons. Before the procedure the patient removes all metal objects as well as credit cards, which can have their magnetic codes erased in the magnetic field. The patient lies on a platform that slides into a tube containing the doughnut-shaped magnet. The patient is instructed to lie very still during the procedure.

During the scan the patient can talk to and hear the staff via a microphone or earphones placed in the scanner. The patient can hear a loud thumping sound as the magnetic coils are pulsed. Ear plugs are available if the patient wishes to use them. The only discomfort associated with this procedure may be that of lying still on a hard surface. A tingling sensation may be felt in teeth containing metal fillings. The duration of the procedure is approximately 30 to 90 minutes. This procedure is performed by a qualified technologist.

A contrast medium called gadolinium (Magnavist) may be used. This is a paramagnetic enhancement agent that crosses the blood-brain barrier. It is especially useful for distinguishing edema from tumors (see Figure 6-16).

Approximately 10 to 20 ml of Magnavist is injected into a vein. Imaging can begin within 3 to 55 minutes after injection. No dietary restrictions are necessary before using this new agent.

Contraindications. This study is contraindicated in the following:

1. Patients who are pregnant, because the long-term effects of MRI are not known at this time
2. Patients requiring continuous life support equipment, because the monitoring equipment cannot be used inside the scanner
3. Patients with implantable metal objects such as pacemakers, aneurysm clips, braces, metal hip prostheses, inner ear implants, and metal fragments in one or both eyes, because the magnet may move the object within the body causing damage

Nursing considerations

Nursing Diagnoses/Collaborative Problems

- Possible knowledge deficit related to test purpose, preparation, and procedure
- Possible anxiety related to unknown sensations of procedure
- Possible alteration in comfort (claustrophobia) related to test procedure

Nursing Implications with Rationale

- Explain the procedure to the patient. Assure the patient that MRI is a safe and painless procedure. Parents may read or talk to a child in the scanning room during the procedure since no risk of radiation from the procedure exists.
- If possible, show the patient a picture of the scanning machine and encourage verbalization of anxieties. Some patients may experience claustrophobia. Instruct the patient and anyone else who enters the scanning room to remove all metal objects (such as jewelry, hair clips) because they create artifacts on the scan. Movement of metal objects within the magnetic field can be detrimental. Therefore, patients with heart valves, orthopedic screws or rods, or aneurysm clips, for example, cannot be scanned by MRI.
- Inform the parents if the child should fast for 4 hours before the test. This is done because children are often sedated. Anxious adults are also sedated.
- Instruct the parents if the child should be sleep-deprived for this study. This is done by keeping the child awake until midnight the night before the study. The child is then awakened for 5 to 10 min every hour beginning at 4 A.M. The child should not be allowed to sleep in the car on the way to the hospital.
- Inform the patient that he or she must lie motionless during this study. Any movement can cause artifacts on the scan.
- Tell the patient that during the procedure he or she will hear a loud thumping sound. Ear plugs are available if the patient wishes to use them.
- No special postprocedure care is needed. The patient can drive to and from the procedure without any assistance.

CASE STUDY 3: HERNIATED DISC

Mr. S., 38 years old, had a 3-year history of low back pain. Although the pain was intermittent and transient, he had lost many work days during the preceding year. In the 2 months before his admission to the hospital, increasing paresthesia (numbness and tingling) had developed in his toes and was associated with mild weakness of his foot. All results of his physical examination were normal except for right-sided lumbar paraspinal muscle spasm. His neurologic examination also indicated hypoesthesia (decreased sensation to pinprick) and anterior tibial muscle weakness.

Studies	Results
Routine laboratory work	WNL
Lumbosacral spinal x-ray study (LS spine)	Normal (no evidence of lumbosacral arthritic degenerative joint disease)
Nerve conduction studies	No abnormalities in the distal sacral nerve or its branches

Studies	Results
Electromyography (EMG)	Decrease in number of muscle fibers contracting in the anterior tibial muscle
Myelography	Narrowing of the radiographic dye column at the area of L4-L5, indicating herniated disc

The normal results of the lumbosacral spinal x-ray study ruled out degenerative joint disease as a cause for this patient's back pain. Nerve conduction studies and electromyography indicated nerve-root compression at L5. Myelography showed that this compression was caused by a herniated lumbar intervertebral disc.

The patient underwent a posterior decompressive laminectomy of the L4 and L5 region. Postoperatively he had only minimal back pain, which did not interrupt his normal physical activities.

DISCUSSION OF TESTS

Lumbosacral spinal x-ray study

(LS spine)

Normal values: normal lumbar and sacral vertebrae

Rationale. The lumbosacral spinal test is an x-ray study of the five lumbar vertebrae and the fused sacral vertebrae. It usually includes anteroposterior, lateral, and oblique views of these structures (Figure 6-17). The most common indication for this study is low back pain. Degenerative arthritic changes of the spine can frequently be seen as calcified spurs extending from the borders of the involved vertebral bodies. Traumatic fractures, spondylosis (stress fracture of the vertebrae), and spondylolisthesis (slipping of one vertebral body on the other) are also detected by x-ray films of this area.

Metastatic tumor invasion of the spine (such as from breast cancer, melanoma, or colorectal cancer) may be seen as abnormal radiolucent spots on the spine or by destruction of the normal structure of the lumbar or sacral vertebral bodies. No complications are associated with this test when it is done selectively.

Procedure. The unsedated patient is taken to the radiology department. The patient's clothing is removed, and a long x-ray gown is placed on the patient. Metal objects must be removed, or they will obscure visualization of the LS spinal area. The patient is then placed on an x-ray table. Anterior, posterior, lateral, and oblique x-ray films are taken of the lumbar and sacral areas. X-ray films are taken by a radiologic technician in only a few minutes. The patient feels no discomfort. Any area of the spine (cervical, thoracic, lumbar, sacral, or coccygeal) can be studied in a similar manner and can reveal the same information as described above.

Contraindications. This test is contraindicated in the uncooperative or pregnant patient.

Nursing considerations

Nursing Diagnoses/Collaborative Problems

See X-ray studies, p. 5.

Nursing Implications with Rationale

- Explain the procedure to the patient.
- Tell the patient that all clothing above and below the waist must be removed for adequate x-ray visualization.
- In a patient with confirmed or suspected spinal fracture, assist the physician in safely moving the patient. Any excess unnecessary movement is avoided until the extent of the damage is determined. Ensure that appropriate care is given during transportation to and from the radiology department and during the x-ray study.
- If the patient is having severe back pain and cannot cooperate, inform the physician and check to see if the patient should be sedated.
- Assess the patient's menstrual status. Be sure that the patient is not pregnant at the time of the study to prevent x-ray exposure to the fetus.

A

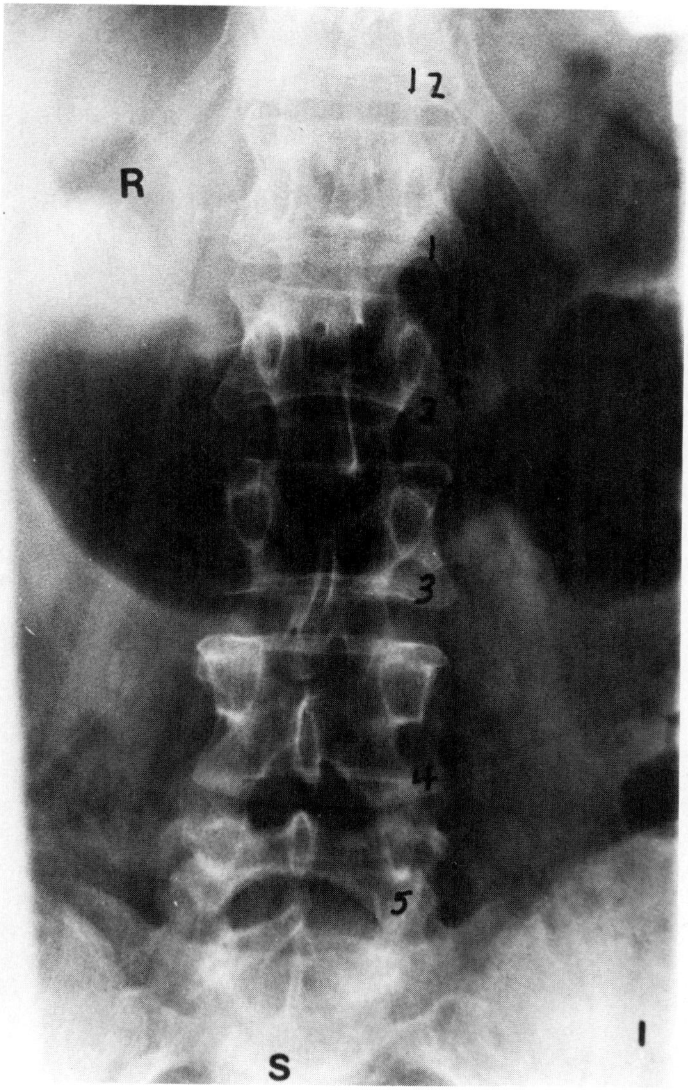

FIGURE 6-17. Normal lumbosacral spine x-ray films. **A,** Anteroposterior view. **B,** Lateral lumbar view. Lumbar vertebral bodies numbered *1* through *5*. **C,** Lateral sacral view. *R,* Rib; *S,* fused sacrum; *I,* iliac bone; *C,* coccyx; *L,* lumbar vertebral bodies. *Continued.*

B

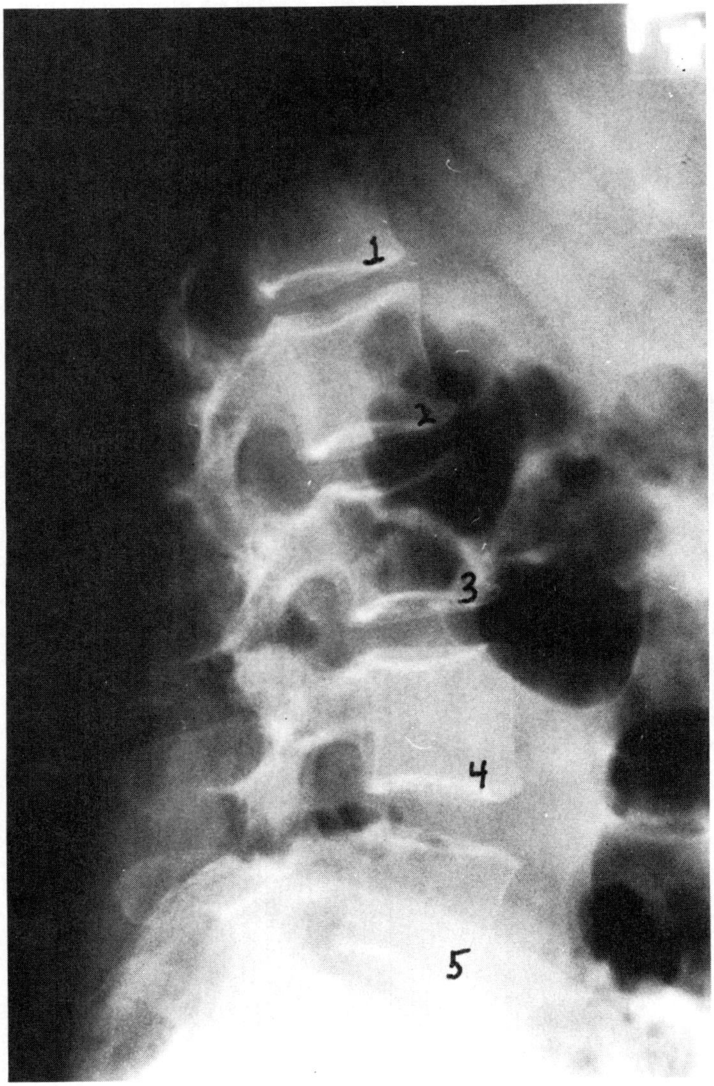

FIGURE 6-17, cont'd. Normal lumbosacral spine x-ray film, lateral view. See p. 207 for legend.

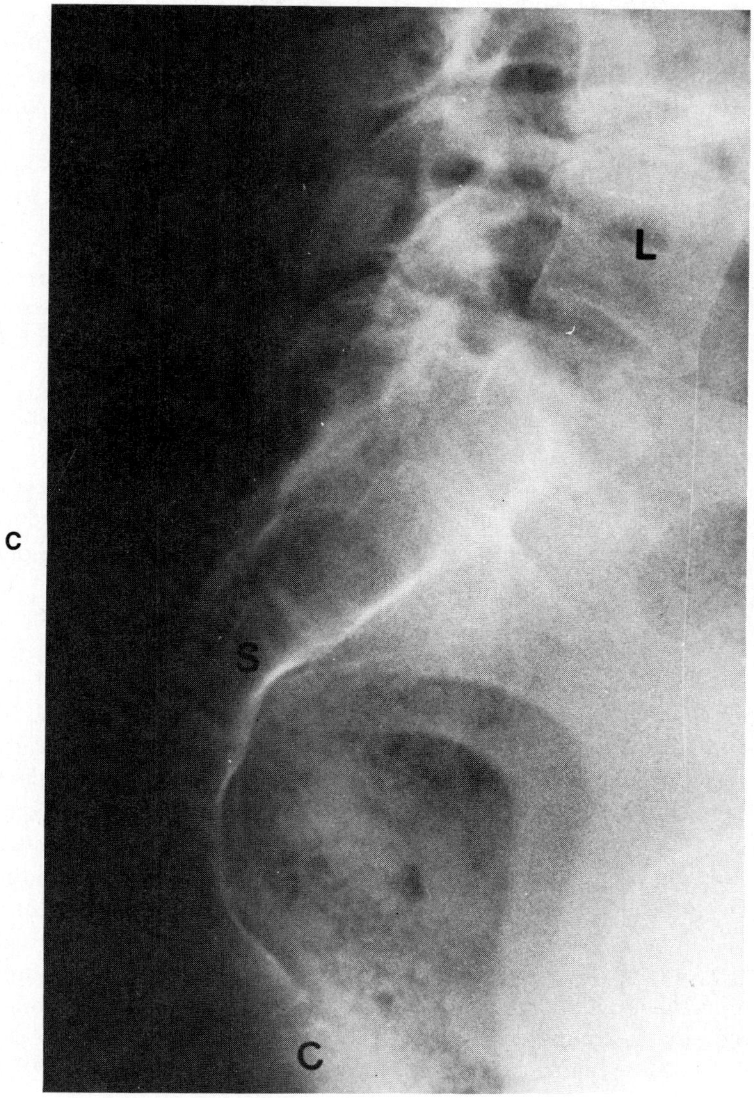

FIGURE 6-17, cont'd. Normal lumbosacral spinal x-ray films. Lateral sacral view. See p. 207 for legend.

Nerve conduction studies

(electroneurography)

Normal value: no evidence of peripheral nerve injury or disease

Rationale. Nerve conduction studies allow for the detection and location of peripheral nerve injury or disease. By initiating an electrical impulse at one site (proximal) of a nerve and recording the time required for that impulse to travel to a second site (distal) of the same nerve, the conduction velocity of any impulse in that nerve can be determined. This study is usually done before electromyography (see the following study) and may be called *electromyoneurography*.

This procedure is performed by placing a shock-emitting device above the area of the nerve to be evaluated and a recording electrode over the muscle innervated by that specific nerve. Both the time from shock to muscle contraction (total latency) and the distance from the stimulating electrode to the recording electrode are precisely measured. The distance per unit of time, measured from the shock to the muscular contraction, is called the *conduction velocity*.

The normal value for conduction velocity varies from one nerve to the next. There is also an individual variation. For these reasons, it is always best to compare the conduction velocity of the suspected side with the contralateral nerve conduction velocity. In general, a range of normal conduction velocity is approximately 50 to 60 m per second.

Traumatic transection or contusion of a nerve usually causes maximum slowing of conduction velocity in the affected side as compared with the normal side. Neuropathies, both local and generalized, also cause a slowing of conduction velocity. A velocity greater than normal does not indicate a pathologic condition.

Because conduction velocity requires contraction of a muscle as an indication of impulse arrival at the recording electrode, primary muscular disorders (such as myotonia and myositis) may cause a falsely slow nerve conduction velocity. This "muscular" variable is eliminated if one evaluates the suspected pathologic muscle group before performing nerve conduction studies. This evaluation can be done by measuring distal latency, that is, the time required for stimulation of the distal end of the nerve (immediately adjacent to the muscle) to cause muscular contraction. The nerve conduction study is then performed normally by stimulating the proximal portion of the nerve bundle. Conduction velocity is determined by the following equation:

$$\text{Conduction velocity (in meters/second)} = \frac{\text{Distance (in meters)}}{\text{Total latency} - \text{Distal latency}}$$

Procedure. No fasting or sedation is required or desired. The patient is taken to the nerve conduction laboratory (in the physiatrist's or neurologist's office, or in the physical rehabilitation department). The machine is portable, enabling the study to also be performed at the bedside.

The patient is placed in whatever position is determined best for studying the area of the specific suspected peripheral nerve injury or disease. A recording electrode is placed on the skin overlying a muscle innervated solely by the relevant nerve. A reference electrode is placed nearby. All skin-to-electrode connections are assured by using electrical paste. The nerve is then stimulated by a shock-emitter device at an adjacent location (Figure 6-18). The time between nerve impulse and muscular contraction (distal latency) is measured in milliseconds on a cathode-ray oscilloscope (electromyograph) (Figure 6-19). Next the nerve is similarly stimulated at a location proximal (that is, more central) to the area of suspected injury or disease (Figure 6-20). The time required for the impulse to travel from the site of initiation to muscle contraction (total latency) is recorded in milliseconds. The distance between the site of stimulation and recording electrode is measured in centimeters. Conduction velocity is con-

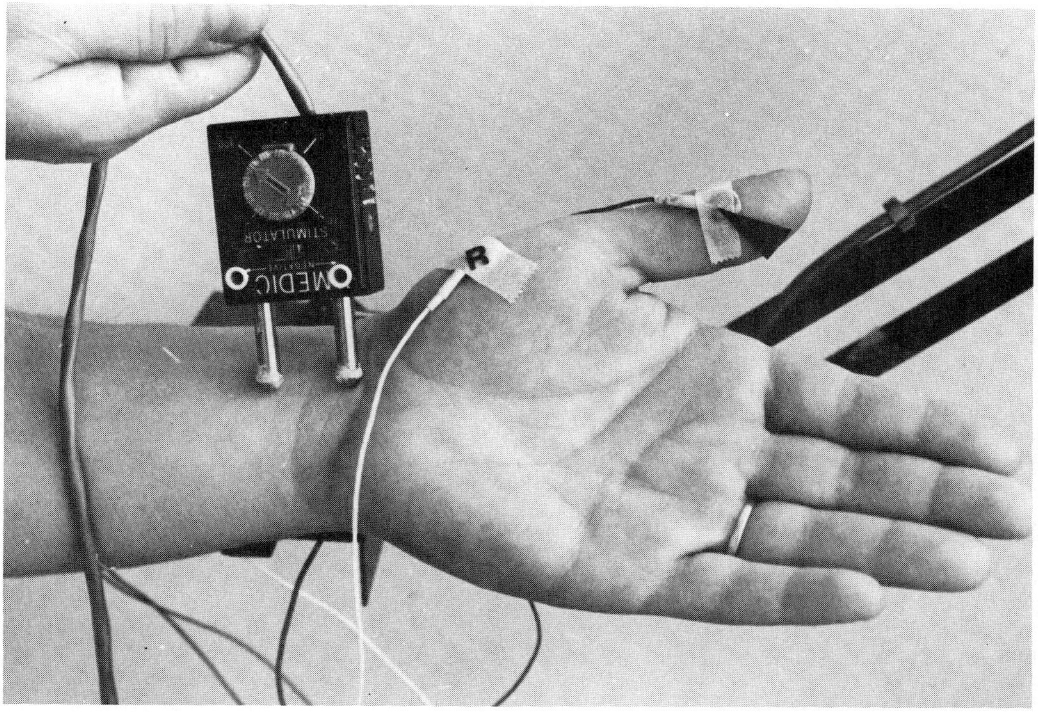

FIGURE 6-18. Nerve conduction studies: measurement of distal latency. Pointer indicates reference electrode. *R,* Recording electrode.

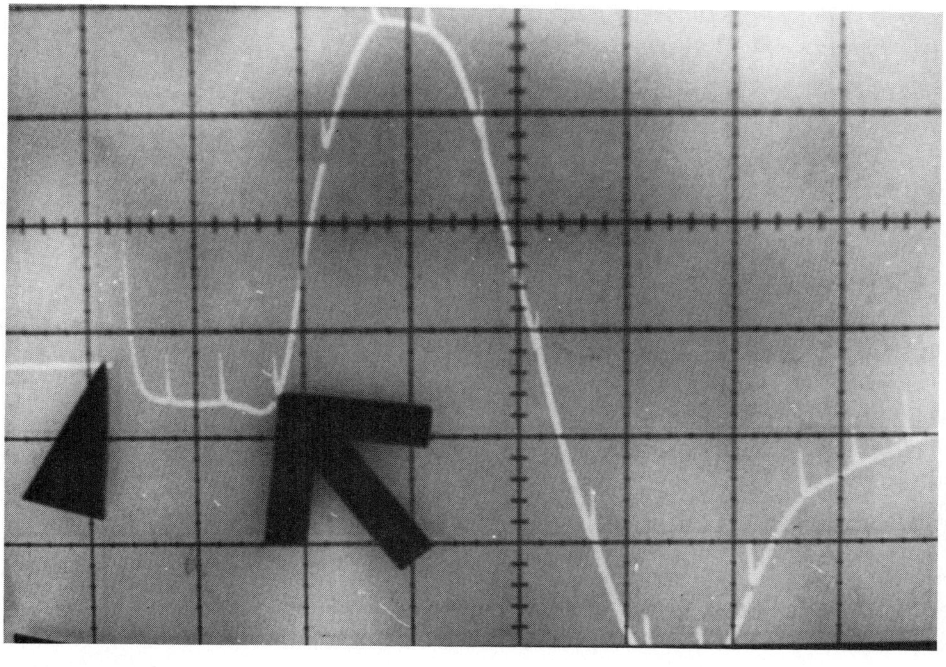

FIGURE 6-19. Nerve conduction studies: electromyogram. Pointer indicates shock stimulation. Arrow indicates initiation of muscular contraction (the wave that follows the arrow). Distal latency is measured from pointer to arrow (1.2 msec).

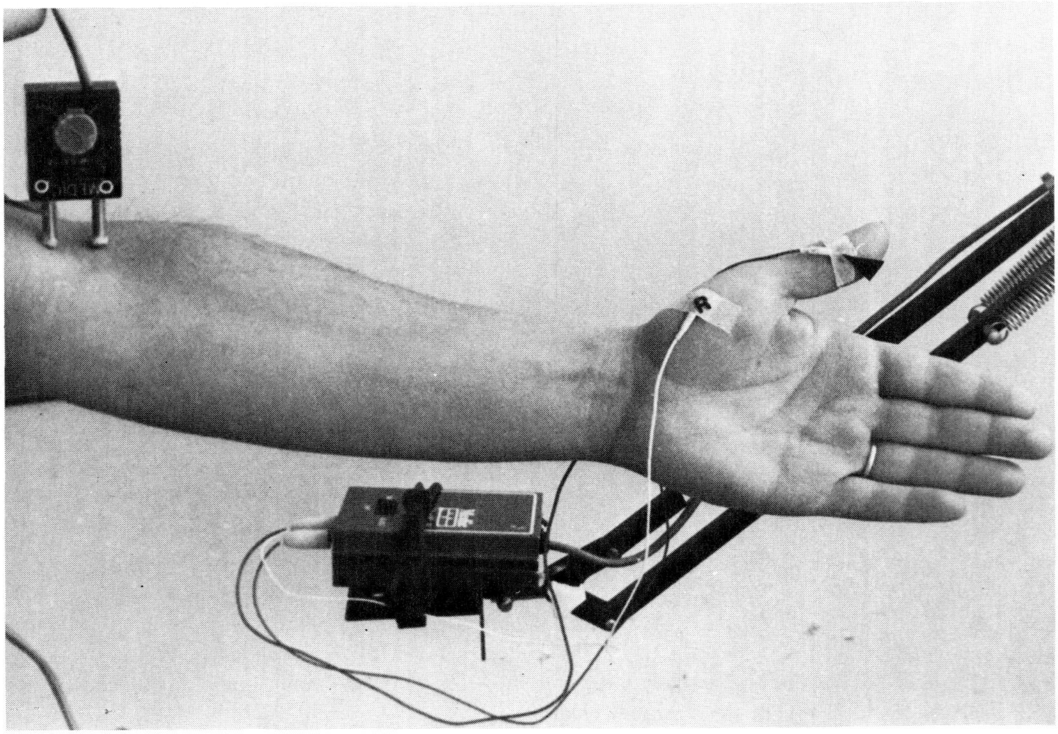

FIGURE 6-20. Nerve conduction studies: measurement of total latency. Pointer indicates reference electrode. *R*, Recording electrode.

verted to meters per second and is computed as in the above equation.

This test is uncomfortable in that a mild electric shock (comparable to that obtained in most household electrical outlet accidents) is required for nerve impulse stimulation. The test is performed by a neurologist, physiatrist, physical therapist, or technician in about 15 minutes. No complications are associated with it.

Contraindications. None.

Nursing considerations

Nursing Diagnoses/Collaborative Problems

- Possible knowledge deficit related to test purpose, preparation, and procedure
- Possible anxiety related to unknown sensations of procedure
- Possible anxiety related to test results
- Possible alteration in comfort related to test procedure

Nursing Implications with Rationale

- Explain the procedure to the patient. Allow the patient to verbalize his or her fears regarding the electrical stimulation (shock) necessary for this study. Provide emotional support.
- After the nerve conduction study is performed, remove the electrode gel from the patient's skin.

Electromyography

Normal value: no evidence of neuromuscular abnormalities

Rationale. Electromyography (EMG) is used to detect primary muscular disorders along with muscular abnormalities caused by other system diseases (such as nerve dysfunction, sarcoidosis, and paraneoplastic syndrome). By placing a recording electrode into a muscle, one can monitor the electrical activity of that muscle in a way very similar to electrocardiography. The electrical activity is displayed on a cathode-ray oscilloscope as an electrical waveform. An audioelectrical amplifier can be added to the system so that both the appearance and the sound of the electrical potentials can be analyzed and compared simultaneously.

EMG records no electrical activity in the normal muscle at rest. As the patient begins to contract the muscle slowly, "normal" electrical waveforms are displayed on the oscilloscope. With stronger contractions, more and more muscle fibers contract, and these waveforms overlie each of the others, causing a disorderly crowd of waveforms on the display. This is referred to as "complete interference pattern" and is representative of a strong, well-functioning skeletal muscle. With audio amplification this may sound like firecrackers or a machine gun popping.

Spontaneous muscle movement, such as fibrillation and fasciculation, can be detected during EMG. When seen, these waves indicate injury or disease of the nerve innervating that muscle or spastic myotonic muscle diseases. Reduced amplitude size of the electrical waveform is indicative of a primary muscle disorder (such as polymyositis, muscular dystrophies, and various myopathies). A progressive decrease in amplitude of the electrical waveform is classic for myasthenia gravis. A decrease in the number of muscle fibers able to contract is seen with peripheral nerve damage.

Although the test requires the insertion of small needles into the muscles being monitored, complications such as hematomas and infection are very rare. This study is usually performed prior to nerve conduction studies (see p. 210) and may be called *electromyoneurography*.

Procedure. No fasting or preparation is required. Premedication or sedation is usually avoided because of the need for the patient to cooperate. Although this study can be done at the bedside, the patient is usually taken to the electromyography laboratory (see Nerve conduction studies). The position the patient is placed in depends on the muscle being studied. A needle that acts as a recording electrode is inserted into the muscle being examined. A reference electrode is placed nearby on the skin surface. The patient is asked to keep the muscle at rest. The oscilloscope display is viewed for any evidence of spontaneous electrical activity, such as fasciculation or fibrillation. Next, the patient is asked to contract the muscle slowly and progressively. The electrical waves produced are examined for their number and form. Maximum muscle contraction against an opposing resistance allows the opportunity to detect a complete interference pattern.

EMG is performed by a physical therapist, physiatrist, or neurologist in about 20 minutes. Results are interpreted by the physician. The test is moderately uncomfortable; pain may occur with the insertion of the needle electrode. The patient may have some muscle soreness after the procedure.

Contraindications. The study is contraindicated in the uncooperative patient, in the patient being given anticoagulant therapy, and in the patient with extensive skin infection.

Nursing considerations

Nursing Diagnoses/Collaborative Problems

- Possible knowledge deficit related to test purpose, preparation, and procedure
- Possible anxiety related to unknown sensations of procedure
- Possible anxiety related to test results
- Possible alteration in comfort related to test procedure

Nursing Implications with Rationale

- Thoroughly explain the procedure to the patient. Assure the patient that the needle will not cause electrocution. Encourage verbalization of the patient's fears.

- After the procedure, observe the needle site for hematoma or inflammation.

Myelography

Normal value: normal spinal canal

Rationale. By placing a radiopaque dye (or air) into the subarachnoid space of the spinal canal, the contents of the canal can be fluoroscopically outlined. Cord tumors, meningeal tumors, metastatic spinal tumors, herniated intravertebral discs, and arthritic bone spurs can readily be detected as indentations of the canal by this study. These lesions present as canal narrowing or as varying degrees of obstruction to the flow of the dye column within the canal (Figure 6-21). The entire canal (from lumbar to cervical area) can be examined. This test is indicated for patients

A

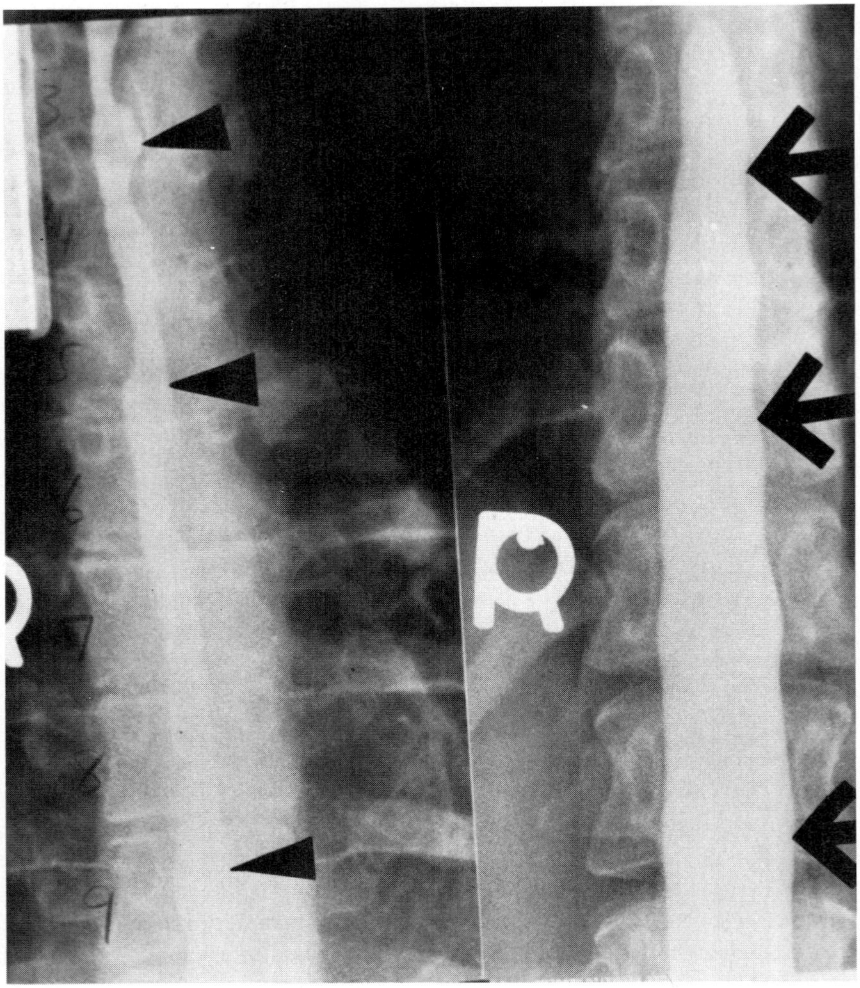

FIGURE 6-21. A, Normal myelograms. Dorsal thoracic myelogram on left and lumbar myelogram on right. Pointers and arrows indicate unobstructed column of radiographic (Pantopaque) dye within subarachnoid space of spinal canal. *Continued.*

with severe back pain or localized neurologic signs that incriminate an area of the spinal cord as the location of injury or disease. Because the test is usually performed by lumbar puncture, all the potential complications of that procedure exist (see p. 178).

Procedure. The patient is usually kept fasting for food and fluids for 4 hours before the myelography. A lumbar puncture (or a cisternal puncture), as described earlier in this chapter, is performed on the nonsedated patient. Fifteen milliliters of CSF is withdrawn, and 15 ml or more of radiographic dye or air is injected into the spinal canal. Since the specific gravity of the dye is greater than that of the CSF, the direction of dye flow depends on the tilt of the table and patient position. With the needle in place, the patient is placed in the prone position on a tilt table with the head tilted down. A foot support and shoulder brace or harness keep the pa-

B

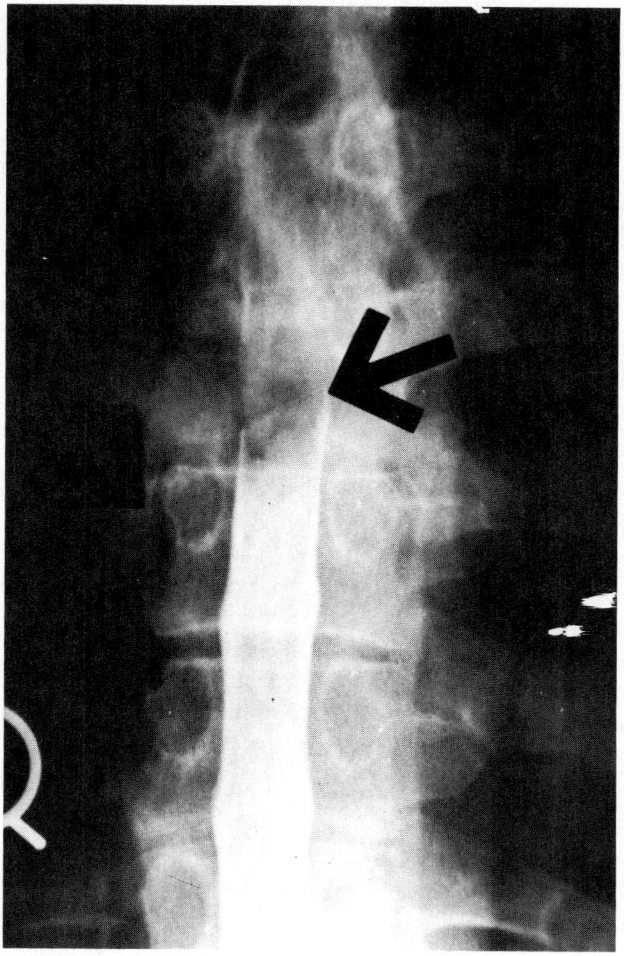

FIGURE 6-21, cont'd. B, Abnormal myelogram. Obstruction of radiographic dye column at high lumbar level *(arrow)* is caused by metastatic tumor compressing the canal. Primary site of tumor is colon.

tient from sliding. The column of dye is followed cephalad under fluoroscopy. Representative x-ray films are taken. Obstructions to the flow of dye are evident, and the level of the lesion is easily determined.

Different types of contrast material can be used for myelography. Pantopaque is most commonly used for the *oil-based* medium. An oil-based dye must be aspirated as much as possible after the procedure before removing the spinal needle. The patient's head is then kept elevated above the level of the spine to prevent upward dispersion of the dye, which could cause irritative meningitis. If the dye is completely removed, the patient may be kept flat for about 12 hours.

A *water-soluble* contrast material, metrizamide (Amipaque), is now commonly used for myelography. This dye is absorbed by the blood and excreted by the kidneys. It has two advantages over the oil-based medium. First, it does not need to be removed at the end of the procedure, since it is water-soluble and is completely reabsorbed. This feature reduces the length of the procedure and minimizes the discomfort associated with the dye removal. Second, metrizamide is less viscous than the iodinated oil-based dye and therefore permits better visualization of small areas (nerves, nerve roots, and sheaths). Also, it can flow freely through narrow canals and afford better differentiation of complete and incomplete spinal blockages. The disadvantage associated with metrizamide is that it may precipitate seizure activity after the procedure. To prevent this the patient should be well hydrated and avoid medications (such as phenothiazines, tricyclics, antidepressants, CNS stimulants, and amphetamines) that could decrease the seizure threshold. A new contrast agent (Omnipaque) has a significantly lower risk of CNS toxicity than does metrizamide. After the procedure the head and thorax should be elevated 30 to 50 degrees for at least 6 to 8 hours to prevent contact of the water-soluble agent with the cerebral meninges, which could precipitate a seizure. Bed rest may be ordered for up to 24 hours. Headache, nausea, and vomiting are often seen 4 to 8 hours after the procedure and may persist for 24 to 36 hours.

To avoid some of the side effects associated with radiopaque substances, some neurosurgeons prefer to perform an *air* myelography. After myelography using air, the patient is positioned with the head lower than the trunk to prevent air from gravitating to the cerebral space and causing headaches. This position is usually maintained for about 48 hours. Most of the air is absorbed by this time, and the head can then be elevated.

After myelography is performed (using an oil-based medium, water-based medium, or air), the needle is removed and a dressing is applied. The patient returns to the unit on a stretcher and is kept on bed rest. Examining time is approximately 45 minutes. Patient response to myelography varies from mild discomfort to severe pain. Many patients having this procedure are already having back pain, which is then exacerbated by the lumbar puncture and dye injection.

Contraindications. See Lumbar puncture, p. 181.

Nursing considerations

Nursing Diagnoses/Collaborative Problems

See Lumbar puncture, p. 182.

Nursing Implications with Rationale

- See Lumbar puncture, p. 182.
- Usually, cease food and fluid to the patient approximately 4 hours before the study to avoid the patient's vomiting during the study.
- Inform the patient that he or she will be tilted into an up-and-down position on a table so that the dye can properly fill the spinal canal and provide adequate visualization of the desired area.
- Proper positioning of the patient (after the

procedure) depends on the type of dye used. Specific positioning (see procedure) should be prescribed by the physician after consultation with the radiologist.

- Observe the patient for signs and symptoms of meningeal irritation (such as fever, stiff neck, occipital headache, or photophobia).
- Monitor the patient's vital signs and his or her ability to void.

QUESTIONS AND ANSWERS

1. **QUESTION:** What role does EEG play in establishing "brain death" before organs can be obtained for transplantation?
   ANSWER: A patient is considered "brain dead" if all of the following conditions apply:
   a. The patient is unaware and unresponsive.
   b. The patient has no natural spontaneous respiration.
   c. The patient has no brainstem reflexes (such as doll's eye, papillary, and oculovestibular).
   d. The patient has not had recent anesthesia, drug overdose, or hypothermia.
   e. The patient registers a flat line on the EEG (isoelectric) twice, being taken 24 hours apart.
2. **QUESTION:** Your patient is scheduled to have CT scanning and is complaining of severe backache. What is the appropriate nursing intervention?
   ANSWER: Because the patient must remain still for long periods during CT scanning, the patient must be comfortable to cooperate. Therefore, you should obtain a physician's order to administer an analgesic to the patient. However, it is important that analgesics or sedatives never be administered to a patient who has an altered level of consciousness. If the analgesic is given and no relief is obtained, the study should be canceled.
3. **QUESTION:** Your patient is admitted for evaluation of a brain tumor. CT scanning is ordered. On the morning of the examination you are informed that the CT scanner is broken indefinitely. What study will probably be ordered at this time?
   ANSWER: Although less sensitive and specific, brain scanning may be adequate in detecting a brain tumor and therefore will probably be ordered.
4. **QUESTION:** Your patient is scheduled for CT scanning, and you find that he has an allergy to iodine dye. Should you cancel the study?
   ANSWER: No. Although the IV injection of iodine enhances the quality and sensitivity of the CT scan, it is not necessary. Usually an adequate study can be obtained without the dye. Be certain that the request form indicates that the patient is allergic to this dye.
5. **QUESTION:** Your patient returns to the floor after having cerebral angiography. He suddenly has right-sided upper and lower extremity weakness and expressive dysphasia. What might be the cause of this patient's problem?
   ANSWER: Thrombotic or atherosclerotic plaques along the cerebral arterial wall may have been dislodged when the angiocatheter was passed, thus creating the stroke syndrome. Cerebral arterial vasospasm also could cause these symptoms, but in such a case the symptoms are usually transient and milder in degree. Assess the patient and report your findings to the physician immediately.
6. **QUESTION:** Your 29-year-old patient is admitted to the floor with the complaint of sudden onset of paralysis of the right hand. While talking with the patient, you uncover the fact that she has severe guilt feelings relating to child abuse of her infant son. You strongly suspect a conversion reaction. Would either nerve conduction studies or electromyography be indicated?
   ANSWER: An accurately performed nerve conduction study of the median, ulnar, and radial nerves can virtually eliminate any possibility of neurologic deficit to the hand. Electromyography would be less helpful, because patient cooperation is required. Therefore, nerve conduction studies should be recommended, along with psychiatric evaluation.
7. **QUESTION:** A 50-year-old patient is admitted to the emergency room and found to be febrile and comatose. The physician prepares for a lumbar puncture. What should be evaluated before this lumbar puncture is performed?
   ANSWER: Before a lumbar puncture is performed on any patient, the presence of increased intracranial pressure must be ruled out. This can be done by visualizing the optic fundi and assessing for the presence of papilledema.
8. **QUESTION:** A 22-year-old army private is being evaluated for meningitis. Several hours after a lumbar puncture is performed, he begins to complain of severe headache when standing erect.

What is the probable cause of this headache, and what are the appropriate nursing interventions?

ANSWER: The most probable cause of this type of headache is a continued leak of the CSF through the puncture site in the dura mater. Appropriate nursing interventions include keeping the patient on bed rest, forcing fluids, and administering analgesics as ordered. This patient should not have been out of bed for at least 12 hours after this procedure. Explain the reasons for bed rest to the patient.

9. **QUESTION:** A 48-year-old patient is admitted to your ward with the diagnosis of possible herniated lumbar disc. Myelography is ordered. During routine physical examination occult blood was found in the patient's stools, and the physician has ordered a barium enema study. In what sequence should these tests be performed?

ANSWER: Myelography should precede the barium enema study. If the barium enema study were done first, visualization of the radiographic (Pantopaque) dye used in myelography would be obscured by the barium used in the lower GI series.

BIBLIOGRAPHY

Antel JP and Arnason BG: Demyelinating diseases. In Wilson J and others, editors: Harrison's priniples of internal medicine, ed 12, New York, 1991, McGraw-Hill.

Bain, L: MRI—safety issues stimulate concern, Science 252:1244, 1991.

Bosch E: Peripheral neuropathies. In Rakel RE, editor: Conn's current therapy, Philadelphia, 1991, WB Saunders.

Chiappa KH and others: Clinical electrophysiology and other diagnostic methods. In Wilson J and others, editors: Harrison's principles of internal medicine, ed 12, New York, 1991, McGraw-Hill.

Chu W and Sangster W: Potential impacts of MRI accidents, Radiol Technol 56(2):139-141, 1987.

Comella CL and Bleck JP: Selecting the right neurologic test for critically ill patients, J Crit Illness 3(9):47-59, 1988.

Comella CL and Bleck JP: The techniques of lumbar puncture, J Crit Illness 3(9):61-66, 1988.

Davis K: Imaging of the nervous system. In Wilson J and others, editors: Harrison's principles of internal medicine, ed 12, New York, 1991, McGraw-Hill.

Deck M: Radiologic imaging techniques. In Wyngaarden JB and others, editors: Cecil textbook of medicine, ed 19, Philadelphia, WB Saunders.

Doolittle ND: Advances in the neurosciences and implications for nursing care, J Neurosci Nurs 23(4):207-210, 1991.

Goldensohn ES: EEG and clinical neurophysiology at the Neurological Institute of New York, J Clin Neurophysiol 8(3):252-260, 1991.

Kistler JP and others: Cerebrovascular disorders. In Wilson J and others, editors: Harrison's principles of internal medicine, ed 12, New York, 1991, McGraw-Hill.

Lehman LB: Neurologic complications of alcoholism, Postgrad Med 90(5):165-172, 1991.

Martin JB and others: The role of private body consciousness and anxiety in the report of somatic symptoms during magnetic resonance imaging, J Behav Ther Exp Psychiatry 22(1):3-7, 1991.

McBride EV and Distefano K: Explaining diagnostic test for MS, Nursing 18(2):68-72, 1988.

Newman F and others: Magnetic resonance imaging: the latest in diagnostic technology, Nursing 17(1):44-47, 1987.

Stalberg E: The value to the clinical neurologist of electromyography in the 1990s, Clin Exp Neurol 27:1-28, 1990.

Victor JD: Neurologic diagnostic procedures. In Wyngaarden JB and others, editors: Cecil textbook of medicine, ed 19, Philadelphia, 1992, WB Saunders.

Chapter 7

DIAGNOSTIC STUDIES USED IN THE ASSESSMENT OF THE URINARY SYSTEM

ANATOMY AND PHYSIOLOGY

The urinary system consists of the kidneys, ureters, bladder, and urethra (Figure 7-1). The *kidneys* are paired organs located on either side of the vertebral column just above the waistline. The blood supply to each kidney comes from the renal arteries, which branch off from the abdominal aorta. The renal veins drain the kidneys and empty blood into the inferior vena cava (Figure 7-1).

The primary function of the kidneys is to regulate the internal environment of the body. Nitrogenous wastes, along with excess fluid and electrolytes, are filtered out by the kidneys. The filtrate (urine) is formed within the kidney's functional units, called *nephrons.* Each kidney is composed of approximately one million of these nephrons. The nephron (Figure 7-2) includes Bowman's capsule, with its invaginated glomeruli, and the renal tubules (proximal and distal convoluted tubules, loop of Henle, and collecting tubules). A *glomerulus* is a tuft of capillaries fed by an afferent arteriole. As blood

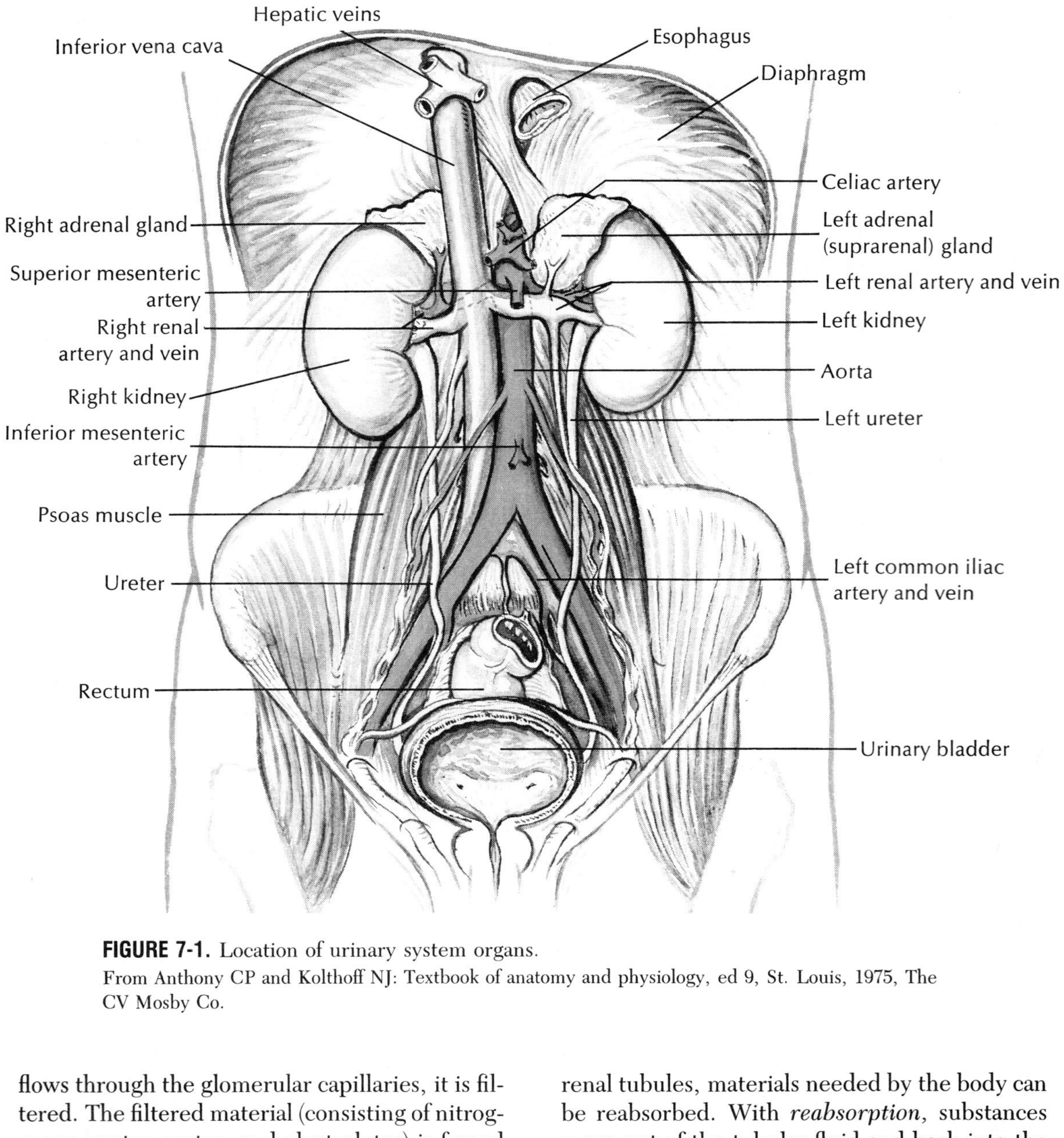

FIGURE 7-1. Location of urinary system organs.
From Anthony CP and Kolthoff NJ: Textbook of anatomy and physiology, ed 9, St. Louis, 1975, The CV Mosby Co.

flows through the glomerular capillaries, it is filtered. The filtered material (consisting of nitrogenous wastes, water, and electrolytes) is forced into Bowman's capsule because of the pressure gradient existing between these two areas. The filtrate then passes into the proximal convoluted tubules, then into the loop of Henle, the distal convoluted tubule, and finally into the collecting tubule. As the filtrate passes through these renal tubules, materials needed by the body can be reabsorbed. With *reabsorption,* substances move out of the tubular fluid and back into the blood by both active and passive transport. A major portion of water, electrolytes (sodium chloride and bicarbonate), and nutrients (glucose and amino acids) is reabsorbed in the proximal tubule. Within the loops of Henle, sodium chloride is reabsorbed. Sodium and water are

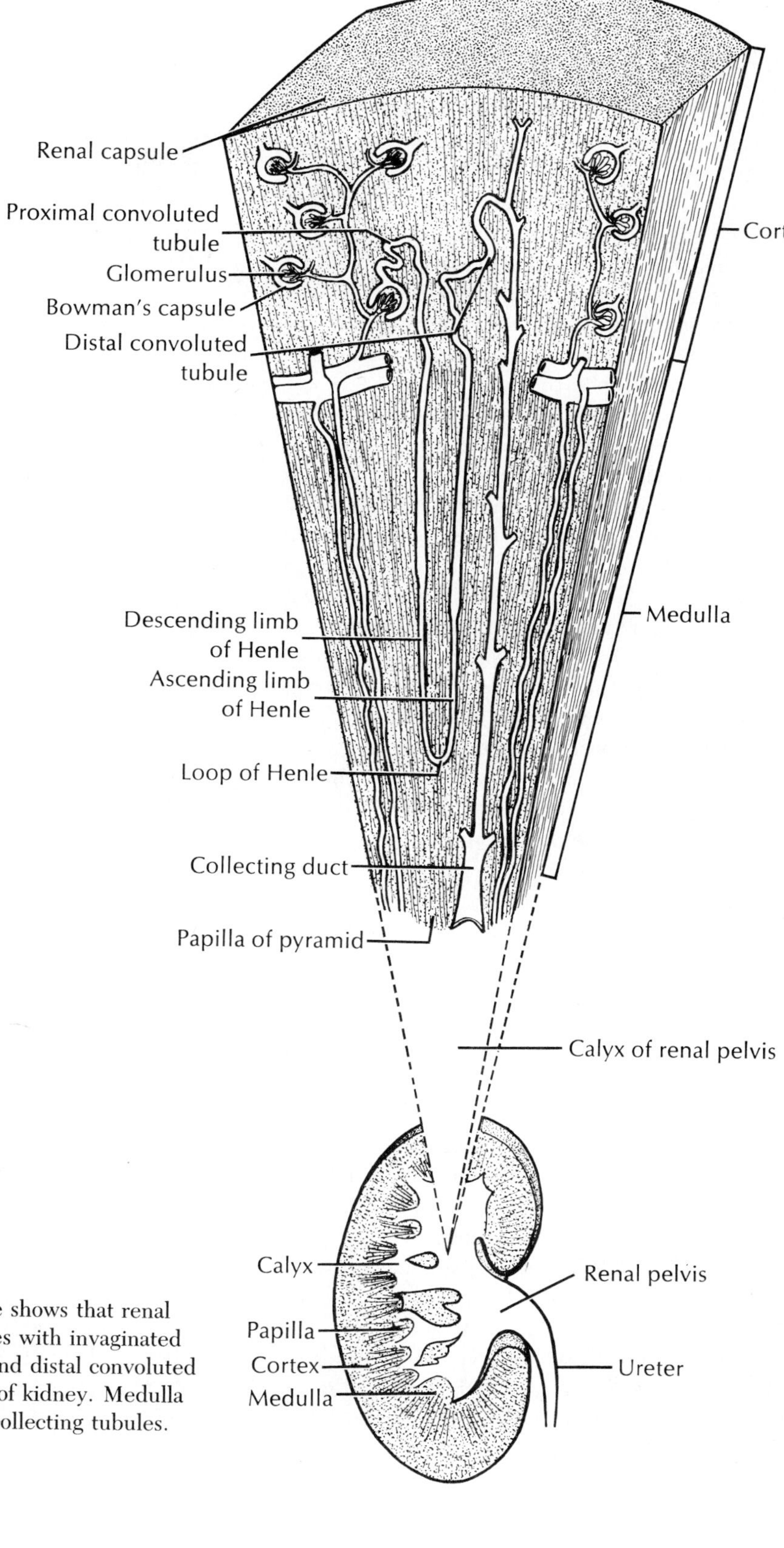

FIGURE 7-2. Magnified wedge shows that renal corpuscles (Bowman's capsules with invaginated glomeruli) in both proximal and distal convoluted tubules are located in cortex of kidney. Medulla contains loops of Henle and collecting tubules.

also reabsorbed in the distal and collecting tubules. Nitrogenous wastes are generally not reabsorbed. Not only can the tubular cells absorb substances, but they can also secrete substances. With tubular *secretion,* substances such as ammonia, potassium, hydrogen, and certain drugs (such as penicillin) move out of the blood and into the tubular fluid by both active and passive transport. Although secretion occurs primarily in the distal and collecting tubules, 90% of hydrogen ion and penicillin secretion occurs in the proximal tubules.

The relatively dilute urine received into the distal convoluted and collecting tubules is either excreted unchanged into the renal calyces or further concentrated, depending on the individual's state of hydration. These calyces then empty the urine into the pelvis of the kidney (Figure 7-2). The urine passes from the pelvis into the *ureters* and finally into the urinary bladder. The *bladder* is a collapsible vesicle located directly behind the symphysis pubis. It serves as a temporary reservoir for urine. The bladder walls consist primarily of smooth muscle (called detrusor muscle) whose contraction is mainly responsible for emptying the bladder during urination (micturition). During micturition the urine is emptied through the *urethra.* In the male the urethra is also the terminal point of the reproductive tract and serves as the conduit for expelling the semen.

Electrolyte and water regulation

The amount of electrolytes and water excreted by the kidney and other sites of insensible loss (such as skin and lung) must equal the daily intake to maintain balance (homeostasis). Sodium and potassium excretion is regulated by aldosterone through the *renin-angiotensin* system (Figure 7-3). When the sodium level falls or when the potassium level rises, specialized cells within the kidney, collectively called the macula densa, stimulate the juxtaglomerular cells (found in the walls of the renal afferent arterioles) to secrete renin into the blood. Within the liver, renin converts angiotensinogen to angiotensin I. In the pulmonary tissue, angiotensin I is converted to angiotensin II. Angiotensin II stimulates the adrenal cortex to secrete *aldosterone.* This final hormone stimulates the renal tubule to reabsorb increased amounts of the sodium and to secrete potassium. When electrolyte levels approach normal, the renin-angiotensin system is turned off.

Regulation of water excretion takes place in the kidney, primarily by way of two regulatory mechanisms: renin-angiotensin and antidiuretic hormone (ADH).

Renin-angiotensin. When the patient is dehydrated, the renal blood flow drops. Specialized, pressure-sensitive cells within the juxtaglomerular apparatus recognize this fall in renal blood pressure. These cells surround the glomerular afferent arteriole in the kidney and secrete renin when renal blood flow decreases. The renin-angiotensin mechanism (as previously described) is activated (Figure 7-3). The end result of sodium reabsorption causes the obligatory reabsorption of water. The patient becomes euhydrated and the renin system is "turned off."

Antidiuretic hormone. When a patient becomes dehydrated, the serum osmolality increases (that is, the amount of solute per unit of water increases). This increase in osmolality stimulates the posterior pituitary gland to release ADH. This hormone stimulates water reabsorption in the renal collecting-tubule cells. The patient becomes euhydrated, osmolality returns to normal, and the feedback system is turned off.

CASE STUDY 1: GLOMERULONEPHRITIS

A 7-year-old boy was brought to his pediatrician because he had developed hematuria, which required hospitalization. About 6 weeks before his admission he had had a severe sore throat but received no treatment for it. Subsequently, he did well except for complaints of mild lethargy and decrease in appetite. For the 10 days before admission he had a temperature of 101° F daily. He complained of minimal bilateral back pain. Physical examination revealed a well-developed young boy with moderate bi-

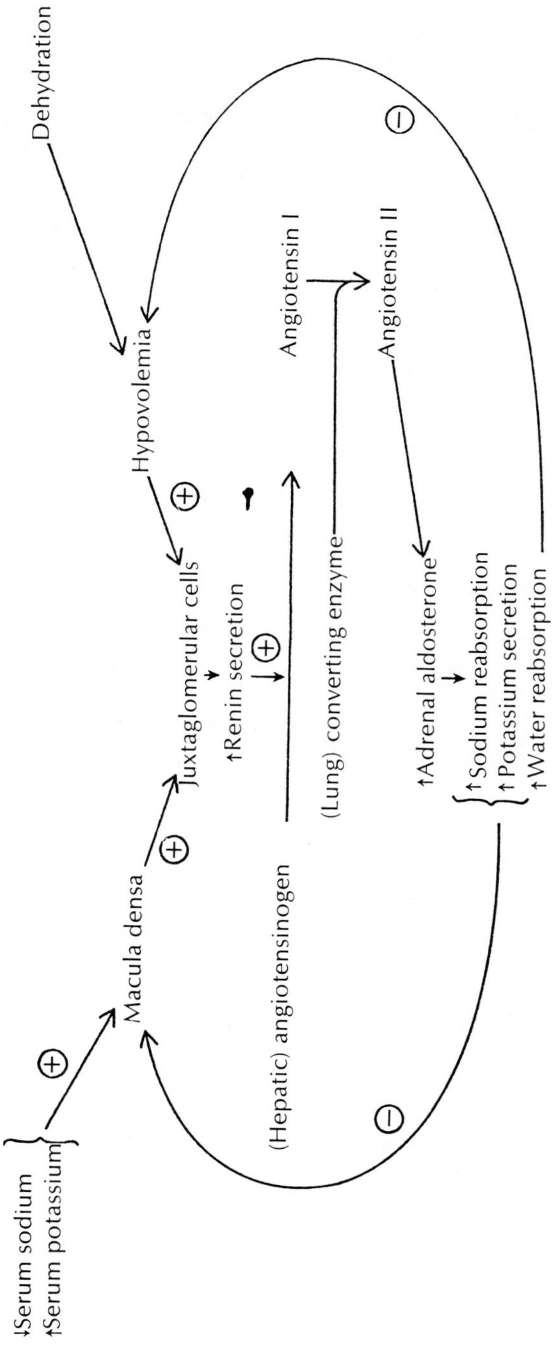

FIGURE 7-3. Renin-angiotensin system of sodium, potassium, and water regulation.

lateral costovertebral angle (CVA) tenderness. The remainder of the physical examination results were negative. His blood pressure was 140/100 mm Hg in both arms and legs.

Studies	Results
Urinalysis	Blood, +4; protein, +1; red blood cell (RBC) casts, positive; specific gravity, 1.025; red-tinged urine (normal: negative for blood, protein, and RBC casts; specific gravity, 1.010-1.025; amber-yellow urine)
Blood urea nitrogen (BUN) and creatinine test	
BUN	42 mg/dl (normal: 7-20 mg/dl)
Creatinine	1.8 mg/dl (normal: 0.7-1.5 mg/dl)
Creatinine clearance test	64 ml/min (normal: approximately 120 ml/min)
Intravenous pyelography (IVP)	Delayed visualization bilaterally; enlarged kidneys, no tumor; no obstruction seen
Renal biopsy	Swelling of glomerular tuft, along with polymorphonuclear leukocyte infiltrates in Bowman's capsule (findings compatible with glomerulonephritis); immunofluorescent staining, positive for IgG
Antistreptolysin O (ASO) titer	210 Todd units/ml (normal: ≤200 Todd units/ml)
Antideoxyribonuclease-B titer (Anti-DNase-B)	200 units (normal: ≤170 units)

The blood, protein, and RBC casts in this child's urine indicated a primary renal disorder. The elevated creatinine and BUN levels indicated that the problem was severe and that it was markedly affecting his renal function. IVP was helpful only in ruling out tumor (Wilms') or congenital abnormality. Renal biopsy was most helpful in suggesting glomerulonephritis. The history of recent pharyngitis, the positive ASO titration, the positive anti-DNase-B titer, and the finding of IgG antibodies on the immunofluorescent stain all suggested poststreptococcal glomerulonephritis.

The patient was placed on a 10-day course of penicillin. He was given antihypertensive medication, and his fluid and electrolyte balance was closely monitored. At no time did his creatinine or BUN level rise to a point requiring dialysis. After 6 weeks, the child's renal function returned to normal (creatinine, 0.7 mg/dl; BUN, 7 mg/dl). His antihypertensive medications were discontinued. He remained normotensive and returned to normal activity.

DISCUSSION OF TESTS

Urinalysis and urine culture

Urinalysis

pH

Normal values: 4.6-8.0 (6.0 average)

Appearance

Normal value: clear

Color

Normal value: amber-yellow

Odor

Normal value: aromatic

Specific gravity

Normal values:

Adult: 1.005-1.030 (usually 1.010-1.025)

Elderly: values decrease with advancing age

Newborn: 1.001-1.020

Protein (albumin)

Normal values: up to 8 mg/dl

50-80 mg/24 hr (at rest)

<250 mg/24 hr (after strenuous exercise)

Glucose

Normal value: none (random specimen)

24 hour specimen: <0.5 g/day or <2.78 mmol/day (SI units)

Ketones

Normal value: none

Blood

Normal values: up to 2 red blood cells (RBCs)

Microscopic examination

RBC: 1-2/low power field

WBC: 0-4/low power field

Casts: negative or occasional hyaline

Crystals: negative

Bacteria: none

Rationale. The urinalysis is a useful urologic screening test. It is an essential component of physical examinations and hospital admission workups. Results may provide a tentative diagnosis, indicate further studies, or monitor the progression of diagnosed disorders. Routine urinalysis includes the following: assessment of appearance, color, and odor; measurement of pH and specific gravity; and determination of the presence of glucose, protein, blood, and ketones. Microscopic examination of the urine sediment is also performed to detect cells, casts, crystals, and bacteria. A discussion of each follows.

Routine urinalysis

pH. The analysis of the pH of a freshly voided urine specimen indicates the acid-base balance of the patient. An alkaline pH is obtained in a patient with alkalemia. This can also be caused by bacteriuria, urinary tract infection (caused by *Pseudomonas* or *Proteus*), or a diet high in citrus fruits or vegetables. An acidic urine is generally obtained in patients with acidemia, which can be a result of metabolic or respiratory acidosis, starvation, diarrhea, or a diet high in meat protein or cranberries.

Appearance. The normal urine specimen should be clear. Cloudy urine may be caused by the presence of pus, RBCs, or bacteria. However, normal urine may also be cloudy due to ingestion of certain food (for example, large amounts of fat), urates, or phosphates.

Color. The color of the urine ranges from pale yellow to amber because of the pigment urochrome. The color indicates the concentration of the urine and varies with the specific gravity. Dilute urine is straw colored, and concentrated urine is deep amber.

Abnormally colored urine can result from a pathologic condition or from the ingestion of certain foods or medicine. For example, bleeding from the kidney produces dark red urine, whereas bleeding in the lower urinary tract produces bright red urine. Dark yellow urine may indicate the presence of urobilinogen or bilirubin. *Pseudomonas* organisms usually produce green urine. Beets may cause red urine. Rhubarb can cause the urine to be brown. Many commonly used drugs affect urine color (Table 7-1).

Odor. The aromatic odor of fresh, normal urine is caused by the presence of volatile acid. The urine of patients in diabetic ketosis has a severe smell of acetone. In infected persons urine has a very unpleasant odor.

Specific gravity. Specific gravity is a measure of the concentration of particles (including wastes and electrolytes) in the urine. A high specific gravity indicates a concentrated urine; a low specific gravity indicates a dilute urine.

The specific gravity is *increased* in patients with the following conditions:

1. Dehydration, because the kidneys are reabsorbing all available free water and the excreted urine is thus very concentrated
2. A pituitary tumor that causes the release of excessive amounts of ADH, resulting in excessive water reabsorption
3. A decrease in renal blood flow (as in heart failure, renal artery stenosis, or hypotension)
4. Glycosuria and proteinuria, because of the increased number of particles in the urine.

The specific gravity is *decreased* in patients with the following conditions:

1. Overhydration
2. Diabetes insipidus, because of inadequate ADH secretion, which causes a decrease in water reabsorption
3. Chronic renal failure, because the kidney has lost its ability to concentrate urine through water reabsorption.

Protein (albumin). Proteinuria is a sensitive indicator of kidney dysfunction. Normally protein is not present in the urine, because the spaces in the normal glomerular membrane are too small to allow its passage. If, as in glomerulonephritis, the glomerular membrane is injured, the spaces become much larger and protein is allowed to seep out into the filtrate and

TABLE 7-1. Commonly Used Drugs that Can Affect Urine Color

Generic and brand names	Drug classification	Urine color
Anisindione (Miradon)	Oral anticoagulant	Red-orange in alkaline urine
Cascara sagrada	Stimulant laxative	Red in alkaline urine; yellow-brown in acid urine
Chloroquine (Aralen)	Antimalarial	Rusty yellow or brown
Chlorzoxazone (Paraflex)	Skeletal muscle relaxant	Orange or purple-red
Danthron (Modane)	Stimulant laxative	Pink or red in alkaline urine
Dioctyl calcium sulfosuccinate (Doxidan, Surfak)	Laxative	Pink to red to red-brown
Furazolidone (Furozone)	Antiinfective, antiprotozoal	Brown
Iron preparations (Ferotran, Imferon)	Hematinic	Dark brown or black on standing
Levodopa	Antiparkinsonian	Dark brown on standing
Methylene blue (Urolene Blue)	Antimethemoglobinemic	Blue-green
Nitrofurantoin (Macrodantin, Nitrodan)	Antibacterial	Brown
Phenazopyridine (Pyridium)	Urinary tract analgesic	Orange to red
Phenindione (Eridione)	Anticoagulant	Red-orange in alkaline urine
Phenolphthalein (Ex-Lax)	Contact laxative	Red or purplish pink in alkaline urine
Phenothiazines (for example, prochlorperazine [Compazine])	Antipsychotic, neuroleptic, antiemetic	Red-brown
Phenytoin (Dilantin)	Anticonvulsant	Pink, red, red-brown
Riboflavin (vitamin B_2)	Vitamin	Intense yellow
Rifampin	Antibiotic	Red-orange
Sulfasalazine (Azulfidine)	Antibacterial	Orange-yellow in alkaline urine
Triamterene (Dyrenium)	Diuretic	Pale blue fluorescence

then the urine. If this persists at a significant rate, the patient can become hypoproteinemic because of the serum protein loss through the kidneys. This decreases the normal capillary oncotic pressure that holds fluid within the vasculature and causes severe interstitial edema, which is known as the *nephrotic syndrome*.

The urine of all pregnant women is routinely checked for proteinuria, which can be an indicator of preeclampsia.

Glucose. In diabetic patients whose condition is not well controlled with hypoglycemic agents, blood glucose levels can become very high. High glucose levels can also be produced artificially by IV administration of dextrose-containing fluids.

When the blood glucose level exceeds 180 mg/dl (the renal threshold), glucose begins to spill over into the urine. As the blood glucose level increases further, the amount of glucose in the urine also increases. (This abnormal presence of glucose in the urine is called glycosuria.)

Other causes of glycosuria include problems such as central nervous system disorders (for example, stroke), Cushing's syndrome, severe stress, infection, and drugs such as ascorbic acid, aspirin, cephalothin (Keflin), epinephrine, and streptomycin.

Ketones. In poorly controlled diabetes (most frequently in juvenile diabetes), there is massive fatty acid catabolism. The purpose of this catabolism is to maintain an energy source at a time when glucose cannot be used because of the lack of insulin. Ketones are the end product of the fatty acid breakdown. Like glucose, when ketones become increased in the blood, they spill over into the urine. Ketonuria can also be seen in nondiabetic patients suffering from dehydration, starvation, or excessive aspirin ingestion.

Blood. Any disruption in the blood-urine barrier, whether at the glomerular or the tubular level, will cause blood cells to enter the urine. This is seen with glomerulonephritis, interstitial nephritis, acute tubular necrosis, pyelonephritis, and renal trauma or tumor. Pathologic conditions involving the mucosa of the collecting system (such as tumor, inflammation, trauma, or abrasion secondary to calculi) also cause hematuria (blood in the urine). This can be detected and semiquantitated by routine analysis.

Microscopic examination

RBC. Normally, only one or two red blood cells are found in the urine sediment on microscopic examination. The finding of more than five red blood cells is an indication of microscopic hematuria, the causes of which have previously been discussed.

WBC. Normally zero to four white blood cells are found in the urine sediment on microscopic examination. The presence of more than five white blood cells indicates a urinary tract infection. A clean-catch urine culture should be done.

Casts. Casts are clumps of material or cells. They are found in the renal-collecting tubule and have the shape of the tubule, hence the name *cast.* On microscopic examination of urine sediment, *white blood cell casts* (clumps of white blood cells) are most frequently found in acute pyelonephritis. White cell casts are also seen with glomerulonephritis and lupus nephritis. *Red cell casts* suggest glomerulonephritis. They may be found in subacute bacterial endocarditis, renal infarct, Goodpasture's syndrome, vasculitis, sickling, and malignant hypertension. *Hyaline casts* are conglomerations of protein and indicate proteinuria. The causes of proteinuria have been previously discussed. A few hyaline casts can be found normally, especially after strenous exercise. *Epithelial casts* are most suggestive of glomerulonephritis. A urine specimen should be checked for casts when fresh because after the specimen sits the casts break up.

Crystals. Crystals found in the urine sediment on microscopic examination indicate that renal stone formation is imminent, if not already present. Urate crystals occur in patients with high serum uric acid levels (gout). Phosphate and calcium oxalate crystals occur in the urine of patients with hyperparathyroidism or malabsorption states. The type of crystal found varies with the urine pH (for example, urate crystals in acid urine and calcium oxalate crystals in alkaline urine).

Bacteria. Demonstration of bacteria on microscopic examination of sediment from an appropriately obtained specimen indicates urinary tract infection (such as pyelonephritis or cystitis).

Procedure. A reliable urinalysis depends on the proper collection of the urine specimen and the immediate performance of the analysis. The first-voided morning specimen is the ideal urine specimen for analysis because of its concentration and characteristic acidity. However, a fresh urine specimen collected at any other time is usually reliable. For a *routine urinalysis,* usually no special preparation of the patient is needed. The patient voids into a clean bedpan, urinal, or preferably, a urine container. This specimen cannot be used for a culture and sensitivity. If a culture and sensitivity test is also required, a *clean-catch,* or *midstream,* specimen is collected. This test requires meticulous cleaning of the perineal area or penis with an iodine preparation to reduce contamination of the specimen by external organisms. Then the cleaning agent must be completely removed, or it will contaminate the urine specimen. The midstream collection is obtained by having the patient begin to urinate into a bedpan, urinal, or toilet, and then stop. (This washes the urine out of the distal urethra.) Then a sterile urine container is correctly positioned, and the patient voids 3 to 4 ounces of urine into the container. The container is then capped. The patient finishes voiding. For patients unable to void, urinary catheterization may be needed; however, this procedure is not commonly performed because of the risk of introducing organisms and because of patient discomfort.

In patients with an indwelling urinary catheter, a specimen can be obtained by attaching a small-gauge needle to a syringe and aseptically inserting the needle into the catheter at a point distal to the sleeve leading to the balloon. Urine is aspirated and then placed into the urine container. Usually the catheter tubing distal to the puncture site needs to be clamped for 15 to 30 minutes before the aspiration of urine to allow urine to fill the tubing. After the specimen is withdrawn, the clamp is removed.

Suprapubic aspiration of urine is a safe method of collecting urine in neonates and infants. For this technique, the abdomen is prepared with an antiseptic, and a 25-gauge needle (attached to a 5 ml syringe) is inserted into the suprapubic area, 1 inch above the symphysis pubis. Urine is aspirated into the syringe and then transferred to a sterile urine container.

Specimens from infants and young children can be collected in a disposable bag called a *U-bag*. This bag has an adhesive backing around the opening to attach to the child.

Composite urine specimens are collected over a time that may range from 2 to 24 hours. Composite specimens are examined for specific components (such as electrolytes, catecholamines, and creatinine). To collect a composite specimen the patient is instructed to void and discard the urine. This is then noted at the start of the test. All subsequent urine is saved in a container for the designated time. At the end of this time period, the patient urinates and adds this urine to the collection container.

Routine examination. The pH and the presence of protein, glucose, ketones, or blood (hemoglobin) can be easily detected by using Multistix reagent strips for urinalysis. Multistix is a plastic stick to which several separate reagent strips are affixed for testing various substances. (See Chapter 4 for urine bilirubin testing.) The reagent strip is completely immersed in the well-mixed urine and removed immediately to avoid dissolving out the reagents. The strip is held in a horizontal position to prevent possible mixing of the chemical reagents and then is compared with the test chart at the time specified.

Test	When to read results	Range of results
pH	Anytime	5-9
Protein	Anytime	Negative-+4 (>2000 mg/dl)
Glucose	10 sec (qualitative)	Negative-+4
	30 sec (quantitative)	Negative-+4 (2%)
Ketones	15 sec	Negative-+3 (large)
Blood	25 sec	Negative-+3 (large)

Specific gravity. Specific gravity is measured in several easy steps by the use of a urinometer. First, the urine is placed in a clean, dry cylinder. Second, a weighted urinometer is suspended (floated) in the cylinder of urine. The concentration of the urine determines the depth at which the urinometer will float. Third, this depth is measured by the calibrated scale on the urinometer and is called the specific gravity.

Specific gravity can also be detected by a newer technique, the refractometer. For this procedure one drop of urine is placed on a slide at the end of the refractometer (a small telescope-like instrument). The density of the urine determines the refractive index.

Microscopic examination. An aliquot (approximately 10 ml) of the urine specimen is placed in a test tube and centrifuged for 3 to 5 minutes. The supernatant liquid is then poured off, and the sediment is resuspended in the last few drops of urine by vigorous agitation of the tube. A drop of the sediment is then placed on a glass slide and covered with a coverslip for low-power microscopic examination. Another drop of the sediment is smeared on a slide for staining. Cells, casts, crystals, and bacteria are then identified.

Contraindications. None.

Nursing considerations

Nursing Diagnoses/Collaborative Problems

See Urine studies, p. 3.

Nursing Implications with Rationale

- Explain the purpose and specific method of urine collection to the patient. Give the patient the proper specimen jars and cleaning agents if necessary. The perianal area should be washed if it is soiled with feces. Most hospitals use commercial kits for a clean-catch specimen; these contain all the necessary equipment and provide directions for obtaining the specimen.
- For collecting a specimen for culture, determine if the patient is capable of obtaining the urine specimen independently. If not, nursing personnel will need to assist the patient.
- If possible, obtain the first-voided specimen of the day, because it is usually more concentrated than other specimens.
- If the specimen cannot be tested immediately, cover and refrigerate it. Refrigeration may reduce the bacterial cell proliferation and retard deterioration of casts and cells. The pH of uncovered specimens becomes alkaline, because CO_2 diffuses into the air.
- If the patient is menstruating, indicate it on the lab slip. Hematuria is then discounted.
- When using dipsticks (Multistix reagent strips) or tablets, read the directions on the bottle or package insert and follow the directions precisely. The color reaction must be compared with the manufacturer's color chart at the *exact* time specified. After removing the dipstick from the bottle, close the bottle tightly to prevent the stick's absorbing moisture and altering future results. Check the expiration date on the bottle before use.
- Inform the patient that toilet paper or feces should not be in the urine container because of contamination.

Blood urea nitrogen and creatinine test

Blood urea nitrogen (BUN)

Normal values:

Adult: 10-20 mg/dl or 3.6-7.1 mmol/L (SI units)

Elderly: may be slightly higher than those of adults

Child: 5-18 mg/dl

Infant: 5-18 mg/dl

Newborn: 3-12 mg/dl

Cord: 21-40 mg/dl

Possible critical values >100 mg/dl (indicates serious impairment of renal function)

Creatinine

Normal values:

Adult: female, 0.5-1.1 mg/dl or 44-97 μmol/L (SI units)

male, 0.6-1.2 mg/dl

Elderly: decrease in muscle mass may cause decreased values

Adolescent: 0.5-1.0 mg/dl

Child: 0.3-0.7 mg/dl

Infant: 0.2-0.4 mg/dl

Newborn: 0.3-1.2 mg/dl

Possible critical values >4 mg/dl (indicates serious impairment in renal function)

Rationale. The tests most commonly used to assess kidney function include the blood urea nitrogen (BUN) and serum creatinine test and the creatinine clearance test (see next study). These tests are referred to as renal function studies.

BUN. The BUN test measures the amount of urea nitrogen in the blood. Urea is formed in the liver as an end product of protein catabolism and is excreted entirely by the kidney. Therefore the blood concentration of urea is directly related to the excretory function of the kidney and serves as an index of this function.

Within the gut, protein is digested to amino acids, which are absorbed. In the liver these amino acids are catabolized, and free ammonia is formed as the end product. This ammonia is combined to form urea. The urea is deposited into the blood and transported to the kidneys, from which it is excreted.

Nearly all primary renal diseases cause inadequate excretion of urea, and the blood concentration rises above normal. These renal diseases include glomerulonephritis, pyelonephritis, acute tubular necrosis, and urinary obstruction from tumor or stones.

Toxins such as gentamycin, tobramycin, myoglobin, and free hemoglobin decrease BUN excretion. In dehydration, shock, and congestive heart failure, there is a physiologic decrease in renal blood flow, which also causes a decrease in the excretion of BUN. With the decreased excretion of the urea nitrogen, its level in the blood rises above normal.

BUN levels may also be elevated in circumstances other than primary renal disease. For example, when excessive amounts of protein are available for hepatic catabolism, large quantities of urea are made. The normal kidneys are overwhelmed and are unable to excrete this sudden load of urea, causing the BUN level to rise. Urea levels may also be increased in GI bleeding disorders (where intestinal blood is reabsorbed and acts as the protein source).

Decreased BUN levels may be associated with overhydration, liver failure, and negative nitrogen balance. Pregnancy, which causes an increase in plasma volume, also reduces the BUN level.

Finally, one must be aware that the synthesis of urea depends on the liver. With combined liver and renal disease (as in hepatorenal syndrome), the BUN level may be normal not because the renal excretory function is good, but rather because the hepatic function is poor and the formation of BUN is decreased.

Creatinine. Creatinine, like BUN, is excreted entirely by the kidneys and is therefore directly proportional to renal excretory function. Unlike BUN, however, it is affected very little by dehydration, malnutrition, or hepatic function. Creatinine is a catabolic product of creatine, which is used in skeletal muscle contraction. The daily production of creatine, and subsequently creatinine depends on muscle mass, which fluctuates very little. It is evident then that with normal renal excretory function, the serum creatinine level should remain constant and normal. Only renal disorders, such as glomerulonephritis, pyelonephritis, acute tubular necrosis, and urinary obstructions, cause an abnormal elevation in creatinine. The normal BUN/creatinine ratio is about 20:1 (some sources use 15:1). When the BUN level rises out of proportion to the creatinine level, this indicates dehydration, GI bleeding, or malnutrition. When both the BUN and the creatinine levels rise, the patient must be assessed for kidney disease or failure. A lower ratio may be found in low protein intake, overhydration, or severe liver failure, which reduces the BUN but not the creatinine levels.

Procedure (BUN and creatinine). One red-top tube of blood is drawn from a peripheral vein and sent to the chemistry laboratory. A multifunctional analysis machine determines the level of both substances.

Contraindications. None.

Nursing considerations

Nursing Diagnoses/Collaborative Problems

See Blood studies, p. 2.

Nursing Implications with Rationale

- Apply pressure or a pressure dressing to the venipuncture site after the procedure is completed. Observe the site for bleeding.

Creatinine clearance test

Normal values:
Adult (<40 years): male, 97-137 ml/min
female, 88-128 ml/min
Values decrease 6.5 ml/min/decade because of decline in glomerular filtration rate (GFR)
Newborn: 40-65 ml/min

Rationale. Creatinine clearance is a measure of the glomerular filtration rate (GFR), that is, the number of milliliters of filtrate made by the kidneys per minute. Urine and serum creatinine levels are assessed, and the clearance rate is calculated.

The amount of filtrate made in the kidney depends on the amount of blood present to be filtered and on the ability of the glomeruli to act as a filter. The amount of blood present for filtration is decreased in renal artery atherosclerosis, dehydration, or shock. The ability of the glomeruli to act as a filter is decreased by diseases such as glomerulonephritis, acute tubular necrosis, and most other primary renal diseases. Obstruction to urinary outflow affects glomerular filtration (creatinine clearance) only after it is severe and long-standing.

When one kidney alone becomes diseased, the opposite kidney, if normal, has the ability to compensate by increasing its filtration rate. Therefore, with unilateral kidney disease or excision, a decrease in creatinine clearance is not expected.

Procedure. The patient's urine is collected in an appropriate specimen container over a 24-hour period. It is then sent to the chemistry laboratory for measurement of volume and quantity of creatinine. No special diet is necessary. During the 24-hour collection period, a serum creatinine level test specimen is drawn and sent to the chemistry laboratory. Creatinine clearance is then computed from the above measurements using the following formula:

$$\text{Creatinine clearance} = \frac{\text{UV}}{\text{P}}$$

U = Number of mg/dl of creatinine excreted in the urine over 24 hours

V = Volume of urine, in ml/min (total volume [in ml] of urine in 24 hours is divided by 1440 minutes to get ml/min

P = Serum creatinine in mg/dl

For example, when U = 96 mg/dl, V = 1800 ml/24 hours, and P = 1.0 mg/dl, the equation would be:

$$\frac{(96\ \text{mg/dl})\ (1800\ \text{ml/24 hours})}{(1.0\ \text{mg/dl})\ (1440\ \text{min})} = 120\ \text{ml/min}$$

Contraindications. None.

Nursing considerations

Nursing Diagnoses/Collaborative Problems

See Blood studies, p. 2 and Urine studies, p. 3.

Nursing Implications with Rationale

- Explain the procedure to the patient. Show the patient where to store the urine specimen. The 24-hour urine specimen for creatinine does not need refrigeration. (Some hospitals prefer that all urine specimens be refrigerated.)
- The 24-hour collection period begins after the patient urinates. Indicate the starting time on the urine container or slip. Discard the first sample. Make sure that all urine passed by the patient during the next 24 hours is collected. Test results are calculated on the basis of a 24-hour output, and results will be inaccurate if any specimens are missed. If one voided specimen is accidentally discarded, the 24-hour collection usually must begin again. However, some hospitals allow the specimen to be sent if the amount of urine discarded is indicated on the lab slip and is less than 250 ml.
- Post the hours for the urine collection on the patient's door, on the bedpan hopper, and in the utility room to prevent accidental discarding of a specimen.
- It is not necessary to measure each urine specimen (24-hour collection of some other specimen may require this measurement).
- Remind the patient to void before defecating so that the urine is not contaminated by feces. Toilet paper should not be placed in the collection container.
- Encourage the patient to drink fluids during the 24-hour period unless this is contraindicated for medical purposes.
- Collect the last specimen as close as possible to the end of the 24-hour period. Remind the patient when the last sample is needed. Indicate the time of the last specimen on the laboratory slip or urine container. Send the specimen to the laboratory when the test is completed.

- Draw a venous blood sample in a red-top tube during the 24-hour collection period.

Intravenous pyelography

(IVP, excretory urography/EUG)

Normal values: normal size, shape, and position of the kidneys, renal pelvis, ureters, and bladder

Rationale. Intravenous pyelography is an x-ray study that uses radiopaque contrast medium to visualize the kidneys, renal pelvis, ureters, and bladder. The dye is injected intravenously, filtered out by the glomeruli, and then passed through the renal tubules. An x-ray film taken at this time will show the kidneys well opacified (visualized). The dye then collects in the renal pelvis, ureters, and bladder. X-ray films taken at this time will show these structures to be well opacified (Figure 7-4).

If the artery leading to one of the kidneys is blocked, the dye cannot enter that part of the renal system and that kidney will not be visualized. If the artery is partially blocked, the length of time required for the appearance of the contrast material will be prolonged.

With primary glomerular disease (such as glomerulonephritis) the glomerular filtrate is reduced, which causes a reduction in the quantity of dye filtered. It will therefore take a longer period of time for enough dye to enter the kidney filtrate and allow for renal opacification. Therefore, a delay in kidney visualization occurs. This provides an estimation of renal function.

Tumor (benign or malignant) or benign renal cyst will distort the bean-shaped contour of the kidney (Figure 7-5). Defects in the dye filling of the renal pelvis, ureters, or bladder are indicative of intrinsic tumors (Figures 7-4 and 7-6) or stones (Figure 7-7). Often these intrinsic tumors and stones, and also extrinsic tumors, cause complete obstruction of the dye flow in the collecting systems (pelvis, ureters, bladder). If the obstruction has been of sufficient duration, the collecting systems proximal to the obstruction are dilated (hydronephrosis). Retroperitoneal and pelvic tumors, aneurysms, and enlarged lymph nodes can also produce extrinsic compression and distortion of the opacified collecting system.

IVP is used to assess the effects of trauma to the urinary system. Renal hematomas distort the renal contour. Renal artery laceration is suggested by nonopacification of one kidney. Lacerations of the kidneys, pelvis, ureters, and bladder often cause urine leaks, which are identified by dye extravasation from the urinary system.

IVP can also assess the patient for congenital absence or malposition of kidneys. Horseshoe kidneys (connection of the two kidneys), double ureters, and pelvic kidneys are common congenital abnormalities.

Complications of IVP include the following:

1. Allergic reaction varying from mild flush, itching, and urticaria to life-threatening anaphylaxis. This, of course, is treated with diphenhydramine (Benadryl), steroids, and epinephrine. If a patient has a known allergy to iodine and yet requires IVP, allergic reaction can be avoided by giving prednisone, 5 mg, four times a day, and diphenhydramine, 25 mg, four times a day, for as many as 3 days before and 3 days following the test.
2. Infiltration of the contrast agent. This is avoided by being certain of the patency of the IV line. The treatment of this infiltration is elevation of the extremity and warm soaks.
3. Renal shutdown and failure. This occurs most frequently in the elderly patient who is dehydrated before the dye injection. The treatment is supportive care. It can be prevented by assuring adequate hydration in these patients.

Procedure. In the afternoon or the evening before the examination, the patient is given a strong laxative (such as castor oil) or a cathartic. No laxatives are usually required in the young child or infant. The patient is kept NPO after midnight. A suppository or enema may be given

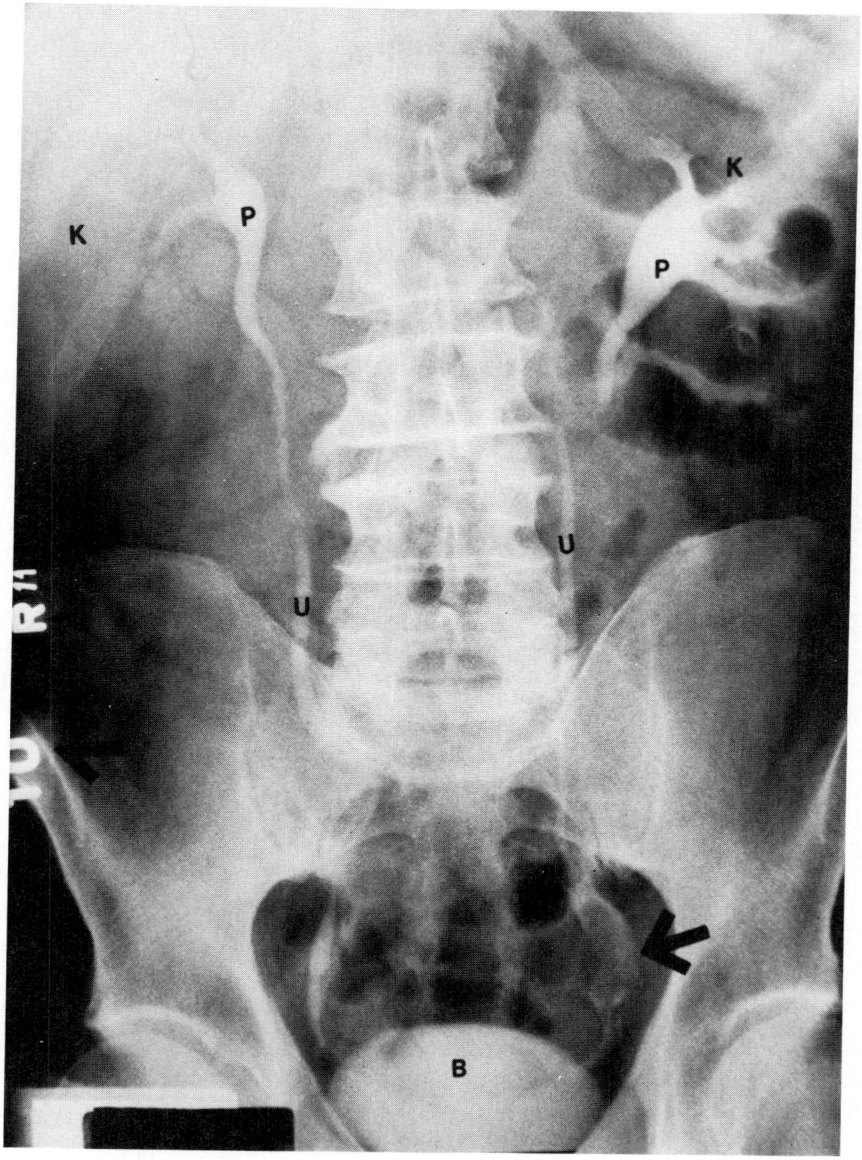

FIGURE 7-4. Intravenous pyelogram. Black arrow at right indicates a left ureteral tumor. *K*, Kidney; *P*, renal pelvis; *U*, ureter; *B*, bladder. Note black arrow at left indicating that x-ray film was taken 10 minutes after injection of dye. The *R* on left side of picture indicates right side of patient.

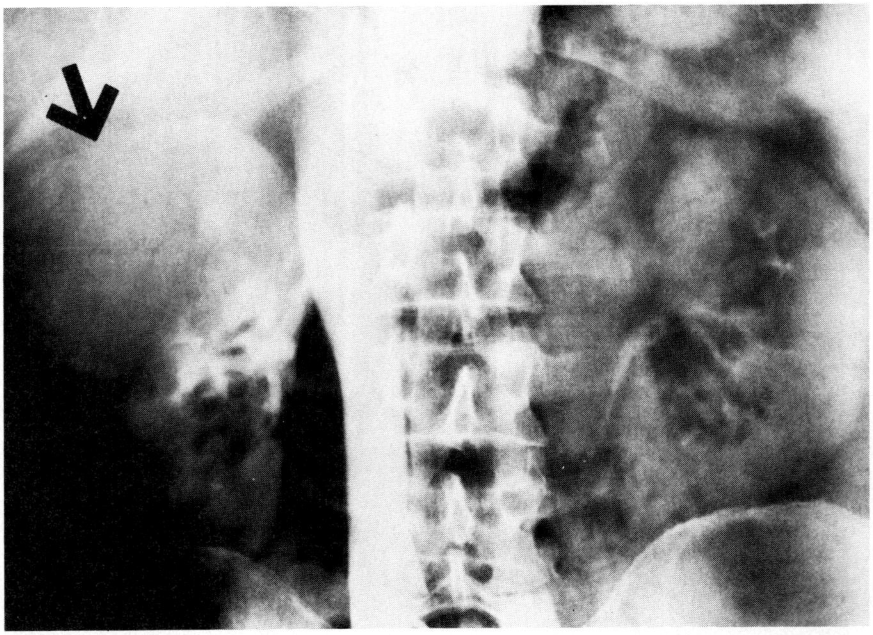

FIGURE 7-5. Intravenous pyelogram. Arrow indicates distortion of upper pole of right kidney by tumor.

on the morning of the examination. The patient is taken to the radiology department and placed in the supine position for this study. A plain film of the patient's abdomen (see KUB, p. 257) is taken to be sure that no residual stool obscures visualization of the renal system. This also screens for calculi in the renal collecting system. Skin testing for iodine allergy is often done. It is important to realize that a negative skin test does not ensure that a reaction will not occur during the IVP. A peripheral IV line (scalp vein in an infant) is started, and as much as 1 ml of contrast dye (diatrizoates such as Hypaque or Renografin) per pound of body weight is given by IV push. In patients whose impaired renal function (BUN >50 mg/dl) prevents adequate visualization of the urinary tract, higher than normal doses of dye are required. Larger doses of dye can be given by an IV infusion drip to produce opacification of the renal parenchyma and complete filling of the urinary tract, which is called an *infusion drip pyelography* or *drip-infusion IVP*.

X-ray films are taken at specified times, usually at 1, 5, 10, 15, 20, and 30 minutes, and sometimes longer to follow the dye course from the cortex of the kidney to the bladder. Tomograms may be taken to identify a mass.

The patient is then taken to the bathroom and asked to void. A postvoid film is taken to assess bladder emptying.

Occasionally it is necessary to occlude the ureters temporarily to get a better fill of the collective system and the upper part of the ureters. This is done by compressing the abdomen with an inflatable rubber tube wrapped tightly around the abdomen slightly below the umbilicus.

Initial IV needle placement and lying on a hard x-ray table are the only discomforts associated with IVP. Occasionally patients become dizzy or have some other idiosyncratic reaction

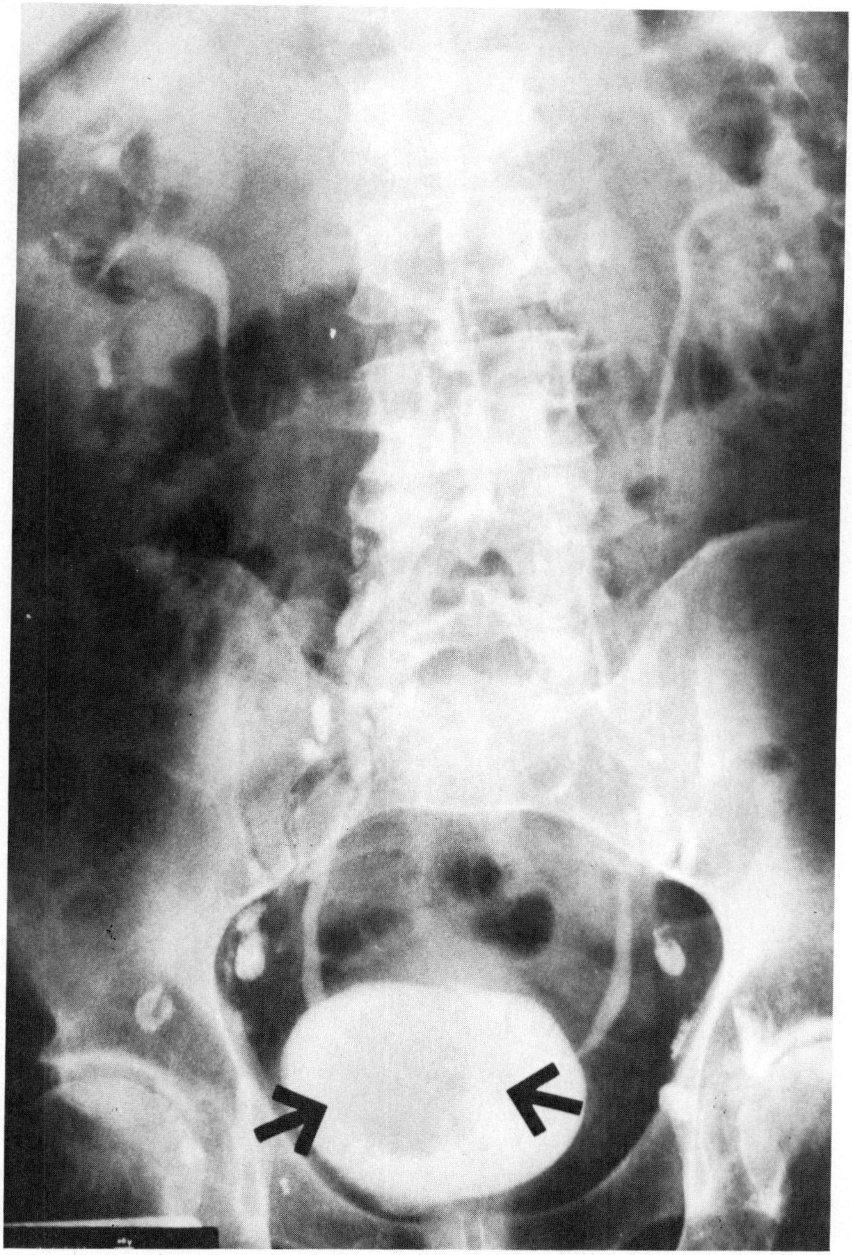

FIGURE 7-6. Intravenous pyelogram. Arrows indicate shadow (filling defect) in the bladder caused by bladder tumor.

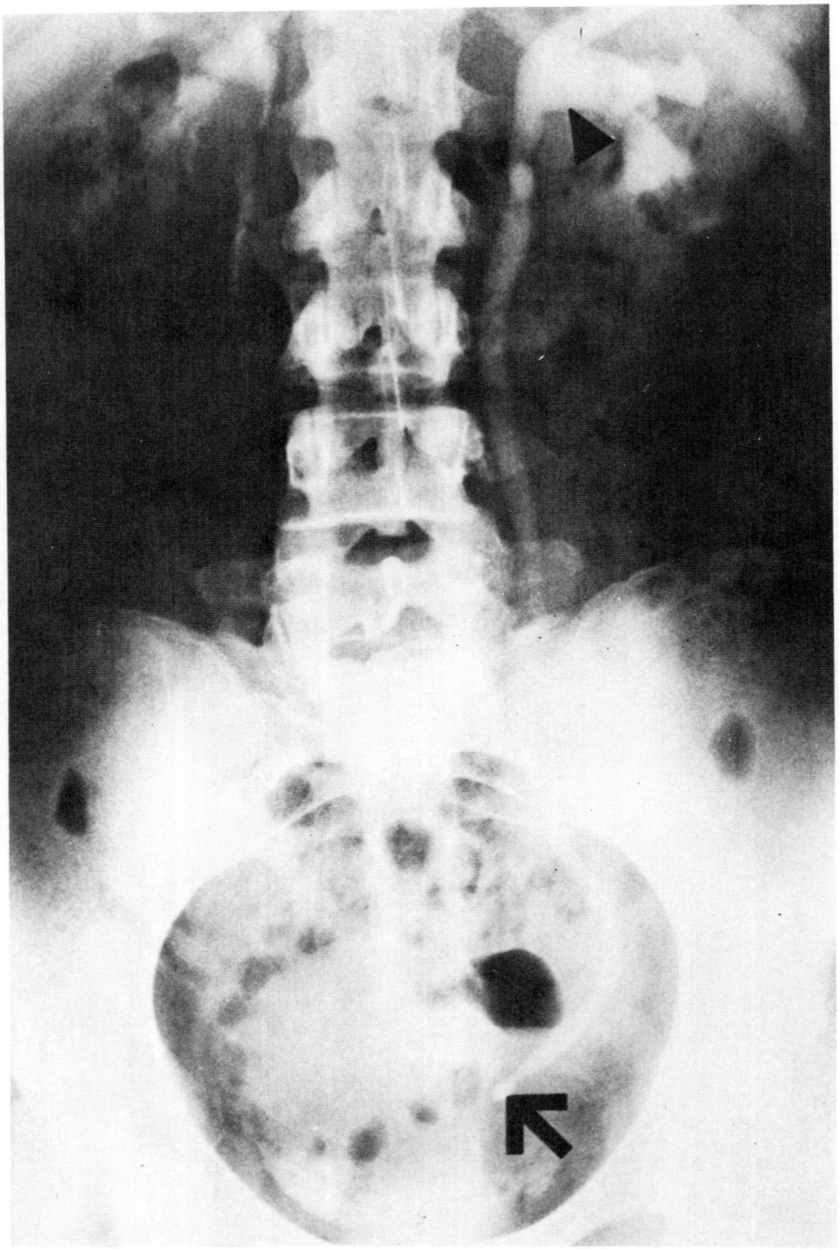

FIGURE 7-7. Intravenous pyelogram. Arrow indicates ureteral stone obstructing left ureter. Pointer indicates dilated proximal ureter and pelvis secondary to obstruction.

with injection of the dye. This test takes approximately 45 minutes and is done by a radiologist.

Contraindications. IVP is contraindicated in the following:

1. Patients who are allergic to shellfish or iodinated dyes and are not properly prepared beforehand with prednisone and diphenhydramine
2. Patients who are severely dehydrated, unless appropriate measures have been taken
3. Patients with renal insufficiency
4. Patients with multiple myeloma.

Nursing considerations

Nursing Diagnoses/Collaborative Problems

See X-ray studies, p. 5.

- Potential complication: renal failure

Nursing Implications with Rationale

- Explain the purpose and procedure of this test to the patient. Written instructions should be given as a reminder.
- Give the patient cathartics or laxatives, as ordered, on the evening before the test. Stool or gas in the bowel may obscure visualization of the renal system. Children and infants are usually not given cathartics.
- Keep the patient NPO after midnight. Moderate dehydration is necessary for the concentration of the contrast dye within the urinary system. The oral fasting time in infants and children varies and will be ordered specifically for each child. The oral fasting time for elderly and debilitated patients also varies according to the patient. If the patient is receiving intravenous fluids, the infusion rate may be decreased for several hours before the study.
- Assess serum BUN and creatinine levels before the test. Abnormal renal function could make the IVP hazardous because the dye is excreted via the kidney.
- Inform the patient that before the study he or she should void to prevent dilution of the contrast medium in the bladder.
- Before the study assess the patient for allergy to iodine dye. If the patient has a history of allergy to iodine dye, administer the prednisone and diphenhydramine, as ordered, for 1 to 3 days before and as many days after the procedure.
- Tell the patient that the dye injection often causes a flushing of the face, a feeling of warmth, and a salty taste in the mouth. The effects are transitory.
- Assess the IV site for infiltration by the contrast agent. Extravasation of iodine can cause sloughing of the tissue. A local injection of hyaluronidase may be used to hasten absorption of iodine and resolution of the reaction.
- After the dye injection, look for signs and symptoms of anaphylaxis, such as respiratory distress, shock, and a drop in blood pressure. Emergency drugs (diphenhydramine, steroids, epinephrine) and equipment (oxygen and endotracheal equipment) should be on hand for immediate use in the event of anaphylaxis.
- After the procedure allow the patient to resume a normal diet. Encourage the patient to drink fluids to counteract the fluid depletion caused by the preparation for this test.
- After the study, assess the elderly and debilitated patient for weakness because of the combination of fasting and catharsis necessary for test preparation. Encourage bed rest and ambulation only with assistance.

Renal biopsy

(kidney biopsy)

Normal value: no pathologic conditions found

Rationale. Biopsy of the kidney affords microscopic examination of renal tissue. Renal biopsy is performed for the following purposes:

1. To diagnose the cause of renal disease (such as poststreptococcal, Goodpasture's syndrome, lupus nephritis)
2. To diagnose or rule out primary and metastatic malignancy of the kidney in patients who are not candidates for surgery

3. To evaluate the amount of rejection that occurs after kidney transplantation, because this information enables the physician to determine the appropriate dose of immunosuppressive agents.

Renal biopsy specimens are most often obtained percutaneously. During this procedure a needle is inserted through the skin and into the kidney to obtain a sample of tissue. The biopsy needle is more accurately placed when guided by ultrasonography or fluoroscopy. These techniques allow more precise localization of the desired kidney tissue. The most common complication of this procedure is hemorrhage from the highly vascular renal tissue. Inadvertent puncture of the liver, lung, bowel, aorta, and inferior vena cava may also complicate this procedure and require surgical repair. Occasionally, open renal biopsy is performed. This involves an incision through the flank and dissection to expose the kidney. With this procedure there is less risk of hemorrhage, but an increased risk of infection. The recovery period is also longer.

Procedure. The patient is kept NPO after midnight on the day of the procedure. No sedative is required. The needle stick may be done at the bedside. If fluoroscopic or ultrasound guidance is to be used, the needle stick is performed in the radiology or ultrasonography department. The patient is placed in a prone position with a sandbag or pillow under the abdomen to straighten the spine. Under sterile conditions, the skin overlying the kidney is infiltrated with a local anesthetic (lidocaine). While the patient holds his or her breath to stop kidney movement, the physician inserts the biopsy needle (the type that he or she is most comfortable using) into the kidney and takes a specimen. After this procedure is completed, the needle is removed and pressure is applied to the site for approximately 20 minutes. A pressure dressing is then applied, and the patient is turned on his or her back and remains on bed rest for about 24 hours. The vital signs, puncture site, and hematocrit values are assessed frequently during this period. The biopsy specimen is placed in a container filled with a fixative solution. This is then sent to the pathology department for appropriate staining and microscopic review.

A renal biopsy can also be done via cystoscopy (see pp. 244-246).

This procedure is uncomfortable, but only minimally if enough lidocaine is used. The procedure is performed in about 10 minutes.

Contraindications. Renal biopsy is contraindicated in uncooperative patients and in patients with:

1. Coagulation disorders, because of the risk of excessive bleeding
2. Operable kidney tumors, because tumor cells may be disseminated during the procedure
3. Hydronephrosis, because the enlarged renal pelvis can easily be entered and cause a persistent urine leak requiring surgical repair
4. Infections, because the needle insertion may disseminate the active infection throughout the retroperitoneum.

Nursing considerations

Nursing Diagnoses/Collaborative Problems

- Possible knowledge deficit related to test purpose, preparation, and procedure
- Possible alteration in comfort related to test procedure
- Possible anxiety related to unknown sensations of procedure
- Potential complication: hemorrhage
- Potential complication: perforation of liver, lung, bowel, aorta, or inferior vena cava

Nursing Implications with Rationale

- Explain the procedure to the patient. Keep the patient NPO in the event that bleeding necessitates surgical intervention. Describe the postprocedure routine also.
- Ensure that written and informed consent for this procedure is obtained by the physician.
- Check the results of the patient's coagulation studies (prothrombin time and partial throm-

boplastin time). The patient's hemoglobin and hematocrit values should also be checked. The patient may also be typed and cross-matched for blood in the event of severe hemorrhage requiring transfusions.

- After the removal of the biopsy specimen, apply pressure to the site of the needle stick. Usually the patient is kept in the prone position for 20 to 30 minutes after the needle stick to minimize bleeding. The patient is then kept on bed rest for 24 hours. Any activity that increases abdominal venous pressure (such as coughing) should be avoided.
- Check the vital signs and puncture site every 15 minutes for the first hour after the needle stick and then with decreasing frequency, as ordered. Assess the patient for signs and symptoms of hemorrhage, such as a decrease in blood pressure, increase in pulse, pallor, backache, shoulder pain, and lightheadedness. Evaluate the abdomen for signs of bowel or liver penetration, such as abdominal pain and tenderness, abdominal muscle guarding and rigidity, and decreased bowel sounds.
- Inspect all urine specimens for gross hematuria. Usually the patient's urine contains blood initially, but this does not usually continue after the first 24 hours. Urine samples may be placed in consecutive chronological order to facilitate comparison for evaluation of hematuria. This is referred to as "rack" or "serial" urines.
- Encourage the patient to drink large amounts of fluid to prevent clot formation and urine retention. (However, an oliguric patient in renal failure could develop pulmonary edema with increased fluid intake.)
- Frequently, you will need to draw blood for a hemoglobin and hematocrit determination 8 hours after removal of the biopsy specimen to assess for active bleeding. One purple-top tube of blood is needed.
- Instruct the patient to avoid, for at least 2 weeks, strenuous activities, such as heavy lifting, contact sports, horseback riding, or any other activity that causes jolting of the kidney. Teach the patient the signs and symptoms of renal bleeding and instruct him or her to call the physician if any of these symptoms occur.
- Instruct the patient to report burning on urination or any temperature elevations. These could indicate a urinary tract infection.

Antistreptolysin O titer

(ASO titer)

Normal values:
Adult/elderly: ≤160 Todd units/ml
Children
Newborn: similar to mother's value
6 mo-2 years: ≤50 Todd units/ml
2-4 years: ≤160 Todd units/ml
5-12 years: 170-330 Todd units/ml

Rationale. The antistreptolysin O (ASO) titer is a serologic procedure that demonstrates the reaction of the body to infection caused by group A streptococci. It is used primarily in the differential diagnosis of poststreptococcal disease, such as glomerulonephritis, rheumatic fever, bacterial endocarditis, and scarlet fever.

The streptococcus organism produces an enzyme called streptolysin O, which has the ability to destroy (lyse) red blood corpuscles. Because streptolysin O is antigenic, the body reacts by producing ASO, a neutralizing antibody. ASO appears in the serum from 1 week to 1 month after the onset of a streptococcal infection. A high titer is not specific for a certain type of poststreptococcal disease but is merely indicative that a streptococcal infection is or has been present. When the ASO elevation is seen in a patient with glomerulonephritis or endocarditis, one can safely assume that the disease was caused by streptococcal infection.

Procedure. Peripheral venipuncture is performed, and one red-top tube of blood is collected. No fasting is required.

Contraindications. None.

Nursing considerations

Nursing Diagnoses/Collaborative Problems

See Blood studies, p. 2.

Nursing Implications with Rationale

- Apply pressure to the venipuncture site after the blood is drawn. Assess the site for bleeding.

SUPPLEMENTAL INFORMATION

Antideoxyribonuclease-B titer

(Anti-DNase-B, ADNase-B)

Normal values:
Preschool: ≤60 units
School age: ≤170 units
Adult: ≤85 units

Rationale. Like the ASO (see previous study) this immunologic test also detects antigens produced by group A streptococci and is elevated in most patients with acute rheumatic fever and poststreptococci glomerulonephritis. This test is often run concurrently with the ASO. Subsequent testing is usually done to detect differences between the acute and convalescent blood samples. A rise in the titer of two or more dilution increments between the acute and convalescent sera is significant and indicates a streptococcal infection has occurred.

Procedure. Peripheral venipuncture is performed, and one red-top tube of blood is collected. No fasting is required.

Contraindications. None.

Nursing considerations

Nursing Diagnoses/Collaborative Problems

See Blood studies, p. 2.

Nursing Implications with Rationale

- Apply pressure to the venipuncture site after the blood is drawn.
- Assess the site for bleeding.

CASE STUDY 2: HEMATURIA

Mr. N. was a 55-year-old white man who developed painless hematuria. He was otherwise completely asymptomatic. The results of his physical examination were within normal limits (WNL).

Studies	Results
Routine laboratory studies	WNL
Urinalysis (see pp. 224-229)	Positive for blood (normal: no blood) Red blood cells: too numerous to count (TNTC) (normal: up to 2) Other components WNL
Intravenous pyelography (IVP) (see pp. 232-237)	1. Distortion of renal outline, compatible with a renal mass 2. Questionable bladder tumor 3. Mild right ureteral dilatation
Nephrotomography	Cystic appearance of renal mass
CT scanning of the mass	Normal kidneys, renal cyst present
Ultrasound-guided cyst aspiration study	Straw-colored fluid, complete disappearance of the cyst
Cystography	Bladder tumor (see Figure 7-8)
Cystoscopy	Bladder tumor seen lying near the right ureteral orifice
Biopsy	Transitional cell carcinoma
Retrograde pyelography	Bladder tumor involving right distal ureter

Urinalysis documented this patient's hematuria. Three distinct abnormalities on IVP could have been responsible for the hematuria. The renal mass could have been a solid tumor or a benign cyst. Nephrotomography, CT scanning, and ultrasonography with aspiration all indicated that the mass was the result of a benign renal cyst and was not the cause of the hematuria.

The questionable bladder tumor seen on IVP was more clearly demonstrated by cystography, and a specimen for biopsy was taken during cystoscopy. The diagnosis was transitional cell carcinoma of the bladder. Right ureteral dilatation (seen on IVP) implied possible ureteral involvement by the bladder tumor. A retrograde pyelography study indicated that this was indeed the situation.

After 2 months of preoperative radiation, the

patient had a total cystectomy and ileal urinary diversion. He died 6 years later of recurrent tumor.

DISCUSSION OF TESTS

Nephrotomography

Normal value: diffusely normal kidney

Rationale. Nephrotomography provides radiographic visualization of the kidney using tomographic technique following the IV injection of a radiopaque dye. This study permits visualization of different tissue planes in the kidney for the purpose of differentiating solid renal and adrenal tumors from benign renal cysts. This test is much less used since the introduction of CT scans.

Procedure. Intravenous pyelography (IVP) is performed, as discussed on pp. 232-237. Tomograms (see pp. 139-140) of the kidney are taken as the contrast dye is excreted through the kidneys, the ureters, and the bladder.

Contraindications. See IVP, p. 237.

Nursing considerations

Nursing Diagnoses/Collaborative Problems

See IVP, p. 237.

Nursing Implications with Rationale

- See IVP, p. 237.

Computed tomography of the kidney

(CT of the kidney)

Normal value: no evidence of abnormality

Rationale. Computed tomography of the kidney is a noninvasive, yet very accurate, x-ray procedure used to diagnose pathologic renal conditions such as tumors, cysts, obstructions, calculi, and congenital anomalies. The technique by which CT scanning provides a cross-sectional image of abdominal organs is described on p. 123 in the discussion of CT of the abdomen (see Figure 4-14).

Procedure. (See also pp. 123-124.) Usually a contrast dye may be administered intravenously to enhance the kidney image. If dye will be administered, the patient should be kept NPO for 4 hours before the test. Acute renal failure can be a complication of dye infusion. However, adequate hydration before the procedure may reduce the likelihood of this complication.

Contraindications. This test is contraindicated in the uncooperative patient.

Nursing considerations

Nursing Diagnoses/Collaborative Problems

See X-ray studies, p. 5.

- Potential complication: renal failure

Nursing Implications with Rationale

- See also p. 124.

Renal ultrasonography

(kidney sonogram)

Normal values: normal size, shape, and position of the kidneys

Rationale. Through the use of reflected sound waves, ultrasonography provides accurate visualization of the kidney structures for many diagnostic purposes. The technique of ultrasonography requires the emission of high-frequency sound waves from the transducer to penetrate the organ being studied. The sound waves are bounced back to the transducer and electronically converted into a pictorial image. A realistic Polaroid picture of the organ studied is then obtained.

Ultrasonography of the kidney is used to diagnose hydronephrosis, locate renal cysts, to differentiate renal cysts from solid renal tumors, to demonstrate renal or pelvic calculi, and to guide a percutaneously inserted needle for cyst aspiration or removal of a biopsy specimen. One advantage of a kidney ultrasound is that it can be performed in patients with impaired renal function and in those with iodine allergy.

Abdominal ultrasonography should not be performed on patients who have recently had barium contrast studies unless they have been given adequate cathartics. Barium distorts the ultrasound image. No complications are associated with ultrasonography.

Procedure. No food or fluid restrictions are necessary. The patient is placed on the ultrasonography table in a prone position. The ultrasonographer (usually a radiologist) applies a greasy conductive paste to the back. This paste is used to enhance sound wave transmission and reception. A transducer is then passed over the skin, and pictures are taken of the reflections. No discomfort is associated with this safe procedure; in fact, it may feel like a back rub. The test is completed in approximately 20 minutes.

Contraindications. None.

Nursing considerations

Nursing Diagnoses/Collaborative Problems

See Ultrasound studies, p. 6.

Nursing Implications with Rationale

- Explain the procedure to the patient. No fasting is required.
- If the patient's abdomen appears distended or if the patient has recently had a barium study, this test should be cancelled. Barium and gas reflect the sound waves and alter the test results.
- After the procedure remove the coupling agent (grease) from the patient's back.
- If a biopsy is done, see the nursing considerations for renal biopsy, pp. 238-239.

Ultrasound-guided cyst aspiration study

Normal values: no evidence of abnormality

Rationale. Occasionally a renal cyst appears to be complex (i.e., with a fluid and solid component). Cystic renal tumors must be excluded. With aspiration of these cysts, fluid can be examined cytologically to see if any malignant cells exist. Ultrasound is used to guide the needle to the cyst and ensure good sampling. (See also discussion of renal ultrasonography, previous study). No complications are associated with ultrasonography, only with the needle insertion. Inadvertent puncture of a blood vessel or bowel may occur; however, this is very rare with ultrasound guidance.

Procedure. The patient is placed on the ultrasonography table in the prone position. The renal cyst is located with a sterile transducer that has a hole in its center. With the transducer held still against the skin, a needle is passed aseptically through the hole in the transducer into the previously anesthetized skin. It is advanced to the cyst with ultrasound guidance. The cyst is aspirated dry, and the fluid is sent to the cytology laboratory to test for cystic tumor.

The procedure is mildly uncomfortable. Adequate local anesthesia should minimize most of the discomfort. An ultrasonographer and a urologist perform the study in approximately 30 minutes.

Contraindications. None.

Nursing considerations

Nursing Diagnoses/Collaborative Problems

See Ultrasound studies, p. 6.

- Potential alteration in comfort related to test procedure
- Potential for anxiety related to unknown sensations of procedure

Nursing Implications with Rationale

- See previous study.

Voiding cystourethrography

(voiding cystogram)

Normal values: normal structure and function of the bladder

Rationale. Filling the bladder with radiopaque contrast material provides visualization of the bladder for radiographic study. Fluoroscopic or x-ray film demonstrates bladder filling and shows excretion of the contrast medium as the patient voids. Filling defects or shadows within the bladder indicate primary bladder tumors (Figure 7-8). Extrinsic compres-

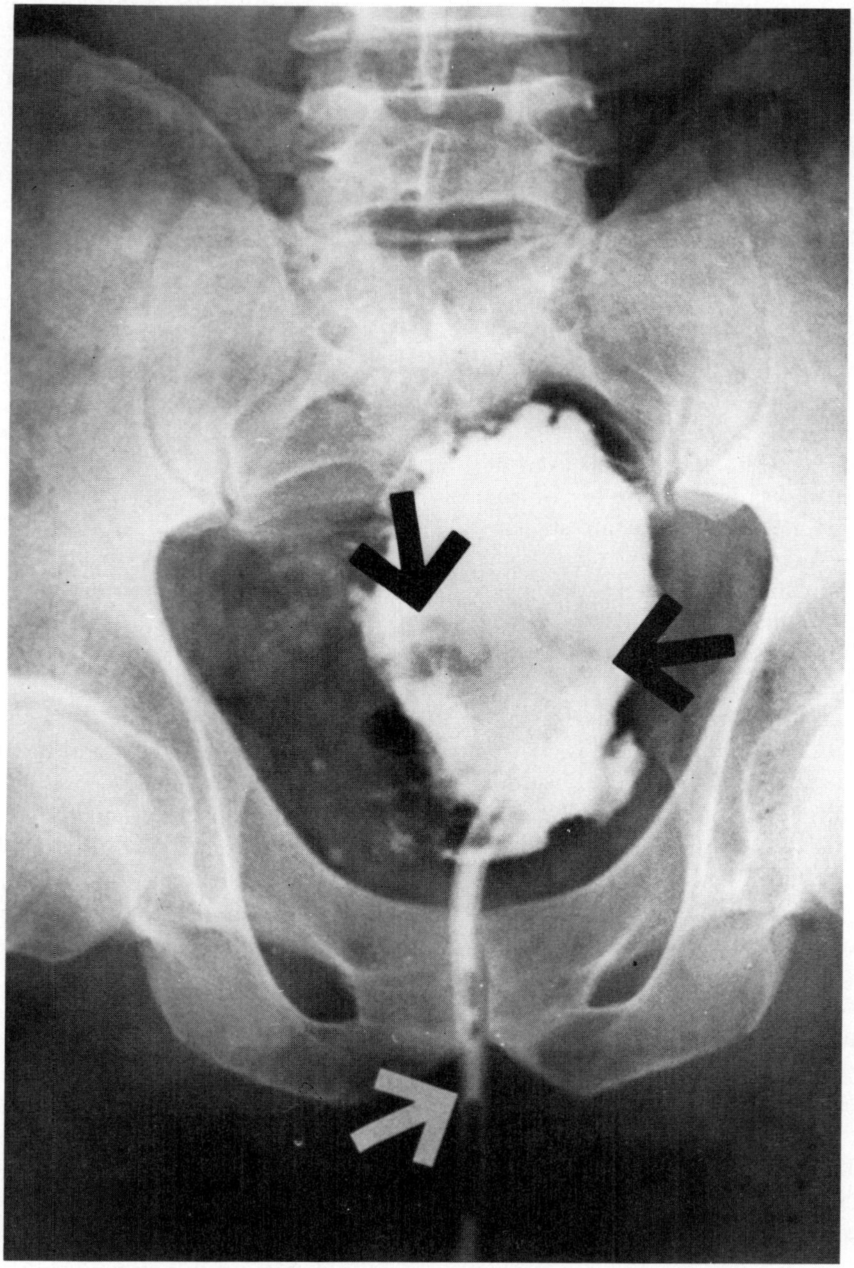

FIGURE 7-8. Cystogram. Black arrows indicate large bladder tumor distorting normal bladder. White arrow indicates Foley catheter in urethra.

sion or distortion of the bladder is seen with pelvic tumors (such as of the rectum, prostate, or cervix) or hematomas (secondary to pelvic bone fractures). Extravasation of dye into the peritoneum is seen with traumatic rupture of the bladder. Vesicoureteral reflux (abnormal backflow of urine from bladder to ureters), which can cause persistent pyelonephritis, may be demonstrated during cystography. Although the bladder is visualized during an IVP, primary pathologic bladder conditions are best studied by cystography. This study may be indicated for children with urinary infections and in adults with recurrent urinary tract infections.

A urinary tract infection may result from the catheter placement required for this test or from the instillation of contaminated contrast material during this study.

Procedure. The patient is given only clear liquids for breakfast on the day of the examination. No cathartics are necessary. The patient is then taken to the radiology department and placed in the supine or lithotomy position. Unless a catheter is already present, one is placed through the urethra and into the bladder. Through the catheter approximately 300 cc of air or radiopaque dye (much less for children) is injected into the bladder, and the catheter is clamped. X-ray films are then taken. If the patient is able to void, the catheter is removed and the patient is asked to micturate. Further x-ray films are then taken.

This test is moderately uncomfortable if bladder catheterization is required. A radiologist performs this study in approximately 15 to 30 minutes.

Contraindications. This study is contraindicated in unstable patients and in patients with urethral or bladder infection or injury.

Nursing considerations

Nursing Diagnoses/Collaborative Problems

See X-ray studies, p. 5.

- Potential complication: urinary tract infection

Nursing Implications with Rationale

- Explain the procedure to the patient. Embarrassment may inhibit the patient's ability to void on command. Assure the patient that he or she will be draped to prevent unnecessary exposure.
- If the patient has a large amount of residual urine, make sure that the patient voids or is catheterized to avoid bladder distention.
- Males should wear a lead shield over the testes to prevent irradiation of the gonads. Female patients cannot be shielded without blocking bladder visualization.
- Assess the patient for signs of urinary tract infection.

Cystoscopy

Normal values: normal structure and function of the urethra, bladder, prostate (males), and ureters

Rationale. Cystoscopy provides direct visualization of the urethra and bladder through the transurethral insertion of a cystoscope (a lighted telescopic tube) into the bladder. Cystoscopy is used diagnostically to allow:

1. Direct inspection and removal of biopsy specimens of the prostate, bladder, and urethra for tumor determination
2. Collection of separate urine specimen directly from each kidney by the placement of ureteral catheters
3. Measurement of bladder capacity and evidence of ureteral reflux
4. Identification of bladder and ureteral calculi
5. Placement of ureteral catheters for the performance of retrograde pyelography (see next study)
6. Identification of the source of hematuria.

Cystoscopy is used therapeutically to permit:

1. Resection of small tumors
2. Removal of foreign bodies and stones
3. Dilation of the urethra and ureters
4. Placement of catheters to drain urine from the renal pelvis

5. Coagulation of bleeding areas
6. Implantation of radium seeds into a tumor
7. Placement of laser optic fibers for stone dissolution.

The cystoscope consists primarily of an obturator and a scope. The obturator is used to insert the cystoscope atraumatically. After the cystoscope is within the bladder, the obturator is removed and the scope lens is passed through the cystoscope. The lens and lighting system of the scope permit adequate visualization of the lower genitourinary tract. Transcopic instruments, such as forceps, scissors, needles, catheters, and electrodes, are used when appropriate.

Complications of cystoscopy include hematuria, perforation of the bladder, and sepsis by seeding the bloodstream with bacteria from infected urine.

Procedure. Cystoscopy is usually performed in a hospital cystoscopy room or in a urologist's office, with the patient under local or general anesthesia. Fluids are forced several hours before the procedure to maintain a continuous flow of urine for urine collection and to prevent bacterial multiplication of organisms that may be introduced during this technique. General anesthetics can be used for children and for the uncooperative or overly anxious adult. If general anesthetics are used, the patient is kept NPO after midnight (or a shorter time period in children). Fluids are given intravenously during the procedure.

Patients are sedated 1 hour before the study. The patient is placed in the lithotomy position with his or her feet in stirrups. The external genitalia are cleaned with an antiseptic solution such as povidone-iodine (Betadine). A local anesthetic is instilled into the urethra. The patient is instructed to lie very still during the entire procedure to prevent trauma to the urinary tract. The patient will have the desire to void as the cystoscope passes the bladder neck. When the procedure is completed, the patient remains on bed rest for a short time.

When done under local anesthesia, this test is uncomfortable, much more so than urethral catheterization. This procedure is performed by a urologist in about 25 minutes.

Contraindications. This test is contraindicated in the clinically unstable patient.

Nursing considerations

Nursing Diagnoses/Collaborative Problems

See Endoscopy procedures, pp. 6-7.

- Potential complication: hematuria
- Potential complication: perforation of bladder
- Potential complication: sepsis

Nursing Implications with Rationale

- Explain the procedure to the patient. Tell the patient that the cystoscope is inserted into the bladder in the same manner as a Foley catheter. Encourage verbalization of the patient's fears. Provide emotional support.
- Ensure that written and informed consent for this procedure is obtained by the physician.
- If enemas are ordered to clear the bowel, assist the patient as needed and record the results.
- If the procedure will be done with the patient under *local anesthesia*, you may give a liquid breakfast. Encourage fluids to provide urine samples as needed and to prevent stasis of urine in the event that bacteria are introduced during cystoscopy.
- If the procedure is performed with the patient under *general anesthesia*, follow routine anesthesia precautions. Keep the patient NPO after midnight. You may give fluids intravenously.
- Administer the preprocedure medications as ordered before the study. In addition to reducing anxiety, the sedatives decrease the spasm of the bladder sphincter, thus decreasing the patient's discomfort. Deep-breathing exercises can also minimize spasms.
- Do not allow the patient to stand or walk alone immediately after his or her legs have been removed from the stirrups. The sudden

change in circulatory blood volume may cause dizziness and fainting.

- Assess the patient's ability to void for at least 24 hours after the procedure. Urinary retention may be secondary to edema caused by instrumentation. If urinary retention does occur, an indwelling catheter may need to be inserted. Record the urine color and test the urine for blood. Pink-tinged urine is common. The presence of bright red blood or clots should be reported to the physician.
- The patient may complain of back pain, bladder spasms, urinary frequency, and burning upon urination. Warm sitz baths and mild analgesics may be ordered and given. Sometimes belladonna and opium (B&O) suppositories are given to relieve bladder spasms. Warm moist heat to the lower abdomen may help relieve pain and promote muscle relaxation.
- Encourage increased intake of fluids. A dilute urine decreases burning upon urination. Fluids also maintain a constant flow of urine to prevent stasis and the accumulation of bacteria in the bladder.
- Check and record the patient's vital signs as ordered. Watch for a decrease in blood pressure and an increase in pulse as an indication of hemorrhage. Observe for signs and symptoms of sepsis (elevated temperature, flush, chills, decreased blood pressure, and increased pulse).
- Occasionally antibiotics are ordered 1 day before and 3 days after the procedure to reduce the incidence of bacteremia that may occur with instrumentation of the urethra and bladder.

Retrograde pyelography

Normal values: normal outline and size of the ureters and bladder

Rationale. Retrograde pyelography refers to radiographic visualization of the urinary tract through ureteral catheterization and the injection of contrast material. The ureters are catheterized during cystoscopy (see previous study). A radiopaque material is injected in the ureters and x-ray films are taken (Figure 7-9). This test can be performed when the patient has an allergy to IV contrast dye. Only a small amount of the dye injected into the ureters is absorbed through the membranes.

Retrograde pyelography is helpful in radiographically examining the ureters in patients where IVP visualization is inadequate. Frequently in patients with unilateral renal disease, the involved kidney and collecting system are not visualized. To rule out ureteral obstruction as a cause of the unilateral kidney disease, retrograde pyelography must be done to examine the ureters. Tumors, benign strictures, stones, and extrinsic compression can cause ureteral obstruction. These lesions can be seen by retrograde pyelography. Occasionally the IVP only poorly demonstrates lesions of the ureters. Retrograde pyelography can frequently provide better visualization of these lesions.

Complications of retrograde pyelography include the possibility of urinary tract infection. Manipulation of the ureters can cause edema, resulting in temporary obstruction to urine flow. Other complications include those associated with cystoscopy (see previous study).

Procedure. The ureteral catheters (Figure 7-10) are passed into the ureters by means of cystoscopy (see previous study). Radiopaque contrast material (Hypaque or Renografin) is injected, and x-ray films are taken. The entire ureter and the renal pelvis are demonstrated. As the catheters are withdrawn, more dye is injected and more x-ray films are taken to visualize the complete outline of the ureter. The study is uncomfortable and is performed by a urologist in approximately 15 minutes. This procedure is usually done in the operating room.

Contraindications. None.

Nursing considerations

Nursing Diagnoses/Collaborative Problems

See X-ray studies, p. 4 and Cystoscopy, p. 245.

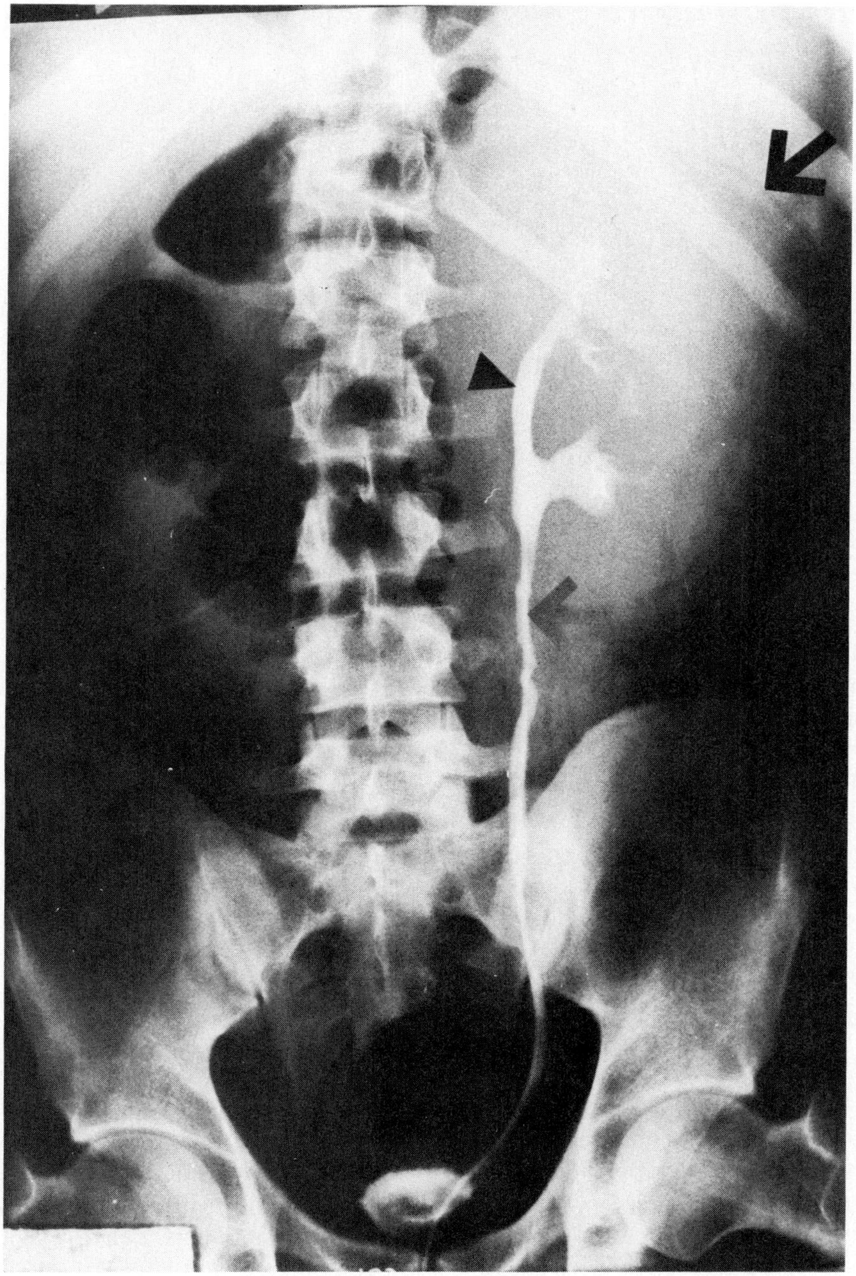

FIGURE 7-9. Retrograde pyelogram. Black arrow indicates Wilms' tumor. Pelvis and ureters did not visualize on intravenous pyelogram. Pointer indicates ureteral catheter within distorted pelvis. Gray arrow indicates ureter.

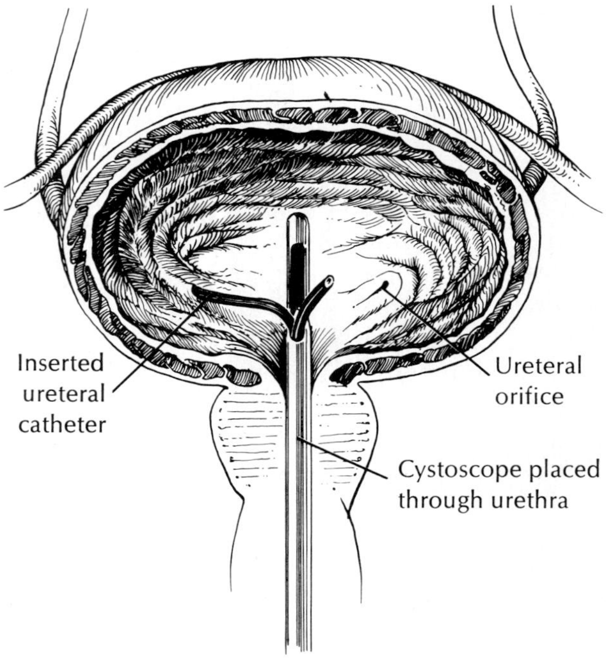

FIGURE 7-10. Ureteral catheterization through cystoscope. Note ureteral catheter inserted into right orifice. Left ureteral catheter is ready to be inserted.
From Phipps WJ, Long BC, and Woods NF, editors: Medical-surgical nursing: concepts and clinical practice, St Louis, 1979, The CV Mosby Co.

Nursing Implications with Rationale

- See Cystoscopy, pp. 245-246.

SUPPLEMENTAL INFORMATION

Antegrade pyelography

Normal values: normal outline, size, and position of the ureters and bladder

Rationale. Occasionally a kidney with very poor opaque excretion cannot be examined by retrograde pyelography because the ureter is impassable from below (such as from obstruction) or because a cystoscopic procedure is clinically contraindicated. For this patient the upper collecting system may be opacified by injection of contrast material via a percutaneous needle puncture of the renal pelvis or calyx. This test is usually done when attempts at retrograde catheterization (see previous study) have been unsuccessful. Antegrade pyelography is specifically indicated in the following conditions:

1. Localization of ureteral obstruction caused by stricture, nonopaque stone, or tumor
2. Evaluation of ureteral obstruction after urinary diversion operation
3. Hydronephrosis in a child with poor opaque excretion to identify ureteropelvic and ureterovesicle obstruction.

Procedure. For antegrade pyelography the patient is placed in a prone position. The renal pelvis is localized by ultrasound or fluoroscopy. Skin overlying the desired site is marked and prepared. Under local anesthesia the skin is incised and a 1.5-inch, 14-gauge needle with a stylet is inserted its full length toward the renal pelvis. With the patient suspending respiration a 20-gauge, thin-walled biopsy needle with a stylet is advanced through the needle into the lumen of the renal pelvis. Flexible tubing connects the syringe to the needle to aspirate urine. Contrast medium is injected to outline the upper collecting system to the point of obstruction below. Posteroanterior, oblique, and anteroposterior x-ray views are taken. Antibiotic drugs are usually recommended for several days afterward because of the instrumentation above the ureteral obstructed area.

The only uncomfortable aspect of this test is the local anesthesia used to numb the skin overlying the pelvis. This test is performed by a radiologist or urologist in less than 1 hour.

Contraindications. None.

Nursing considerations

Nursing Diagnoses/Collaborative Problems

See X-ray studies, p. 4.

- Potential complication: hemorrhage

Nursing Implications with Rationale

- Explain the purpose and procedure of this test to the patient. Allow time for verbalization of questions regarding this procedure.
- After the test apply a small pressure dressing to the incisional site. Assess the site for bleeding.
- Because the kidney is a highly vascular area, check the vital signs as ordered to detect any evidence of bleeding.

Endourology

Normal values: no abnormalities of the bladder and urethra

Rationale. Endourology is an endoscopic procedure that allows for visualization of the bladder and the urethra. It is more comprehensive than cystoscopy (see p. 244) because it includes a detailed visualization of the urethra. This test is important in the evaluation of hematuria, chronic infection, suspected stone, and radiographic filling defects within the lower urinary tract. The urethra on inspection may show inflammation or structural causes of the obstruction (such as stricture, neoplasia, prostatic hypertrophy). If the obstruction is functional (such as detrusor/bladder neck dyssynergia) rather than structural, the site of obstruction will not be demonstrated by endoscopy.

Procedure. See Cystoscopy, p. 245. In addition to visualization of the bladder, the urethra is evaluated.

Contraindications. See Cystoscopy, p. 245.

Nursing considerations

Nursing Diagnoses/Collaborative Problems

See Endoscopic procedures, pp. 6-7.

Nursing Implications with Rationale

- See Cystoscopy, pp. 245-246.

CASE STUDY 3: RENOVASCULAR HYPERTENSION

Mr. V. was a 65-year-old man who had a 2-year history of hypertension. He had been treated with antihypertensive medications. Recently he came to the emergency room with complaints of headache and mild chest pain. The results of his physical examination were essentially normal, except for a blood pressure reading of 210/120 mm Hg and an S4 heart sound heard on auscultation. He was admitted to the hospital for evaluation; the following studies were conducted.

Studies	Results
Routine laboratory work	WNL
Chest x-ray study	Normal
EKG (see Chapter 2)	Mild left ventricular hypertrophy
IVP (see pp. 232-237)	Delayed visualization of the right kidney
Urine test (24-hour) for vanillylmandelic acid (VMA) and catecholamines	VMA: 6 mg/24 hours (normal: 1-9 mg/24 hours) Catecholamines Epinephrine: 16 μg/24 hours (normal: 5-40 μg/24 hours)

Studies	Results
	Norepinephrine: 28 μg/24 hours (normal: 10-80 μg/24 hours)
	Metanephrine: 53 μg/24 hours (normal: 24-96 μg/24 hours)
	Normetanephrine: 128 μg/24 hours (normal 73-375 μg/24 hours)
17-Hydroxycorticosteroids test (see pp. 299-300)	8.3 mg/24 hours (normal 5.5-14.5 mg/24 hours)
Renal scanning	Delayed visualization of the right kidney
Renal angiography	Stenosis of right renal artery (see Figure 7-11)
Renal vein renin assay	Right renal vein: 80 μg Left renal vein: 40 μg (normal: renin ratio of involved kidney to uninvolved kidney <1.4)

The normal values for VMA, catecholamines, and 17-hydroxycorticosteroids ruled out the possibility of pheochromocytoma and Cushing's syndrome as causes of the hypertension. The IVP, renal scanning, renal angiography, and renin assay indicated that right renal artery stenosis was the cause of the patient's increased blood pressure. The patient underwent an aorta-to-renal artery bypass of the stenotic area. Postoperatively, his blood pressure returned to normal, and he required no antihypertensive medication.

DISCUSSION OF TESTS

Twenty-four-hour urine test for vanillylmandelic acid and catecholamines

(VMA and epinephrine, norepinephrine, metanephrine, normetanephrine, dopamine)

Normal values:

VMA
- Adult/elderly: 2-7 mg/24 hr or 10-35 μmol/24 hr
- Newborn: <1.0 mg/24 hr
- Infant: <2.0 mg/24 hr
- Child: 1-3 mg/24 hr
- Adolescent: 1-5 mg/24 hr

Epinephrine
- Adult/elderly: 0.5-20 μg/24 hr
- Child: 0-1 years: 0-2.5 μg/24 hr
  - 1-2 years: 0-3.5
  - 2-4 years: 0-6.0
  - 4-7 years: 0.2-10
  - 7-10 years: 0.5-14

Norepinephrine
- Adult/elderly: 15-80 μg/24 hr
- Child: 0-1 years: 0-10 μg/24 hr
  - 1-2 years: 0-17
  - 2-4 years: 4-29
  - 4-7 years: 8-45
  - 7-10 years: 13-65

Dopamine
- Adult/elderly: 65-400 μg/24 hr
- Child: 0-1 years: 0-85 μg/24 hr
  - 1-2 years: 10-140
  - 2-4 years: 40-260
  - Over 4 years: 65-400

Metanephrine: 24-96 μg/24 hr
Normetanephrine: 75-375 μg/24 hr

Rationale. 24-hour urine test for VMA and catecholamines is primarily performed to diagnose hypertension secondary to pheochromocytoma. A pheochromocytoma is an adrenal tumor that frequently secretes abnormally high levels of epinephrine and norepinephrine. These hormones then result in episodic or persistent hypertension by causing arterial vasoconstriction. Dopamine is the precursor of epinephrine and norepinephrine. Metanephrine and normetanephrine are catabolic products of epinephrine and norepinephrine, respectively. VMA is the product of catabolism of both metanephrine and normetanephrine. In patients with pheochromocytoma, one or all of the above substances will be present in excessive quantities in a 24-hour collection of urine.

Elevated levels of VMA and catecholamines are also seen in patients with neuroblastomas, ganglioneuromas, and ganglioblastomas. Severe stress, strenuous exercise, and acute anxiety can cause elevated catecholamine levels.

Procedure

VMA. For 2 or 3 days before the 24-hour urine collection and throughout the collection period, the patient is placed on a VMA-restricted diet. Generally the foods restricted include coffee, tea, bananas, chocolate, cocoa, licorice, citrus fruit, all foods and fluids containing vanilla, and also aspirin. Dietary restrictions may vary among different laboratories. Antihypertensive medications, and sometimes all medications, are also prohibited during this period and possibly even longer (depending on the laboratory). A 24-hour urine specimen is collected using a preservative.

Catecholamines. A 24-hour urine specimen is collected and sent to the chemistry laboratory for measurement of catecholamine levels. No special diet is needed.

Contraindications. None.

Nursing considerations

Nursing Diagnoses/Collaborative Problems

See Urine studies, p. 3.

Nursing Implications with Rationale

- Explain the procedure to the patient. Show the patient where to store the urine specimen. The 24-hour urine specimen for VMA requires a preservative.
- See the Nursing considerations regarding a 24-hour urine collection under the creatinine clearance test (pp. 230-231, except for the first and last considerations given).
- After the 24-hour collection for VMA is completed, allow the patient to have the foods and drugs that have been restricted in preparation for the test.
- Excessive physical exercise and emotion can alter catecholamine test results by causing an increased secretion of epinephrine and norepinephrine. Therefore, identify and minimize factors contributing to patient stress and anxiety.

Renal scanning

(kidney scan, radiorenography, radionuclide renal imaging, nuclear imaging of the kidney)

Normal values: normal size, shape, and function of the kidney

Rationale. This nuclear medicine procedure provides visualization of the urinary tract after the IV administration of an isotope. The distribution of the radioactive material is scanned or mapped. Scans do not interfere with the normal physiologic process of the kidney. The resultant image (scan) indicates distribution of the radionuclide within the kidney.

Each tracer is handled by the kidney in a different manner. For example, technetium DTPA is excreted by glomerular filtration. Technetium DMSA is taken up by the tubular cells and not appreciably excreted. ^{131}I is both filtered by the glomerulus and secreted by the tubules.

Various agents can be used for the scanning. Technetium-99m can be tagged to compounds such as DTPA or DMSA to permit static views of the kidney *structures* or to assess dynamic *perfusion* of the kidneys. Orthoiodohippurate can be tagged with ^{131}I to evaluate *excretory* function by measuring the time necessary for the radioisotope to travel through the cortex and pelvis of each kidney. Two IV injections may be given to evaluate perfusion, structure, excretory function of the kidney. This is sometimes called a triple renal study.

The time of uptake, transit, and excretion of the radioisotope by each kidney is plotted on a graph called a *renogram* curve (isotope renography). This can be compared to a normal reference curve to aid in the detection of abnormalities in either kidney (such as tubular disease, urinary obstruction, pyelonephritis, renal vascular hypertension, and absence of kidney function).

Renal scanning is used to:

1. Detect renal infarctions. The infarcted area is shown as a nonperfused defect in an otherwise homogeneous renal pattern.

2. Detect renal arterial atherosclerosis or trauma. The renal uptake of the radionucleated material is delayed or absent on the affected side(s).
3. Monitor rejection of a transplanted kidney. In chronic rejection the uptake and excretion of the nuclear material are delayed.
4. Detect primary renal disease (such as glomerulonephritis or acute tubular necrosis). The uptake and excretion of the nuclear material are delayed.
5. Detect pathologic renal and ureteral obstructive conditions in patients who cannot have IVP because of dye allergies.
6. Detect tumors, abscesses, or cysts. These appear as "cold spots" in the kidney because these abnormalities do not take up the nuclear material.
7. Detect and monitor renovascular hypertension. There is decreased uptake on the side of the arterial occlusion.

Procedure. The unsedated, nonfasting patient is taken to the nuclear medicine department. A peripheral IV injection of a radionuclide is given. It takes only minutes for the radioisotope to be concentrated in the kidneys. While the patient assumes a supine, prone, or sitting position, a gamma-ray detecting device is passed over the kidney area, and records the radioactive uptake on either x-ray or Polaroid film.

For a *Lasix renal scan* or a *diuretic renal scan,* the patient is imaged with DTPA. Images are obtained for 20 minutes. Then 40 mg of Lasix is administered intravenously and another 20 minutes of images are obtained.

The patient feels no pain or discomfort during this procedure. The patient must lie still during the study. The duration of this test varies from 1 to 4 hours depending on the specific information required. Perfusion scans are done in approximately 20 minutes and functional scans in less than 1 hour. Static structure scans require anywhere from 20 minutes to 4 hours for completion. This study is performed by a nuclear medicine technologist. Because only tracer doses of radiosotopes are used, no precautions need to be taken against radioactive exposure.

Contraindications. This test is contraindicated in pregnant patients.

Nursing considerations

Nursing Diagnoses/Collaborative Problems

See Nuclear scanning, p. 5.

Nursing Implications with Rationale

- Explain the procedure to the patient. Encourage verbalization of the patient's fears.
- Assure the patient that the exposure is not to large amounts of radioactivity, because only tracer doses of isotopes are used. The radioactive substance is usually excreted from the body within 6 to 24 hours.

Renal angiography

(renal arteriography)

Normal value: normal renal vasculature

Rationale. Through the injection of radiopaque contrast material into the renal arteries, renal angiography permits visualization of the large and small renal vasculature. This permits evaluation of blood flow dynamics, demonstration of abnormal blood vessels, and differentiation of primary renal cysts (avascular) from tumors (very vascular). Atherosclerotic narrowing (stenosis) of the renal artery is best demonstrated with this study (Figure 7-11). The angiographic location of the stenotic area is helpful to the vascular surgeon considering repair. Complete transection of the renal artery by blunt or penetrating trauma will be seen as a total vascular obstruction. Highly vascular renal tumors produce a "blush" of contrast material during angiography (Figure 7-12).

As in all studies that use iodinated contrast material, anaphylaxis is a potential complication. Also, an atherosclerotic plaque may be dislodged from the aorta and travel to any abdominal organ or to the legs. Organ ischemia and infarction may be the result. Finally, persistent

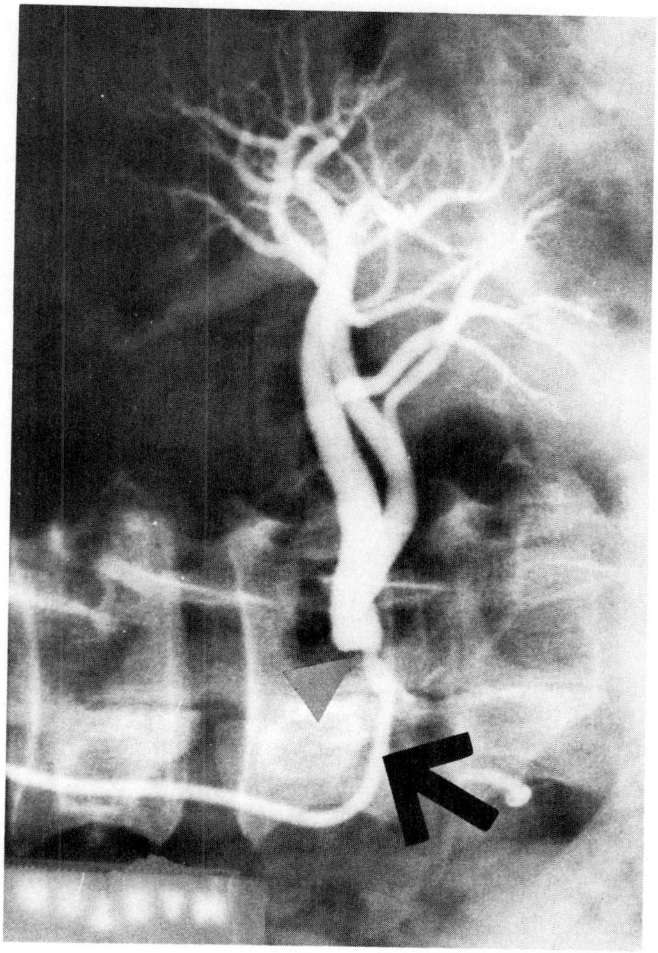

FIGURE 7-11. Right renal angiogram. Arrow indicates catheter in renal artery. Pointer indicates area of renal artery narrowing.

hemorrhage from the puncture site used for arterial access may occur.

Procedure. A cathartic may be given the evening before the test to eliminate fecal material from the bowel. The patient is kept NPO after midnight on the day of the examination. Because the contrast medium is an osmotic diuretic, the patient should void immediately before the test to avoid developing an overdistended bladder. The patient is usually sedated with meperidine and atropine. In the angiography room, located in the radiology department, the patient is placed on an x-ray table in the supine position. Since access to the renal arteries is usually achieved through the femoral artery, the groin is prepared and draped in a sterile manner. The catheter is passed into the femoral artery and advanced into the aorta. With fluoroscopic visualization (motion picture x-ray images displayed on a television monitor) the catheter is manipulated into the renal artery. Dye is injected and x-ray films are taken in timed sequence over several seconds. This allows all portions of the injection to be photographed.

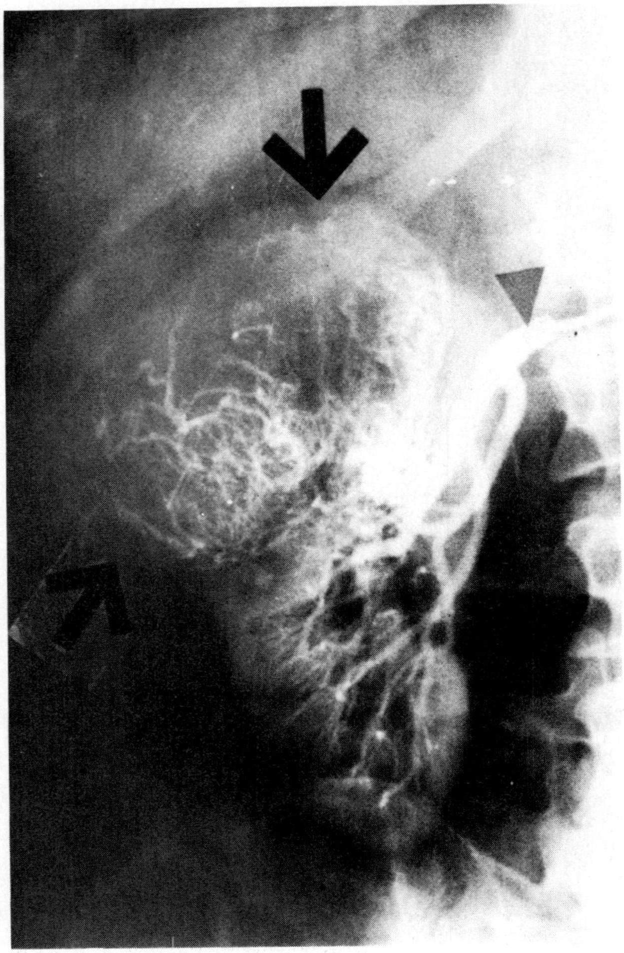

FIGURE 7-12. Renal angiogram. Black arrows indicate arterial "blush" of renal tumor. Pointer indicates renal artery.

Delayed films may be taken to visualize subsequent filling of the renal vein. After the x-ray films are taken, the catheter is removed and a pressure dressing is applied to the puncture site. The procedure is usually performed by an angiographer (radiologist) in about 1 hour. During the dye injection the patient may feel an intense burning flush throughout the body, but this is transient and gone in seconds. The only other discomfort is the groin puncture necessary for arterial access.

Contraindications. This study is contraindicated in:

1. Patients with dye allergies
2. Patients with atherosclerosis
3. Patients whose vital signs are unstable
4. Patients who are pregnant
5. Patients with bleeding disorders.

Nursing considerations

Nursing Diagnoses/Collaborative Problems

- Possible knowledge deficit related to test purpose, preparation, and procedure
- Possible anxiety related to unknown sensation of procedure

- Possible anxiety related to possible test results
- High risk for alteration in comfort related to test procedure
- Possible injury related to effects of sedatives
- Potential complication: adverse reaction/allergy
- Potential complication: bleeding
- Potential complication: cardiac arrhythmias
- Potential complication: perforation
- Potential complication: stroke or myocardial infarction
- Potential complication: peripheral arterial problems
- Potential complication: infection

Nursing Implications with Rationale

- Explain the procedure to the patient. Tell the patient where the catheter will be inserted (usually the femoral artery). Inform the patient that a warm flush will be felt when the dye is injected. Encourage verbalization of the patient's feelings regarding angiography. This test is frightening for most patients.
- Ensure that the written and informed consent for this procedure is in the chart.
- Assess the patient for allergies to iodine dye.
- Determine if the patient has been taking anticoagulants.
- Keep the patient NPO after midnight on the day of the study.
- Administer cathartics as ordered. The presence of feces or gas in the GI tract may impair clarity of the x-ray films and hinder the test result interpretation.
- Mark the patient's peripheral pulses with a pen before catheterization. This permits quicker assessment of the pulses after the procedure. Note and record the quality of the pulses as baseline data.
- Administer the preprocedure medications as ordered. Have the patient void before this study because the dye acts as an osmotic diuretic. Bladder distention may cause patient discomfort during this study.
- After the procedure observe the arterial puncture site frequently for hematoma, hemorrhage, or absence of pulse. Assess the extremity for signs of ischemia (numbness, tingling, pain, absence of peripheral pulses, and loss of function). Compare with the preprocedure baseline values. The color and temperature of the extremity are compared with those of the uninvolved extremity.
- Assess the pulses and vital signs frequently (every 15 minutes for four times, then every 30 minutes for four times, and then every hour for four times, and then every 4 hours), because embolism or bleeding requires immediate intervention. Notify the physician of any abnormalities.
- Keep the patient on bed rest for 12 to 24 hours after the procedure to allow complete sealing of the arterial puncture.
- Apply cold compresses to the puncture site if these are needed to reduce discomfort and swelling.
- Force fluids after the study to prevent diuretic-induced dehydration caused by the dye.

Renal vein assays for renin

Normal value: renin ratio of involved kidney to uninvolved kidney <1.4

Rationale. Renin is an enzyme released by the juxtaglomerular apparatus of the kidney into the renal veins in response to sodium depletion and hypovolemia (see Figure 7-13). It activates the renin-angiotensin system, which results in angiotensin II, a powerful vasoconstrictor that also stimulates aldosterone production from the adrenal cortex. Angiotensin and aldosterone increase the blood pressure.

These mechanisms when abnormally overactive can cause hypertension (Figure 7-13). Renal vein assays are used to diagnose renovascular hypertension. By injection of radiopaque dye into the inferior vena cava, the renal veins can be identified. A catheter is placed into each renal vein, and blood is drawn from each vein. Radioimmunoassay is used to determine the renin quantity in each. If hypertension is caused by renal artery stenosis, the renal vein renin level

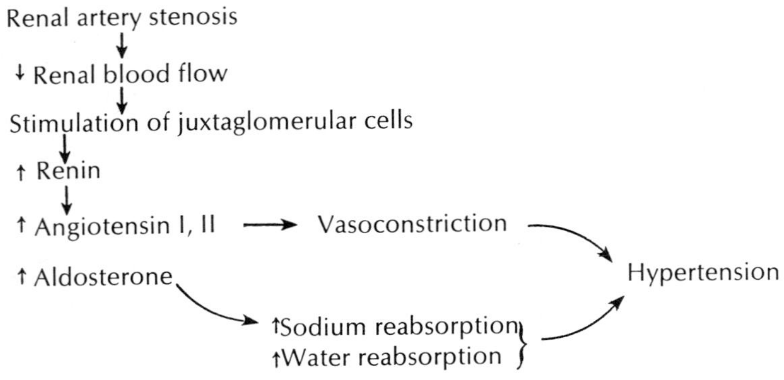

FIGURE 7-13. Physiology of renovascular hypertension.

of the affected kidney should be 1.4 or more times greater than that of the unaffected kidney. If the levels are the same, the hypertension is not caused by renal artery stenosis (any stenosis present is not severe enough to cause renin-related hypertension). Another cause for the patient's elevated blood pressure must be investigated.

Procedure. To obtain minimum renin stimulation, the patient is placed on a "no added salt" diet and diuretics for 3 days before the examination. The patient is asked to stay in the upright position for 2 hours before the test. The fasting patient is premedicated with meperidine and atropine and is taken to the radiology department. There the patient is placed on the fluoroscopy table in the supine position. The patient's groin is prepared and draped in a sterile manner then anesthetized. The femoral vein is punctured, and a catheter is placed into the vein and advanced into the inferior vena cava. Fluoroscopy is used to monitor the catheter placement. Dye is injected and the renal veins are identified. The catheter is placed into one renal vein at a time, and separate blood specimens are withdrawn.

The catheter is removed, and a pressure dressing is applied to the puncture site. The blood is usually sent to a commercial laboratory for analysis. This procedure is usually performed by a radiologist in less than 1 hour. The groin puncture needed for arterial access is uncomfortable.

Contraindications. This test is contraindicated in patients with allergies to iodine dye.

Nursing considerations

Nursing Diagnoses/Collaborative Problems

See Renal angiography, p. 254.

Nursing Implications with Rationale

- Explain the procedure to the patient. Encourage the patient to discuss feelings and fears regarding this study.
- See Nursing considerations for renal angiography (previous study).
- Assess the patient for allergies to iodine.
- Ensure that written and informed consent for this procedure is obtained by the physician.
- Keep the patient in the upright position for 2 hours before the test because the renin level is at its maximum when the patient is in this position.
- Give the preprocedure medications as ordered, usually 1 hour before the procedure.
- Be sure that the blood specimens are correctly labeled.
- After the procedure assess the patient for bleeding. Check the patient's urine for blood.
- Assess the patient for renal vein thrombosis, which may occur 1 to 7 days after the procedure and is manifested by costovertebral an-

gle (CVA) tenderness, hematuria, and elevated creatinine levels.

SUPPLEMENTAL INFORMATION

X-ray study of kidneys, ureters, and bladder

(KUB)

Normal value: no evidence of abnormality

Rationale. The KUB is a *flat plate,* or simple x-ray film of the lower abdomen. It is referred to as a *plain film,* or *scout film* of the abdomen or an *obstruction series* (see p. 84). It can be done to demonstrate the size, shape, and location of the kidneys and bladder. The KUB can also be used to identify calculi in these organs and in the ureters (Figure 7-14). It is often one of the first studies done to diagnose other intraabdominal diseases such as intestinal obstruction, soft tissue masses, and a ruptured viscus. It is useful in detecting abnormal accumulations of gas and of ascites within the GI tract. This study involves no contrast medium and poses no risk to the patient.

Procedure. No fasting or sedation is necessary. In the radiology department the patient is placed in the supine position with the arms extended overhead. X-ray films are taken of the patient's lower abdomen. Other films can be taken with the patient standing up and turned to the side. No discomfort is associated with this study. KUB is performed by a radiologic technician in a few minutes. A KUB should be taken before IVP or GI studies.

Contraindications. This study is contraindicated in the pregnant patient.

Nursing considerations

Nursing Diagnoses/Collaborative Problems

See X-ray studies, p. 4.

Nursing Implications with Rationale

- Explain the procedure to the patient.
- For adequate visualization, ensure that this test is scheduled before any barium studies.
- Ensure that the male patient has a lead shield over his gonads to prevent irradiation of the testes. The female ovaries cannot be shielded because of their proximity to the kidneys, ureters, and bladder.

Plasma renin activity

Normal values:

Adult/elderly: upright position, sodium *depleted* (sodium-restricted diet)
ages 20-39: 2.9-24 ng/ml/hr
>40: 2.9-10.8 ng/ml/hr

Adult/elderly: upright position, sodium *repleted* (normal sodium diet)
ages 20-39: 0.1-4.3 ng/ml/hr
>40: 0.1-3.0 ng/ml/hr

Child: 0-3 years: <16.6 ng/ml/hr
3-6 years: <6.7 ng/ml/hr
6-9 years: <4.4 ng/ml/hr
9-12 years: <5.9 ng/ml/hr
12-15 years: <4.2 ng/ml/hr
15-18 years: <4.3 ng/ml/hr

Rationale. The plasma renin activity (PRA) test is a screening procedure for the detection of essential, renal, or renovascular hypertension. It is usually supplemented by other tests, such as renal vein assay for renin (see p. 255). A determination of the PRA and a measurement of the plasma aldosterone level (see next study) are used in the differential diagnosis of primary versus secondary hyperaldosteronism. Patients with primary hyperaldosteronism have an increased aldosterone production associated with a decreased renin activity. Patients whose hyperaldosteronism is secondary to arterial occlusion have increased aldosterone and increased renin activity.

Elevated renin levels may occur in essential hypertension, malignant and renovascular hypertension, Addison's disease, cirrhosis, hypokalemia, hemorrhage, and renin-producing renal tumors (Bartter's syndrome).

Decreased levels are associated with salt-retaining steroid therapy and antidiuretic hormone therapy.

Procedure. Random samples of PRA are useless because of marked fluctuations in renin activity caused by salt intake, time of the day, and

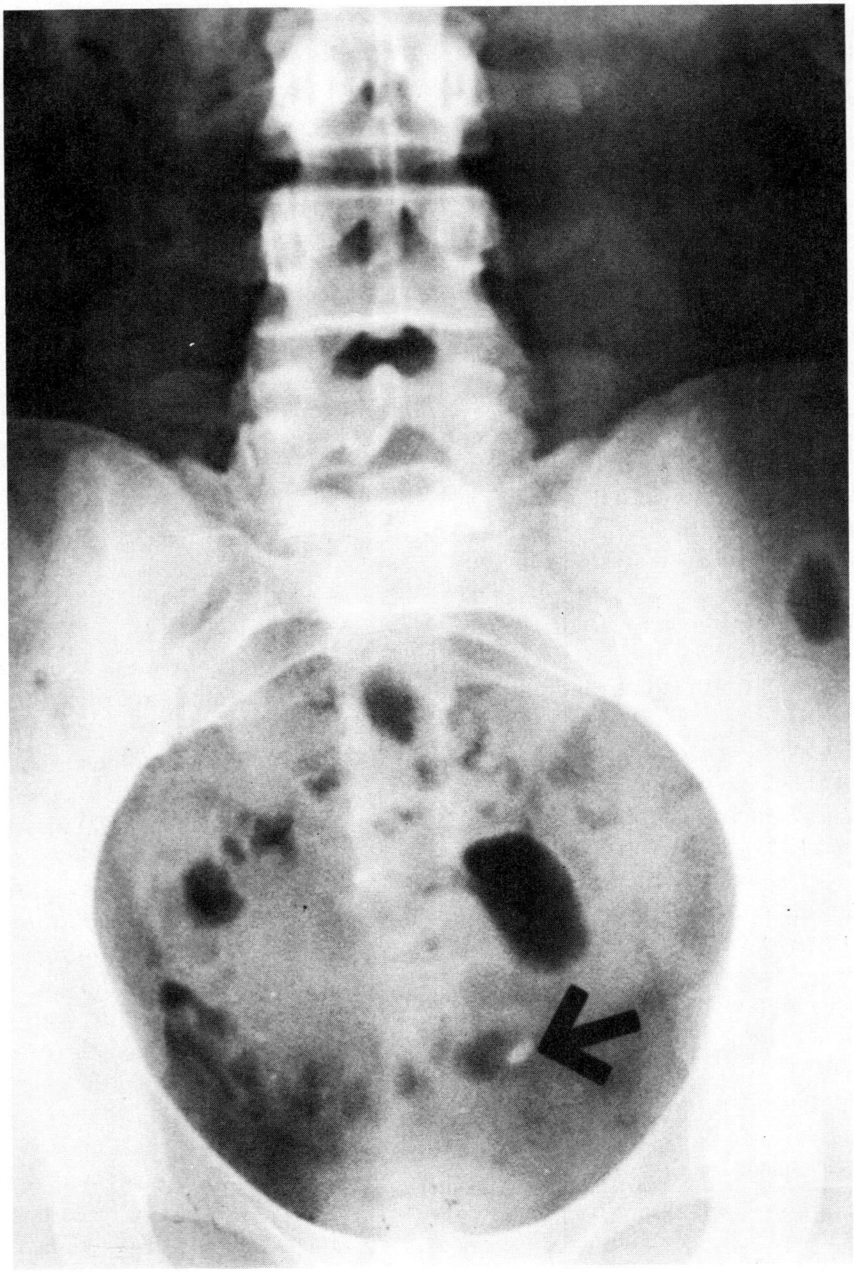

FIGURE 7-14. KUB. Plain film of the abdomen demonstrating abnormalities in the kidneys, ureters, and bladder. Arrow indicates radiopaque calcified stone in the left ureter.

positioning. For this reason the patient must maintain a normal diet with a restricted amount of sodium (approximately 3 g/day) for 3 days before the test. (A high sodium diet causes a decrease in renin.) Medications (such as diuretics, antihypertensives, vasodilators, and oral contraceptives) and licorice are usually discontinued 2 to 4 weeks before the test. Positioning influences renin secretion, with a change from the patient in the recumbent to the upright position causing increased renin secretion. Having the patient in the upright position is usually ordered. For this test the patient must stand or sit upright for 2 hours before the blood is drawn. If a recumbent sample is ordered, the patient should remain in bed in the morning until the blood sample has been obtained.

Because the renin values are higher in the morning, a fasting blood sample is usually drawn. Approximately 7 to 12 ml of peripheral venous blood is obtained and placed in a chilled lavender-top tube with EDTA as an anticoagulant. The tube should be gently inverted to allow adequate mixing of the blood sample and the anticoagulant. The tube of blood is then placed on ice and immediately sent to the laboratory. The PRA is measured by radioimmunoassay.

The blood sample is collected in a few minutes. The only discomfort is that of the venipuncture. Usually after the test a normal diet may be resumed, and medications that were withheld before the test may be reordered.

Contraindications. Renin levels are affected by pregnancy and many drugs (such as antihypertensives, levodopa, estrogens, diuretics, and vasodilators). Results will therefore be inaccurate if influenced by any of these factors.

Nursing considerations

Nursing Diagnoses/Collaborative Problems

See Blood studies, p. 2.

Nursing Implications with Rationale

- Explain the test to the patient. Renin levels are affected by failure to observe diet restrictions before the test. A high sodium diet causes a decrease in renin activity. Improper patient positioning before the test also affects the results. The renin levels are decreased in supine patients. The test is usually ordered for the patient to be in the upright position.
- Be certain the patient has discontinued diuretics, oral contraceptives, antihypertensives, vasodilators, and licorice as ordered. These can all affect the plasma renin levels.
- Chill the collection tube (containing EDTA) before withdrawing the blood sample. After the blood is drawn, the tube is gently inverted and then placed on ice. If these measures are not taken, renin breakdown occurs because the enzyme is very unstable.
- After the test apply pressure to the site and check the venipuncture site for bleeding.
- Record the position of the patient and the time of the day on the lab slip. Note any medications that the patient may be currently taking.

Aldosterone assay

Normal values:

Blood

Supine: 3-10 ng/dl or 0.08-0.3 nmol/L (SI units)

Upright: female—5-30 ng/dl or 0.14-0.8 nmol/L (SI units)

male—6-22 ng/dl or 0.17-0.61 nmol/L (SI units)

Newborn: 5-60 ng/dl

1 week-1 year: 1-160 ng/dl

1-3 years: 5-60 ng/dl

3-5 years: <5-80 ng/dl

5-7 years: <5-50 ng/dl

7-11 years: 5-70 ng/dl

11-15 years: <5-50 ng/dl

Urine

2-80 µg/24 hr or 5.5-72 nmol/24 hr (SI units)

Rationale. Aldosterone, a hormone produced by the adrenal cortex, is a potent mineralocorticoid. Production of this enzyme is regulated by adrenocorticotropic hormone (ACTH), plasma sodium or potassium concentration, and the renin-angiotensin system (Figure 7-3). Aldosterone stimulates the renal tubules to reabsorb increased amounts of sodium (which causes water retention) and to secrete potassium. It regulates sodium, potassium, and water balance based on the body's needs.

Increased aldosterone is the major diagnostic finding in primary aldosteronism (where a tumor of the adrenal cortex or bilateral adrenal hyperplasia causes an increased production of aldosterone). The typical laboratory pattern for primary aldosteronism (Conn's syndrome) is an increased aldosterone level and a decreased renin level (see previous study). The renin level is low in compensatory response to the increased serum sodium and blood volume. Patients with primary aldosteronism characteristically have hypertension and hypokalemia. Aldosterone levels may be elevated in certain nonadrenal conditions (secondary aldosteronism) such as hyponatremia, hyperkalemia, physical stress, recovery after surgery, Cushing's syndrome, malignant hypertension, generalized edema (from congestive heart failure, nephrotic syndrome, cirrhosis), renal ischemia, and Bartter's syndrome (a renin-producing renal tumor). Pregnancy and oral contraceptives can also increase aldosterone levels. Some diuretics (e.g., lasix and spironolactone) and steroids promote sodium excretion and may raise aldosterone levels.

Decreased aldosterone levels are seen in patients consuming a high sodium diet and in patients with hypokalemia. Addison's disease and eclampsia are also associated with low aldosterone levels. Some antihypertensives (e.g., captopril) may reduce aldosterone levels because they promote sodium and water retention. Licorice is aldosterone-like in activity. Therefore, when large quantities are ingested, serum aldosterone levels are decreased in compensation.

Procedure. Aldosterone assay can be done on 24-hour urine specimens or on a plasma blood sample. The advantage of the 24-hour urine sample is that short-term fluctuations are eliminated. (Lower values occur in the afternoon; having the patient in an upright position greatly increases the plasma aldosterone levels.) Plasma values are more convenient to sample, but they are affected by the short-term fluctuations. Therefore, 24-hour urine collection is more reliable. Levels of both urine and plasma are increased by low sodium diets and are decreased by high sodium diets. Hypokalemia inhibits aldosterone secretion.

Blood collection. The patient should maintain a normal sodium diet (approximately 3 g/day) for at least 2 weeks before the blood collection. Excess salt should not be consumed before the test. Drugs that alter sodium, potassium, and fluid balance (such as diuretics, antihypertensives, steroids, oral contraceptives) should be withheld at least 2 weeks before the test. Renin inhibitors (such as propranolol) should not be taken 1 week before the test. Licorice should be avoided at least 2 weeks before the test because of its aldosterone-like effect.

A fasting blood test is withdrawn with the patient in a supine position. The blood is collected in a red-top tube and sent to the laboratory. Four hours later a second sample is sometimes drawn with the patient in the standing position and after he or she has been up and about.

Urine collection. A normal sodium diet (approximately 3 g/day) should be followed 2 weeks before the test. During the 24-hour collection period the patient should avoid strenuous exercise and stressful situations. Any medication restrictions that applied to the blood test also apply for the urine test. Keep urine specimen refrigerated. The normal values for urine depend on total urinary sodium.

Contraindications. None.

Nursing considerations

Nursing Diagnoses/Collaborative Problems

See Blood studies, p. 2 and Urine studies, p. 3.

Nursing Implications with Rationale

Blood

- Indicate on the lab slip if the patient was supine or standing during the venipuncture.
- Give the patient written dietary and medication restriction instructions. Failure to ob-

serve the dietary and medication limitations may interfere with the test results.

- Handle the blood sample gently. Rough handling may cause hemolysis and alter the test results.

Urine

- Explain the procedure for collecting a 24-hour urine sample. Follow the nursing considerations for a 24-hour creatinine clearance test (p. 231), except for the first and last considerations. A preservative is used in the 24-hour collection. Keep the specimen on ice or refrigerate during the 24-hour period.
- Ensure that the patient avoids strenuous exercise and stress because both can stimulate adrenocortical secretions and increase aldosterone levels.
- After the urine or blood test is completed, check that the patient's normal diet is resumed and any restricted medications reordered.

Acid phosphatase

(prostatic acid phosphatase [PAP])

Normal values:
Adult/elderly: 0.11-0.60 U/L (Roy, Brower, Hayden; 37° C) or 0.11-0.60 U/L (SI units)
Child: 8.6-12.6 U/ml (30° C)
Newborn: 10.4-16.4 U/ml (30° C)

Rationale. The enzyme acid phosphatase is found in highest concentrations in the prostate gland. The prostatic component is separated from total acid phosphatase by immunoassay. This component is called prostatic acid phosphatase. The determination of prostatic acid phosphatase is primarily used to diagnose and stage prostatic carcinoma and to monitor the efficacy of treatment. Elevated levels are seen in patients with prostatic cancer that has metastasized beyond the capsule to other parts of the body, especially the bone. If the tumor is successfully treated by surgery, the acid phosphatase levels decrease in several days. If the tumor is treated by estrogen therapy, the enzyme levels return to normal in several weeks. Rising levels of acid phosphatase may indicate prostatic tumor progression.

Acid phosphatase is also found in high concentrations in seminal fluid. For this reason, prostatic acid phosphatase tests may be done on vaginal secretions to investigate alleged acts of rape.

Elevated levels of total acid phosphatase are also seen in patients with the following conditions: multiple myeloma, Paget's disease, hyperparathyroidism, sickle cell crisis, Gaucher's disease, renal impairment, cancer of the breast and bone, cirrhosis, thrombocytosis, and any cancer metastasis to the bone.

Falsely high levels of acid phosphatase may occur after a rectal examination and after instrumentation of the prostate gland (such as cystoscopy) because of prostatic stimulation. Hemolysis of the specimen also fictitiously increases serum levels. Drugs that may cause elevations of this enzyme include androgens (in females) and clofibrate (Atromid-S). Decreased levels may be caused by fluorides, phosphates, heparin, oxalates, and alcohol.

Procedure. No food or drink restrictions are associated with this test. Peripheral venipuncture is performed, and 5 to 10 ml of blood is collected in a red-top tube. Hemolysis should be avoided. The test should be performed without delay, or the specimen should be frozen.

The enzyme can be fractionated to specify the amount secreted by the prostate gland in contrast to the total enzyme activity, which is also present in the bone, liver, kidney, red blood cells, platelets, and spleen.

Contraindications. None.

Nursing considerations

Nursing Diagnoses/Collaborative Problems

See Blood studies, p. 2.

Nursing Implications with Rationale

- Explain the purpose of the test to the patient.
- Note on the lab slip if the patient has had a prostatic examination or instrumentation of the prostate gland (such as cystoscopy) within

24 hours. Prostatic manipulation may elevate the serum acid phosphatase level.

- Some laboratories request that they be notified before the blood sample is drawn so that immediate attention (<1 hour) can be given to the sample. The activity of the enzyme in the specimen will be decreased if the specimen is left at room temperature for as little as 1 hour because the enzyme is heat and pH sensitive.

Prostate-specific antigen (PSA)

Normal values: <4 ng/ml

Rationale. PSA is a glycoprotein (part carbohydrate, part protein) normally found in the cytoplasm of prostatic epithelial cells. This antigen can be detected in all men. However, its level is greatly increased in patients who have prostatic cancer. Although PSA was originally measured by histochemical techniques, radioimmunoassay (RIA) techniques have recently increased its accuracy.

Elevated PSA levels are associated with prostate cancer. The higher the levels, the greater is the tumor burden. Further, the PSA assay is a sensitive test for monitoring response to therapy. Successful surgery, radiation, or hormone therapy is associated with a marked reduction in the PSA blood level. Subsequent significant elevation in PSA indicates the recurrence of prostatic cancer.

PSA is more sensitive and more specific than other prostatic tumor markers, such as prostatic acid phosphatase (PAP, see p. 261). Also, PSA is more accurate than PAP in monitoring response and recurrence of tumor after therapy. PSA (and PAP) levels may also be elevated in patients with benign prostatic hypertrophy and prostatitis.

Procedure. No food or drug restrictions are associated with this test. Peripheral venipuncture is performed and 5 ml of blood is collected in red-top tube.

Contraindications. None.

Nursing considerations

Nursing Diagnoses/Collaborative Problems

See Blood studies, p. 2.

Nursing Implications with Rationale

- Explain the purpose of the test to the patient.
- Apply pressure or a pressure dressing to the venipuncture site.
- Observe the venipuncture site for bleeding.

Transrectal ultrasonography

(prostate sonogram)

Normal values: normal size, shape and consistency of the prostate gland

Rationale. Through the use of reflected sound waves, ultrasonography provides accurate visualization of the prostate for many diagnostic purposes. The technique of ultrasonography requires the emission of high-frequency sound waves from the transducer to penetrate the organ being studied. The sound waves are bounced back to the transducer and electronically converted into a pictorial image. A realistic Polaroid picture or x-ray film of the organ studied is obtained.

Ultrasound examination of the prostate is valuable in the diagnosis of prostatic cancer. This procedure can be used to evaluate prostate tissue, seminal vesicles, and surrounding tissues. Small tumors may be identified using this technique. Ultrasonography is also used to evaluate palpable nodules and as a guide for biopsy.

Procedure. No food or fluid restrictions are necessary. However, 1 hour before the test an enema is administered to eliminate feces from the rectum. The patient is then placed on the ultrasonography table on the left side with the knees bent toward the chest. The ultrasonographer applies a greasy conductive paste to the probe. A digital rectal exam usually precedes insertion of the rectal transducer. After insertion of the lubricated rectal probe, water may be introduced into the sheathes surrounding the transducer. Scans are performed in various planes by a slight rotation of the transducer.

This procedure is mildly uncomfortable because of the rectal examination and the rectal insertion of the transducer. Patients may also complain of slight pressure when water is inserted during the procedure. This procedure is performed by an ultrasonographer or urologist in approximately 30 minutes.

Contraindications. None.

Nursing considerations

Nursing Diagnoses/Collaborative Problems

See Ultrasound studies, p. 6.

- Possible alteration in comfort related to test procedures.
- Possible anxiety related to unknown sensations of the procedure.

Nursing Implications with Rationale

- Explain the procedure to the patient. No fasting is required; however, the patient must administer an enema 1 hour prior to the study in order to eliminate feces from the bowel.
- After the procedure, the lubricant is removed from the rectal area.

CASE STUDY 4: URINARY OBSTRUCTION

Mr. M.P., 57 years old, noted a decrease in his force of urinary stream and urinary hesitancy for several months. It had progressively become worse. His physical examination was essentially negative except for an enlarged prostate, which was bulky and soft.

Studies	Results
Routine laboratory studies	WNL
IVP (see p. 232)	Mild indentation of the interior aspect of the bladder, indicating an enlarged prostate
Uroflowmetry with total voided flow of 225 ml	8 ml/sec (normal: >12 ml/sec)
Cystometry	Resting bladder pressure: 35 cm H_2O (normal: <40 cm H_2O) Peak bladder pressure: 50 cm H_2O (normal: 40-90 cm H_2O)
Electromyography of the pelvic sphincter muscle	Normal resting bladder with a positive tonus limb
Cystoscopy (see p. 244)	Benign prostatic hypertrophy (BPH)

Because of the patient's symptoms, bladder outlet obstruction was highly suspected. Physical examination indicated an enlarged prostate. IVP studies corroborated that finding. The reduced urine flow rate indicated an obstruction distal to the urinary bladder. Because the patient was found to have a normal total voided volume, one could not say that the reduced flow rate was the result of an inadequately distended bladder. Rather, the bladder was appropriately distended and, despite that, the flow rate was decreased. This indicated outlet obstruction. The cystogram indicated that the bladder was capable of mounting an effective pressure and was not an atonic bladder compatible with neurologic disease. The tonus limb again indicated the bladder had the capability of contracting. The peak bladder pressure of 50 cm of H_2O is normal, again indicating appropriate muscular function of the bladder. From these studies the patient was diagnosed with a urinary outlet obstruction. Cystoscopy documented that finding, and the patient was appropriately treated by transurethral prostatectomy (TURP). This patient did quite well postoperatively and had no major problems.

DISCUSSION OF TESTS

Urine flow studies

(uroflowmetry)

Normal values: dependent on the patient's age, sex, and volume voided

Age	Minimum volume (ml)	Male (ml/sec)	Female (ml/sec)
4-13	100	>10-12	>10-15
14-45	200	>21	>18
46-65	200	>12	>15
66-80	200	>9	>10

Rationale. Uroflowmetry is the simplest of the

urodynamic techniques, being noninvasive and requiring simple and relatively inexpensive equipment. This study measures the volume of urine expelled from the bladder per second. This test is indicated to investigate dysfunctional voiding or suspicious outflow tract obstruction and before and after any procedure designed to modify the function of the urinary outflow tract.

Procedure. This test should be performed when the patient has a normal desire to void and in conditions suitable for privacy. The bladder should be adequately full. If urine samples are needed for another test, there should be a separate voiding. Essentially all the patient has to do is urinate into the flowmeter. Several different types of flowmeters are available. The position of the patient, the method of filling the bladder (it should be natural), and whether or not the study was part of another evaluation should be recorded.

The urine flow rate is highly dependent on the volume of urine voided. The flow rates are highest and most predictable in the urine volume range of 200 to 400 ml. Over 400 ml, the efficiency of the bladder muscle is markedly decreased. Nomograms of maximum flow versus voided volume can be used for accurate test result interpretation, taking into account sex and age. If the flow rates are abnormally low, the test should be repeated to check for accuracy.

Modern urine flowmeters provide a permanent graphic recording. If flowmeters are not available, the patient can time the urinary stream with a stopwatch and record the voided volume. From this the average flow is calculated.

In some cases it is more valuable to analyze several voided volumes and flow rates rather than a single flow rate. If this is to be done, the patient is taught to use a flowmeter on the first day, and on the second day the flowmeter is used with each voiding. On the third day the client is asked to refrain from voiding as long as possible and then void into the flowmeter. A graph of flow versus volume is then plotted. This, together with clinical observation, provides very valuable additional information on the severity of the patient's problem, the likelihood of urinary retention, and the state of compensation or decompensation of the detrusor muscle.

Contraindications. None.

Nursing considerations

Nursing Diagnoses/Collaborative Problems

- Possible knowledge deficit related to test purpose, preparation, and procedure
- Possible anxiety related to possible test results

Nursing Implications with Rationale

- Explain the procedure to the patient; ensure that the patient knows how to void into the urine flowmeter. Ensure privacy during voiding.
- Determine the number of flow rates that are needed.
- If a series of flow rates are needed, explain this procedure to the patient.
- Record the position of the patient, the method of filling the bladder, and whether or not this study was part of another evaluation. Uroflowmetry is usually the first of the urodynamic investigations performed. In many instances, urine flow studies alone allow for a confident urodynamic diagnosis.

Cystometry

(cystometrogram)

Normal values:
- Normal sensations of fullness and temperature
- Normal pressures and volumes
- Maximal cystometric capacity:
  - male, 350-750 ml
  - female, 250-550 ml
- Intravesical pressure when bladder is empty: usually <40 cm H_2O
- Detrusor pressure: <10 cm H_2O

Rationale. The purpose of cystometrogram is to evaluate the motor and sensory function of the bladder when incontinence is present or when there is suspicion of neurologic bladder dysfunction. A graphic recording of pressure exerted at varying phases of the filling of the urinary bladder is produced. A pressure/volume relationship of the bladder is made. This urodynamic study assesses the neuromuscular function of the bladder by measuring the efficiency of the detrusor muscle, intravesical pressure and capacity, and the bladder's response to thermal stimulation.

Cystometry can determine whether bladder dysfunction is caused by neurologic, infectious, or obstructive disease. Cystometry is indicated to elucidate the cause for frequency and urgency, especially before surgery on the urinary outflow tract. Cystometry is also part of the evaluation for the following: incontinence, persistent residual urine, vesicoureteric reflux, neurologic disorders, sensory disorders and the effect of certain drugs on bladder function.

Procedure. No food or fluid restrictions are necessary for cystometry. The test is usually performed in a urologist's office or in a special procedure room. The test begins with the patient being asked to void. The amount of time required to initiate voiding, and the size, force, and continuity of the urinary stream are recorded. The amount of urine, the time of voiding, and the presence of any straining, hesitancy, and terminal urine dribbling are also recorded.

The patient is then placed in a lithotomy or supine position. A retention catheter is inserted through the urethra and into the bladder. (The catheter can also be inserted suprapubically.) Residual urine volume is measured and recorded.

Thermal sensation is evaluated by the installation of approximately 30 ml of room-temperature sterile saline solution or water into the bladder, followed by an equal amount of warm water. The patient reports any sensations. This fluid is then withdrawn from the bladder.

The urethral catheter is then connected to a cystometer (a tube used to monitor bladder pressure); sterile water, normal saline solution, or carbon dioxide gas is slowly introduced into the bladder at a controlled rate. The patient is usually placed in a sitting position for this. Patients are then asked to indicate the first urge to void (usually after 100 to 200 ml has been instilled) and then the feeling when they must void (approximately 350 to 450 ml). The bladder is full at this point. The pressures and volumes are plotted on a graph. The patient is asked to void, and the maximal intravesical voiding pressure is recorded. The bladder is then drained for any residual urine. If no additional studies are to be done, the urethral catheter is removed. Throughout the study the patient should report any sensations such as pain, flushing, sweating, nausea, bladder filling, and an urgency to void.

Certain drugs may be administered during the cystometric examination to distinguish between underactivity of the bladder because of muscle failure and underactivity associated with denervation. Cholinergic drugs (such as bethanechol [Urecholine]) may be given to enhance the tone of a flaccid bladder. Anticholinergic drugs (such as atropine) may be given to promote relaxation of a hyperactive bladder. If these drugs are to be given, the catheter is left in place. The drugs are given and the examination is repeated 20 to 30 minutes later, using the first test as a control value.

This test is performed by a urologist in about 45 minutes. Discomfort associated with this study is similar to urethral catheterization.

Contraindications. Cystometry is contraindicated in patients with urinary tract infections because of false readings, which may be caused by uninhibited contractions of the bladder, and because of the potential for pyelonephritis and septic shock.

Nursing considerations

Nursing Diagnoses/Collaborative Problems

- Possible knowledge deficit related to test purpose, preparation, and procedure

- Possible alteration in comfort related to test procedure
- Possible anxiety related to possible test results
- Potential complication: sepsis

Nursing Implications with Rationale

- Explain the purpose and the procedure to the patient. Many patients are embarrassed by this procedure. Assure them that they will be draped to ensure privacy.
- Assess the patient for signs and symptoms of urinary tract infection, which would make the examination contraindicated because of the possibility of false results and the potential for the spread of infection.
- Instruct the patient not to strain while voiding because the results can be skewed.
- If the patient has a spinal cord injury, ensure that he or she is transported to the test on a stretcher. The test will then be performed with the patient on the stretcher.
- After the test suggest a warm sitz bath or tub bath, which may be comforting to the patient.
- After the cystometry observe the patient for any manifestations of infection (such as elevated temperature or chills), which may indicate sepsis.
- After the test examine the urine for hematuria. Notify the physician if the hematuria persists after several voidings.

Pelvic floor sphincter electromyography

(pelvic floor sphincter EMG)

Normal values: increased EMG signal during bladder filling; silent EMG signal on voluntary micturition; increased EMG signal at end of voiding

Rationale. This urodynamic test uses the placement of electrodes in the pelvic floor musculature of the anal and urethral sphincter to evaluate the neuromuscular function of the lower urinary tract. The main benefit of this study is to evaluate external sphincter (skeletal muscle) activity during voiding. This test is also used to evaluate the bulbocavernous reflex and voluntary control of external sphincter or pelvic floor muscles. It also aids in the investigation of "functional" or psychologic disturbances of voiding.

Procedure. Three electrodes are used for this procedure. Recordings may be made from surface or needle electrodes within the muscle. Surface electrodes are most commonly used. Two electrodes (which may be pediatric surface electrocardiographic electrodes) are placed at the 2 o'clock and 10 o'clock positions on the perianal skin and monitor the pelvic floor muscular activity during voiding. The third electrode is usually placed on the thigh and serves as a grounding plate. These electrodes allow for observation of and change in the muscle activity before and during voiding.

This test begins by recording the electrical activity with the bladder empty and the patient relaxed. Reflex activity is then evaluated by asking the patient to cough and by stimulating the urethra and trigone by gently tugging the Foley catheter (bulbocavernous reflex). Voluntary activity is then evaluated by asking the patient to contract and relax the sphincter muscle. The bladder is filled at 100 ml/min with sterile water at room temperature. The EMG responses to filling and detrusor hyperreflexia (if present) are recorded. Finally, when the bladder is full and the patient is in voiding position, the filling catheter is removed and the patient is asked to urinate. In the normal patient the EMG signals build during bladder filling and cease promptly on voluntary micturition, remaining silent until the pelvic floor contracts at the end of voiding. The electrical waves produced are examined for their number and form.

This study is slightly more uncomfortable than urethral catheterization. A urologist performs this study; the duration of the study is less than 30 minutes.

Contraindications. This test is contraindicated in the uncooperative patient.

Nursing considerations

Nursing Diagnoses/Collaborative Problems

- Possible knowledge deficit related to test purpose, preparation, and procedure
- Possible alteration in comfort related to test procedure
- Possible anxiety related to possible test results

Nursing Implications with Rationale

- Explain the purpose and procedure of pelvic floor sphincter electromyography to the patient. Patient cooperation is essential. If the patient does not cooperate, the interpretation of the test results will be difficult.
- If the perianal area is soiled, ensure that it is washed before the placement of the electrodes.
- If needle electrodes were used, after the test observe the needle site for hematoma or inflammation.

SUPPLEMENTAL INFORMATION

Urethral pressure measurements

(urethral pressure profile/UPP)

Normal values: maximum urethral pressures in normal patients (cm H_2O)

Age	Male	Female
<25	37-126	55-103
25-44	35-113	31-115
45-64	40-123	40-100
>64	35-105	35-75

Rationale. The UPP indicates the intraluminal pressure along the length of the urethra with the bladder at rest. Indications for this urodynamic investigation include the following:

1. Assessment of prostatic obstruction
2. Assessment of stress incontinence in females
3. Assessment of postprostatectomy problems
4. Assessment of the adequacy of external sphincterotomy
5. Analysis of the effects of drugs on the urethra
6. Analysis of the effects of stimulation on urethral flow
7. Assessment of adequacy of implanted artificial urethral sphincter devices.

Procedure. No fasting or sedation is required for this test. A catheter is passed into the bladder and withdrawn slowly through the urethra. Fluids (or gas) are instilled through the catheter, which is withdrawn while the pressures along the urethral wall are obtained. A constant infusion of the fluids or gas is maintained by a motorized syringe pump. The catheter is removed, and the test is completed in less than 15 minutes. This test is slightly more uncomfortable than urethral catheterization. This test is usually performed by a urologist.

Contraindications. This study is contraindicated in patients with urinary tract infections.

Nursing considerations

Nursing Diagnoses/Collaborative Problems

- Possible knowledge deficit related to test purpose, preparation, and procedure
- Possible alteration in comfort related to test procedure
- Possible anxiety related to possible test results
- Potential complication: urinary tract infection

Nursing Implications with Rationale

- Explain the procedure to the patient. Many patients are embarrassed by this procedure. Assure them that they will be draped to ensure privacy.
- After the study suggest a warm tub bath or a sitz bath, which may be comforting to the patient.

QUESTIONS AND ANSWERS

1. **QUESTION:** IVP is ordered for a trauma patient whose vital signs are stable. After the injection of the iodinated dye, the patient becomes flushed,

hypotensive, and develops severe bronchospasms. What should be done?

ANSWER: This patient is having an anaphylactic reaction to the dye. You should reassure the patient and do the following:

a. Place the patient in the Trendelenburg position.
b. Increase the IV rate to treat the hypotension.
c. Administer oxygen by mask or nasal cannula.
d. Notify the physician. The physician will most probably order epinephrine, 0.3 ml subcutaneously (SQ), methylprednisolone sodium succinate (Solu-Medrol), 2 g IV, and diphenhydramine, 25 mg IV or intramuscularly (IV).
e. Draw blood for a hemoglobin and hematocrit determination to be certain that the hypotension is not related to unrecognized, trauma-induced intraabdominal bleeding.
f. The patient may require endotracheal intubation for respiratory support. Dopamine may be required for circulatory support.

2. **QUESTION:** Your patient is scheduled for IVP. His creatinine level is 2.4 mg/dl and his BUN level is 49 mg/dl. Will the kidneys be visualized by IVP?

   ANSWER: Yes. Even with the decreased renal function, the kidneys will be visualized. It will just require more time for visualization. (For example, instead of seeing the kidney on a 5-minute film, you may not see anything for 15 minutes.)

3. **QUESTION:** Your patient has had a renal biopsy. Shortly afterward, he develops severe back and leg pain on the side of the biopsy. He begins to have nausea and vomiting. His blood pressure drops from 140/100 mm Hg to 100/68 mm Hg. What should be done for this patient?

   ANSWER: An expanding retroperitoneal hematoma secondary to inadvertent puncture of a blood vessel is probably causing the back and leg pain and also the hypotension. The nausea and vomiting is a result of the paralytic ileus that usually occurs with retroperitoneal hematoma. You should reassure the patient and do the following:

   a. Monitor the vital signs every 15 minutes and notify the physician. Ask the physician to come to the ward and examine the patient.
   b. Start an IV, because the patient will require fluid volume replacement.
   c. Draw blood for a hemoglobin and hematocrit determination to document the bleeding.
   d. Type and cross-match the patient for several units of blood, as ordered. Transfusion may become necessary.
   e. Determine prothrombin time and partial thromboplastin time to be sure that the patient has the clotting ability to plug the puncture hole in the vessel.
   f. Keep the patient NPO; surgical repair may be required if the hypotension persists. The physician will probably order an x-ray film of the abdomen because these clinical symptoms could also occur with inadvertent puncture of the bowel. In that case, free air may be seen on the x-ray film.

4. **QUESTION:** What precautions are necessary before CT scanning of the kidneys in a patient who is allergic to iodinated dyes is performed?

   ANSWER: Frequently for CT scanning of the kidney, the patient is injected with an iodinated contrast material to aid in renal visualization. The physician should be notified of the patient's allergy. If the patient requires CT scanning with iodinated contrast material, he will need a diphenhydramine-prednisone preparation (see p. 232). Of course, CT scanning without contrast material can be done without any precautions.

5. **QUESTION:** Your patient returns to the floor after having had transcystoscopic biopsy-specimen removal. A Foley catheter is in place. On his return, you note gross hematuria and blood clots. Two hours later you notice that the patient has not produced any urine. He begins to complain of lower abdominal midline pain and is mildly hypotensive. What are the appropriate interventions for this patient?

   ANSWER: Obviously the hematuria and blood clots indicate postprocedure bleeding. The clots should have concerned you because urine is a mild anticoagulant and clotting occurs only with brisk urinary bleeding. Probably a clot has occluded the catheter and caused acute urinary retention (resulting in the lower abdominal pain). You should reassure the patient and do the following:

   a. Flush the Foley catheter with a premeasured amount of sterile saline solution, using sterile technique.
   b. After patency is established, monitor the urine output.
   c. Notify the physician.
   d. Increase the rate of the IV infusion, as ordered.

This is done to increase urine output, which will flush out the bladder. Maintain accurate intake and output.

e. Begin Foley irrigation, as ordered, to attempt to clear the bladder of clots.

f. Draw blood for a hemoglobin and hematocrit determination to measure the severity of the blood loss.

g. Draw, type, and cross-match blood, as ordered, in the event that a transfusion is required. Surgery or recystoscopy may be necessary to terminate the bleeding.

6. **QUESTION:** Your patient is scheduled to receive a nephrotoxic drug. She has no suspected renal disease or injury, yet her creatinine clearance is only 52 ml/min. What should be done?

   ANSWER: Do not administer the drug. In a young adult who has no suspected renal disease or injury, the most likely cause of the abnormal creatinine clearance is error in the collection (such as not all of the urine samples being collected). The creatinine clearance test should be repeated. If the results are within the normal range, administer the drug. If the results still indicate 52 ml/min., the renal function is truly impaired and the drug should not be given. A complete workup will be required to elucidate the patient's renal problem.

7. **QUESTION:** A 28-year-old woman who is menstruating comes to the emergency room complaining of a sudden onset of colicky, left-sided back pain with radiation to the groin. A ureteral calculus (stone) is suspected. The physician orders a urinalysis. What should be done?

   ANSWER: You should remind the physician that the patient is menstruating, and suggest that the patient be catheterized for urine specimen. Red blood cells are diagnostic of a ureteral stone. However, one has to expect red blood cells in a quantity too numerous to count in a voided specimen from a menstruating patient. The only way to obtain an adequate specimen is by urethral catheterization.

8. **QUESTION:** Your patient develops bleeding from a peptic ulcer. His routine laboratory studies indicate a BUN level of 68 mg/dl and a creatinine level of 1.0 mg/dl. Does this patient have renal disease?

   ANSWER: No. The creatinine level is normal. The BUN level is elevated because there is an increased GI absorption of protein (blood), which is metabolized to urea. Patients with normal renal function who develop GI bleeding will have elevated BUN levels. The BUN level returns to normal as soon as the GI hemorrhage ceases.

BIBLIOGRAPHY

Andreoli TE: Approach to the patient with renal disease. In Wyngaarden JB and others, editors: Cecil textbook of medicine, ed 19, Philadelphia, 1992, WB Saunders.

Barrett DM and Wein AJ: Flow evaluation and simultaneous external sphincter electromyography in clinical urodynamics, J Urol 125:538-541, 1981.

Brenner BM, Milford EL, and Seifter JL: Urinary tract obstruction. In Wilson J and others, editors: Harrison's principles of internal medicine, ed 12, New York, 1991, McGraw-Hill.

Brenner BM and Rector FC, editors: The kidney, ed 4, Philadelphia, 1991, Ardmore Medical Books.

Coe FL and Brenner BM: Approach to the patient with diseases of the kidneys and urinary tract. In Wilson J and others, editors: Harrison's principles of internal medicine, ed 12, New York, 1991, McGraw-Hill.

Couser WG: Glomerular disease. In Wyngaarden JB and others, editors: Cecil textbook of medicine, ed 19, Philadelphia, 1992, WB Saunders.

Cronin RE: Renal cell carcinoma, Am J Med Sci 302(4):249-259, 1991.

Demmler RW: Urinary incontinence. In Rakel RE, editor: Conn's current therapy, Philadelphia, 1991, WB Saunders.

Freeman NJ and others: Elevated prostate markers in metastatic small cell carcinoma of unknown primary, Cancer 68(5):1118-1120, 1991.

Glassock RJ and Brenner BM: The major glomerulopathies. In Wilson J and others, editors: Harrison's principles of internal medicine, ed 12, New York, 1991, McGraw-Hill.

Groggel GC. Glomerular disorders. In Rakel RE, editor: Conn's current therapy, Philadelphia, 1991, WB Saunders.

Johnson CP and others: Evaluation of renal transplant dysfunction using color Doppler sonography, Surg Gynecol Obstet 173(4):279-284, 1991.

Mayo ME: Value of sphincter electromyography in urodynamics, J Urol 122:357-360, 1979.

Pak CY: Renal calculi. In Wyngaarden JB and others, editors: Cecil textbook of medicine, ed 19, Philadelphia, 1992, WB Saunders.

Ujiie K and others. Angiotensin-converting enzyme activity as a prognostic factor in acute renal failure, Nephron 58(4):443-449, 1991.

Williams RD: Tumors of the kidney, ureter, and bladder. In Wyngaarden JB and others, editors: Cecil textbook of medicine, ed 19, Philadelphia, 1992, WB Saunders.

Chapter 8

DIAGNOSTIC STUDIES USED IN THE ASSESSMENT OF THE
ENDOCRINE SYSTEM

PITUITARY GLAND
Anatomy and physiology
- Disorders of the pituitary gland

Case study 1: Partial growth hormone deficiency
Discussion of tests
- Growth hormone
- Somatomedin C
- Growth hormone stimulation test

THYROID GLAND
Anatomy and physiology
- Production, storage, and secretion of thyroid hormone
- Regulation of thyroid hormone production
- Thyroid disorders

Case study 2: Thyroid nodule
Discussion of tests
- Serum thyroxine test
- Serum triiodothyronine test
- Radioactive iodine uptake test
- Thyroid scanning
- Ultrasound examination of the thyroid

Supplemental information
- Free thyroxine index
- Thyrotropin-releasing hormone test
- T_3 resin uptake test
- Thyroid-stimulating hormone test
- TSH stimulation test
- Antithyroglobulin antibody test
- Antithyroid microsomal antibody test
- Long-acting thyroid stimulator

PARATHYROID GLANDS
Anatomy and physiology
- Calcium metabolism

Case study 3: Hyperparathyroidism
Discussion of tests
- Serum calcium test
- Serum parathyroid hormone test
- Cortisone administration test
- Serum phosphate (phosphorus) concentration test
- Tubular phosphate reabsorption test

Supplemental information
- Urine calcium test

ADRENAL GLANDS
Anatomy and physiology
- Glucocorticoid secretion
- Mineralocorticoid secretion
- Androgen and estrogen secretion
- Epinephrine secretion
- Diseases affecting the adrenal glands

Case study 4: Cushing's syndrome
Discussion of tests
- Urine tests for 17-hydroxycorticosteroids and 17-ketosteroids
- Plasma cortisol test
- Dexamethasone suppression test
- Serum adrenocorticotropic hormone test
- Adrenocorticotropic hormone stimulation test
- Metyrapone test
- X-ray study of the sella turcica
- Adrenal angiography

Supplemental information
- Adrenal venography
- Computed tomography of the adrenal glands
- Androstendione

ENDOCRINE PANCREAS
Anatomy and physiology
Case study 5: Adolescent with diabetes mellitus
Discussion of tests
- Serum glucose test
- Two-hour postprandial glucose test
- Glucose tolerance test
- Glycosylated hemoglobin test
- Serum osmolality test

Supplemental information
- Urine test for glucose and acetone
- Plasma insulin assay
- C-Peptide
- Blood glucose self-monitoring

Questions and answers

The endocrine system functions to maintain homeostasis of the body's internal environment. Endocrine glands are different from exocrine glands. Endocrine glands secrete their products directly into the bloodstream, in contrast to exocrine glands (such as salivary glands), whose secretions travel through a duct to the site of use. The endocrine system secretes chemical substances called *hormones*. Figure 8-1 shows the anatomy and location of the endocrine glands.

The concentration of most hormones is maintained at an appropriate level in the bloodstream by a "feedback-control mechanism." If the hormone concentration increases, further production of the hormone is inhibited. When the hormone concentration decreases, production of that hormone is then stimulated.

Hormones are the main regulators of metabolism, growth and development, reproduction, and stress response. Excess or deficiency of the

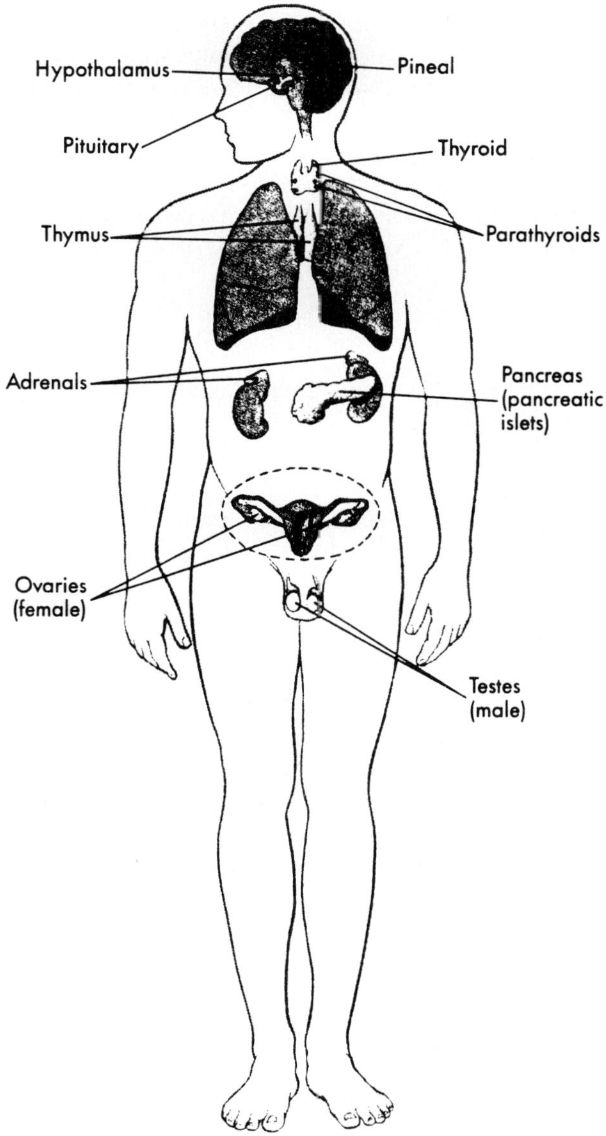

FIGURE 8-1. Location of endocrine glands.
From Thibodeau GA: Anthony's textbook of anatomy and physiology, ed 14, St Louis, 1994, Mosby–Year Book, Inc.

hormones causes various types of abnormalities. This chapter focuses on the diagnostic studies related to the pituitary, thyroid, parathyroid, and adrenal glands, and the endocrine pancreas. The anatomy and physiology of each gland are discussed briefly before the relevant case study to facilitate better use of the tables and figures included in each discussion.

PITUITARY GLAND

ANATOMY AND PHYSIOLOGY

The pituitary gland is a small gland located at the base of the brain within the bony cavity called the sella turcica. Because of its position under the hypothalamus, it is also called the *hypophysis*. The pituitary gland is divided into regions that function as distinct and separate endocrine glands. This gland consists of an anterior lobe (also called the *adenohypophysis*), a smaller posterior lobe (also called the *neurohypophysis*), and a poorly developed intermediate lobe *(pars intermedia)* lying between the anterior and posterior lobes.

The anterior pituitary gland (adenohypophysis) (Figure 8-2) has multiple functions, and because it regulates the functions of many other glands, it is also known as the "master gland." Seven anterior pituitary hormones have been identified (Table 8-1). The posterior gland (neurohypophysis) stores two hormones, antidiuretic hormone and oxytocin. The only known secretion of the intermediate lobe is melanocyte-stimulation hormone (MSH) which does not seem to be of major importance in skin pigmentation of humans. See Table 8-1 for a brief overview of pituitary hormones, target organs, and principal functions.

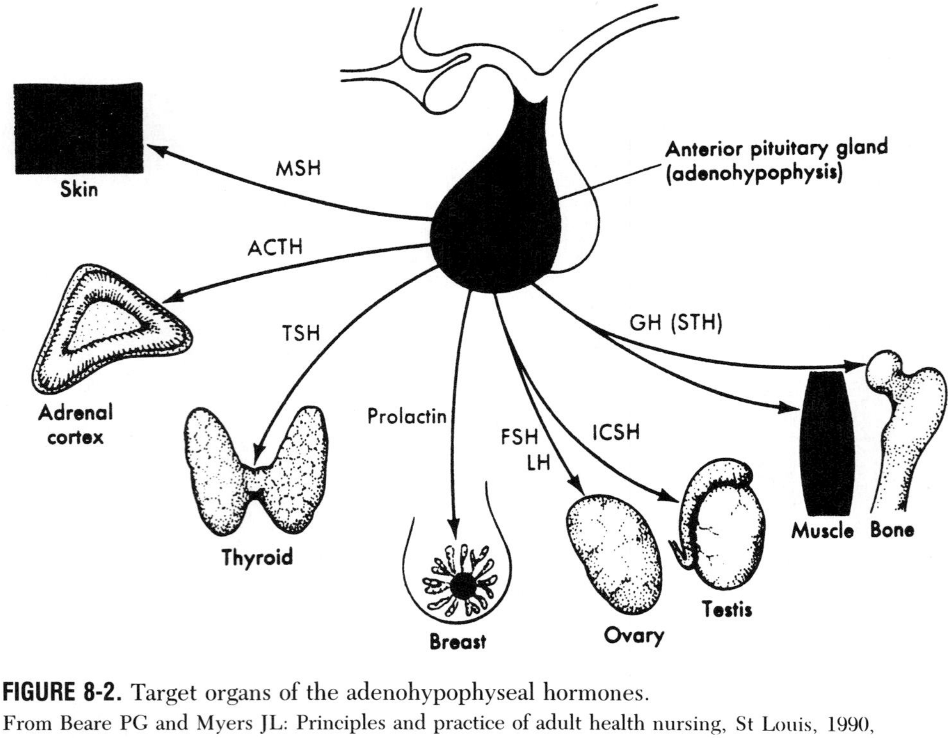

FIGURE 8-2. Target organs of the adenohypophyseal hormones.
From Beare PG and Myers JL: Principles and practice of adult health nursing, St Louis, 1990, Mosby–Year Book, Inc.

Disorders of the pituitary gland

Growth hormone is the only hormone secreted by the anterior pituitary that has no specific target organ. All body cells are affected by growth hormone. Growth hormone is regulated by release hormones from the hypothalmus and by somatomedins, which are synthesized in the liver. The action of growth hormone is influenced by many other hormones (such as thyroid hormone, insulin, steroids, and androgens). Nutritional status, exercise, stress, sleep, and diurnal rhythm also affect growth hormone secretion.

Overproduction of growth hormone, which is usually from a benign pituitary adenoma, causes gigantism or acromegaly. *Gigantism* occurs when growth hormone excess occurs before the closure of the epiphyses while the long bones are still capable of longitudinal growth. The excessive growth usually occurs proportionally. These children can grow as tall as 8 feet.

Symptoms of *acromegaly* usually occur insidiously in the third and fourth decades of life. Because growth occurs after epiphyses closure, bones increase in thickness and width. Physical features include the enlargement of hands, feet, and paranasal and frontal sinuses. Deformities of the spine and mandible also result. The therapeutic goal for treating patients with gigantism and acromegaly is to return growth hormone level to normal by surgery, irradiation, drug therapy, or some combination of these three treatment modes.

Hyposecretion of growth hormone during childhood results in growth retardation, or dwarfism. Individuals with severe short stature should undergo evaluation as illustrated in case study #1 (p. 274). Replacement therapy for

TABLE 8-1. Pituitary Gland Hormones

Hormones	Target organ or tissue	Principal function
Anterior Pituitary		
Growth hormone (Somatotropin)	General	Accelerates rate of body growth, regulates organic metabolism
Thyroid-stimulating hormone (TSH, thyrotropin)	Thyroid gland	Synthesis and release of thyroid hormone, promotes bone growth
Adrenocorticotropic hormone (ACTH)	Adrenal cortex	Growth of adrenal cortex, secretion of cortisol
Follicle-stimulating hormone (FSH)	Ovaries, testes	Stimulates growth of ovarian follicle in women; spermatogenesis in men
Luteinizing hormone (LH)	Ovaries, testes	Promotes maturation of ovaries, ovulation, and secretion of progesterone in women; stimulates development of the testes and secretion of androgens in men
Prolactin (luteotropic hormone, mammotropin)	Mammary	Proliferation of breast tissue, initiation of milk secretion
Interstitial cell–stimulating hormone (ICSH)	Male development	Promotes secretion of testosterone
Posterior Pituitary		
Antidiuretic hormone (ADH, vasopressin)	Renal tubules, arterioles	Facilitates water reabsorption, produces vasoconstriction
Oxytocin	Uterus	Contracts pregnant uterus

growth hormone deficiency can be given to prepubertal children to facilitate normal growth.

Other hormonal disorders of the pituitary glands are described in this book in the sections where the target organs (such as thyroid, adrenal, and uterus) are discussed.

CASE STUDY 1: PARTIAL GROWTH HORMONE DEFICIENCY

E.L. is a 14-year-old girl who was 4 feet 9 inches tall with no signs of pubertal development. Her parents were both tall. Because of her drop on the growth chart for both height and weight, her pediatrician ordered a complete workup to investigate her short stature.

Studies	Results
Routine laboratory studies (CBC and urinalysis)	WNL
Growth hormone	5.1 ng/ml (normal: 0-10 ng/ml)
Somatomedin C	98 ng/ml (normal: 96-256 ng/ml)
Wrist and hand x-ray film (see p. 424)	Bone age of 11½ years (normal: similar to chronological age)
Serum thyroxine (see p. 280)	6.3 μg/dl (normal: 4-11 μg/dl)
MRI (see p. 201)	No evidence of craniopharyngioma or other central nervous system lesion
Serum calcium (see p. 291)	9.2 mg/dl (normal: 8.8-10.8 mg/dl)
Serum phosphate (see p. 294)	5.2 mg/dl (normal: 4.5-6.5 mg/dl)
Carbon dioxide content (see p. 475)	24 mEq/L (normal: 23-30 mEq/L)
Blood urea nitrogen (BUN) (see p. 229)	12.2 mg/dl (normal: 5-18 mg/dl)
Erythrocyte sedimentation rate (sed rate) (see p. 444)	8 mm/hr (normal: ≤10 mm/hr)
Chromosomal karyotype	No evidence of sex chromatin abnormality
GH stimulation test	8 ng/ml (normal: ≥10 ng/ml)

The thyroxine level ruled out the possibility of hypothyroidism. An adequate thyroid level is a prerequisite for normal growth. The MRI ruled out a craniopharyngioma, which could have resulted in impaired secretion of growth hormone. The calcium level excluded the possibility of pseudohypoparathyroidism. The normal phosphate eliminated vitamin D–resistant rickets. Renal tubular acidosis was ruled out by the normal carbon dioxide level. The possibility of renal failure was excluded based on the normal BUN. The normal sedimentation rate eliminated the possibility of inflammatory bowel disease. The normal chromosomal karyotype excluded Turner's syndrome and other genetic abnormalities. The low-normal levels of growth hormone and somatomedin C suggested the possibility of a partial deficiency of growth hormone. The growth hormone stimulation test confirmed the diagnosis. The child was placed on daily subcutaneous injection of growth hormone for 2 years. She eventually reached the height of 5 feet 4 inches and began her menses at the age of 16.

DISCUSSION OF TESTS

Growth hormone

(GH, human growth hormone [HGH], somatotropin hormone [SH])

Normal values:
- Men: <5 ng/ml or <5 μg/L (SI units)
- Women: <10 ng/ml or <10 μg/L
- Children: 0-10 ng/ml or 0-10 μg/L
- Newborn: 10-40 ng/ml or 10-40 μg/L

Rationale. Growth hormone (somatotropin) is secreted by the anterior pituitary gland and plays a central role in the modulation of growth from birth until the completion of puberty. In the total absence of growth hormone, linear growth occurs at one half to one third the normal rate. Growth hormone also plays a role in the control of body anabolism throughout life by increasing protein synthesis, increasing the breakdown of fatty acids in adipose tissue, and increasing the blood glucose level. The secretion of growth hormone is increased by stress, exercise, and low blood glucose. If secretion of growth hormone is insufficient during childhood, limited growth and dwarfism may result. Conversely, overproduction of growth hormone during childhood results in gigantism with a person reaching nearly 7 to 8 feet in height. An excess of growth hormone during adulthood results in acromegaly, a condition characterized by an increase in bone thickness and width, but no increase in height.

Growth hormone tests are used to confirm hypo- or hyperpituitarism. Because growth hormone secretion is episodic, random measurements are not adequate determinants of growth hormone deficiency. Screening for insulin-like growth factor (IGF-1), or somatomedin C (see p. 275), provides a more accurate reflection of the mean plasma concentration of growth hormone. Growth hormone stimulation tests (see p. 276) can be done to evaluate the ability of the body to produce growth hormone. Since about two thirds of the total production of growth hormone occurs during sleep, growth hormone secretion can also be measured during hospitalization by obtaining blood samples during sleep.

Elevated levels of GH may occur with gigantism, acromegaly, diabetes mellitus, anorexia nervosa, stress, and major surgery. Decreased levels occur with pituitary insufficiency and dwarfism.

Procedure. Peripheral venipuncture is performed and one red-top tube of blood is collected. It is preferred that the patient be fasting and well rested. The patient should not be under physical or mental stress since this can increase growth hormone levels.

Contraindications. None.

Nursing considerations

Nursing Diagnoses/Collaborative Problems

See Blood studies, p. 2.

Nursing Implications with Rationale

- Indicate the patient's fasting status and time blood is obtained on the lab slip. Remember random levels do not permit a firm diagnosis to be established.
- Apply pressure to the venipuncture site after the blood is drawn. Assess the site for bleeding.

Somatomedin C

(insulin-like growth factor, IGF-1)

Normal values:

Adults: 42-110 ng/ml

Children:	*Girls*	*Boys*
Age 0-8	7-110 ng/ml	4-87 ng/ml
9-10	39-186	26-98
11-13	66-215	44-207
14-16	96-256	48-255

Rationale. Because growth hormone (see p. 274) secretion is episodic, random measurements of plasma growth hormone are not adequate tests of growth hormone deficiency. Measuring somatomedin C is a good screening test for growth hormone deficiency since most patients with growth hormone deficiency have low somatomedin levels. The amount of somatomedin provides an indirect measure of the amount of growth hormone present. Somatomedins (also known as insulin-like growth factor) are the "middlemen" in the growth process. The majority of growth producing actions are mediated by somatomedin. Growth hormone stimulates the liver and other body tissues to produce somatomedin, which then induces growth.

Because somatomedin peptides are tightly bound to plasma proteins and have half-lives of hours rather than minutes, a random measurement provides an accurate reflection of mean plasma concentrations. Therefore, measurement of somatomedin C provides a reasonable screen for growth hormone deficiency. Low levels of somatomedin C should lead to a more extensive evaluation (such as growth hormone stimulation tests, see p. 276). Decreased levels also occur with Laron dwarfism, inactive growth hormone, and resistance to somatomedins. Increased concentrations are used to diagnose acromegaly and to evaluate tall stature.

Procedure. A peripheral venipuncture is performed and one lavender- or red-top tube of blood is collected. An overnight fast is preferred.

Contraindications. None.

Nursing considerations

Nursing Diagnoses/Collaborative Problems

See Blood studies, p. 2.

Nursing Implications with Rationale

- Apply pressure to the venipuncture site after the blood is drawn. Assess the site for bleeding.

Growth hormone stimulation test

(GH provocation test, insulin tolerance test [ITT])

Normal values: Growth hormone levels of 10 μg/L (10 ng/ml)

Rationale. Because growth hormone (see p. 274) secretion is episodic, random measurements of plasma growth hormone (GH) are not adequate tests of growth hormone deficiency. In order to diagnose growth hormone deficiency, growth hormone stimulation tests are indicated. One of the most reliable growth hormone stimulators is insulin-induced hypoglycemia in which the blood glucose declines to less than 40 mg/dl. Other growth hormone stimulants include vigorous exercise, and drugs such as arginine, glucagon, levodopa, and clonidine. For children, usually a double stimulated test is performed using an arginine infusion followed by insulin-induced hypoglycemia. A growth hormone concentration of >10 μg/L after stimulation effectively excludes growth hormone deficiency.

Procedure. Various agents such as insulin, arginine, glucagon, levodopa, and clonidine can be used to stimulate growth hormone production. For these tests, the patient remains NPO except for water after midnight on the morning of the test. A heparin lock intravenous line is inserted for the administration of medications and the withdrawal of frequent blood samples. Baseline blood levels are obtained for GH, glucose, and cortisol. Venous samples for growth hormone are obtained at 0, 60, and 90 minutes after injection of insulin or arginine. Blood glucose levels are monitored at 15- to 30-minute intervals with a glucometer. The blood sugar should drop to less than 40 mg/dl for effective measurement of GH reserve. The patient is monitored for signs of hypoglycemia, postural hypotension, and somnolence. At the end of the test, the patient receives cookies and punch or an intravenous glucose infusion.

Growth hormone can also be stimulated by vigorous exercise. This entails running or stairsteps for 20 minutes. Blood samples of growth hormone are obtained at 0, 20, and 40 minutes.

Contraindications. GH stimulation should not be performed on patients with epilepsy, cerebrovascular disease, myocardial infarction, and low basal plasma cortisol levels.

Nursing considerations

Nursing Diagnoses/Collaborative Problems

See Blood studies, p. 2.

Nursing Implications with Rationale

- Explain the procedure very carefully to the patient and parents, if appropriate. Most patients and their families are anxious regarding the possible diagnosis of growth hormone deficiency.
- Instruct the patient to remain NPO after midnight except for water on the morning of the test.
- During the test, monitor the patient for diaphoresis, nervousness, somnolence, and hypotension. Ice chips are often given during the test for patient comfort.
- After the test, observe the venipuncture site for bleeding.
- After the test, inform the patient and family that the results are generally not available for approximately 10 to 14 days. Most laboratories only run growth hormone tests once per week.

THYROID GLAND

ANATOMY AND PHYSIOLOGY

The thyroid gland (Figure 8-3) is located in the neck anterior to the thyroid-laryngeal cartilage. It is bilobal, with a narrow strip (isthmus) of glandular tissue connecting the lateral lobes and giving the gland an H-shaped appearance. Often a second narrow strip of tissue—the pyramidal lobe—extends upward from the isthmus. Embryologically the thyroid originates near the foramen cecum of the tongue and descends cau-

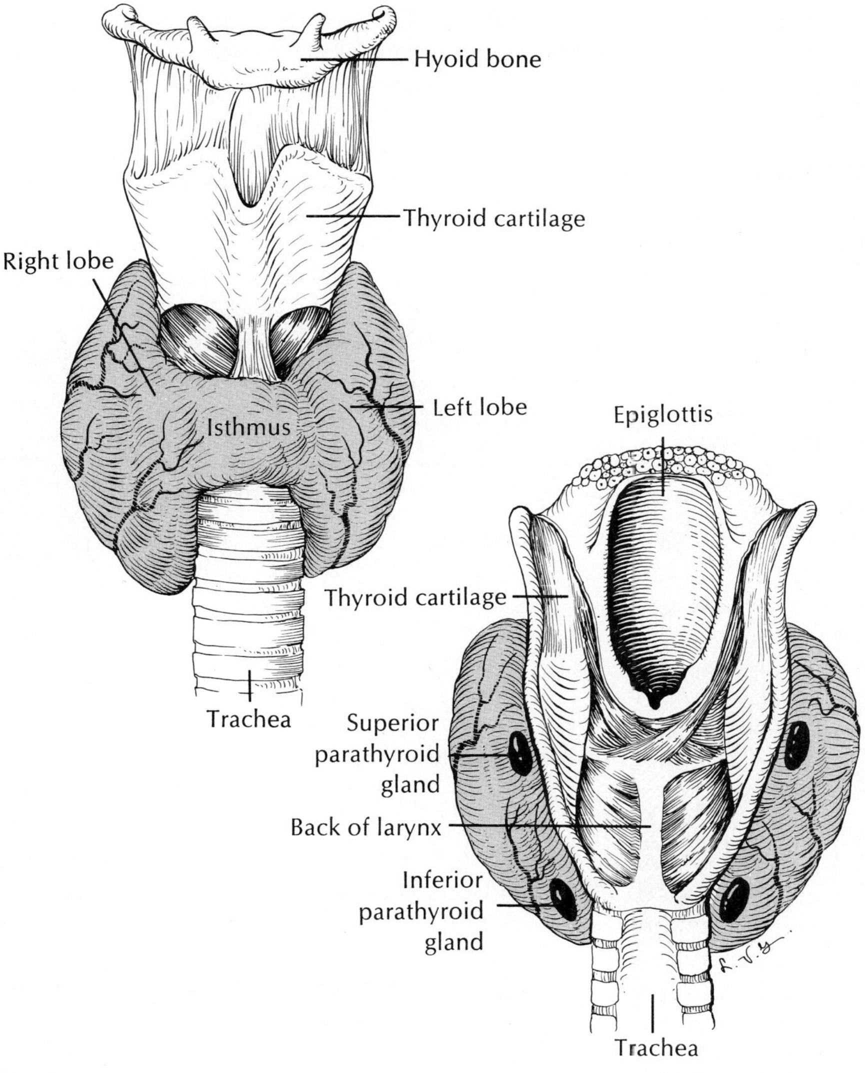

FIGURE 8-3. Anterior *(left)* and posterior *(right)* views of anatomical relationship of thyroid and parathyroid glands.

From Schottelius BA and Schottelius DD: Textbook of physiology, ed 18, St Louis, 1978, The CV Mosby Co.

dally to its place in the neck. Not infrequently ectopic thyroid tissue is found along that tract of descent or even more distally in the chest.

Microscopically the thyroid is composed of follicles lined by cuboidal-shaped epithelial cells. In the center of these follicles is a colloidal material (thyroglobulin) where thyroid hormones are stored. These follicular cells produce T_3 and T_4 hormones. Next to these follicular cells are parafollicular cells, or C cells. These C cells probably produce calcitonin, a calcium-lowering hormone (see p. 290).

Production, storage, and secretion of thyroid hormone

Dietary ingestion of iodine provides the iodide necessary for thyroid hormone synthesis. The plasma iodide is actively transformed to its organic form, I_2, which immediately becomes bound to thyroglobulin. The tyrosine radical of the thyroglobulin molecule combines with the organic iodine and becomes monoiodotyrosine or diiodotyrosine. A complicated coupling of a monoiodotyrosine and a diiodotyrosine makes triiodothyronine (T_3). A similar coupling of two diiodotyrosines makes thyroxine (T_4). T_4 contains four iodine atoms in each molecule, whereas T_3 contains only three. The hormones, still bound to thyroglobulin, are stored in their inactive states. When secretion is required, the thyroglobulin is broken off by proteinases secreted by the thyroid cells, and the free hormone is secreted into the plasma (Figure 8-4). The ratio of T_4 to T_3 in the serum is 20:1. Most

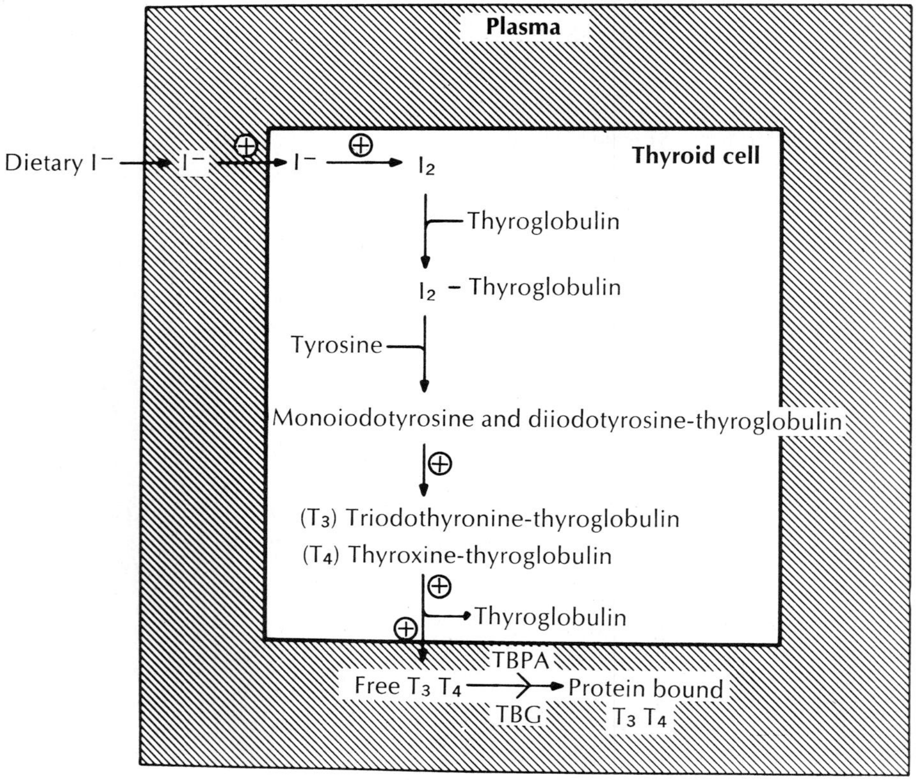

FIGURE 8-4. Thyroid hormone synthesis. Plus signs indicate steps that are enhanced or stimulated by thyroid-stimulating hormone. *TBPA*, Thyroid-binding prealbumin; *TBG*, thyroid-binding globulin.

of the T_4 (and some of the T_3) becomes bound to thyroid-binding globulin (TBG) and thyroid-binding prealbumin (TBPA). T_3 is the active form of the thyroid hormone.

Regulation of thyroid hormone production

When the blood levels of T_4 and T_3 fall, thyrotropin-releasing factor (TRF) or thyrotropin-releasing hormone (TRH) is secreted by the hypothalamus. TRH stimulates the anterior pituitary gland to secrete thyroid-stimulating hormone (TSH). TSH enhances many of the chemical reactions that occur during thyroid hormone synthesis (Figure 8-4). When the blood levels of T_3 and T_4 return to normal, the secretion of TRH is inhibited by a negative feedback mechanism. This feedback system promotes hormone regulation in a normal (or euthyroid) person.

In a normally functioning thyroid regulation system, one would expect the following:

1. When T_3 and T_4 levels are decreased, TRH and TSH levels should be increased unless the pituitary is not functional (as in panhypopituitarism or cretinism).
2. When T_3 and T_4 levels are increased, TRH and TSH levels should be decreased.

When adenomas or carcinomas of the thyroid are present, this regulatory function may be lost.

Thyroid disorders

Hyperthyroidism, or thyrotoxicosis, is the hypermetabolic state that occurs with excessive production of thyroid hormone. The most common cause of hyperthyroidism is Graves' disease. Other causes of hyperthyroidism include nodular toxic goiter (Plummer's disease), overtreatment with thyroid drugs, thyroid adenoma or carcinoma, and excessive secretion of TSH by a pituitary adenoma.

Hypothyroidism results when the thyroid gland produces too little of either or both of its hormones (T_3 and T_4). Major causes of hypothyroidism include:

1. Cretinism (a disorder of infancy and childhood caused by insufficient thyroid hormone during fetal or neonatal life). Newborn screening programs for the diagnosis of hypothyroidism include assays of T_4 and TSH.
2. Myxedema (the deficient synthesis of thyroid hormone in the adult).
3. Surgical removal of all thyroid tissue.
4. Radioactive iodine ablation of the thyroid.
5. Autoimmune destruction of the thyroid.

The most commonly used tests to evaluate *thyroid function* include the T_3, T_4, free thyroxine index, TSH assay, and the radioactive iodine uptake (RAIU) test. Tests used to evaluate *homeostatic controls and feedback mechanisms* include the thyroid-stimulating hormone test (TSH stimulation test) and the thyrotropin-releasing hormone test (TRH stimulation test). Many other laboratory tests are less commonly used but are of historical interest; tests no longer performed are deliberately excluded from this chapter.

CASE STUDY 2: THYROID NODULE

Mrs. H., 43 years old, went to her doctor complaining of a lump on her neck. She was asymptomatic. Physical examination revealed a mass in the lower pole of the left lobe of the thyroid gland.

Studies	Results
Routine laboratory work	WNL
T_4 test	8 μg/dl (normal: 4-11 μg/dl)
T_3 radioimmunoassay	115 ng/dl (normal: 110-130 ng/dl)
Radioactive iodine uptake (RAIU) test	20% (normal: 8% to 30%)
Thyroid scanning	Cold nodule in lower lobe of thyroid (normal: no nodules)
Ultrasound examination of thyroid	Mixed pattern of solid and cystic components (normal: normal size, shape, and position of the thyroid)

The normal values of T_3, T_4, and RAIU testing indicated that the patient was euthyroid (that is, not hyperthyroid or hypothyroid). This eliminated thyroid toxic adenoma or nodular goiter as a cause of the mass. The thyroid scan detected a nonfunctioning nodule in the thyroid, which could have been caused by cancer, cyst, or nontoxic goiters. Ultrasonography eliminated the possibility that this was merely a cyst. Surgery was performed to exclude cancer.

A left thyroid lobectomy was performed, with the patient under general anesthesia. Microscopic examination of the tissue indicated that the mass was a benign, nontoxic, multinodular goiter. Postoperatively the patient was given suppressive doses of thyroid extract and had no further problems.

DISCUSSION OF TESTS

Serum thyroxine test

(T_4 test)

Normal values:
- Murphy-Pattee technique:
  - Neonate: 10.1-20.0 μg/dl
  - 1-4 months: 7.5-16.5 μg/dl
  - 4-12 months: 5.5-14.5 μg/dl
  - 1-6 yr: 5.6—12.6 μg/dl
  - 6-10 yr: 4.9-11.7 μg/dl
  - >10 yr: 4-11 μg/dl
- Radioimmunoassay: 5-10 μg/dl

Rationale. The serum thyroxine study is a direct measurement of the total amount of T_4 present in the patient's blood. Greater than normal levels would indicate hyperthyroid states, as seen in Graves' disease, Plummer's disease, overdosage of thyroid medication, or toxic thyroid adenoma. Subnormal values are seen in hypothyroid states, such as cretinism or myxedema. Newborns are screened by T_4 tests to detect hypothyroidism.

This is a very reliable test of thyroid function. It is, however, affected by thyroid-binding globulin (TBG). Because T_4 is bound by serum proteins, any increase in these proteins (as in pregnant women and in patients taking oral contraceptives) will cause elevated levels of T_4 and to some extent T_3. The levels of these carrier proteins (such as TBG) can be measured by T_3 resin uptake studies (see following studies). This must be considered in interpreting T_4 test results. No complications are associated with this test.

Procedure. No special preparation is required. A peripheral venous blood specimen is obtained in a red-top tube and sent to the chemistry laboratory. A heel stick is done on newborns.

Two commonly used methods of determining T_4 concentrations in serum are competitive binding techniques and radioimmunoassay. The first is the Murphy-Pattee technique, in which the patient's serum (containing T_4) is mixed with a solution containing a known standard amount of tracer, or labeled, T_4. TBG is added to the mixture, and the two T_4 solutions compete for uptake by the TBG carrier protein. The greater the quantity of T_4 in the patient's serum, the smaller the quantity of tracer T_4 that can attach to the TBG. Therefore, by measuring the amount of free tracer T_4 and comparing it with a standard curve, the amount of T_4 in the patient's serum can be accurately estimated.

A second, more accurate, method of determining the quantity of T_4 in the blood is by radioimmunoassay. Antibodies to T_4 are produced by injecting T_4 into an animal. These antibodies are then tagged with a radioactive tracer and added to the patient's serum for binding. All T_4-bound antibodies are then separated out, measured, and compared with a curve, thus allowing for accurate estimation of the quantity of T_4 present in the patient's blood.

Contraindications. None.

Nursing considerations

Nursing Diagnoses/Collaborative Problems

See Blood studies, p. 2.

Nursing Implications with Rationale

- Explain the procedure to the patient.
- Evaluate the patient. Determine whether the patient is pregnant or taking any oral contraceptives, since these conditions will alter serum T_4 concentrations as a result of increased

amounts of estrogen. Also, be sure that the patient is not taking exogenous thyroxine medication, since this will affect the results. Notify the physician of any findings that may alter the accuracy of the study.

- After drawing the blood, apply pressure or a pressure dressing to the venipuncture site. Observe the site for bleeding.

Serum triiodothyronine test

(T_3 test)

Normal values:
Adult/elderly: 110-230 ng/dl or 1.2-1.5 nmol/L (SI units)
Newborn: 90-170 ng/dl
Child (6-12 yr): 115-190 ng/dl

Rationale. Like the T_4 test (see previous study), the serum T_3 test is an accurate measure of thyroid function. T_3 is less stable than T_4 and occurs in minute quantities in the active form. Generally when the T_3 level is below normal, the patient is in a hypothyroid state. The T_3 determination is clinically important in the patient who has a normal T_4 level but has all of the symptoms of hyperthyroidism. In this patient high T_3 levels may identify T_3 thyrotoxicosis.

Procedure. No special patient preparation is required. A peripheral venous sample is obtained in a red-top tube and sent to the chemistry lab. Radioimmunoassay with an antibody to T_3 is used for the determination (see radioimmunoassay of T_4). No complications are associated with this study.

Contraindications. None.

Nursing considerations

Nursing Diagnoses/Collaborative Problems

See Blood studies, p. 2.

Nursing Implications with Rationale

- Explain the procedure to the patient. Determine whether the patient is taking exogenous triiodothyronine medication, since this will affect the results.
- After the blood is drawn, apply pressure or a pressure dressing to the site. Observe the site for bleeding.

Radioactive iodine uptake test

(RAIU test)

Normal values:
2 hours: 4%-12% absorbed by thyroid
6 hours: 6%-15% absorbed by thyroid
24 hours: 8%-30% absorbed by thyroid

Rationale. The RAIU or radioactive iodine uptake test is a useful guide to thyroid function. It is based on the ability of the thyroid gland to trap and retain iodine. In this procedure a known quantity of radioactive iodine (^{131}I) or technetium is given orally to the patient. A gamma-ray detector (as is used in most nuclear scanning) determines the quantity or percentage of radioactive iodine taken up by the gland over a specific period of time.

Performing the measurement at different times after the iodine is given allows several aspects of thyroid function to be evaluated. Uptake determination at 30 minutes reflects the ability of the thyroid to trap iodine. When uptake is measured at 6 hours, the ability of the thyroid gland to organically bind iodine is evaluated. Maximum iodine uptake is observed within 24 hours. Determination of iodine uptake after this time measures the ability of the gland to release the iodine in the form of thyroid hormone. Routinely the RAIU test is performed 24 hours after iodine injection. Increased thyroid uptake of radioactive iodine is seen in hyperthyroid states, and decreased uptake occurs in hypothyroid conditions.

Several factors may artificially influence the results of this study. If the patient is iodine-deficient, the uptake will be markedly increased because the thyroid-trapping mechanism is maximally effective. Rebound thyroid stimulation after discontinuation of suppressive doses of thyroid extract or antithyroid drugs also falsely increases RAIU levels. Estrogen, phenothiazines, and lithium can fictitiously raise RAIU. Artificially decreased RAIU levels can be seen in patients taking suppressive doses of thyroid extract or antithyroid drugs. Similarly, previous intake of iodine (such as radiopaque dye) increases the iodine pool and relatively decreases the uptake of the radioactive iodine by the thyroid. Patients with diarrhea have decreased absorption of tracer doses in the gastrointestinal tract, thereby decreasing RAIU levels in test results.

Radioactive exposure to the thyroid is the only complication to this procedure. This is minimized when ^{123}I or ^{125}I is used instead of ^{131}I.

Procedure. The patient is asked to eat a light breakfast and to report to the nuclear medicine laboratory. (Some laboratories prefer the patient fasts overnight.) A short history including dietary habits, recent medications, and previous x-ray contrast study results is obtained. A tasteless, standard dose of radioactive iodine (usually ^{123}I) is given by mouth. If RAIU is to be determined at 2 hours, the iodine must be administered intravenously. The patient is then asked to return to the laboratory anywhere from 2 to 24 hours later (usually 24 hours). On return, the patient lies in the supine position, and a counter is placed over him or her. The amount of radioactive iodine accumulated in the thyroid is calculated. The uptake of the iodine is expressed as a percentage of the thyroid uptake compared with the total of the administered dose.

$$\text{RAIU} = \frac{\text{Neck count of patient}}{\text{Standard dose given}} \times 100\%$$

The test is not uncomfortable and takes only 30 minutes to perform. A technician performs the study and computes the uptake. The physician interprets the results.

Contraindications. The RAIU test is contraindicated in the following:

1. Patients who have taken thyroid or antithyroid drugs
2. Patients who have had recent x-ray dye studies
3. Pregnant patients
4. Patients taking exogenous iodine preparations because this iodine increases the body's iodine pool and decreases uptake by the gland
5. Patients who have recently had radioactive studies.

Nursing considerations

Nursing Diagnoses/Collaborative Problems

See Nuclear scanning, p. 5.

Nursing Implications with Rationale

- Explain the procedure to the patient. Be sure that the patient understands the exact time that he or she must return to the laboratory. Question the patient concerning his or her intake of iodine or thyroid hormones. Assess the patient's intake of large amounts of iodine in food (fish, shellfish), drugs (saturated solution of potassium iodine, Lugol's solution, tolbutamide), antiseptics containing iodine, and iodinated contrast materials used in x-ray studies. Note the usage of thyroid or antithyroid drugs, TSH, estrogen, or barbiturates. These iodine and thyroid preparations should be restricted for 1 week before testing. Inform the physician of any pertinent findings.
- Advise the patient of restrictions necessary before the study. Some hospitals prefer the patient be in the fasting state before taking the tracer dose. The patient is allowed to eat 45 minutes later.
- Assure the patient that the dose of radioiodine used in this test is minute and therefore harmless. No isolation is necessary.

Thyroid scanning

(thyroid scintiscan)

Normal values: normal size, shape, position, and function of the thyroid gland; no areas of decreased or increased uptake

Rationale. The thyroid scanning test allows the size, shape, position, and anatomic function of the thyroid gland to be determined with the use of radionuclear scanning (Figure 8-5). A radioactive substance (such as iodine or prefera-

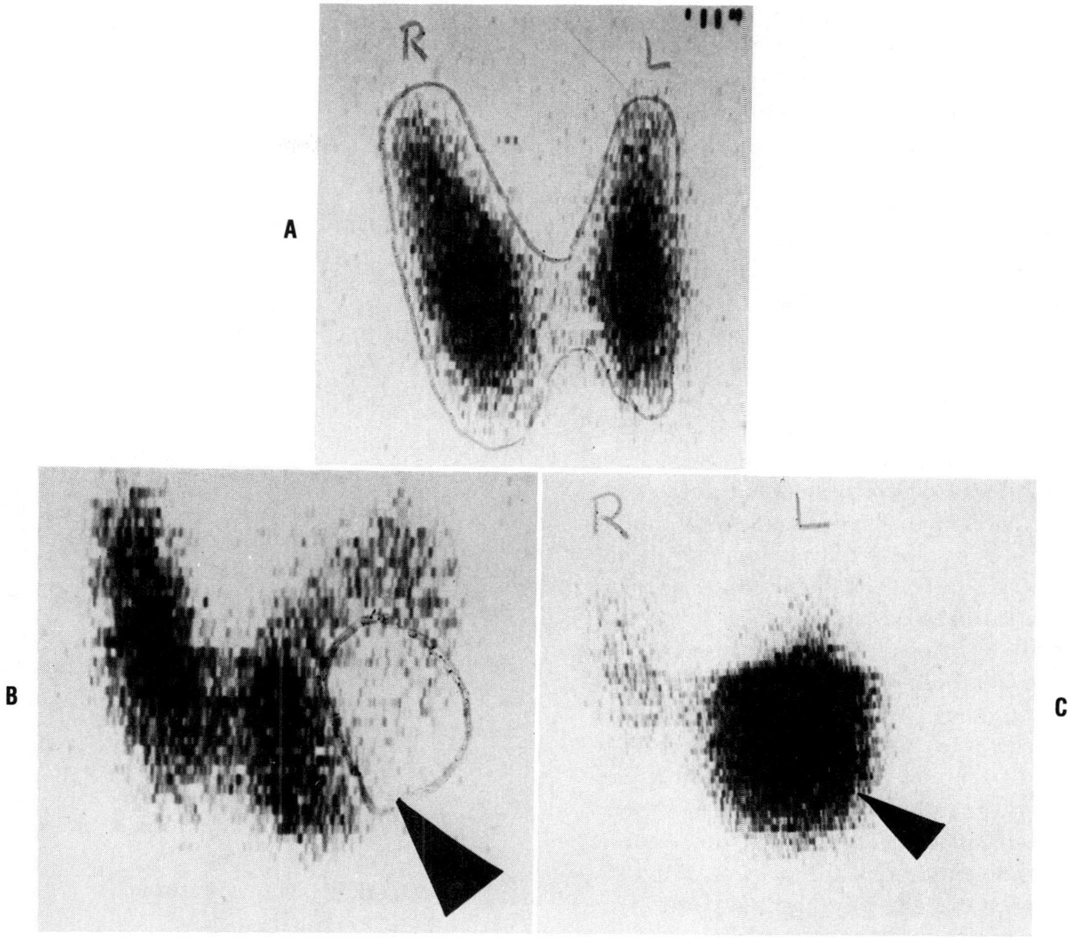

FIGURE 8-5. **A,** Normal thyroid scan. **B,** "Cold" area *(pointer)* on thyroid scan. **C,** "Hot" area *(pointer)* on thyroid scan.

bly technetium) is given to the patient to demonstrate uptake or lack of uptake by the thyroid gland. A scanner is passed over the neck area, making a graphic record, as a photograph or an x-ray film, of the radiation emitted. Areas of increased or decreased uptake are demonstrated.

Thyroid nodules are easily detected by this technique. Nodules are classified as functioning (warm/hot) or nonfunctioning (cold), depending on the amount of radionuclide taken up by the nodule. A functioning nodule could represent benign adenoma or localized toxic goiter. A nonfunctioning nodule, on the other hand, may represent a cyst, carcinoma, nonfunctioning adenoma or goiter, lymphoma, or localized area of thyroiditis.

Scanning is useful in:

1. Patients with a neck mass or substernal mass. Scanning can determine whether the mass is arising from within or outside of the thyroid.
2. Patients who have a thyroid nodule. Scanning indicates the nodule's function, thereby narrowing its possible causes. Thyroid cancers are almost always nonfunctioning (cold) nodules.

3. Patients who have hyperthyroidism. Scanning assists in differentiating the two forms of hyperthyroidism: Graves' disease (diffusely enlarged hyperfunctioning thyroid gland) or Plummer's disease (nodular hyperfunctioning gland). Scanning is also useful in evaluating the success of medical therapy. With successful treatment the gland is expected to get smaller.
4. Patients who have evidence of metastatic tumor without a known primary site. Scanning may demonstrate a primary thyroid tumor.
5. Patients who have a well-differentiated form of thyroid cancer. Areas of metastasis show up on a subsequent nuclear scan of the body because the metastatic tumor retains its ability to trap iodine or technetium.

Radiation-induced oncogenesis is the only complication associated with this study. This complication is eliminated if technetium is used instead of iodine.

Procedure. No patient preparation is required. The patient is taken to the nuclear medicine department. A history concerning previous IV contrast x-ray studies, nuclear scanning, or intake of any thyroid suppressive or antithyroid drugs is taken. As in the RAIU test, recent intake of these agents markedly affects the outcome of the scanning. A standard dose of radioactive iodine or technetium is given by mouth. The capsule is tasteless. Scanning is performed 24 hours later. If technetium is used, scanning is performed 2 hours later. A rectilinear gamma-ray detector is passed over the thyroid area, and the radioactive counts are recorded and displayed in the image of the thyroid gland. The image appears as a photograph or an x-ray film, depending on the technique used. This study is performed by a technician, and the results are interpreted by a physician. No discomfort is associated with this study, which is performed in approximately 30 minutes.

Contraindications. See RAIU test, p. 282.

Nursing considerations

Nursing Diagnoses/Collaborative Problems

See Nuclear scanning, p. 5.

Nursing Implications with Rationale

- See RAIU test, pp. 281-282.

Ultrasound examination of the thyroid

(thyroid echogram)

Normal values: normal size, shape, and position of the thyroid.

Rationale. As with other ultrasound studies, a nonfunctioning thyroid nodule can be evaluated with the use of reflected sound waves (see p. 104). Ultrasound examination of the thyroid is valuable for distinguishing cystic from solid nodules. If the nodule is found to be purely cystic and fluid filled, the fluid can simply be aspirated. Surgery is avoided. However, if the nodule has a mixed or solid appearance, carcinoma is a good possibility and surgery may be necessary for diagnosis and treatment.

This study may also be repeated at intervals to determine the response of a thyroid mass to medical therapy. No complications are associated with this study. It is a test of choice for pregnant patients, since radioactive iodine is harmful to the fetus.

Procedure. The nonfasting, unsedated patient is taken to the ultrasonography department (usually in the radiology department) and placed in the supine position. Gel is applied to the patient's neck. An ultrasound technician passes a sound transducer over the nodule. Photographs are taken of the image displayed, and these are evaluated by the ultrasound physician. No discomfort is associated with this study. It is usually performed in about 15 minutes.

Contraindications. None.

Nursing considerations

Nursing Diagnoses/Collaborative Problems

See Ultrasound studies, p. 6.

Nursing Implications with Rationale

- Explain the procedure to the patient. Assure the patient that no discomfort is associated with this study. Tell the patient that breathing and swallowing will not be affected by the placement of a transducer on the neck.
- Tell the patient that a liberal amount of lubricant will be applied to the neck to ensure effective transmission and reception of the sound waves.
- After the study help the patient remove the lubricant from his or her neck.

SUPPLEMENTAL INFORMATION

Free thyroxine index

(FTI)

Normal values: 0.8-2.4 ng/dl or 10-31 pmol/L (SI units)

Rationale. The free thyroxine index study measures the amount of free T_4, which is only a fraction of the total T_4. The free T_4 is the unbound T_4 that enters the cell and is metabolically active. The diagnostic value of measuring the free T_4 level is that it is not affected by TBG abnormalities; therefore, it correlates more closely with the true hormonal status than T_4 or T_3 determinations do.

To determine the FTI, the T_3 uptake is measured and multiplied by the measured serum T_4 concentration. This simple mathematical computation corrects the estimated total T_4 assay for the effects of TBG protein alterations.

This index is useful in diagnosing hyperthyroidism and hypothyroidism, especially in persons with abnormalities in TBG levels. High FTI calculations suggest hyperthyroidism; low FTI values suggest hypothyroidism. The FTI study also aids in the evaluation of the thyroid status of pregnant women and patients who have abnormal TBG levels and are being treated with certain drugs (such as estrogen, phenytoin, salicylates).

Procedure. T_3 uptake multiplied by T_4 equals FTI.

Contraindications. None.

Nursing considerations

Nursing Diagnoses/Collaborative Problems

See T_3, RAIU, and T_4 tests, pp. 280-282.

Nursing Implications with Rationale

- See serum T_3, RAIU, and T_4 tests.

Thyrotropin-releasing hormone test

(TRH test, thyrotropin-releasing factor test, TRF)

Normal value: prompt rise in serum TSH level to approximately twice the baseline level by 30 minutes after the dose of an IV bolus of TRH (response is normally greater in women)

Rationale. The TRH, or thyrotropin-releasing hormone test, assesses the responsiveness of the anterior pituitary gland via its secretion of thyrotropin-stimulating hormone (TSH) to an IV injection of thyrotropin-releasing hormone (TRH). After the TRH injection, the normally functioning pituitary gland should secrete TSH. In addition to assessing the responsiveness of the anterior pituitary gland, this study aids in the detection of primary, secondary, and tertiary hypothyroidism.

In hyperthyroidism either a slight increase or no increase in the TSH level is seen, because pituitary TSH production is suppressed by the direct effect of excessive circulating T_4 and T_3 on the pituitary. A normal result is considered reliable evidence for excluding the diagnosis of thyrotoxicosis. The TRH test is one of the most reliable confirmatory procedures for hyperthyroidism. (Other tests are often compared to it to detect their accuracy.) In primary hypothyroidism (thyroid gland failure) the increase in the TSH level is two or more times the normal result. This may make this test useful in patients with equivocal symptoms and equivocal serum TSH levels. With secondary hypothyroidism (anterior pituitary failure) there is no TSH response. Tertiary hypothyroidism (hypothalamic failure) may be diagnosed by a delayed rise in the TSH level. Multiple injections of TRH may be needed to induce the appropriate TSH response in this case.

Certain conditions (such as psychiatric primary depression, acute starvation and old age, especially in men) and medications (aspirin, levodopa, or adrenocorticosteroids) depress the TSH response to TRH. Thyroid preparation should be discontinued 3 to 4 weeks before a TRH test.

TRH may also be useful in differentiating primary depression from manic-depressive psychiatric illness and from secondary types of depression. In primary depression the TSH response is blunted in the majority of patients, while patients with other types of depression have a normal TRH-induced TSH response.

Procedure. No fasting or sedation is required. A 500 μg bolus of TRH is given intravenously. Venous blood samples are obtained at intervals and measured for TSH levels. The maximum response usually occurs in 20 minutes. The TSH concentration should return to normal within 2 hours.

Contraindications. None.

Nursing considerations

Nursing Diagnoses/Collaborative Problems

See Blood studies, p. 2.

Nursing Implications with Rationale

- Explain the procedure to the patient. Check with your laboratory for the specific protocol for carrying out this test.
- Indicate on the lab slip if the patient is pregnant. The TSH response to TRH is increased during pregnancy.
- Assess the patient for medications currently being taken. T_4, antithyroid drugs, estrogens, corticosteroids, or levodopa can modify the TSH response.

T_3 resin uptake test

(RT_3U test, triiodothyronine uptake test)

Normal values: 25% to 35%

Rationale. The T_3 resin uptake (RT_3U) test allows the quantity of thyroid-binding globulin (TBG) and thyroid-binding prealbumin (TBPA) to be measured indirectly in the blood. Pregnancy, birth control pills, and some genetic disorders tend to raise inappropriately the quantity of these carrying proteins. As a result, T_4 and T_3 levels may be artificially elevated, and yet the patient may be euthyroid. Similarly, androgenic hormones, intercurrent serious illness, and nephrotic syndromes tend to lower the quantity of these proteins, thereby causing falsely low T_3 and T_4 levels in euthyroid patients. Therefore, accurate assessment of the patient's thyroid status requires measurement of the TBG and TBPA levels, as RT_3U testing does.

In this procedure a blood sample is obtained, and radiolabeled T_3 is added to the patient's serum. A particulate material (resin) capable of binding T_3 is also added. The labeled T_3 apportions itself to the binding proteins (resin) in the same ratio as the patient's own T_3 does. The percentage of labeled T_3 absorption by the resin is then calculated. The more protein-binding sites available (that is, TBG and TBPA) for T_3, the less labeled T_3 is found on the resin. Thus the proportion of labeled hormone taken up by the resin varies inversely with the quantity of TBG and TBPA present in the patient's serum.

Procedure. This test requires only peripheral venous blood collection in a red-top tube. At present TBG and TBPA levels can be directly and accurately measured in the patient's serum, thereby obviating the need for the RT_3U test in most cases.

Contraindications. None.

Nursing considerations

Nursing Diagnoses/Collaborative Problems

See Blood studies, p. 2.

Nursing Implications with Rationale

- Assess the venipuncture site for bleeding.

Thyroid-stimulating hormone test

(TSH test, thyrotropin hormone)

Normal values:
Adult: 2-10 U/ml or 2-10 mU/L (SI units)

Newborn: 3-18 U/ml or 3-18 mU/L (SI units)
Cord: 3-12 U/ml or 3-12 mU/L (SI units)
Values vary between laboratories

Rationale. The TSH concentration aids in differentiating "primary" from "secondary" hypothyroidism. As described in the section on anatomy and physiology of the thyroid, pituitary TSH secretion is stimulated by hypothalamic TRH. Low levels of T_3 and T_4 are the underlying stimuli for TRH and TSH. Therefore, there is a compensatory elevation of TRH and TSH in patients in primary hypothyroid states, such as surgical or radioactive thyroid ablation; patients with burned-out thyroiditis, thyroid agenesis, or congenital cretinism; or patients taking antithyroid medications.

In secondary hypothyroidism, the function of the hypothalamus or pituitary is faulty (because of tumor, trauma, or infarction). Therefore, TRH and TSH cannot be secreted, and plasma levels of these hormones consequently decline to near zero.

The TSH test is also used to evaluate and monitor exogenous thyroid replacement in patients with primary hypothyroidism. This test is also done on newborns who have low screening T_4 levels for the detection of primary hypothyroidism. TSH and T_4 levels are frequently measured to differentiate pituitary from thyroid dysfunction. A decreased T_4 and normal or elevated TSH level can indicate a thyroid disorder. A decreased T_4 with a decreased TSH can indicate a pituitary disorder.

Procedure. Five milliliters of peripheral venous blood is collected in a red-top tube. A heel stick is done on newborns.

Contraindications. None.

Nursing considerations

Nursing Diagnoses/Collaborative Problems

See Blood studies, p. 2.

Nursing Implications with Rationale

- Explain the purpose of the test to the patient or to the mother of the newborn.
- No food or drink restrictions are necessary.
- Assess the venipuncture site for bleeding.

TSH stimulation test

(thyroid-stimulating hormone stimulation test)

Normal value: increased thyroid function with administration of exogenous TSH

Rationale. The TSH stimulation test is used to differentiate "primary," or thyroidal, hypothyroidism from "secondary," or hypothalamic-pituitary, hypothyroidism (see p. 279). Healthy persons and patients with hypothalamic-pituitary hypothyroidism are capable of increasing thyroid function when exogenous TSH is given. However, patients with primary thyroidal hypothyroidism are not. Their thyroid is inadequate and cannot function no matter how much stimulation it receives.

Procedure. Baseline levels of RAIU and T_4 (or protein-bound iodine) are obtained. Five to 10 units/day of TSH is administered intramuscularly for 3 days. Patients with less than a 10% increase in RAIU or less than a 1.5 μg/dl rise in T_4 are considered to have a primary cause for their hypothyroid state. If the initially low uptake is caused by inadequate pituitary stimulation of an intrinsically normal thyroid (that is, if the patient's condition is secondary hypothyroidism), the RAIU level should increase at least 10% and the T_4 level should rise 1.5 μg/dl or more.

Contraindications. None.

Nursing considerations

Nursing Diagnoses/Collaborative Problems

See RAIU and T_4, p. 280.

Nursing Implications with Rationale

- Attain the baseline levels of RAIU or T_4 as indicated.
- Administer the TSH intramuscularly for 3 days and then obtain repeat levels of the RAIU or T_4.
- After the blood is drawn, assess the venipuncture site for bleeding.

Antithyroglobulin antibody test

(thyroid autoantibody test)

Normal value: titer <1:100

Rationale. The serum antithyroglobulin titer evaluation detects the presence of thyroid antibodies formed in response to the thyroglobulin released from the thyroid gland in certain destructive thyroid disorders. These autoantibodies combine with thyroglobulin and cause inflammation of the thyroid gland. These thyroid antibodies indicate the existence of an autoimmune disease and may be responsible for further destruction of the thyroid gland.

This test is primarily used in the differential diagnosis of thyroid diseases such as Hashimoto's thyroiditis. The level must be extremely high to confirm the diagnosis of Hashimoto's thyroiditis. Increased antithyroglobulin antibodies are also seen with rheumatoid-collagen disease, pernicious anemia, thyrotoxicosis (Graves' disease), and lupus erythematosus.

Procedure. Peripheral venipuncture is performed, and approximately 3 to 5 ml of blood is obtained in a red-top tube.

Contraindications. None.

Nursing considerations

Nursing Diagnoses/Collaborative Problems

See Blood studies, p. 2.

Nursing Implications with Rationale

- Assess the venipuncture site for bleeding.

Antithyroid microsomal antibody test

(antimicrosomal antibody test, microsomal antibody)

Normal value: titer <1:100 (present in 5% to 10% of healthy people)

Rationale. The antithyroid microsomal antibody test measures for the detection of thyroid microsomal antibodies, which are found in the majority of patients with Hashimoto's thyroiditis. Microsomal antibodies are produced in response to microsomes escaping from the epithelial cells surrounding the thyroid follicle. These escaped microsomes then act as antigens and give rise to antibodies, which have cytotoxic effects on the thyroid follicle.

In addition to Hashimoto's thyroiditis, elevated titers are seen in patients with myxedema, thyroid carcinoma, granulomatous thyroiditis, lupus erythematosus, rheumatoid arthritis, autoimmune hemolytic anemia, and nontoxic nodular goiter.

Procedure. Venipuncture is performed, and approximately 3 to 5 ml of venous blood is obtained.

Contraindications. None.

Nursing considerations

Nursing Diagnoses/Collaborative Problems

See Blood studies, p. 2.

Nursing Implications with Rationale

- Assess the venipuncture site for bleeding.

Long-acting thyroid stimulator

(LATS)

Normal value: normally long-acting thyroid stimulator does not appear in serum

Rationale. The long-acting thyroid stimulator antibody is an immunoglobulin directed against some aspect of the thyroid cell plasma membrane. LATS mimics the action of TSH. It stimulates the thyroid gland to produce and secrete excessive amounts of thyroid hormones. It inhibits TSH secretion through the normal negative feedback mechanism. This factor is found in the blood of some hyperthyroid patients. Assessment for LATS is important in the evaluation of some patients with thyroid disease, especially patients with malignant exophthalmos and Graves' disease. Because LATS crosses the placenta, it may be found in neonates whose mothers have Graves' disease.

Procedure. No fasting or special preparation is required. A peripheral venipuncture is made, and approximately 5 ml of blood is drawn in a red-top tube and sent to the laboratory for analysis. The laboratory should be notified if ^{131}I has been administered to the patient within the preceding 2 days.

Contraindications. None.

Nursing considerations

Nursing Diagnoses/Collaborative Problems

See Blood studies, p. 2.

Nursing Implications with Rationale

- Assess the patient to see if he or she has had radioactive iodine within the past 2 days, since this may affect the test results.
- Handle the blood sample gently. Hemolysis may interfere with test result interpretation.

PARATHYROID GLANDS

ANATOMY AND PHYSIOLOGY

Most people have four parathyroid glands, with a pair located behind each lobe of the thyroid gland (Figure 8-3). The location of the parathyroids is not constant, although in most people, all four glands are found in the neck. The parathyroid glands can, however, occur anywhere from the base of the tongue to the mediastinum. This sometimes presents a surgical problem when the surgeon attempts to locate these tiny (7 mm) glands.

Microscopically the glands are composed of oxyphil cells, chief cells, and water-clear cells. The first are considered by some to be inactive, whereas the other cells actively secrete parathormone (parathyroid hormone) (PTH). This hormone is one of the major factors in the control of calcium metabolism (see following section). PTH increases serum calcium levels by causing:

1. Increased bone resorption
2. Increased calcium absorption from the intestines
3. Increased tubular reabsorption of calcium in the kidney
4. Increased phosphate excretion, which indirectly raises the serum calcium level

The most potent stimulus to PTH secretion is low serum calcium levels. As the serum calcium level decreases, the parathyroids are stimulated to secrete PTH. This in turn raises the serum calcium level. The increased calcium level then acts as a negative feedback inhibitor and "turns off" PTH secretion, thus maintaining normal calcium levels.

So-called primary hyperparathyroidism can be the result of parathyroid hyperplasia or tumor (adenoma or carcinoma). In these diseases both the serum calcium and serum PTH levels are high (Figure 8-6).

"Secondary" hyperparathyroidism occurs in patients with a buildup of serum phosphates (for example, because of renal failure). The phosphate levels vary inversely with calcium levels; this chronic increase in phosphate levels causes a chronically low serum calcium level. The resulting hypocalcemia acts as a powerful stimulus for PTH secretion and causes the parathyroids to become maximally stimulated to produce PTH, resulting in compensatory parathyroid hyperplasia. Thus in patients with renal failure, the serum calcium level is usually low despite the high serum PTH level. The patient experiences very severe bone weakening.

The phosphate and calcium levels return to normal when the patient is no longer in renal failure (because of transplant, dialysis, or healing of the primary renal injury or disease). However, the parathyroids are occasionally unable to decrease their overstimulation despite the new (normal) calcium levels. Therefore, they continue to secrete high levels of PTH. This is called "tertiary" hyperparathyroidism. It results in hypercalcemia and high PTH levels, much the same as in primary hyperparathyroidism.

Tumor of the lung, thymus, kidney, or pancreas can secrete a PTH-like substance that can cause severe hypercalcemia (paraneoplastic syndrome). Patients with this disorder will also have increased levels of calcium and PTH.

The most common cause of hypoparathyroidism is infarction or removal of the parathyroid during thyroid or parathyroid surgery. Autoim-

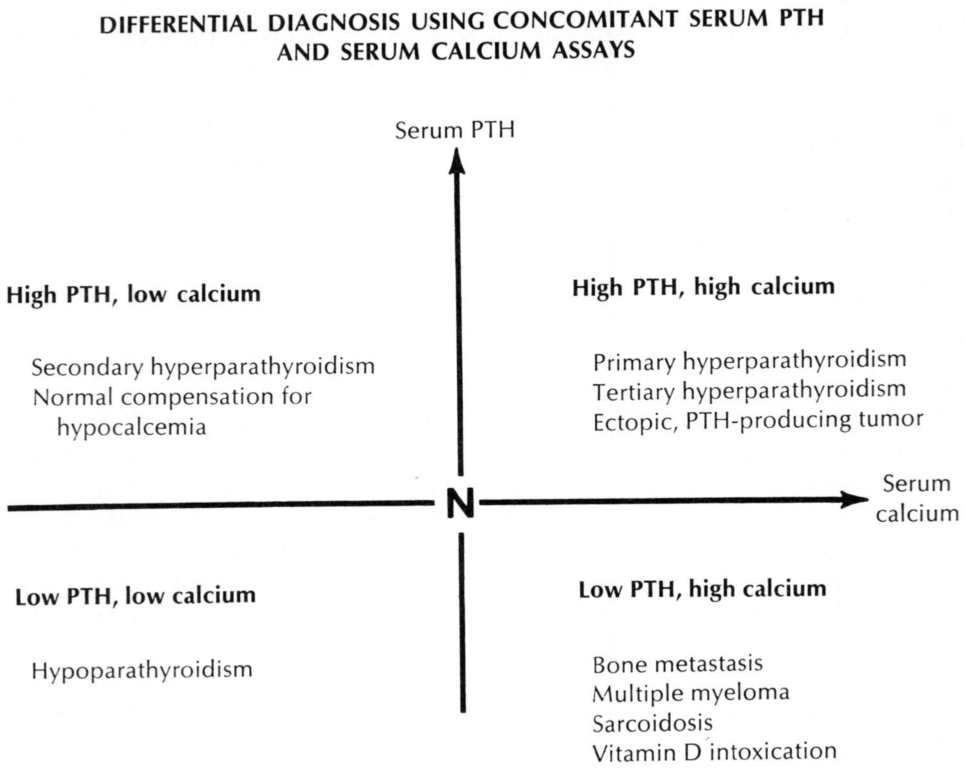

FIGURE 8-6. Graph showing various disease entities associated with concomitantly abnormal PTH and calcium levels. *N*, Normality, which is marked by eucalcemia and a normal PTH level.

mune destruction has rarely been reported. (This is seen only in young patients when it does occur.)

Calcium metabolism

Ingested calcium is actively absorbed by the intestinal mucosa. This absorption is facilitated by the action of activated vitamin D and PTH. Calcium exists in the blood in a free ionized form and in a bound (to albumin) form. The ionized calcium is the physiologically active form used in nerve conduction and in skeletal and cardiac muscle contractility. There are large stores of calcium in the bone. PTH can mobilize these stores by stimulating bone resorption, thus raising serum calcium levels. Calcitonin (secreted by the parafollicular cells of the thyroid glands) lowers the serum calcium and phosphate levels by inhibiting bone resorption, thus acting as an antagonist to PTH. Calcium is excreted in the urine and stool. Here again PTH acts to increase serum calcium levels.

Vitamin D is another principal factor in calcium homeostasis. Vitamin D is produced by sunlight irradiation of the skin. This inactive form of the vitamin is then hydroxylated, first in the liver and then in the kidney. The hydroxylated form is the active form that increases intestinal absorption of calcium. Patients with renal failure are unable to hydroxylate vitamin D, which contributes to their hypocalcemia.

Hypercalcemia can be caused by many disorders other than hyperparathyroidism. These include metastatic and primary tumors of the bone; nonparathyroid, ectopic, PTH-producing tumors; vitamin D intoxication; sarcoidosis; and milk-alkali syndrome. These disorders can be differentiated by determinations of concomitant serum calcium and PTH levels (Figure 8-6).

Symptoms of hypercalcemia vary from complete absence of symptoms to nausea, vomiting, anorexia, polyuria, dehydration, muscle weakness, coma, and death. Hypercalcemia is considered to be a contributing factor in pancreatitis, peptic ulcers, renal stone formation, and pathologic fractures. With the widespread use of multichannel serum-testing machines, more asymptomatic patients are being recognized.

Hypocalcemia is most frequently caused by renal disease, hypoparathyroidism, or low serum albumin levels (see p. 99). Symptoms of hypocalcemia include increased neuromuscular excitability (tetany, carpal pedal spasms, convulsions, or laryngeal spasms). Milder forms may present as paresthesia, muscle cramps, numbness, dysphagia, or dysarthria.

CASE STUDY 3: HYPERPARATHYROIDISM

Mr. O., 42 years old, was found to have hypercalcemia after a blood test taken during a routine physical examination at work. He was completely asymptomatic, and the results of a physical examination were negative.

Studies	Results
Routine laboratory work	Normal except for: Serum calcium: 12.8 mg/dl (normal: 9.0-10.5 mg/dl) Phosphorus: 1.4 mg/dl (normal: 2.5-4.5 mg/dl)
Serum parathormone (PTH) test	4020 pg/ml (normal: <2000 pg/ml)
Cortisone administration test (Dent test)	No change in calcium
Serum phosphorus	1.8 mg/dl (normal: 2.5-4.5 mg/dl)
Tubular phosphate reabsorption	65% (normal: 80%-90%)
X-ray study of skull and hands	Normal: no bone resorption
Intravenous pyelography (see Chapter 7)	Normal: no renal calculi

Although the patient was completely asymptomatic, he had significant hypercalcemia. Concomitantly elevated PTH levels indicated that his hypercalcemia was the result of primary hyperparathyroidism. The cortisone administration test reinforced this diagnosis, as did the serum phosphorus and the tubular phosphate reabsorption test. X-ray films of the skull and hands (the most common locations of bone resorption caused by hyperparathyroidism) were negative, indicating that the hyperparathyroidism was not of long duration. A normal IVP excluded the possibility of a PTH-producing renal tumor and ruled out renal stone formation.

The patient underwent extensive neck exploration, and only three small parathyroid glands were found. No further surgery was performed.

Postoperatively neck and chest venous PTH assays were performed. PTH levels in all neck veins were below 2000 pg/ml. However, the PTH in the superior vena cava was 8654 pg/ml. This indicated that a fourth parathyroid gland was still encased in the chest. The patient underwent exploration of the mediastinum. A large parathyroid benign adenoma was found and excised. Postoperatively the patient had no difficulties, and his calcium level returned to normal.

DISCUSSION OF TESTS

Serum calcium test

(total serum calcium)

Normal values:
- Adult (total): 9.0-10.5 mg/dl or 2.25-2.75 mmol/L (SI units)
  (ionized): 4.5-5.6 mg/dl or 1.05-1.30 mmol/L (SI units)
- Elderly: values slightly decreased
- Child (total): 8.8-10.8 mg/dl or 2.2-2.7 mmol/L (SI units)
- Newborn (total): 9.0-10.6 mg/dl or 2.3-2.65 mmol/L (SI units)
- Umbilical cord (total): 9.0-11.5 mg/dl or 2.25-2.88 mmol/L (SI units)

Possible critical values:
- <6 mg/dl (may lead to tetany)
- >14 mg/dl (may lead to coma)

Rationale. The serum calcium test is used to evaluate parathyroid function and calcium metabolism by directly measuring the total amount of calcium in the blood. Total calcium exists in the blood in its free (ionized) form and in its protein-bound form (with albumin). The serum calcium level is a measure of both. As a result, when the serum albumin level is low, the serum calcium level is also low and vice versa. As a rule of thumb, the total serum calcium level decreases by approximately 0.8 mg for every 1 g decrease in the serum albumin level.

When the serum calcium level is elevated on three separate determinations, the patient is said to have hypercalcemia. The causes of hypercalcemia include metastatic tumor to the bone, hyperparathyroidism, nonparathyroid PTH-producing tumors (such as lung and renal carcinomas), vitamin D intoxication, sarcoidosis, and excessive ingestion of concentrated milk or calcium-containing antacids. Thiazide diuretics, hydralazine, and lithium may cause hypercalcemia. It is important to differentiate these disorders. Hyperparathyroidism can be confirmed by a serum parathormone blood level determination (Figure 8-6).

Hypocalcemia is seen in patients who have hypoparathyroidism (usually following parathyroid surgery) and in those with renal failure or rickets. Anticonvulsants, aspirin, steroids, heparin, loop diuretics, oral contraceptives, and magnesium salts can lower calcium levels. Because calcium and phosphorus exist in the blood in an inversely proportional relationship, hyperphosphatemia secondary to renal failure is associated with hypocalcemia. In these patients, serum PTH levels are elevated (Figure 8-6). There are no complications that are associated with this test.

The ionized form of calcium can also be measured (normal values: 4.5-5.6 mg/dl at a pH of 7.4). An advantage of measuring the ionized calcium is that it is unaffected by changes in serum albumin levels, just as the total serum calcium is. Some physicians consider the measurement of the ionized calcium as more sensitive and reliable than that of the total calcium level in the detection of primary hyperparathyroidism. However, there is not total agreement on this. Most laboratories do not have the equipment to perform the ionized calcium assay.

Procedure. Approximately 7 ml of peripheral venous blood is obtained from a nonfasting patient and placed in a red-top tube. The blood is then transported to the clinical chemistry laboratory. Usually the serum calcium determinations are part of a multiple-chemical analysis done automatically by a machine (see Chapter 14). The patient may be kept fasting for multichannel examinations.

The only discomfort associated with this test is that of the venipuncture.

Contraindications. None.

Nursing considerations

Nursing Diagnoses/Collaborative Problems

See Blood studies, p. 2.

Nursing Implications with Rationale

- Explain the test to the patient. If fasting is required (for multichannel determinations), inform the patient. Assess the patient for concurrent use of thiazide diuretics, which can cause hypercalcemia.
- Perform a peripheral venipuncture and draw the blood. Apply pressure or a pressure dressing to the site, and observe the site for bleeding.
- Usually this test is done on a multichannel laboratory machine that is only in operation during working hours from Monday through Friday. If a calcium determination is needed on a weekend, be certain that the laboratory is aware of this and prepared to perform the serum calcium test separately.

Serum parathyroid hormone test

(PTH test, parathormone test)

Normal value: <2000 pg/ml

Rationale. The serum parathyroid hormone test measures the quantity of parathyroid hormone (PTH) within the blood. PTH is the only hormone secreted by the parathyroid gland. It is one of the major factors in calcium metabolism (see anatomy and physiology). Increased levels are seen in patients with hyperparathyroidism; patients with nonparathyroid, ectopic, PTH-producing tumors (as in lung and kidney carcinoma); or as a normal compensatory response to hypocalcemia in patients with renal failure or vitamin D deficiency (Figure 8-6). Drugs such as anticonvulsants, steroids, phosphates, lithium, and rifampin cause fictitiously high PTH levels. Decreased levels are seen in patients with hypoparathyroidism (as from surgery) or as a response to hypercalcemia in patients with metastatic bone tumors, sarcoidosis, vitamin D intoxication, or milk-alkali syndrome (Figure 8-6). Commonly used drugs, such as cimetidine (Tagamet) and propranolol (Inderal), are associated with reduced PTH levels. PTH is associated with a normal circadian rhythm. Highest values usually occur around 4 P.M. Baseline levels exist around 8 A.M.

Procedure. The procedure of acquiring blood for this study varies according to the laboratory performing the study. Peripheral venous blood is obtained from the fasting patient (usually in the morning). Some laboratories require 15 ml of blood in an iced plastic syringe; others require only 7 ml in a red-top tube placed on ice. The blood is then taken to the chemistry lab, where it is often sent out to a commercial lab, a procedure requiring several days for the results. Testing is done by radioimmunoassay. The serum calcium level determination (see p. 291) should be obtained at the same time that the PTH specimen is drawn.

The only discomfort associated with this study is the venipuncture.

Contraindications. None.

Nursing considerations

Nursing Diagnoses/Collaborative Problems

See Blood studies, p. 2.

Nursing Implications with Rationale

- Explain the procedure to the patient. Keep the patient NPO except for water after midnight on the day of the test.
- Perform a venipuncture and draw the blood as required by the specific laboratory.
- Obtain a serum calcium level determination at the same time, if ordered. The serum PTH and serum calcium levels are important in differential diagnosis.
- After drawing the blood, apply a pressure dressing to the venipuncture site. Check the site for bleeding.

Cortisone administration test

(Dent test)

Normal value: depend on baseline levels

Rationale. The cortisone administration test is used to aid in differentiating the causes of hypercalcemia. Oral administration of cortisone for 10 days lowers the serum calcium level in patients who have hypercalcemia resulting from causes other than hyperparathyroidism (such as sarcoidosis, vitamin D intoxication, or bone metastasis). Cortisone does not lower calcium levels in hyperparathyroid patients. This fact can differentiate the hyperparathyroid patient from the patient with hypercalcemia resulting from other causes.

No complications are associated with this test.

Procedure. A baseline serum calcium level determination is obtained. The patient is then given 100 to 150 mg of cortisone acetate orally for 10 days while on a regular diet. The serum calcium level determination is repeated at the end of the 10-day period. If no change occurs in the calcium level, the patient is hyperparathyroid. A decreased serum calcium level indicates that the hypercalcemia is caused by sarcoidosis or some other disorder, such as those previously mentioned.

This is not an uncomfortable test. It requires only two venipunctures; however, it takes a long time (10 days) to perform. This study is rarely used today, since serum PTH assays are so easily performed. The PTH level is even more helpful than the Dent test in determining the cause of hypercalcemia.

Contraindications. None.

Nursing considerations

Nursing Diagnoses/Collaborative Problems
See Blood studies, p. 2.

Nursing Implications with Rationale

- Explain the procedure to the patient. Assure the patient that no complications are associated with the 10-day administration of cortisone. Stress the importance of maintaining the patient's usual diet. An increase or decrease in dietary calcium can affect the results of the test.
- Administer the cortisone acetate orally with milk or with an antacid (if ordered) to protect the patient from gastric irritation. Note that glucose intolerance can occur in diabetics and higher blood pressure readings can occur in hypertensives taking steroids.
- Obtain a baseline calcium level determination before the test and a second calcium level determination after the 10-day course of cortisone (see Serum calcium test, p. 291).

Serum phosphate (phosphorus) concentration test

Normal values:
Adult: 3.0-4.5 mg/dl or 0.97-1.45 mmol/L (SI units)
Elderly: values slightly lower than adult
Child: 4.5-6.5 mg/dl or 1.45-2.1 mmol/L (SI units)
Newborn: 4.3-9.3 mg/dl or 1.4-3.0 mmol/L (SI units)
Possible critical values <1 mg/dl

Rationale. Most of the body's phosphorus is combined with calcium within the skeleton. However, approximately 15% exists in the blood as a phosphate salt. Dietary phosphorus is absorbed in the small bowel. The absorption is very efficient, and only rarely is hypophosphatemia caused by gastrointestinal malabsorption. Antacids, however, can bind phosphorus and decrease intestinal absorption. Renal excretion of phosphorus should equal dietary intake to maintain a normal level of serum phosphate (PO_4^-).

Phosphorus levels are determined by calcium metabolism (see pp. 290-291), parathormone (PTH), and, to a lesser degree, intestinal absorption. Because an inverse relationship exists between calcium and phosphorus, a decrease in one mineral results in an increase in the other. Serum phosphorus levels therefore depend on calcium metabolism and vice versa.

Regulation of phosphate by PTH is such that PTH tends to decrease phosphate reabsorption in the kidney. However, PTH and vitamin D tend to weakly stimulate phosphate absorption within the gut.

Hyperphosphatemia can be caused by hypoparathyroidism, renal failure, vitamin D intoxication, diabetes with ketosis, malignant hyperthermia, cirrhosis, acidosis, or increased dietary or intravenous intake. Symptoms are few. However, calcium phosphate deposits in soft tissue may occur with chronic and persistent elevations of phosphate levels.

Hypophosphatemia may occur with inadequate dietary ingestion of phosphorus, steatorrhea, renal tubular acidosis, acute alcoholism, sepsis, rickets, alkalosis, chronic antacid ingestion, hyperparathyroidism, and hypercalcemia resulting from other causes. Symptoms of hypophosphatemia may include retarded skeletal growth in children; anorexia; dizziness; muscular weakness; waddling gait; skeletal and cardiac myopathies; decreased red blood cell (RBC) oxygen transport because of a decrease in 2,3-diphosphoglyceric acid (a phosphate-containing enzyme); and RBC hemolysis caused by a lack of adenosine triphosphate (ATP), which results in a lack of RBC-membrane pliability.

Procedure. This test is usually included in a multiphasic automated system's analysis of serum. Some hospitals require the patient be fasting. Usually for these multiphasic analyses, two red-top tubes are filled with peripheral venous blood. Hemolysis must be avoided, because if it occurs intracellular phosphate can be released, which would artificially raise the phosphate level. The test is done in the chemistry laboratory. The only discomfort associated with this test is that of the peripheral venipuncture.

Contraindications. None.

Nursing considerations

Nursing Diagnoses/Collaborative Problems

See Blood studies, p. 2.

Nursing Implications with Rationale

- Explain the procedure to the patient.
- Perform the peripheral venipuncture. Apply pressure to the site and assess it for bleeding.
- Indicate on the lab slip the time that the blood was obtained because often a serum glucose determination is performed simultaneously in the multiphasic test.
- Prevent hemolysis of the blood specimen.

Tubular phosphate reabsorption test

(TPR, parathyroid function test, tubular reabsorption of phosphate, TRP)

Normal value: 80% to 90%

Rationale. The tubular phosphate reabsorption test indirectly measures PTH by estimating its effects on renal phosphate reabsorption. It is mostly done to detect primary hyperparathyroidism. This value is calculated using the serum creatinine level, the serum phosphorus concentration, and the creatinine clearance rate. Values less than 80% indicate diminished renal tubular reabsorption of phosphate and suggest primary hyperparathyroidism. Decreased values may also be associated with sarcoidosis, myeloma, and hypercalcemia caused by malignancy.

Procedure. The patient should be on a normal phosphate diet (>500 mg/day and <3000 mg/day). A low phosphate diet raises TPR values, and a high phosphate diet lowers values. This test can be done using a 24-hour urine sample or by taking hourly samples.

For the *24-hour urine test,* the patient is kept NPO, except for water, for 8 hours before drawing the blood sample. A 24-hour urine sample is collected. (The patient is not kept NPO during the entire time of the 24-hour period, only until the blood sample is drawn.) The blood is usually drawn early in the collection period.

The *hourly test* begins with the patient drinking several 8-ounce glasses of water and voiding completely. This marks the beginning of the test. One hour later a blood specimen is drawn for phosphorus and creatinine measurements. One hour later (2 hours after beginning the test) the patient voids, and the urine volume and the urine concentration of creatinine and phosphorus are determined. The creatinine measurement and the filtration rate of phosphorus by the glomeruli are calculated. The amount of phosphorus reabsorbed by the tubules is then determined from these values.

Contraindications. None.

Nursing considerations

Nursing Diagnoses/Collaborative Problems

See Blood studies, p. 2, and Urine studies, p. 3.

Nursing Implications with Rationale

- Find out which method of testing will be used from the laboratory performing the test. Give the patient written dietary instructions. High or low phosphate diets skew the test results.
- Collect the urine and blood samples as needed, and mark each specimen with the time it was collected.

SUPPLEMENTAL INFORMATION

Urine calcium test

Normal values:

Normal diet: 100-300 mg/day or
2.50-7.5 mmol/day (SI units)

Low-calcium diet: 50-150 mg/day or
1.25-3.75mmol/day(SI units)

Rationale. This quantitative test measures the amount of calcium excreted in the urine within a 24-hour period. (This differs from the qualitative Sulkowitch test, which is rarely performed today.) Excretion of calcium in the urine is increased in the majority of patients with primary hyperparathyroidism. Hypercalciuria may also be seen in patients with the following: idiopathic hypercalciuria, Cushing's syndrome, milk-alkali syndrome, osteoporosis, osteolytic bone diseases (e.g., metastatic breast or bladder cancer), Paget's disease, renal tubular acidosis, sarcoidosis, and vitamin D intoxication. Values are decreased in patients with hypoparathyroidism, malabsorption disorders, vitamin D deficiency, and dilute urine. Anticonvulsants, carbonic anhydrase inhibitors, and diuretics tend to increase urine calcium levels. Steroids and oral contraceptives decrease calcium in the urine.

Procedure. Disagreement exists as to whether the specimen should be collected with the patient on a normal diet, a normal diet except for milk products, or a controlled 100 to 200 mg calcium diet. The reference values vary according to the type of diet. The 24-hour urine specimen is collected and stored at room temperature using a preservative.

Contraindications. None.

Nursing considerations

Nursing Diagnoses/Collaborative Problems

See Urine studies, p. 2.

Nursing Implications with Rationale

- Explain the procedure to the patient. Find out the diet regimen recommended by the specific laboratory. Give the patient a written copy indicating any dietary restrictions or particulars.
- Collect the 24-hour specimen. See Chapter 7, pp. 230-231, nursing considerations for the creatinine clearance test (except for the first and last considerations) for 24-hour urine collection.

ADRENAL GLANDS

ANATOMY AND PHYSIOLOGY

The adrenal glands (see Figure 7-1) lie in the retroperitoneum, immediately superior to the kidneys. Because of this anatomic relationship, any significant enlargement in the adrenals displaces the kidneys (as can be seen during IVP). The arterial supply to the glands is variable and multiple. The venous drainage is more constant. The right adrenal vein enters the inferior vena cava directly, whereas the left adrenal vein enters the left renal vein directly. Microscopically the adrenal glands are composed of an inner medulla and an outer cortex, which has three layers (zona glomerulosa, zona fasciculata, and zona reticularis).

The adrenal glands have the ability to secrete many hormones. Glucocorticoids, mineralocorticoids, androgens, and estrogens are secreted by the adrenal cortex. See Table 8-2 for the action of each hormone. The adrenal medulla is responsible for production of epinephrine and norepinephrine.

Glucocorticoid secretion

Cortisol is the primary and physiologically the most important glucocorticoid. Normally, the hypothalamus secretes corticotropin-releasing factor (CRF), which travels down to the anterior pituitary gland by way of the pituitary portal blood system. Adrenocorticotropic hormone (ACTH) secretion from the anterior pituitary is then stimulated by CRF. ACTH directly stimulates the adrenals to produce and secrete cortisol and, to a lesser degree, aldosterone. Cortisol then acts as described in Table 8-2. As the levels of cortisol increase, CRF secretion is inhibited by a negative feedback mechanism to maintain appropriate levels of cortisol.

With any physical or emotional stress, such as trauma, infection, chronic illness, or high levels of anxiety, this negative feedback cortisol control system can be overcome by other central nervous system mechanisms. Therefore, CRF and ACTH can be secreted despite high levels of cortisol. These elevated cortisol levels are apparently protective, supplying the body with extra sources of glucose as well as other substances.

Normally, there is diurnal variation in the secretion of CRF and ACTH and therefore in cortisol secretion. This is a basic biologic circadian

TABLE 8-2. Action of Adrenal Hormones and Symptoms of Excess and Deficiency

Hormone	Function	Excess	Deficiency
Cortisol	Glycogenesis	Diabetes, polyuria	Hypoglycemia, asthenia, weakness
	Mobilization of protein	Destruction of protein material in bone, connective tissue, and muscle Muscle weakness, osteoporosis, back pain, pathologic fractures, cutaneous striae, ease in bruisability	
	Mobilization and redeposition of adipose tissue	Buffalo hump, moon facies, truncal obesity	
	Increased reabsorption of sodium	Hypertension, edema, plethora	Orthostatic hypotension
	Increased potassium excretion	Hypokalemic alkalosis	Hyperkalemic acidosis
	Reduction of inflammation	Increased susceptibility to infection	
	Maintenance of integrity of personality	Emotional lability	Irritability
	Suppression of ACTH		Excess ACTH (MSH-like hyperpigmentation)
Androgen	Secondary male sex characteristics	Hirsutism Acne Precocious puberty Baldness In women: Amenorrhea Deepening of voice Atrophy of uterus Atrophy of breast Enlargement of clitoris Increased sex drive	In men: Lack of body hair Decreased sex drive
Estrogen	Secondary female sex characteristics	In men: Gynecomastia Reduction of body hair Increased subcutaneous fat	
		In women: Uterine bleeding Uterine cancer Precocious puberty Cystic breast	In women: Hot flashes Amenorrhea
Aldosterone	Increased water reabsorption	Hypertension, edema	
	Increased sodium reabsorption	Hypernatremia	Hyponatremia
	Increased potassium excretion	Hypokalemia	Hyperkalemia

rhythm. As a result, cortisol is maximally secreted about 6 to 8 AM, and the level falls to its nadir around midnight. An important feature of Cushing's syndrome (adrenal hyperfunction) is failure of this circadian rhythm and resultant variation in cortisol levels.

Mineralocorticoid secretion

Aldosterone is the mineralocorticoid of primary physiologic importance. Of this hormone secretion, 25% to 30% is influenced by ACTH, whereas the majority depends on the renin-angiotensin system, as described in Chapter 7, p. 222.

Androgen and estrogen secretion

The quantity of these hormones produced by the adrenals (in contrast to the gonads) is a subject of ongoing debate. However, it should be sufficient to say that adrenal production of these hormones is secondary to gonadal production. In men the adrenal gland is the primary source of estrogen, and in women the adrenal gland is the primary source of androgen. After menopause, the adrenals become the only source of estrogen production in women.

Epinephrine secretion

Epinephrine is secreted by the adrenal medulla. This hormone affects smooth muscle and cardiac muscle, along with many other tissues. Epinephrine is sympathomimetic. Increased secretion of epinephrine is one of the body's first responses to physical and emotional stress.

Diseases affecting the adrenal glands

Many diseases affect the adrenals. Cushing's syndrome is the result of adrenal gland hyperfunction. Bilateral adrenal hyperplasia (Cushing's *disease*), adrenal adenomas and carcinomas, and nonadrenal ACTH-producing tumors (such as of the lung or thymus) can all produce Cushing's syndrome. One must also be aware that exogenously administered pharmacologic doses of steroids can also cause the signs and symptoms of cortisol excess (Table 8-2).

Addison's disease is the result of adrenal gland hypofunction and can be caused by destruction of the adrenal gland by hemorrhage, infarction, metastatic tumor invasion, or autoimmunity. Congenital enzyme deficiency and enzyme blockers such as metyrapone and o'p-DDD also cause adrenal hypofunction. Pituitary hypofunction may result not only in adrenal hypofunction but also in a decrease in thyroid growth and sexual function. Addison's disease is most commonly found in patients who have had their adrenal glands surgically removed and are taking inadequate cortisol replacement. The tests described in this section are used not only to diagnose adrenal hyperfunction or hypofunction but also to differentiate the disease entities causing the adrenal dysfunction.

CASE STUDY 4: CUSHING'S SYNDROME

Ms. D., a 22-year-old nurse, complained of weakness, tiredness, easy bruising, leg edema, recent acne, and hirsutism. Her menses became irregular. Her family commented that she was emotionally labile. They also believed that her face had become fuller. On physical examination she was found to be mildly hypertensive with a moon facies, buffalo hump, truncal obesity, diffuse cutaneous striae, and +2 pitting pretibial edema. The results of a recent chest x-ray study performed at work were reported as normal.

Studies	Results
Routine laboratory work	WNL except glucose: 240 mg/dl (normal: 60-120 mg/dl)
Urine test for 17-hydroxycorticosteroids (17-OHCS)	28 mg/24 hours (normal: 5.0-13.5 mg/24 hours)
Urine test for 17-ketosteroids (17-KS)	14 mg/24 hours (normal: 6-12 mg/24
Plasma cortisol test	
8 AM	88 μg/dl (normal: 6-28 μg/dl)
4 PM	78 μg/dl (normal: 2-12 μg/dl)

Studies	**Results**
Dexamethasone suppression test	
Plasma cortisol level after 2 mg/day	60 μg/dl (normal: <10 μg/dl)
Plasma cortisol level after 8 mg/day	8 μg/dl (normal: <10 μg/dl)
Plasma ACTH test	140 pg/ml (normal: 15-100 pg/ml)
Plasma cortisol level after ACTH stimulation test	140 μg/dl (normal: >40μg/dl, <60 μg/dl)
Urine 17-OHCS level after metyrapone stimulation test	Baseline excretion of 17-OHCS tripled (normal: doubled excretion)
X-ray study of sella turcica	Normal
Adrenal angiography	Bilaterally enlarged adrenal gland; no tumor neovascularity seen (normal: no enlargement or tumor)

The patient had the classic signs and symptoms of Cushing's syndrome (adrenal gland hyperactivity). Her elevated urinary 17-OHCS level and the elevation and loss of normal diurnal variation in her plasma cortisol levels substantiated the diagnosis. The underlying pathologic condition causing the adrenal gland hyperfunctioning had to be determined to permit appropriate therapy. The causes could have been bilateral adrenal hyperplasia, adrenal adenoma or carcinoma, a pituitary tumor, or an ACTH-secreting tumor. Lack of adrenal gland suppression with 2 mg of dexamethasone combined with complete suppression with 8 mg of dexamethasone strongly indicated that adrenal hyperplasia rather than an adrenal tumor was causing the Cushing's syndrome. The patient's elevated levels on the plasma ACTH, metyrapone suppression, and ACTH stimulation tests were all consistent with bilateral adrenal hyperplasia. The x-ray study of the sella turcica and the adrenal angiography eliminated the possibility of pituitary and adrenal tumors.

The patient underwent bilateral adrenalectomy and became asymptomatic. She was given physiologic steroid-replacement medications and had no further difficulties.

DISCUSSION OF TESTS

Urine tests for 17-hydroxycorticosteroids and 17-ketosteroids

17-Hydroxycorticosteroids (17-OHCS)

Normal values:

Male

Under age 8 years: <1.5 mg/24 hr
Under age 12 years: <4.5 mg/24 hr
Adult: 4.5-10 mg/24 hr
Elderly: values lower than for adult

Female

Under age 8 years: <1.5 mg/24 hr
Under age 12 years: <4.5 mg/24 hr
Adult: 2.5-10 mg/24 hr
Elderly: values lower than for adult

17-Ketosteroids (17-KS)

Normal values:

Male: 8-15 mg/24 hr
Female 6-12 mg/24 hr
Elderly values decrease with age
Child: under 12 years, <5 mg/24 hr
12-15 years, 5-12 mg/24 hr

Rationale. This urine study is used to assess adrenal cortical function by measuring the cortisol (17-OHCS) and testosterone or estrogen (17-KS) metabolites in a 24-hour urine collection. Elevated levels of 17-OHCS are seen in patients with hyperfunctioning of the adrenal gland (Cushing's syndrome), whether this condition is caused by pituitary or adrenal tumor, bilateral adrenal hyperplasia, or ectopic ACTH-producing tumor. Low values of 17-OHCS are seen in patients who have a hypofunctioning adrenal gland (Addison's disease). Addison's disease can result from destruction of the adrenals (by hemorrhage, infarction, metastatic tumor, or autoimmunity), surgical removal of adrenals without appropriate steroid replacement, congenital enzyme deficiency, hypopituitarism, or adrenal suppression after prolonged exogenous steroid ingestion.

Elevated 17-KS levels are frequently seen in patients with congenital adrenal hyperplasia and testosterone- or estrogen-secreting tumors of the adrenals, ovaries, or testes. Low levels of 17-KS occur in Addisonian patients (mentioned previously), in those who have undergone removal of the ovaries or testes, and in menopausal women.

Testing the urine for these hormone precursors is only an indirect measurement of adrenal function. It is far more accurate to measure urine and plasma levels of cortisol (see next study), testosterone, or estrogen.

This study is without complications. Many drugs can affect the results of these urine tests. Aspirin, acetaminophen, morphine, barbiturates, reserpine, furosemide, and thiazides artificially decrease measurements. Paraldehyde, monoamine oxidase inhibitors, spironolactone, cloxacillin, and licorice artificially raise these levels.

Procedure. Urine is collected over a 24-hour period in a 1-gallon urine container. A preservative is necessary for the 17-KS. The urine specimen is refrigerated or kept on ice during the entire collection period. At the end of the collection period, the urine is sent to the chemistry laboratory. The test is usually performed using a calorimetric technique.

Contraindications. None.

Nursing considerations

Nursing Diagnoses/Collaborative Problems

See Urine studies, p. 3.

Nursing Implications with Rationale

- Explain the procedure to the patient. Be sure that the patient knows what is expected so that no urine is discarded. Valid interpretation of adrenal function depends on a complete 24-hour urine collection.
- See Chapter 7, pp. 230-231, nursing considerations for the creatinine clearance test (except for first and last implications), for 24-hour urine collection.
- Be certain that none of the drugs previously mentioned are administered during the collection period because they may interfere with the chemical determination of the urinary steroids. List any medications the patient is taking on the lab slip.
- Deliver the completed 24-hour urine specimen to the lab, preferably during the 7 A.M. to 3 P.M. shift so that it can be evaluated immediately during routine laboratory working hours.
- Emotional stress and physical stress (such as infection) may cause increased adrenal activity. These complications alter the test results. Report any evidence of stress noted in the patient to the physician. In such a case the test should be rescheduled.
- Encourage the patient to have foods and fluids during the 24-hour collection period, unless these are contraindicated for medical reasons.

Plasma cortisol test

(hydrocortisone)

Normal values:
Adult/elderly: 8 AM—6-28 μg/dl or 170-625 nmol/L (SI units)
4 PM—2-12 μg/dl or 80-413 nmol/L (SI units)
Child: 8 AM—15-25 μg/dl
4 PM—5-10 μg dl
Newborn: 1-24 μg/dl

Rationale. Cortisol is a potent glucocorticoid released from the adrenal cortex in response to adrenocorticotropic hormone (ACTH) stimulation. The best method of evaluating adrenal activity is direct measurement of plasma cortisol levels. Normally cortisol levels rise and fall during the day, which is called the diurnal variation. Cortisol levels are highest around 6 to 8 A.M., and gradually fall during the day to their lowest point around midnight. Sometimes the earliest sign of adrenal hyperfunction is the loss of this diurnal variation, even though the cortisol levels are not yet elevated. For example, individuals with Cushing's syndrome often have top-normal plasma cortisol levels in the morning and do not exhibit a decline as the day proceeds. High cortisol levels occur in Cushing's disease, adrenal adenoma or carcinoma, ectopic

ACTH production or significant physical stress. Low levels of plasma cortisol are suggestive of Addison's disease (see preceding study), adrenogenital syndromes, and hypopituitarism. Cortisol can also be detected and measured in the urine. Either plasma or urine values can be used in evaluating adrenal function. This study has no complications.

Procedure. At 8 AM, after the patient has had a good night's sleep, 7 to 10 ml of peripheral blood is obtained in a red-top tube. It is then sent to the chemistry laboratory for analysis. A second specimen is usually taken later in the day to identify the normal diurnal variation of the plasma cortisol levels. Although the level is at its nadir at midnight, this is a very inconvenient time for the staff, patient, and lab. Therefore, the blood is obtained in a manner similar to the 8 AM collection at around 4 PM. One would expect the 4 PM value to be one third to two thirds of the 8 AM value. Normal values may be transposed in individuals who have worked during the night and slept during the day for long periods of time.

The cortisol is usually measured by a radioimmunoassay technique. It is important that very little anxiety be associated with the venipuncture. As stated earlier, physical and emotional stress can artificially elevate the cortisol level.

Contraindications. None.

Nursing considerations

Nursing Diagnoses/Collaborative Problems

See Blood studies, p. 2.

Nursing Implications with Rationale

- Explain the procedure to the patient to minimize anxiety. Stress causes elevated cortisol levels and complicates the test interpretation. Assess the patient for signs of physical stress (such as infection or acute illness) or emotional stress, and report these to the physician.
- Obtain a specimen, causing minimal trauma to the patient. Indicate the time of the venipuncture on the request slip. After the venipuncture, apply pressure or a pressure dressing to the site. Observe the site for bleeding.

Dexamethasone suppression test

(prolonged/rapid DST, cortisol suppression test, ACTH suppression test)

Prolonged method:
- Expected values (normal)
  - Low dose: >50% reduction of plasma cortisol and 17-OHCS levels
  - High dose: >50% reduction of plasma cortisol and 17-OHCS levels
- Cushing's syndrome
  - Bilateral adrenal hyperplasia
    - Low dose: no change
    - High dose: >50% reduction of plasma cortisol and 17-OHCS levels
  - Adrenal adenoma or carcinoma
    - Low dose: no change
    - High dose: no change
  - Ectopic ACTH-producing tumor
    - Low dose: no change
    - High dose: no change

Rapid method:
- Normal: nearly 0 cortisol levels

Rationale. The dexamethasone test is an important test for diagnosing adrenal hyperfunction (Cushing's syndrome). It also enables one to distinguish hyperplastic from neoplastic causes of adrenal hyperfunction.

As described in the discussion of the physiology of the adrenals, pituitary ACTH secretion is dependent on plasma cortisol levels. That is, as plasma cortisol levels increase, ACTH secretion is suppressed; as cortisol levels decrease, ACTH secretion is stimulated. This important feedback system does not function properly in patients with Cushing's syndrome. In Cushing's syndrome caused by bilateral adrenal hyperplasia, the pituitary gland is reset upward and responds only to high plasma levels of cortisol steroids. In Cushing's syndrome caused by an adrenal adenoma or cancer, the tumor is autonomous and continues to secrete cortisol despite a decrease in ACTH. Finally, when Cushing's syndrome is caused by an ectopic ACTH-producing tumor (as in lung cancer) that tumor is also considered autonomous and continues to secrete ACTH despite high cortisol levels. Knowledge of these defects in the normal cortisol-ACTH feedback system is the basis for understanding the dexamethasone suppression test.

Dexamethasone is a potent synthetic glucocorticoid, much like cortisol. In normal patients, even low doses of exogenously administered dexamethasone inhibit ACTH secretion and results in reduced stimulation to the adrenals and ultimately a drop of 50% or more in plasma cortisol and 17-OHCS levels.

In patients whose Cushing's disease is caused by bilateral adrenal hyperplasia, the pituitary is accustomed to high levels of glucocorticoids, and ACTH is not suppressed. Therefore, there is no reduction in plasma or urinary steroid levels on low-dose dexamethasone suppression. In Cushingoid patients who have autonomous adrenal tumors, pituitary ACTH already is suppressed, and the tumor secretes high levels of cortisol despite the dexamethasone. Therefore, there is no reduction in plasma and urine steroid levels with low-dose dexamethasone suppression in these patients either.

If, however, dexamethasone is administered in high enough doses to a patient with adrenal hyperplasia, pituitary ACTH production is suppressed and plasma and urinary steroid levels would be expected to fall. However, in patients with adrenal tumors or ectopic ACTH-producing tumors, there is no plasma or urine steroid level reduction even with high-dose suppression.

The dexamethasone suppression test also can identify depressed persons likely to respond to electric shock therapy or antidepressants rather than to psychologic or social interventions. ACTH production is not suppressed after administration of low-dose dexamethasone in these patients.

The *prolonged* dexamethasone suppression test can be performed over a 6-day period on an outpatient basis. No complications are associated with it.

The *rapid* dexamethasone test is an easily and rapidly performed test used mostly as a screening test to diagnose Cushing's syndrome. It is less accurate and less informative than the prolonged dexamethasone suppression test, but when its results are normal, the diagnosis of Cushing's syndrome can safely be excluded. The ease with which this test can be performed makes it useful in clinical medicine.

For the rapid dexamethasone test, cortisol levels are determined in the morning after low- or high-dose of dexamethasone administration on the previous night. In normal patients the plasma cortisol levels fall to nearly zero. Cortisol levels in patients with Cushing's syndrome (despite the cause) are > 6 μg/dl.

Procedure. In the *prolonged* test, urinary 17-OHCS levels are usually measured. However, with the increased ease in obtaining plasma cortisol levels, this measurement is gradually replacing the urine determination. Specific protocols vary among laboratories performing this test. Nevertheless, a classic dexamethasone suppression test will be described.

Day 1: A baseline 24-hour urine test for corticosteroids (urinary 17-OHCS or urinary cortisol) is done.

Day 2: Same as Day 1.

Day 3: A low dose (0.5 mg) of dexamethasone is given by mouth every 6 hours, for a total of 2 mg/day. A 24-hour urine test for corticosteroids is done (as on Days 1 and 2).

Day 4: Same as Day 3.

Day 5: A high dose (2.0 mg) of dexamethasone is given by mouth every 6 hours, for a total of 8 mg/day. A 24-hour urine test for corticosteroids is done.

Day 6: Same as Day 5.

The creatinine content should be measured in all 24-hour urine collections to demonstrate the accuracy and adequacy of the collection period. Creatinine excretion varies very little from day to day. The urine sample for cortisol and 17-OHCS should not contain a preservative. The specimen is kept refrigerated or on ice during the collection period and is sent to the chemistry laboratory at the end of each 24-hour period.

For the *rapid* dexamethasone suppression test, 1 mg of dexamethasone is given to the patient by mouth at 11 P.M. The patient is also sedated with a barbiturate to ensure a good night's sleep. At 8 A.M. the next morning the patient's plasma cortisol level is determined before he or she gets out of bed, as described on p. 300. If there is no cortisol suppression after 1 mg of dexamethasone, a higher dose (8 mg) may be given to suppress ACTH production. This is often referred to as the *overnight 8 mg dexamethasone suppression test.*

Contraindications. None.

Nursing considerations

Nursing Diagnoses/Collaborative Problems

See Blood studies, p. 2, and Urine studies, p. 3.

Nursing Implications with Rationale

- Explain the procedure to the patient, and allow plenty of time to answer questions so that anxiety (stress) is diminished as much as possible. Stress can cause ACTH release and obscure the interpretation of test results.
- Administer the dexamethasone orally at the exact time it is ordered, with milk or an antacid (if ordered) to prevent gastric irritation. Administer a hypnotic, if ordered, to ensure the patient a good night's rest.
- See pp. 230-231 for the nursing implications associated with a 24-hour urine collection for 17-OHCS. In studies such as the dexamethasone suppression test, when six continuous 24-hour urine collections are needed, no urine specimens are discarded except for the first one, after which the collection begins.
- Assess the patient for steroid-induced side effects by monitoring the patient's weight daily, checking the urine for glucose and acetone, assessing serum potassium levels, and evaluating the patient for evidence of gastric irritation.
- See nursing implications for serum cortisol determinations (preceding study).

Serum adrenocorticotropic hormone test

(serum ACTH)

Normal values:
AM: 15-100 pg/ml or 10-80 ng/L (SI units)
PM: <50 pg/ml or <50 ng/L (SI units)

Rationale. The serum adrenocorticotropic hormone study is a test of anterior pituitary function that affords the greatest insight into the causes of either Cushing's syndrome or Addison's disease. In the patient with Cushing's syndrome an elevated level of ACTH can be caused by bilateral hyperplasia, a pituitary ACTH-producing tumor (rare), or a nonpituitary (ectopic) ACTH-producing tumor (usually in the lung, pancreas, thymus, or ovary). ACTH levels >200 pg/ml usually indicate ectopic ACTH production. If the ACTH level is below normal in a cushingoid patient, an adrenal adenoma or carcinoma is most probably the cause of the hyperfunction.

In a patient with Addison's disease, an elevated ACTH level indicates primary adrenal gland failure (as in adrenal gland destruction caused by infarction, hemorrhage, or autoimmunity; surgical removal of the adrenals; congenital enzyme deficiency; or adrenal suppression after prolonged ingestion of exogenous steroids). If the ACTH level is below normal in a patient with Addison's disease, hypopituitarism is most probably the cause of the hypofunction.

One must be aware that there is a diurnal variation to ACTH levels. Evening samples are usually one half to two thirds of the morning specimen.

No complications are associated with this study.

Procedure. A chilled, plastic, heparinized syringe is used to collect 20 ml of peripheral venous blood. The blood is placed on ice and sent immediately to the chemistry laboratory for radioimmunoassay. A fasting sample of blood is drawn, usually between 8 and 10 A.M. As with cortisol, stress of any kind can artificially increase the ACTH level. Therefore, one must try to minimize the psychologic trauma of venipuncture.

Contraindications. None.

Nursing considerations

Nursing Diagnoses/Collaborative Problems

See Blood studies, p. 2.

Nursing Implications with Rationale

- See the Nursing implications for the plasma cortisol test, pp. 300-301.

Adrenocorticotropic hormone stimulation test

(ACTH stimulation test)

Normal values: >40 μg/dl after 24-hour infusion
Rapid test: increase of >7 μg/dl above baseline

Rationale. In this test, exogenous ACTH is given to the patient, and the ability of the adrenals to respond to ACTH stimulation is measured by plasma cortisol levels. In normal patients after a 24-hour ACTH infusion, the plasma cortisol level should increase and exceed 40 μg/dl. Cushingoid patients with bilateral adrenal hyperplasia have an exaggerated response to the ACTH stimulation. Because hyperfunctioning adrenal tumors are autonomous and relatively insensitive to changes in ACTH levels, there is little or no cortisol increase above baseline in these patients.

This test is even more valuable in the patient suspected of having Addison's disease (adrenal insufficiency). If after a 24-hour infusion of ACTH plasma, cortisol levels are between 10 and 40 μg/dl, this shows that the adrenal gland is capable of function if stimulated. The cause of the adrenal insufficiency lies within the pituitary (hypopituitarism), and the patient thus has secondary adrenal insufficiency. If either little or no rise in cortisol levels occurs, the adrenal gland cannot secrete cortisol (primary adrenal insufficiency) due to adrenal destruction caused by hemorrhage, infarction, autoimmunity, metastatic tumor, surgical removal of the adrenals, or congenital adrenal enzyme deficiency.

No complications are associated with this study.

Procedure. After a baseline plasma cortisol level (see p. 300) is obtained, an intravenous infusion of synthetic alpha-ACTH (cosyntropin) in 1 L of normal saline solution is administered at the rate of 2 units/hour for 24 hours. Peripheral venous blood for plasma cortisol level determination is again obtained 24 hours later and sent to the chemistry laboratory. This test can also be performed by comparing the baseline urine hydroxysteroid excretion with stimulated hydroxycorticosteroid excretion. In normal patients, stimulated hydroxysteroid excretion should exceed 25 mg/day.

The ACTH stimulation test can also be performed by intravenous administration of 25 units of cosyntropin over an 8-hour period on 2 to 3 consecutive days. The response seen at the end of the second and third 8-hour period should approximate that seen after the continuous 24-hour infusion.

For the sake of convenience, the most widely used test is the *rapid ACTH stimulation test,* which is done by giving an intramuscular injection of 25 units (0.25 mg) of cosyntropin and measuring plasma cortisol levels before and at 30- and 60-minute intervals after drug administration. Normal patients have an increase of cortisol of more than 7 μg/dl above baseline values.

This test is only as uncomfortable as the ACTH injection and the venipuncture. It takes about 24 hours to complete.

Contraindications. None.

Nursing considerations

Nursing Diagnoses/Collaborative Problems

See Blood studies, p. 2.

Nursing Implications with Rationale

- See nursing implications for plasma cortisol test, pp. 300-301.
- Accurately administer the cosyntropin as ordered. Perform the venipuncture for cortisol level determination or obtain a urine specimen at the exact time indicated.

Metyrapone test

Normal values: baseline excretion of urinary 17-OHCS should be more than doubled

Rationale. This test is useful in differentiating adrenal hyperplasia from adrenal tumor by determining whether the pituitary-adrenal feedback mechanism is intact. Metyrapone (Metopirone) is a potent blocker of an enzyme involved in cortisol production. When this drug is given, the resulting fall in cortisol production should stimulate pituitary secretion of ACTH by way of a negative feedback mechanism. However, since cortisol itself cannot be synthesized because of the metyrapone inhibition of the 11-beta-hydroxylation step, an abundance of cortisol precursors are formed, which can be detected in the urine when urinary 17-OHCS is measured. This test is similar to the ACTH stimulation test.

In patients with adrenal hyperplasia the urinary levels of 17-OHCS are markedly increased, even more than in normal patients. There is no response (no increase in urinary 17-OHCS levels) to metyrapone in patients whose Cushing's syndrome results from adrenal adenoma or carcinoma because the tumors are autonomous and therefore insensitive to changes in ACTH secretion. This test has no significant advantage over the ACTH stimulation test in the differential diagnosis of Cushing's disease.

Chlorpromazine (Thorazine) interferes with the response to metyrapone and therefore should not be administered during the testing period. Because metyrapone inhibits cortisol production, Addison's disease (adrenocortical insufficiency) and addisonian crisis are potential complications of this study.

Procedure. Before this study is performed, a baseline 24-hour urine specimen for 17-OHCS (see pp. 299-300) should be collected. A 24-hour urine collection for 17-OHCS is also obtained during and again 1 day after the oral administration of 500 to 750 mg of metyrapone, which is given every 4 hours for 24 hours. The 24-hour excretion of 17-OHCS on the last day of collection should at least double the baseline excretion.

Contraindications. None.

Nursing considerations

Nursing Diagnoses/Collaborative Problems

See Urine studies, p. 3.

Nursing Implications with Rationale

- Explain the test. Be certain that the patient knows how to collect the three 24-hour urine specimens required for this study.
- See pp. 299-300 for the 24-hour collection procedure for urinary 17-OHCS.
- Because metyrapone inhibits cortisol production, assess the patient for impending signs of addisonian crisis (muscle weakness, mental and emotional changes, anorexia, nausea, vomiting, hypotension, hyperkalemia, and vascular collapse). Addisonian crisis is a medical emergency that must be treated vigorously. Basically the immediate treatment includes replenishing steroids, reversing shock, and restoring blood circulation.

X-ray study of the sella turcica

Normal value: no abnormalities

Rationale. This study involves taking an x-ray film of the sella turcica (see Figure 6-3), which contains the pituitary gland. ACTH-producing tumors of the pituitary can cause Cushing's syndrome.

One can diagnose these tumors easily if erosion or destruction of the normal sella turcica exists. This test is easily performed and is without complications. Computerized tomography is usually done if a pituitary tumor is suspected.

Procedure. See the procedure for a skull x-ray study, Chapter 6, p. 177.

Nursing considerations

Nursing Diagnoses/Collaborative Problems

See X-ray studies, p. 4.

Nursing Implications with Rationale

- See the nursing implications for a skull x-ray study, p. 178.

Adrenal angiography

(adrenal arteriography)

Normal value: normal adrenal artery vasculature

Rationale. In this study the adrenal gland and its arterial system are visualized by the injection of radiopaque dye into the adrenal arteries. Both benign and malignant tumors of the adrenals (such as pheochromocytomas, adrenal adenomas, and carcinomas) can be detected easily by this technique. Bilateral adrenal hyperplasia can also be diagnosed.

The major complication of this test is anaphylaxis secondary to allergy to the iodinated dye. In patients with a pheochromocytoma (catecholamine-producing tumor of the adrenal medulla), a fatal episode of severe hypertension can be precipitated. Precautionary measures are necessary to prevent this complication. Propranolol (Inderal), which is a beta-adrenergic blocker, and phenoxybenzamine (Dibenzyline), which is an alpha-adrenergic blocker, are given for several days before the study to avoid the precipitation of a malignant hypertensive episode. Other complications include hemorrhage from the puncture site used for the arterial access and extremity ischemia or infarction from the dislodgement of an atherosclerotic plaque.

Occasionally arteriography (and venography) can induce serious hemorrhage within the adrenal. This may cause necrosis of the glands, leading to Addison's disease. In the event that an adrenal tumor is subsequently found and requires operative removal, the surgical procedure is technically more difficult after hemorrhage or infarction.

Procedure. The procedure used in adrenal angiography is similar to that of renal angiography (see Chapter 7, pp. 252-254). The only difference is that in adrenal angiography the inferior adrenal artery, a branch of the renal artery, must be cannulated for dye injection.

Contraindications. See the contraindications for renal angiography, p. 254.

Nursing considerations

Nursing Diagnoses/Collaborative Problems

See Renal angiography, pp. 254-255.

- Potential complication: severe hypertension
- Potential complication: Addison's disease

Nursing Implications with Rationale

- See the nursing implications for renal angiography, p. 255.
- If the patient is suspected of having a pheochromocytoma, administer propranolol and phenoxybenzamine as ordered before the study to prevent precipitation of an episode of malignant hypertension.

SUPPLEMENTAL INFORMATION

Adrenal venography

Normal values: normal adrenal veins and normal adrenal vein hormone assay

Rationale. Adrenal venography is a radiologic test performed to detect and lateralize unilateral adrenal pathology which produces hormones. Once the vein is identified, a catheter can be placed in the vein and blood can be selectively obtained from each adrenal.

In patients with Cushing's syndrome, the blood is analyzed for plasma cortisol. If the plasma cortisol level in the blood obtained from one side is markedly higher than that of the other, a unilateral adrenal tumor is causing the Cushing's syndrome. If, on the other hand, levels of plasma cortisol are bilaterally elevated, one can safely conclude that the cause of the Cushing's syndrome is bilateral adrenal hyperplasia.

In patients with a pheochromocytoma, the adrenal venous blood is analyzed for catecholamines. If the catecholamine level on one side is markedly higher than that of the other, a unilateral pheochromocytoma exists on the side of the elevated levels. If blood obtained from both sides is equally elevated, the patient most probably has bilateral adrenal pheochromocytomas (this occurs more frequently in children and with the familial type of pheochromocytomas). If the adrenal venous blood samples are not elevated on either side in a patient who has elevated peripheral blood catecholamine levels, the pheochromocytoma exists outside the adrenal gland (extraadrenal pheochromocytoma).

The venous blood can also be evaluated for aldosterone, androgens, and other substances. The complications associated with this study are allergy to iodinated x-ray contrast material and also adrenal hemorrhage or necrosis caused by the pressure of the dye injection. This may cause Addison's disease. If adrenalectomy is subsequently indicated, the adrenal surgery would be technically more difficult to perform in the presence of adrenal hemorrhage or necrosis.

Procedure. The fasting patient is brought to the special studies angiography laboratory (usually in the radiology department). The patient is placed in the supine position on the x-ray table. The patient's groin is prepared in a sterile manner. After the venipuncture site is locally anesthetized, the femoral vein is catheterized. The catheter is passed into the adrenal vein. Dye is injected to visualize the adrenal veins and to ensure that the catheter is indeed in the adrenal vein. Blood is obtained and sent to the chemistry laboratory for assays.

In a patient suspected of having a pheochromocytoma, appropriate pharmacologic beta- and alpha-adrenergic blocking agents are administered, propranolol (Inderal) and phenoxybenzamine (Dibenzyline), respectively. This prevents the occurrence of a catecholamine-initiated malignant hypertensive episode.

The duration of the study is approximately 1 hour. Venous catheterization is as uncomfortable as any cutaneous needle stick. A burning sensation is associated with the dye injection.

Contraindications. This study is contraindicated in the uncooperative patient and in those allergic to iodinated dye. However, the patient who is allergic to iodine can receive this study if he or she is given prednisone, 5 mg four times a day, and diphenhydramine (Benadryl), 25 mg four times a day, for 3 days before and 3 days after the test.

Nursing considerations

Nursing Diagnoses/Collaborative Problems

See X-ray studies, p. 5.

- Potential complication: severe hypertension
- Potential complication: cellulitis
- Potential complication: thrombophlebitis
- Potential complication: bacteremia
- Potential complication: embolism

Nursing Implications with Rationale

- Explain the procedure to the patient and allay the patient's fears regarding venography. Provide emotional support.
- Ensure that written and informed consent for this procedure is obtained by the physician before the study.
- Assess the patient for allergies to dye. Administer a steroid and antihistamine preparation, if this has been ordered, to the patient allergic to dye (see Contraindications).
- Administer propranolol and phenoxybenzamine as ordered.
- After the study assess the patient's vital signs frequently (normally every 15 minutes for four times, then every 30 minutes for four times, then every hour for four times, and then every 4 hours). Assess the patient suspected of having a pheochromocytoma for signs and symptoms of a hypertensive epi-

sode. If such an episode occurs, notify the physician immediately, to obtain an order for appropriate alpha- and beta-adrenergic blocking agents.

- After the study assess the groin site for redness, pain, swelling, and bleeding with each vital sign check.

Computed tomography of the adrenal glands

(CT scan of the adrenals)

Normal value: no evidence of abnormality

Rationale. Computed tomography (CT) of the adrenal glands is a noninvasive and yet very accurate method of detecting even very small tumors (adenomas, carcinomas, and pheochromocytomas) of the adrenal glands. Some radiologists feel capable of diagnosing even the type of adrenal tumor on the basis of the density coefficients shown on the CT scan (see p. 123). The density coefficients of the normal adrenal gland can be used to detect bilateral adrenal hyperplasia.

Adrenal hemorrhage causing Addison's disease can also be detected with this highly refined recent advance in radiographic tomography. No complications are associated with this study. The amount of patient radiation is minimal.

Procedure. See also the procedure for CT of the abdomen, p. 123. No fasting is required. A contrast agent may be administered orally to outline the gut or intravenously to enhance visualization of the kidney.

Contraindications. See Contraindications for CT of the abdomen, p. 124.

Nursing considerations

Nursing Diagnoses/Collaborative Problems

See X-ray studies, p. 5.

Nursing Implications with Rationale

- See the nursing implications for CT of the abdomen, p. 124.
- No fasting is required for CT of the adrenal glands.

Androstendione

Normal values: <250 ng/dl.
Possible critical value: >1000 ng/dl.

Rationale. Androstendione is one of the major adrenal androgens produced by women in the ovaries and, to a lesser extent, in the adrenals. The release of this adrenal hormone is stimulated by ACTH (not by gonadotropins) and suppressed by exogenous glucocorticoid administration. Part of androstendione is secreted into the plasma, and the remainder is converted to estrogen in granulosa cells of the ovary or to testosterone in the interstitium. In the peripheral tissues this hormone can also be converted to testosterone and estrogens.

This hormone is useful in evaluating conditions characterized by hirsutism, including Stein-Leventhal syndrome, and other virilizing conditions. Values >1,000 ng/dl suggest a virilizing adrenal tumor. Values are also highly elevated in congenital adrenal hyperplasia.

Procedure. Peripheral venipuncture is performed and one red-top tube of blood is collected. The specimen should be collected 1 week before or after the menstrual period.

Contraindications. None.

Nursing considerations

Nursing Diagnosis/Collaborative Problems

See Blood studies, p. 2.

Nursing Implications with Rationale

- Indicate the date of the last menstrual period on the laboratory form.
- Assess the venipuncture site for bleeding.

ENDOCRINE PANCREAS

ANATOMY AND PHYSIOLOGY

The pancreas, located in the abdomen (see Figure 4-1), has both exocrine (digestive enzymes) and endocrine functions. The islets of Langerhans are clusters of endocrine-secreting cells embedded in the pancreatic tissue. Many different and distinct cells make up the islets of

Langerhans: alpha cells secrete glucagon; beta cells secrete insulin; gamma cells (or C cells) secrete gastrin; and delta cells secrete vasoactive intestinal polypeptide (VIP).

The major action of insulin is to lower the blood glucose level by facilitating the movement of glucose out of the bloodstream and into the cells of the liver, muscle, or other tissue, where glucose is either used for immediate energy or stored as glycogen for later energy requirements. Insulin also promotes the storage of fat in adipose tissue and aids in the synthesis of body proteins.

In the absence of insulin, serum glucose levels rise because glucose cannot enter the cells. When the levels of glucose reach about 180 mg/dl (renal threshold), glucose spills over into the urine. Diabetes mellitus is both a chronic metabolic disorder involving glucose metabolism and a disturbance of fat and protein metabolism, since these substances are catabolized and used as a source of immediate energy instead of glucose. Patients with diabetes have more than just a deficiency of insulin quantitatively; they also have a disturbance in the production, action, or metabolic use of insulin.

Glucagon, on the other hand, tends to raise the blood glucose level, primarily by promoting the conversion of glycogen to glucose in the liver. Glucagon is secreted by the pancreas in response to a fall in the serum glucose level. Gastrin is a hormone that affects the gastrointestinal tract. It stimulates gastric acid secretion, intestinal motility, and sphincter contraction. VIP, also an active gastrointestinal hormone, is thought to be responsible for a watery diarrhea syndrome.

A detailed discussion of diabetes mellitus can be found in most medical or surgical textbooks. Referring to other texts for a better understanding of the pathophysiology and sequelae of diabetes mellitus is suggested.

CASE STUDY 5: ADOLESCENT WITH DIABETES MELLITUS

Mike F., a 16-year-old high-school football player, was brought to the emergency room in a coma. His mother said that during the past month he had lost 12 pounds. She said that he had also had excessive thirst associated with voluminous urination that often required voiding several times during the night. There was a strong family history of diabetes mellitus. The results of physical examination were essentially negative except for sinus tachycardia and Kussmaul respirations.

Studies	**Results**
Serum glucose test (on admission)	1100 mg/dl (normal: 60-120 mg/dl)
Arterial blood gases test (on admission) (see Chapter 5)	
pH	7.23 (normal: 7.35-7.45)
P_{CO_2}	30 mm Hg (normal: 35-45 mm Hg)
HCO_2	12 mEq/L (normal: 22-26 mEq/L)
Serum osmolality test	440 (mOsm/kg) (normal: 275-300 mOsm/kg)
Serum glucose test (fasting blood sugar)	250 mg/dl (normal: 70-115 mg/dl)
Two-hour postprandial glucose test (2-hour PPG)	500 mg/dl (normal: <140 mg/dl)
Glucose tolerance test (GTT)	
Fasting blood sugar (glucose)	150 mg/dl (normal: 70-115 mg/dl)
30 minutes	300 mg/dl (normal: <200 mg/dl)
1 hour	325 mg/dl (normal: <200 mg/dl)
2 hours	390 mg/dl (normal: <140 mg/dl)
3 hours	300 mg/dl (normal: 70-115 mg/dl)
4 hours	260 mg/dl (normal: 70-115 mg/dl)
Glycosylated hemoglobin	9% (normal: 2.2%-4.8%)

The patient's symptoms and diagnostic studies were classic for hyperglycemic ketoacidosis associated with diabetes mellitus. The glycosylated hemoglobin showed that he had been hyperglycemic over the last several months. The results of his blood gases test on admission indicated metabolic acidosis with some respiratory compensation. He was treated in the emergency room with intravenous regular insulin and intravenous fluids.

During the first 72 hours of hospitalization, the patient was monitored by frequent serum glucose determinations. Insulin was administered according to results of these studies. The patient's condition was eventually stabilized on 40 units of neutral protamine Hagedorn (NPH) insulin daily. Comprehensive patient instruction regarding self-blood glucose monitoring (see p. 318), insulin administration, diet, exercise, foot care, and recognition of the signs and symptoms of hypoglycemia and hyperglycemia was given.

DISCUSSION OF TESTS

Serum glucose test

(blood sugar, fasting blood sugar, FBS)

Normal values:
- Cord: 45-96 mg/dl or 2.5-5.3 mmol/L (SI units)
- Premature infant: 20-60 mg/dl or 1.1-3.3 mmol/L
- Neonate: 30-60 mg/dl or 1.7-3.3 mmol/L
- Infant: 40-90 mg/dl or 2.2-5.0 mmol/L
- Child <2 years: 60-100 mg/dl or 3.3-5.5 mmol/L
- Child >2 years to adult: 70-105 mg/dl or 3.9-5.8 mmol/L
- Elderly: increase in normal range after age 50

Possible critical values:
- Adult male: <50 and >400 mg/dl
- Adult female: <40 and >400 mg/dl
- Infant: <40
- Newborn: <30 and >300 mg/dl

Rationale. The serum glucose test is helpful in diagnosing many metabolic diseases. Serum glucose levels must be evaluated according to the time of the day they are performed. For example, a glucose level of 135 mg/dl may be abnormal if the patient is in the fasting state. However, it would be within normal limits if the patient had eaten a meal within the last hour.

In general, true glucose elevations indicate diabetes mellitus. However, one must be aware of other possible causes of hyperglycemia. These include:

1. Acute stress response (such as to surgery), mediated through epinephrine and glucocorticosteroid secretion
2. Cushing's disease (see p. 298), which causes hyperglycemia by elevating glucocorticoid levels (Table 8-2)
3. Pheochromocytoma, a tumor causing increased levels of epinephrine
4. Hyperthyroidism, which is associated with increased levels of catecholamines
5. Adenoma of the pancreas, which causes pancreatic secretion of glucagon (a hyperglycemic agent) only
6. Pancreatitis, in which there is destruction of islet cells (where insulin is produced)
7. Diuretics (such as furosemide and thiazides), which suppress insulin release by inducing hypokalemia
8. Corticosteroid therapy, which causes a chemically induced diabetes
9. IV administration of dextrose
10. Drugs associated with elevated glucose levels, including steroids, isoniazid, tricyclic antidepressants, beta-blockers, and phenothiazines.

Similarly, hypoglycemia (that is, low serum glucose levels) has many causes. The most common cause, however, is insulin overdose. Glucose determinations must be performed frequently in new diabetics to monitor constantly the dosage of insulin administered to the patient. Other causes of hypoglycemia include:

1. Insulinoma, an insulin-producing tumor of the pancreatic islet cells
2. Hypothyroidism, as a result of decreased levels of thyroid hormones
3. Hypopituitarism, as a result of decreased levels of glucose-elevating hormones (growth hormone, thyroid hormone, and ACTH)
4. Addison's disease as a result of cortisol deficiency (Table 8-2)
5. Extensive liver disease, as a result of the inability of the liver to produce glycogen (a storage form of glucose)

6. An overdose of insulin or oral hypoglycemic agents. Other drugs, such as MAO inhibitors and acetaminophen, and alcohol are associated with decreased serum glucose levels.

No complications are associated with this study.

Procedure. For an FBS, the patient is kept fasting for at least 8 hours, usually from the midnight before the test. Water is permitted. The patient should not fast longer than 16 hours before the study is performed to prevent starvation effects, which may artificially raise the glucose level. A peripheral venipuncture is performed, and approximately 7 ml of venous blood is placed in a red- or gray-top tube and taken to the chemistry laboratory. The blood should be obtained before insulin or hypoglycemic agents are administered.

For diabetic patients being regulated on intermediate-acting insulins, fasting and 3 P.M. blood glucose tests are usually performed. Serum glucose levels should be obtained on any diabetic patient suspected of having an insulin reaction. The blood should be obtained before treatment with oral or intravenous glucose administration. Glucose determinations are now a part of most multichannel specimen analyses (see Chapter 14). Self-blood glucose monitoring is widely done today (see p. 318).

Contraindications. None.

Nursing considerations

Nursing Diagnoses/Collaborative Problems

See Blood studies, p. 2.

Nursing Implications with Rationale

- Explain the procedure to the patient. Be certain that the patient understands the timing of the test in relation to meals. If fasting is required, tell the patient that breakfast will be held until the blood is obtained. Place a "hold breakfast" sign at the bedside or on the patient's door.
- Explain to the diabetic patient that insulin or oral hypoglycemics will be withheld until after the blood is obtained because these drugs lower the blood glucose level.
- If the patient will have repeated blood glucose determinations (for example, daily fasting and 3 P.M. blood glucose tests), explain the reasoning for this. Allow the patient time to verbalize his or her feelings regarding repeated venous punctures.
- Apply pressure or a pressure dressing to the venipuncture site after the blood is obtained. Observe the site for bleeding.
- Be certain that the patient receives a meal after the blood is obtained.

Two-hour postprandial glucose test

(2-hour PPG, 2-hour postprandial blood sugar, 2-hour PPBS)

Normal values:
0-50 years: 70-140 mg/dl or <7.8 mmol/L (SI units)
50-60 years: 70-150 mg/dl
60 years and older: 70-160 mg/dl

Rationale. The 2-hour postprandial glucose test is a measurement of the amount of glucose in the patient's blood 2 hours after a meal (postprandial) is ingested. For this study a meal acts as a glucose challenge to the body's metabolism. In normal patients, insulin is secreted immediately after a meal in response to the elevated blood glucose level, thus causing the level to return to the premeal range within 2 hours. In diabetic patients the glucose level is usually still elevated 2 hours after the meal.

This is an easily performed screening test for diabetes mellitus. If the results of this test are abnormal, a glucose tolerance test may be performed to confirm the diagnosis. No complications are associated with this study.

Procedure. The patient is given a routine meal, consisting of at least 75 g of carbohydrates. Two hours after the meal, 7 ml of peripheral venous blood is obtained in a gray- or red-top tube and taken to the chemistry laboratory for glucose determination.

Contraindications. None.

Nursing considerations

Nursing Diagnoses/Collaborative Problems

See Blood studies, p. 2.

Nursing Implications with Rationale

- Explain the procedure to the patient. Instruct the patient to eat the entire meal and then not to eat anything else until the blood is drawn. Smoking is also prohibited, since it may increase the blood sugar level.
- Draw the blood at the appropriate time, and apply pressure or a pressure dressing to the venipuncture site after the blood is obtained. Observe the site for bleeding.

Glucose tolerance test

(GTT, oral glucose tolerance test, OGTT)

Normal values:
Serum test
Fasting: 70-115 mg/dl or <6.4 mmol/L (SI units)
30 minutes: <200 mg/dl or <11.1 mmol/L
1 hour: <200 mg/dl or <11.1 mmol/L
2 hours: <140 mg/dl or <7.8 mmol/L
3 hours: 70-115 mg/dl or <6.4 mmol/L
4 hours: 70-115 mg/dl or <6.4 mmol/L
Urine test: negative

Rationale. In the glucose tolerance study, the patient's ability to tolerate a standard oral glucose load is evaluated by obtaining serum and urine specimens for glucose level determination before glucose administration, and then at 30 minutes, 1 hour, 2 hours, 3 hours, and sometimes 4 hours after the glucose administration. Patients with appropriate insulin response are able to tolerate the dose quite easily, with only a minimal and transient rise in serum glucose levels within 1 hour after the ingestion. In normal patients glucose will not spill over into the urine.

Diabetic patients, who have a deficiency of active insulin (glucose-lowering hormone), are unable to tolerate this load. As a result, their serum glucose levels are markedly elevated for 1 to 5 hours (Figure 8-7). Also, glucose can usually be detected in their urine.

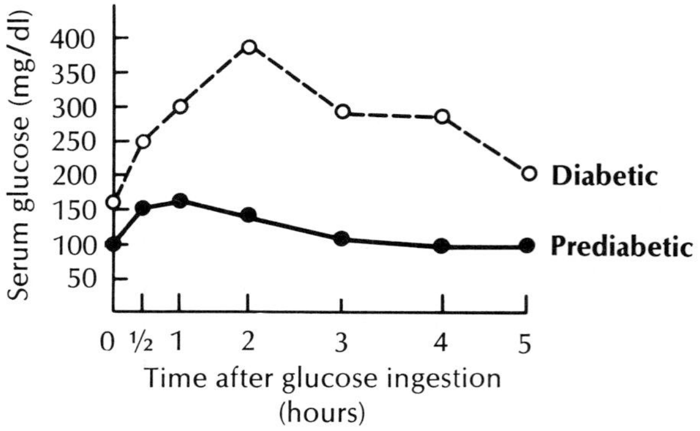

FIGURE 8-7. Glucose tolerance test curve for a diabetic and a prediabetic patient.

Persistent hyperglycemia after glucose loading can also be seen in nondiabetic patients with hyperthyroidism, acromegaly, infection, or ongoing chronic illness (such as cancer). Pregnant or obese patients may also show elevations. Drugs such as nicotine, aspirin, steroids, thiazides, and oral contraceptives may also cause glucose intolerance in nondiabetic patients.

During the GTT, the patient may occasionally have dizziness, tremors, anxiety, sweating, euphoria, or fainting. These complications are rarely serious and can be treated if necessary.

Procedure. After at least 3 days of consuming a high-carbohydrate diet (at least 200 to 300 g), the patient is kept NPO except for water after midnight on the day of the test. A specimen for a fasting blood glucose test is obtained, and the patient's urine is tested for glucose and acetone. The patient is then given a 100 g carbohydrate load, usually in the form of a carbonated sugar beverage (Glucola) or a cherry-flavored gelatin (Gel-a-dex). If these commercial preparations are unavailable, 100 g of glucose is dissolved in water and flavored with lemon juice to increase its palatability. The entire glucose load must be ingested by the patient, since the GTT normal values are based on consumption of the standard 100 g of glucose. For children weighing less than 100 pounds, 1 g of glucose/pound of body weight is given.

Serum and urine specimens for glucose level determination are obtained at 30 minutes, 1 hour, 2 hours, 3 hours, and 4 hours after the patient's ingestion of the carbohydrate load. Sometimes specimens are also obtained at 5 hours. All specimens must be clearly marked with the time they were obtained. During the testing period (approximately 5 hours) the patient is not permitted to eat or smoke. The patient is encouraged to drink water, however, so that urine specimens can be obtained more easily. Coffee and tea are not permitted. Patients should rest during the entire procedure. Any exercise (including walking) can affect glucose levels.

During the testing period, especially between the second and third hours, the patient should be assessed for reactions such as dizziness, sweating, weakness, and giddiness. These reactions are usually transient. The time of the reactions should be recorded.

The patient should not take insulin or oral hypoglycemics before or during the testing period. This study can be performed in the outpatient department or in the patient's hospital room. The serum glucose specimens are drawn by the nurse or by a technician. The patient is responsible for providing the urine specimens unless nursing assistance is needed. The duration of this study is approximately 5 hours.

Occasionally, a patient is unable to absorb the oral glucose load (for example, patients with prior gastrectomy, short bowel syndrome, or malabsorption). In these instances, an *intravenous glucose tolerance test (IV-GTT)* can be performed as follows: a specimen of fasting blood glucose level determination is obtained; a 50% glucose solution (or glucose, 0.33 g/kg of ideal body weight in adults, or 0.5 g/kg body weight of children) is administered intravenously over a 3- to 4-minute period. Blood samples are obtained as indicated by the laboratory. Usually these are at 30 minutes, 1-, 2-, and 3-hour intervals. The values for the IV-GTT differ slightly from those for the oral-GTT, since the intravenous glucose is absorbed faster.

Both the oral and intravenous GTTs are uncomfortable because of the number of venipunctures required for blood glucose determinations. Other than that, patients may complain only of boredom.

Contraindications. A GTT should not be performed on those patients with serious concurrent illness, endocrine disorders, or infections, because glucose intolerance will usually be observed even though the patient may not be diabetic.

Nursing considerations

Nursing Diagnoses/Collaborative Problems

See Blood studies, p. 2 and Urine studies, p. 3.

Nursing Implications with Rationale

- Explain the entire procedure to the patient. Allow the patient ample time to express his or her fears concerning this study and the potential diagnosis of diabetes mellitus. Many patients are very anxious regarding the procedure for this study, since approximately six venipunctures are required in a 4- to 5-hour period. Outpatients who feel faint during blood withdrawal should be placed on a bed or stretcher in the supine position during venipuncture.
- Give the patient written instructions explaining the pretest dietary requirements. An inadequate diet before the GTT may diminish carbohydrate tolerance and cause high glucose levels, simulating diabetes mellitus.
- Encourage the patient to bring reading material or craft work to alleviate some of the boredom associated with this study.
- Obtain the blood specimens as needed. Rotate the venipuncture sites used. Apply pressure to the sites and check them for bleeding.
- Give the patient the necessary urine containers, and write down the times at which specimens are needed. Encourage the patient to drink water to help obtain the urine specimens.
- Do not permit the patient to have anything

by mouth during the study except for water. Tobacco, coffee, and tea are not allowed, because they cause physiologic stimulation, which can alter the test results.

- Be certain that no drugs that alter GTT results are given to the patient during the test.
- If the patient has tremors, dizziness, euphoria, or other reactions during the study, obtain a blood specimen immediately. If the glucose level is too high, the test may need to be stopped and insulin administered.
- After the study allow the patient to eat and drink normally. Insulin or oral hypoglycemics may be administered, if ordered, after the study.

Glycosylated hemoglobin test

(HbA_{1c}/glycohemoglobin)

Normal values: vary with laboratory method employed
- Adults/elderly: 2.2%-4.8%
- Children: 1.8%-4.0%
- Good diabetic control: 2.5%-6%
- Fair diabetic control: 6.1%-8%
- Poor diabetic control: over 8%

Rationale. The glycosylated hemoglobin test provides an accurate long-term index of the patient's average blood glucose control by measuring the patient's glycohemoglobin or glycosylated hemoglobin. Glycohemoglobin is one of the types of minor hemoglobin A_1 components. These components (hemoglobin A_{1a}, A_{1b}, and A_{1c}), which make up about 4% to 8% of the total hemoglobin, are glycosylated—that is, they have glucose attached to them. Hemoglobin A_{1c} is usually measured. (If hemoglobin A_1 is measured, its value is always 2.4% higher than that of the A_{1c} component.)

As the red blood cell (RBC) circulates, it combines some of its hemoglobin with some of the glucose in the bloodstream to form glycohemoglobin. This glycosylation is irreversible. The amount of glycosylated hemoglobin depends on the amount of glucose available in the bloodstream over the RBCs 120-day life span. Since old RBCs are constantly being destroyed and new ones being formed, determination of the glycosylated hemoglobin value reflects the average blood sugar level for the 100- to 120-day period *before* the test. The more glucose the RBC was exposed to, the greater the glycosylated hemoglobin percentage is. One important advantage of this test is that the sample can be drawn at any time because it is not affected by short-term variations (such as food intake, exercise, stress, hypoglycemic agents, patient cooperation, or accuracy).

The glycosylated hemoglobin test is particularly beneficial for the following reasons:

1. Evaluating the success of diabetic treatment, which consists of hypoglycemic agents, dietary therapy, insulin pumps, or patient education programs
2. Comparing and contrasting the success of old and new forms of diabetic therapy
3. Aiding in the determination of the duration of hyperglycemia in newly diagnosed diabetics
4. Providing a sensitive estimate of glucose imbalance in patients with mild cases of diabetes
5. Individualizing diabetic control regimens
6. Providing a feeling of reward for many patients when the test shows achievement of good diabetic control. This further encourages patients to follow their control regimen and to be more active in their self-care

Procedure. No fasting is required. Peripheral venipuncture is performed, and approximately 3 to 5 ml of blood is obtained.

Contraindications. Falsely low values occur in patients with sickle cell anemia and in pregnant women. Falsely elevated values occur when the RBC life span is lengthened (as in thalassemia).

Nursing considerations

Nursing Diagnoses/Collaborative Problems

See Blood studies, p. 2.

Nursing Implications with Rationale

- Explain to the patient what the glycohemoglobin test is and how it helps monitor his or her therapy. This test motivates most patients to follow their control regimen and to take a more active part in their self-care.

- Tell the patient why fasting is not indicated. Most diabetics are accustomed to fasting for blood tests.
- After the blood is drawn, apply pressure to the venipuncture site and assess it for bleeding and hematoma formation.

Serum osmolality test

Normal values:
Adult/elderly: 285-295 mOsm/kg H_2O
Child: 275-290 mOsm/kg H_2O
Possible critical values:
<265 mOsm/kg H_2O
>320 mOsm/kg H_2O

Rationale. The serum osmolality test is a measure of the number of particles per kilogram of the patient's serum. When the number of particles within the blood increases, serum osmolality is elevated. In diabetic patients the number of glucose particles in the serum increases markedly, thus raising serum osmolality to levels as high as 400 mOsm/kg. Patients whose serum osmolality values reach this level are usually comatose. Hypernatremia, ketosis, dehydration, hypercalcemia, and diabetes insipidis can also cause increased serum osmolality. Low serum osmolality usually results from fluid overload, adrenocortical insufficiency, and inappropriate secretion of antidiuretic hormone (ADH).

No complications are associated with this test.

Procedure. Seven milliliters of peripheral venous blood is obtained in a red-top tube from a nonfasting patient and sent to the chemistry laboratory for serum osmolality measurement. This test is only as uncomfortable as the venipuncture.

Contraindications. None.

Nursing considerations

Nursing Diagnoses/Collaborative Problems

See Blood studies, p. 2.

Nursing Implications with Rationale

- Apply pressure or a pressure dressing to the venipuncture site after the blood is obtained. Assess the site for bleeding.

SUPPLEMENTAL INFORMATION

Urine test for glucose and acetone

(urine sugar & acetone, fractional urine)

Normal values: negative for both glucose and acetone

Rationale

Glucose. Glucose is filtered into the urine when blood glucose levels exceed 180 mg/dl (the renal threshold). As the blood glucose level increases, the amount of glucose in the urine also increases. Renal threshold varies according to renal function. Patients with renal disease may have a lower renal threshold than patients with normal renal function (that is, glucose may spill into their urine at lower serum glucose levels).

Acetone (ketones). In a poorly controlled diabetic who is hyperglycemic, there is massive fatty acid catabolism. The purpose of this catabolism is to provide an energy source when glucose cannot be transferred into the cell because of an insufficiency of insulin. Ketones (beta-hydroxybutyric acid, acetoacetic acid, and acetone) are the end product of this fatty acid breakdown. Like glucose, ketones spill over into the urine when their levels are elevated in the blood. (Nondiabetic causes of ketonuria are described in Chapter 7 under urinalysis.)

Because urine glucose and acetone determinations are easily performed, painlessly obtained, and accurately reflective of serum glucose levels, they were used in monitoring insulin therapy in diabetic patients. However, this is being supplanted by self-monitoring of blood glucose (see p. 318). It is important to know that negative results for glucose and acetone are not necessarily indicative of a stabilized condition. Although these results would rule out hyperglycemia, the patient could be hypoglycemic. Because of this, many physicians prefer that juvenile diabetic patients show a trace of glucose in the urine. This is because glucose levels in young diabetic patients are very difficult to regulate and often swing rapidly from hyperglycemic to hypoglycemic.

Procedure. Fractional urine tests for glucose and acetone are performed at specified times during the day, generally before meals and at bedtime. Test results are used to determine the patient's insulin requirements.

Because accuracy is necessary, the urine specimen for testing should contain "fresh" urine only. Stagnant urine that has been in the patient's bladder for several hours does not accurately reveal the amount of glucose and acetone in the urine at the time of the testing because such a specimen may contain a mixture of glucose-free and glucose-containing urine. For this reason a "double-voided" specimen is preferred. This is obtained by collecting a urine specimen 30 to 40 minutes before the time the test specimen is actually needed. This first specimen is discarded, and the patient is given a glass of water (approximately 8 ounces) to drink. A second specimen is then obtained at the required time and tested for glucose and acetone. The result obtained from this double-voided, or second, specimen accurately reflects the amount of glucose in urine that had recently been filtered by the kidney.

Urine glucose and acetone are easily detected by using a Keto-diastix or Multistix reagent strip. The reagent strip is completely immersed in a well-mixed urine specimen and removed immediately to avoid diluting out the reagents. The strip is held in a horizontal position to prevent possible mixing of the chemical reagents and, at the time indicated, is compared with the test chart located on the jar of reagent strips. The ketone reading is made at exactly 15 seconds and the glucose reading at exactly 30 seconds. The ketone results vary from negative to 3+ (large). The glucose results range from negative to 4+, or 2%.

Urine testing for glucose can also be performed quickly and easily by the Clinitest method (a copper-reducing method). For this study a test tube, medicine dropper, Clinitest tablet, and color chart are required. Five drops of well-mixed urine are placed in a test tube containing 10 drops of water. After the Clinitest tablet is placed into the test tube, boiling ensues for a few seconds. The resultant color change (pea green to yellow-green to yellow or brown) permits estimation of the approximate content of sugar up to 2%. This test can be modified to allow estimation of sugar concentrations up to 5% by using 2 (instead of 5) drops of urine and 10 drops of water. A special color chart is used, with a scale ranging from 0% to 5%. This modification is particularly useful in children, in whom marked glycosuria may escape recognition by the standard (5-drop) procedure.

Acetone in the urine can be detected by Acetest tablets. For this test, a drop of urine is placed on an Acetest tablet. If acetone is present, varying shades of lavender appear; these can be compared with a color chart after the time period indicated in the instructions.

Contraindications. None.

Nursing considerations

Nursing Diagnoses/Collaborative Problems

See Urine studies, p. 3.

Nursing Implications with Rationale

- Explain the purpose of testing the urine for glucose and acetone. Teach the diabetic patient how to perform this test accurately.
- Read the directions on the bottle or container of the reagent strips. Compare the color reaction with the manufacturer's color chart at the *exact* time specified. Check the expiration date on the bottle before use. Tightly close the bottle after removing the reagent strips to prevent them from absorbing moisture and altering future results.
- Read the directions on the Clinitest and Acetest bottles before use. Be certain that the patient and the entire staff know whether the Clinitest should be performed with 2 or 5 drops of urine. Check the expiration date on

the bottle before use. Tightly close the reagent bottle after removing a Clinitest or Acetest tablet, because the tablets attract moisture and lose their potency.

- If the patient is receiving cephalothin (Keflin) intravenously or cephalexin (Keflex) orally, do not use Clinitest tablets, because false-positive results can be obtained. Vitamin C, probenecid, chloramphenicol, levodopa, methyldopa, sulfonamides, tetracyclines, nalidixic acid, and high-dose salicylates also cause false-positive results with Clinitest tablets. Therefore, use reagent strips for these patients.

Plasma insulin assay

Normal values:
Adult: 5-24 μU/ml or 36-179 pmol/L (SI units)
Newborn: 3-20 μU/ml
Possible critical value: >30 μU/ml

Rationale. The hormone insulin can now be measured successfully by radioimmunoassay in most larger laboratories. Insulin (see Anatomy and physiology, p. 309) regulates blood glucose levels by facilitating the movement of glucose out of the bloodstream. Insulin secretion is primarily determined by the blood glucose level. Normally, as the blood glucose level increases, the insulin level also increases, and as the glucose level decreases, insulin release stops.

This test is used to diagnose insulinoma and to evaluate abnormal lipid and carbohydrate metabolism. Currently, plasma insulin levels are not used in the diagnosis of diabetes mellitis.

Some investigators believe that measuring the ratio of the blood sugar and the insulin levels together on the same specimen during the oral GTT is more reliable than measuring the insulin levels alone. The insulin assay when compared with the oral GTT can show characteristic curves in certain situations. For example, juvenile diabetics have low fasting insulin levels and display GTT flat curves because of little or no increase in insulin levels. Patients who are mildly diabetic have normal fasting insulin levels and display GTT curves with a delayed rise.

After the patient fasts 12 to 14 hours, the insulin-glucose ratio should be <0.3. Patients with insulinoma have ratios greater than this.

Procedure. After the patient is kept NPO for 8 hours except for water, a fasting blood sample is obtained by peripheral venipuncture. If the serum insulin level is to be measured during the GTT, the blood samples should be drawn before the oral ingestion of the glucose load.

Contraindications. None.

Nursing considerations

Nursing Diagnoses/Collaborative Problems

See Blood studies, p. 2.

Nursing Implications with Rationale

- Explain the procedure to the patient. This test is usually done concurrently with the oral GTT (p. 312).

C-Peptide

(connecting peptide insulin, insulin C-peptide, proinsulin C-peptide)

Normal values: 0.78-1.89 ng/ml or 0.26-0.62 nmol/L (SI units)

Rationale. C-peptide is formed in the islet of Langerhans of the pancreas during the conversion of proinsulin to insulin and C-peptide. C-peptide is released into the portal vein in a 1:1 ratio of insulin. Because it has a longer half-life than insulin, more of it exists in the peripheral circulation. C-peptide levels correlate with insulin levels in the blood, except in islet-cell tumors and possibly in the obese patient. The capacity of the beta cells of the pancreas to secrete insulin can be evaluated by measuring insulin or by measuring C-peptide. Thus, C-peptide is a by-product of *endogenous* insulin synthesis and a marker for endogenous insulin production with or without exogenous insulin injections.

C-peptide is not affected by the presence or absence of insulin antibodies. Therefore, residual beta-cell function can be evaluated in the diabetic patient treated with insulin who may have insulin antibodies. This occurs most often in patients treated with bovine or pork insulin.

C-peptide values are high in patients with insulinoma. In these patients C-peptide concentrations parallel the plasma insulin values.

This test is also useful in evaluating patients with hypoglycemia and identifying patients with fictitious hypoglycemia due to surreptitious injection of insulin. These patients have high circulating levels of insulin with a suppressed C-peptide value because *exogenous* insulin suppresses *endogenous* insulin release. This suppression does not occur in insulinoma. C-peptide levels and insulin concentration are both elevated by the ingestion of sulfonylureas. Normal C-peptide levels occur in diabetics who are in remission.

Procedure. After an 8-10 hour fast from food and medications, venipuncture is performed and 1 red-top tube of blood is collected.

Contraindications. None.

Nursing considerations

Nursing Diagnosis/Collaborative Problems

See Blood studies, p. 2.

Nursing Implications with Rationale

- Instruct the patient to fast for 8 to 10 hours before the test. Only water is permitted.
- After the test assess the venipuncture site for bleeding.

Blood glucose self-monitoring

Today blood glucose self-monitoring is now replacing urine testing for many diabetic patients. Blood monitoring is important because it *directly* reflects the *current* serum glucose level. This is in contrast to urine testing (see pp. 315-317), which indirectly assesses the serum glucose level of several hours previously and which is affected by factors such as fluid volume and renal threshold. Self-monitoring of glucose is especially important in the detection of hypoglycemia, which is not detected on urine specimens. A diabetic can test his or her blood independently whenever hypoglycemia is suspected.

To benefit from blood glucose self-monitoring, the diabetic patient must learn how to correctly perform the blood test, how to keep accurate records, and how to interpret the test results. Having written guidelines describing any alteration in his or her diabetic regimen is also essential. The correct method for accurately monitoring the current blood glucose level follows:

1. Wash both hands with soap and water.
2. Let one arm hang below the level of the heart, and "milk" the finger to be used for the blood sample.
3. Prick the side of the finger rather than the middle of the finger to minimize pain and increase blood flow. A lancet or a needle may be used, but a device such as an Autolet, Autoclix, Hemalet, Monojet, or Penlet that has a spring-loaded lancet and a platform to control the depth of penetration is easier.
4. "Milk" the finger until a ¼ inch-wide drop of blood hangs from the finger.
5. Hold the finger over the reagent strip, and touch the reagent area of the strip to the drop of blood. The drop must cover the entire reagent area.
6. Begin timing the moment the blood touches the strip. Carefully follow the exact instructions on the package of the product used.

There are two types of self-glucose monitoring—the visually read tests and the reflectance meters. Examples of the *visually read test*, which allows the diabetic to make the glucose determination by sight, include Chemstrip bG, Dextrostix, and Visidex. The advantage of this first type of monitoring is that it does not require expensive machinery, machinery calibration, or controlled testing. The disadvantage is that the patient must visually interpret the test results. The color of the reagent strip must be compared to the color chart on the bottle from which it came—*not* from another bottle even of the same brand. If the color falls between two reference blocks, the patient must interpolate (estimate) the results.

The second type of self-glucose monitoring is the *reflectance meters*. Product examples include the Dextrometer, Glucometer, AccuChek bG, Glucoscan-II, and the Stat Tek. Although these meters may improve the accuracy of the blood glucose determination, the process is far more complex. The machine must first be calibrated, then a control test must be done to check the accuracy of the calibration, and finally the test is performed using the patient's blood.

QUESTIONS AND ANSWERS

1. **QUESTION:** Your patient is scheduled to have thyroid scanning. In obtaining a medical history of the patient you find that he had an IVP 1 week ago to evaluate a urologic complaint. Should thyroid scanning be cancelled?
   ANSWER: Yes. The iodine load that the patient received during his IVP will inhibit thyroidal uptake of any radioactive material for at least 4 weeks. Therefore, the results of the scanning would be less than adequate. The physician should be informed, and the test should be cancelled. Occasionally an ^{127}I urine excretion test can be performed by giving the patient a standard dose of ^{127}I by mouth. If the urine excretion of iodine is greater than 1 mg/day, there is still excess iodine in the blood that is blocking the thyroid uptake of ^{127}I and that will also block uptake of any scanning material.
2. **QUESTION:** Your patient is scheduled to have an RAIU test to rule out hyperthyroidism. One of the symptoms of hyperthyroidism is diarrhea, and this patient is having four loose bowel movements per day. Should the test be performed?
   ANSWER: No. The results of this test require gastrointestinal absorption of the orally administered radioactive iodine. If the patient has diarrhea, only a small portion of the iodine will be absorbed and this will bias the results of the test. It is best not to perform the test with orally administered iodine. However, iodine may be given intravenously and the uptake measured at 2 hours (in contrast to the 24 hours required for the orally administered iodine).
3. **QUESTION:** On a routine evaluation for lower back pain, a 54-year-old woman is found to have hypercalcemia. Her serum PTH level is below normal. What might elucidate the cause of this patient's problems?
   ANSWER: The most common cause of hypercalcemia and a concomitantly low PTH level in a postmenopausal woman is bone metastasis from a primary breast cancer. Therefore, mammography and a lumbosacral spinal x-ray study are indicated. (Primary and tertiary hyperparathyroidism were eliminated as causes in light of the low PTH level.)
4. **QUESTION:** A patient is transferred to your floor 2 days after having a complete workup for an adrenal tumor. This workup included a dexamethasone suppression test, adrenal angiography, adrenal venography, and ACTH assay. You notice that over the next 24 hours this patient becomes progressively more obtunded. All laboratory tests are normal except for a low sodium level and a high potassium level. Although the physician orders appropriate IV fluids, the patient dies 48 hours after transfer to your floor. What might have been attempted to reverse the progressive deterioration of this patient?
   ANSWER: Adrenal gland hemorrhage and infarction are complications of adrenal venography. This should have been considered, and the patient should have been given cortisone intravenously. This cortisone certainly would not have hurt. In this patient, autopsy did indeed demonstrate bilateral adrenal gland hemorrhage.
5. **QUESTION:** Your patient, who is suspected of having an adrenal tumor, returns to the floor after having adrenal angiography. On physical assessment of the patient, blood pressure is 280/140 mm Hg, pulse rate is 145 beats/minute, oral temperature is 101° F, and respirations are 38/minute. Is this patient having an allergic reaction to the dye?
   ANSWER: No. Most patients having a serious allergic reaction to iodinated dye are hypotensive. Allergy would also be highlighted by urticaria and wheezing. This patient is most probably having a serious hypertensive episode caused by a pheochromocytoma and induced by the arteriography. The physician should be notified immediately and venous access should be obtained. The physician

will most probably request phenoxybenzamine (an alpha-adrenergic blocker) and propranolol (a beta-adrenergic blocker). The patient should be closely monitored in a quiet, darkened, intensive care facility.

6. **QUESTION:** Your patient is scheduled for a 24-hour urine collection for 17-KS. Why should creatinine also be measured in the urine specimen?

   ANSWER: Excretion of creatinine is relatively constant. If the creatinine concentration in the 24-hour urine collection is less than normal (male, 20-26 mg/kg; female, 14-22 mg/kg), one must suspect that the specimen does not represent a complete 24-hour collection. Perhaps some of the urine has been discarded. This will bias the results for 17-KS or other urine components. Urine collection should be repeated.

7. **QUESTION:** Your patient is having a GTT performed. Thirty minutes after ingestion of the glucose, the patient vomits. What should be done?

   ANSWER: After assessing the patient's vital signs, a blood glucose specimen should be obtained to ensure that the patient is not dangerously hyperglycemic or hypoglycemic. The GTT should then be cancelled because its results are based on the ingestion and digestion of all of the glucose load. Incomplete absorption of the glucose load will bias the results. If the patient cannot tolerate the ingestion of the glucose load, then an intravenous glucose tolerance test can be performed.

8. **QUESTION:** Your patient is admitted to the hospital for evaluation of signs and symptoms suggesting Cushing's syndrome. The doctor has requested that you begin collecting a 24-hour urine specimen for 17-OHCS. In your initial assessment of the patient, you discover that she has a severe upper respiratory tract infection. Should the test be performed?

   ANSWER: No. The ongoing acute upper respiratory tract infection acts as a physical stress to the patient. As a result, the adrenal gland may be appropriately hyperfunctioning, and elevated urine 17-OHCS levels would be expected even in normal patients. For that reason, you should notify the physician of the upper respiratory tract infection. The physician will most probably want to cancel the planned evaluation and treat the patient's respiratory tract infection.

BIBLIOGRAPHY

Barsano CP: Hypothyroidism. In Rakel RE, editor: Conn's current therapy, Philadelphia, 1991, WB Saunders.

Beierwaltes WH: Endocrine imaging: parathyroid, adrenal cortex, and medulla, and other endocrine tumors, Part II, J Nucl Med 32(8):1627-1639, 1991.

Colagiuri R and others: The quality of self-monitoring of blood glucose. Diabetic Med 7(9):800-804, 1990.

Daniels GH and Martin JB: Neuroendocrine regulation and diseases of the anterior pituitary and hypothalamus. In Wilson J and others, editors: Harrison's principles of internal medicine, ed 12, New York, 1991, McGraw-Hill.

Foster DW: Diabetes mellitus. In Wilson J and others, editors: Harrison's principles of internal medicine, ed 12, New York, McGraw-Hill.

Griffin JE: Dynamic tests of endocrine function. In Wilson JD and Foster DW, editors: Williams textbook of endocrinology, ed 8, Philadelphia, 1992, WB Saunders.

Gross MD and others: Scintigraphic imaging of the thyroid, parathyroid, and adrenal glands. Curr Opin Radiol 2(6):851-859, 1990.

Landin-Olsson M and others: Islet cell antibodies and fasting C-peptide predict insulin requirement at diagnosis of diabetes mellitus. Diabetologia 33(9):561-568, 1990.

Makita Z and others: Radioimmunoassay for the determination of glycated haemoglobin. Diabetologia 34(1):40-45, 1991.

Orth DN: The adrenal cortex. In Wilson JD and Foster DW, editors: Williams textbook of endocrinology, ed 8. Philadelphia, 1992, WB Saunders.

Posen S: Hyperparathyroidism and hypoparathyroidism. In Rakel RE, editor: Conn's current therapy, Philadelphia, 1991, WB Saunders.

Rumley AG and others: Within-clinic glycosylated haemoglobin measurement. Diabetic Med 7(9):838-840, 1990.

Schottelius BA and Schottelius DD: Textbook of physiology, ed 18, St Louis, 1978, CV Mosby.

Sherman B and Johanson A: Hypopituitarism. In Rakel RE, editor: Conn's current therapy, Philadelphia, 1991, WB Saunders.

Thibodeau GA: Anatomy and physiology, St Louis, 1987, CV Mosby.

Thorner MO and others: The anterior pituitary. In Wilson JD and Foster DW, editors: Williams textbook of endocrinology, ed 8, Philadelphia, 1992, WB Saunders.

Tsang WM and others: Glycated haemoglobin measurement in uraemic patients. Ann Clin Biochem 28(pt 4):414-416, 1991.

Tsuji A and others: Recent progress in neonatal mass screening for congenital hypothyroidism and adrenal hyperplasia using enzyme immunoassays. Adv Clin Chem 28:109-143, 1990.

Wartofsky L and Ingbar SH: Diseases of the thyroid. In Wilson J and others, editors: Harrison's principles of internal medicine, ed 12, New York, 1991, McGraw-Hill.

Williams GH and Dluhy RG: Diseases of the adrenal cortex. In Wilson J and others, editors: Harrison's principles of internal medicine, ed 12, New York, 1991, McGraw-Hill.

Wilson JD: Hormones and hormone action. In Wilson J and others, editors: Harrison's principles of internal medicine, ed 12, New York, 1991, McGraw-Hill.

Yalow RS: Radioimmunoassay of hormones. In Wilson JD and Foster DW, editors: Williams textbook of endocrinology, ed 8, Philadelphia, 1992, WB Saunders.

Chapter 9

DIAGNOSTIC STUDIES USED IN THE ASSESSMENT OF THE REPRODUCTIVE SYSTEM

ANATOMY AND PHYSIOLOGY

This discussion of anatomy and physiology of the reproductive system deals only with material relevant to the diagnostic studies included in this chapter. A detailed discussion of this complex system can be found in many textbooks (see Bibliography).

Male generative organs

The testes (Figure 9-1) are located in the scrotum, which is ideally suited to provide the appropriate temperature required for sperm pro-

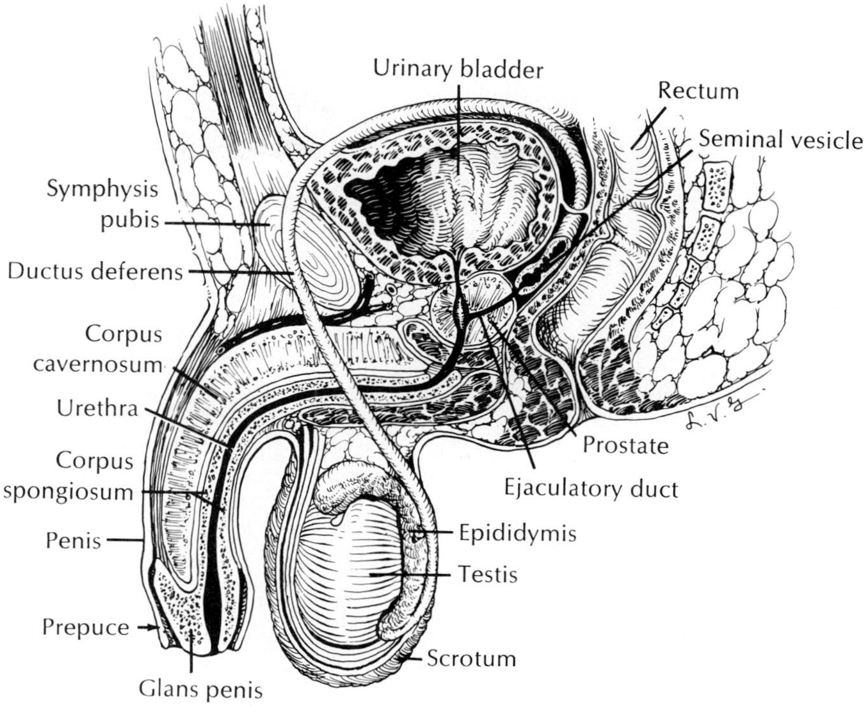

FIGURE 9-1. Male genital organs.
From Schottelius BA, Schottelius DD: Textbook of physiology, ed 18, St Louis, 1978, Mosby–Year Book.

duction (spermatogenesis). The epithelial cells lining the seminiferous tubules within the testes give rise to the spermatozoa, or sperm cells. Sperm production is one of the major functions of the testes. Genital ducts, which include the epididymides, vas deferens, ejaculatory duct, seminal vesicles, and the urethra (Figure 9-1), provide a conduit for transport of the sperm cells.

The other major function of the testes is secretion of testosterone, which is the major androgen (male hormone). Testosterone is secreted by the interstitial cells of the testes. It stimulates development of part of the genital tract as well as development of secondary male sexual characteristics.

Female reproductive organs

The ovaries are the essential sex organs in the female reproductive system (Figure 9-2). Like the testes, the ovaries are multifunctional. They are responsible for ovulation (production of ova) and the secretion of the female hormones (estrogen and progesterone). The fallopian tubes (oviducts) arise from the uterus and terminate adjacent to the ovary (Figure 9-2). These oviducts transport the ovum to the uterus. Fertilization of the ovum by the sperm usually occurs within these ducts.

The uterus (Figure 9-2) is a muscular organ whose inner cavity is lined with a specialized mucosa called the endometrium. The endometrium undergoes cyclic (menstrual) structural changes in preparation for conception and pregnancy. Events occurring in the ovary and uterus during the menstrual cycle are shown in Figure 9-3.

There are three phases of the menstrual cycle: the menstrual phase, the proliferative phase, and the secretory phase. The average

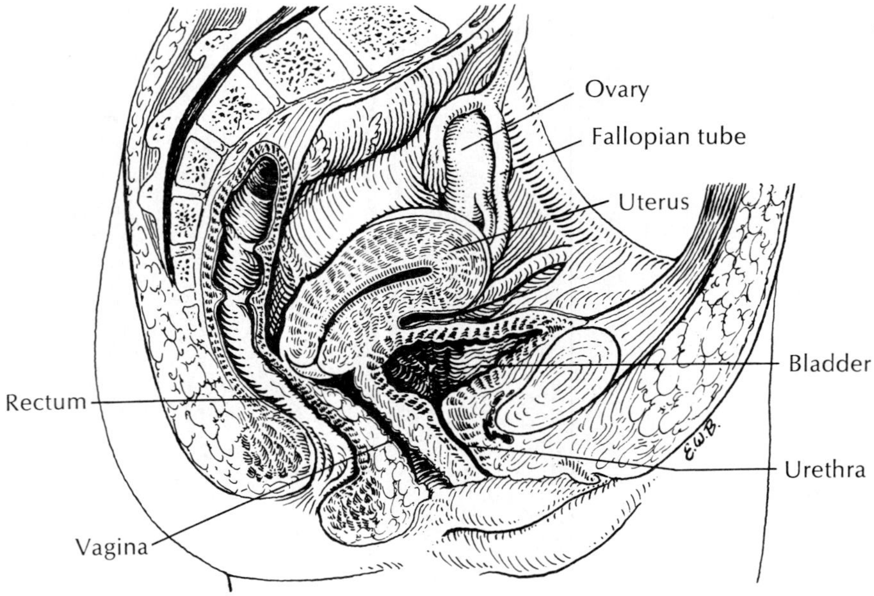

FIGURE 9-2. Female genital organs.
From Schottelius BA, Schottelius DD: Textbook of physiology, ed 18, St Louis, 1978, Mosby–Year Book.

menstrual cycle is 28 days and begins with the first day of vaginal blood flow. During the menses (menstrual phase) the endometrium undergoes degenerative change so that the superficial layer of the endometrium sloughs and is discharged in the menstrual flow. After the blood flow ceases, there is a gradual growth of the endometrium (proliferative phase), which is stimulated by ovarian estrogen. At approximately the fourteenth day of the cycle (Figure 9-3), the graafian follicle, within the ovary, ruptures, and the ovum is expelled (ovulation) into the fallopian tubes. The ruptured ovarian follicle is then called a corpus luteum. Large amounts of progesterone and some estrogen are secreted by the corpus luteum and cause the endometrial glands to thicken and mature. This is called the endometrial secretory phase (Figure 9-3). The submucosal layers become extremely vascular and edematous. The purpose of the secretory phase is to prepare the uterine lining to receive (nidation) and nourish a fertilized ovum. If fertilization does not take place, the corpus luteum degenerates and the endometrium sloughs, leading to vaginal bleeding, which occurs at approximately the twenty-eighth day of the cycle.

Pregnancy

When fertilization does occur, the zygote (fertilized ovum) moves through the fallopian tubes and into the prepared uterine cavity. On coming into contact with the endometrial mucosa, the exposed cells on the outside (trophoblast) of the developing embryonic cell mass (blastocyst) begin to digest a portion of the mucosa. This allows the so-called trophoblast to sink into the mucosa (implant) and absorb nutrition from the uterine glands until the placenta forms. The trophoblast and later the placenta produce human chorionic gonadotropin (HCG), which maintains the corpus luteum's existence. The corpus luteum continues to secrete the progesterone required to maintain the pregnancy. Through continued growth, the embryo be-

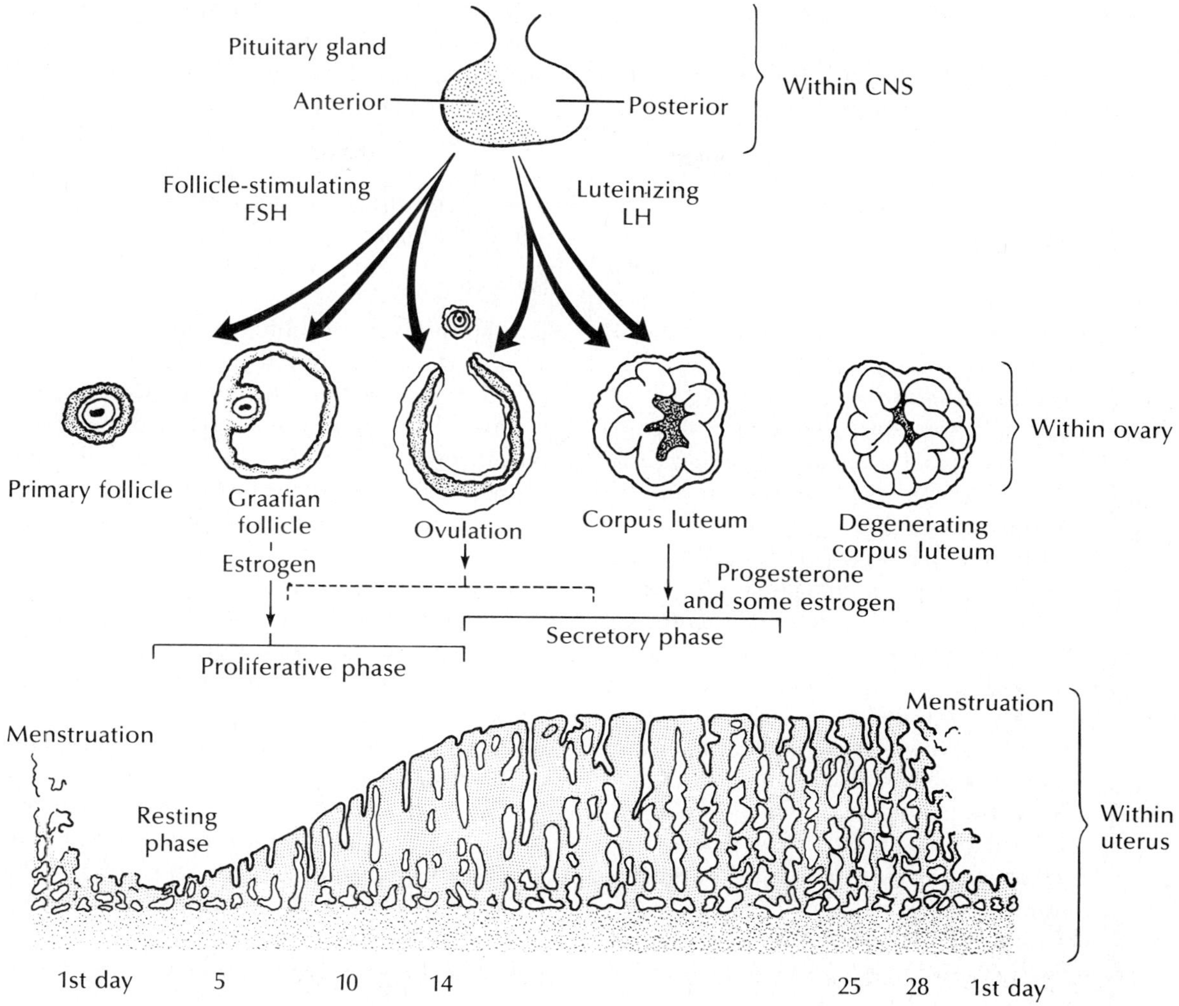

FIGURE 9-3. Hormonal control of menstrual cycle.
From Jensen MD, Benson RC, Bobak IM: Maternity care: the nurse and the family, St Louis, 1977, Mosby–Year Book.

comes surrounded by two membranes: the amnion (inner layer of the fetal membrane) and the chorion (outer layer of the fetal membrane). The space between the embryo and the amnion, the amniotic cavity, is filled with amniotic fluid.

At approximately 8 weeks from the last menstrual period the embryo is completely developed and is called a fetus. For the remaining 32 weeks the fetus grows on the nutritional support provided by the mother through the placenta. Toward the end of pregnancy HCG and progesterone levels decrease, perhaps as a result of placental deterioration. Uterine contractions begin in an effort to expel the fetus vaginally.

High-risk pregnancy

Many disease states can jeopardize the normal events associated with pregnancy, labor, and delivery. When such threats are recognized beforehand, the pregnancy is considered "at high risk" and is monitored more closely than usual. A few examples of situations that are responsible for high-risk pregnancy include the following factors in the patient's history or current status:

1. Advanced maternal age—35 years or older
2. Past or current history of primary idiopathic hypertension
3. Two or more spontaneous or induced abortions in the past
4. Previous stillbirths
5. Previous premature deliveries
6. Previous infant with Rh isoimmunization
7. Previous infant with genetic or familial disorders
8. Previous infant with congenital anomaly
9. Previous small-for-status infant or present small-for-status fetus (intrauterine growth retardation)
10. Multiple pregnancy
11. Genital tract anomalies (such as incompetent cervix, cervical malformation, or uterine malformation)
12. Medical conditions such as hypertension, diabetes mellitus, heart disease, renal disease, cancer, or thyroid dysfunction
13. Social problems (such as teen pregnancy, drug or tobacco use, or poor nutrition)

Infertility

Infertility can be diagnosed whenever a woman is unable to conceive during at least 1 year of regular, unprotected intercourse. Ninety percent of couples are able to achieve a pregnancy within a 1-year period. Normal fertility is dependent on many factors in both the man and the woman. The man must be able to produce a sufficient number of normal, motile spermatozoa that can be ejaculated through a patent pathway (vas deferens) into the vagina. The spermatozoa then must be able to survive in the cervical environment and ascend through the cervix, uterus, and fallopian tubes. The woman must be able to produce an ovum that remains in the fallopian tubes until it is fertilized by sperm. To begin normal development, the products of conception must be allowed to move into the uterus and implant themselves in an endometrium capable of sustaining life. Any defect in these processes will result in infertility.

Male infertility

Problems in male fertility are the sole factor or an important contributing factor in 30% to 40% of infertile marriages. These problems usually involve defects in spermatogenesis or in insemination. Male infertility may be caused by one or more of the following:

1. Spermatozoal abnormalities. These include reduction in the quantity of spermatozoa (<50 million/ml), reduction of the ejaculatory volume (<3.4 ml), abnormal sperm quality (such as too dilute), and abnormally shaped spermatozoa (such as two-headed or tailless).
2. Sperm antibodies (autoimmunization). Autoantibodies may be responsible for interference with normal spermatogenesis or may affect the spermatozoa and prevent pregnancy.
3. Testicular abnormalities, such as complete absence or inappropriate development of the testes. Infections, particularly suppurative orchitis, which may accompany mumps, can destroy the epithelium of the seminiferous tubules. Abnormal testicular location (cryptorchidism), testicular trauma, irradiation, prolonged exposure to high temperatures, or varicocele may result in inadequate spermatogenesis.
4. Abnormalities of the penis. If the penis is abnormally short, buried in fat, or malformed (as in hypospadias), semen emission may take place outside of the vagina.
5. Faulty sperm transmission. Insemination may be inhibited because of scarring that

obstructs the epididymis, vas deferens, or urethra. Postgonorrheal scarring is the most frequent cause.

6. Prostate and seminal vesicle abnormalities. The number or quality of sperm may be reduced or altered by chronic prostatitis or seminal vesiculitis.
7. Advanced nutritional deficiency. This condition alters the function of all organ systems, including the gonads.
8. Emotional factors. These may induce impotence or premature ejaculation.

Female infertility

Ovulation occurs between the twelfth and sixteenth day of most menstrual cycles. Unprotected intercourse must take place within 12 to 24 hours of ovulation. Often failure to conceive is the result of incorrect timing of ovulation. Other causes of female infertility include:

1. Cervical abnormalities. Alterations in cervical mucosa caused by either hormonal deficiency or cervicitis interferes with sperm passage. Obstructions in the cervical canal caused by polyps, fibroids (leiomyomas), atresia, or suppurative discharge impair the transit of the spermatozoa.
2. Vaginal disorders. Absence or incomplete formation of the vagina prevents vaginal penetration by the penis and sperm. Inflammation of the vagina alters the pH, which may destroy or inactivate sperm.
3. Endocrine abnormalities. The abnormal function of the hypothalamus, anterior pituitary, ovaries, thyroid, or adrenal glands can result in anovulation.
4. Uterine disorder. Scarring (after dilation and curettage), malformation, malposition, or tumors of the uterus may prevent nidation of the fertilized ovum into the uterine mucosa or cause early abortion.
5. Tubal disorders. Partial or complete occlusion of the fallopian tubes occurs in a large number of women who fail to conceive. The most common cause of tubal obstruction is scarring (as a result of pelvic inflammatory disease, or PID). Appendicitis and other pelvic infections, along with pelvic endometriosis, may result in adhesions that subsequently can partially or completely obstruct the tubes.
6. Ovarian disorders. Ovarian agenesis or incomplete development can cause anovulation. Tumors, infections, or endometriosis can also disrupt ovarian function transiently or permanently.
7. Severe nutritional deficiencies and chronic disease states. These conditions reduce or inhibit ovulation.
8. Advancing age. Fertility in women reaches a peak at about 20 to 25 years of age and slowly declines until menopause.
9. Emotional factors. Vaginismus (painful spasm of the vagina that prevents coitus) and dyspareunia (pain during coitus) may be the result of psychologic disturbances.
10. Immunologic reactions to sperm. Unexplained infertility may be caused by female production of antisperm antibodies.
11. Drugs. Nearly all ovulating women cease to ovulate while on antineoplastic chemotherapy and many psychotropic drugs.
12. Radiation. Ovulation is permanently obliterated by exposure of the ovaries to radiation levels greater than 800 rad.

Since one or many factors may be the cause of infertility, the man and the woman must both be evaluated. A systematic investigation of infertility is described after Case study 1. During the diagnostic course it is important to allow the couple the opportunity to express feelings of isolation, guilt, depression, or anger that often accompany infertility. Therapy for infertility may require correction of faulty coital techniques, attention to proper timing, surgery to correct a malfunction or anatomic anomalies, or recognition and correction of emotional factors. If the infertility persists, the condition is then referred to as *sterility*. Approximately one out of ten American couples is truly "barren."

CASE STUDY 1: INFERTILITY

After 1 year of unsuccessfully trying to conceive, Mr. and Mrs. S., both age 28, were referred to an infertility specialist. The history and physical examination results were negative, and a diagnostic evaluation was scheduled and performed.

Studies	Results: Husband	Results: Wife
Basic laboratory procedures		
Urinalysis (see Chapter 7)	WNL	WNL
Complete blood count (CBC) (see Chapter 10)	WNL	WNL
Serologic test for syphilis (STS)	Negative	Negative
	(normal: negative)	
Culture for *Ureaplasma* and *Chlamydia*		Negative
Blood type and Rh factor (see Chapter 10)	B+	A+
Thyroid function studies (see Chapter 8)	WNL	WNL
Evaluation of semen (semen analysis)		
Volume	5 ml (normal: 2-5 ml)	
Sperm count	105 million/ml (normal: 20-200 million/ml)	
Motility	62% actively motile (normal: 60%-80% actively motile)	
Sperm morphology	75% normally shaped (normal: 70%-90% normally shaped)	

Studies	Results
Evaluation of tubal patency	
Hysterosalpingography (uterotubography)	Normal passage of radioactive material through the tubes and into the peritoneal area
Evaluation of ovulation	
Cervical mucus test	Ovulation confirmed by "ferning"
Endometrial biopsy	Ovulation confirmed by presence of "late secretory phase" endometrium
Basal body temperature (BBT) measurement	Normal biphasic curve
24-hour urine test for pregnanediol	1.2 mg/24 hours (normal: >1.0 mg/24 hours)
Evaluation of cervical factors	
Sims-Huhner test	Normal (cervical mucus adequate for sperm survival, transmission, and penetration); 12 active sperm per high-power field
Laparoscopy	Normal-appearing fallopian tubes

Because the results of all of these studies were normal, laparoscopy was performed. The normal findings led the physician to suspect that antisperm antibodies were the cause of infertility. Although the husband wore condoms during coitus for several months to decrease his wife's level of antisperm antibodies and permit conception, a pregnancy still did not occur within the next year. The couple initiated adoption procedures.

DISCUSSION OF TESTS

Semen analysis

Volume

Normal value: 2-5 ml

Liquefaction time

Normal value: <20-30 minutes after collection

pH

Normal value: 7.12-8.00

Sperm count (density)
Normal value: 50-200 million/ml
Sperm motility
Normal value: 60% to 80% actively motile
Sperm morphology
Normal value: 70% to 90% normally shaped

Rationale. The semen analysis is one of the most important aspects of the infertility workup, since the cause of the woman's inability to conceive often lies within the man. After 2 to 3 days of sexual abstinence, sperm is collected and examined for volume, sperm count, motility, and morphology.

The freshly collected semen is first measured for volume. After liquefaction of the white, gelatinous ejaculate, a sperm count is done. Men with very low or very high counts are likely to be infertile. The motility of the sperm is then evaluated. At least 60% of the sperm should show progressive motility. Morphology is studied by staining a semen preparation and calculating the number of normal versus abnormal sperm forms.

A simple sperm analysis, especially if it indicates infertility, is inconclusive, because the sperm count varies from day to day. A semen analysis should be done at least twice. Men with aspermia (no sperm) or oligospermia (<20 million) should be evaluated endocrinologically for pituitary, thyroid, adrenal, or testicular aberrations.

A normal semen analysis alone does not accurately assess the male factor, unless the effect of the partner's cervical secretion on sperm survival is also determined (see Sims-Huhner test). In addition to its value in infertility workups, semen analysis is also helpful in documenting adequate sterilization after a vasectomy. It is usually performed 6 weeks after the surgery. If any sperm are seen, the adequacy of the vasectomy must be questioned.

Procedure. After 2 to 3 days of the patient's sexual abstinence, a semen specimen is collected by ejaculation into a clean container. For best results this specimen should be collected in the physician's office or laboratory by masturbation. Less satisfactory specimens can be obtained in the patient's home by coitus interruptus or masturbation. These home specimens must be delivered to the laboratory within 1 hour after collection. Excessive heat and cold should be avoided during transportation of the specimen.

If, for religious reasons, the couple cannot obtain a specimen by masturbation or coitus interruptus, a plastic condom can be used. Rubber condoms should not be used, because the powders and lubricants used in their manufacture may be spermicidal.

Contraindications. None.

Nursing considerations

Nursing Diagnoses/Collaborative Problems

- Possible knowledge deficit related to test purpose, preparation, and procedure
- Possible anxiety related to test results

Nursing Implications with Rationale

- Explain the procedure to the patient. Be certain that the patient knows that a 2 to 3 day period of sexual abstinence is necessary. Prolonged abstinence before the collection should be discouraged, since the quality of the sperm cells, and especially their motility, may diminish.
- Give the patient the proper container for the sperm collection. The collection and delivery of the semen to the laboratory may be embarrassing to the patient. Do not add to his embarrassment. Be matter-of-fact about the specimen collection and delivery.
- If the specimen is obtained at home, be certain that the patient is told that the specimen must be brought to the laboratory for testing within 1 hour after collection and that it should be kept at room temperature. Exposure to heat or cold during the transportation may alter sperm cell motility. Record the date of the previous semen emission, along with the collection time and date of the fresh spec-

imen. The laboratory will refer to these dates.

- Allow time for the patient to discuss any questions or fears regarding the results of this study. Instruct the patient about when and how to obtain the test results. Abnormal results may have a devastating effect on the patient's sexuality.

Hysterosalpingography

(uterotubography, uterosalpingography, hysterogram)

Normal values: patent fallopian tube; no defects in uterine cavity

Rationale. In hysterosalpingography, the uterine cavity and fallopian tubes are radiographically visualized after the injection of contrast material through the cervix. Uterine tumors (such as leiomyomas), intrauterine adhesions, and developmental anomalies (such as uterus bicornis) can be seen. Tubal obstruction caused by internal scarring, tumor, or kinking (resulting from pelvic adhesions) can also be seen. A possible therapeutic effect of this test may be that the passage of dye through the tubes clears mucous plugs, straightens kinked tubes, or breaks up adhesions.

This test may also be used to document adequacy of surgical tubal ligation. Potential complications include allergy to the iodinated contrast material and infection of the endometrium (endometritis) or fallopian tube (salpingitis) caused by using contaminated dye.

Procedure. This procedure is best performed 4 to 5 days after the completion of menstruation, because debris may trap or transiently occlude the fallopian tubes. At this time the risk of inducing abortion if an unknown pregnancy exists is also avoided.

This test is usually performed on an outpatient basis in the radiology department by a gynecologist. A radiologist interprets the x-ray films. A laxative is given the night before the test. An enema or suppository is administered on the morning of the study. Immediately before the study, a plain film of the abdomen is taken to ensure that the preparation adequately eliminated gastrointestinal gas and feces.

After voiding, the patient is placed on the fluoroscopy table in the lithotomy position (as for pelvic examination). A bivalve speculum is inserted into the vagina, and the cervix is visualized and cleansed. A sterile cannula is inserted into the cervix and held in place by a tenaculum. A 2-minute rest period is necessary to allow for relaxation of tubal spasm associated with cervical dilatation. A few milliliters of dye is injected through the cannula during fluoroscopy, and x-ray films are taken. More dye is then injected so that the entire upper genital tract (uterus and tubes) can be filled. This study can be considered satisfactorily performed only if the uterus and the tubes are distended to their maximum capacity or if fluid flows through the fallopian tubes (Figure 9-4).

The duration of this procedure is about 15 minutes. The patient may feel occasional transient menstrual type cramping. Mild sedatives or antispasmodics are sometimes used. The patient may complain of shoulder pain caused by subphrenic irritation from the dye as it leaks into the peritoneal cavity. Cramping and dizziness may occur following this study. A vaginal discharge (sometimes bloody) may be present 1 to 2 days after the test.

Contraindications. This procedure should not be performed in:

1. Patients with infections of the vagina, cervix, or fallopian tubes, for fear of extending the infection. If the woman has PID, the test is rescheduled for 2 to 3 months later and she is treated with antibiotics.
2. Patients with uterine bleeding, since contrast material might enter the open blood vessels.
3. Patients with suspected pregnancy, because the contrast material might induce abortion.
4. Patients having any severe systemic illness that would make patient cooperation difficult.

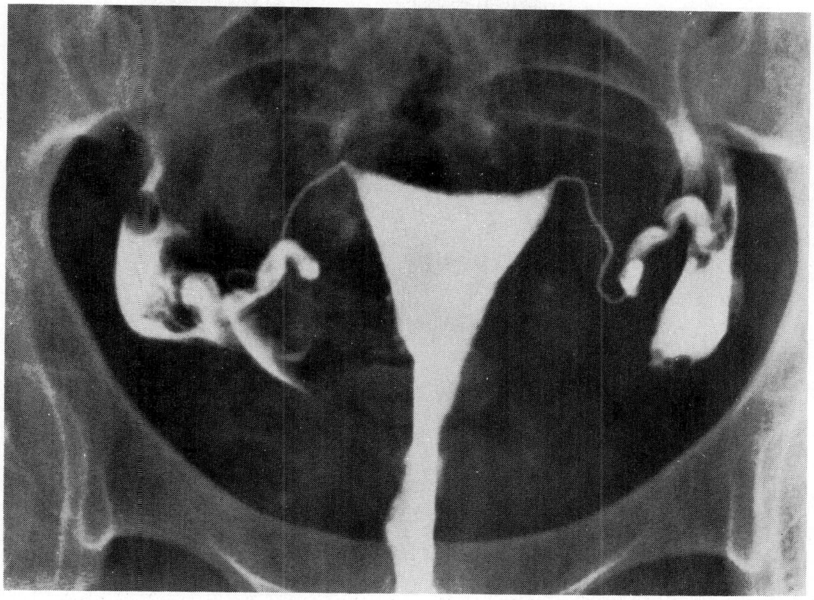

FIGURE 9-4. Normal tubogram (hysterosalpingogram) showing passage of radiopaque material through fimbriated ends of tubes and peritoneal "spill."
From Willson JR, Carrington ER: Obstetrics and gynecology, ed 6, St Louis, 1979, Mosby–Year Book.

Nursing considerations

Nursing Diagnoses/Collaborative Problems

See X-ray studies, p. 5.

- Potential complications: salpingitis, endometritis

Nursing Implications with Rationale

- Explain the procedure thoroughly to the patient. Written instructions are helpful, since the procedure is usually scheduled on an outpatient basis at a later time.
- Encourage the patient to verbalize her feelings regarding this test. Many patients are very fearful that the results of this study may markedly affect their sexuality and fertility.
- Tell the woman what sensations she may be expected to feel during the test. An apprehensive patient will feel more pain and is more likely to show spastic obstruction of the fallopian tubes than a relaxed woman.
- Administer mild sedatives or antispasmodics, if ordered, before this study.
- Be certain that the patient took the cathartic and enema as ordered to prevent gas shadows from obscuring the x-ray film.
- Assess the patient for allergy to iodinated dye. After the study observe the patient for sensitivities to the dye.
- After the study, advise the patient to wear a perineal pad, because radiopaque material may stain her underclothing.
- Patients whose results indicate tubal obstruction are usually very upset after testing. Encourage them to verbalize their fears. Provide emotional support.

Cervical mucus test

(fern test)

Normal value: arborization, or ferning, of cervical mucus during midcycle

Rationale. The cervical mucus can be examined near midcycle and just before menstruation to detect ovulation. Ovulation requires a

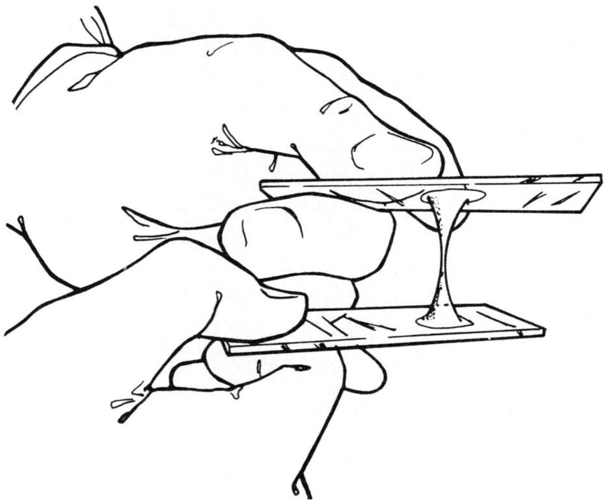

FIGURE 9-5. Spinnbarkheit (elasticity).

surge of estrogen during midcycle (Figure 9-3). Without this surge, ovulation does not occur. Because pregnancy is impossible without ovulation, this study is used in the evaluation of infertility to predict the day of ovulation and to determine whether ovulation occurs.

The cervical mucus at ovulation (the time of maximum estrogen effect) is clear, abundant, watery, and elastic. This elasticity or *spinnbarkheit* (Figure 9-5) increases at ovulation. Excellent spinnbarkheit occurs when the mucus can be stretched at least 5 to 6 cm.

When the cervical mucus is spread on a clean glass slide and allowed to dry, a pattern of "arborization," or "ferning," occurs (Figure 9-6). This is due to the increased level of salt and water interacting with the glycoproteins in the mucus during ovulation. This pattern is correlated with estrogen activity and is therefore present in all ovulatory women at midcycle. When the cervical mucus is checked again immediately before menstruation, no ferning is found because of progesterone activity. Therefore during a normal ovulatory cycle, the ferning of cervical mucus occurs at midcycle and no ferning occurs before menstruation.

Besides its absence in anovulatory premenopausal patients, ferning of the cervical mucus is also absent in postmenopausal or castrated women because very little estrogen exists. Because of the presence of fern-inhibiting progesterone in pregnant women, ferning does not occur.

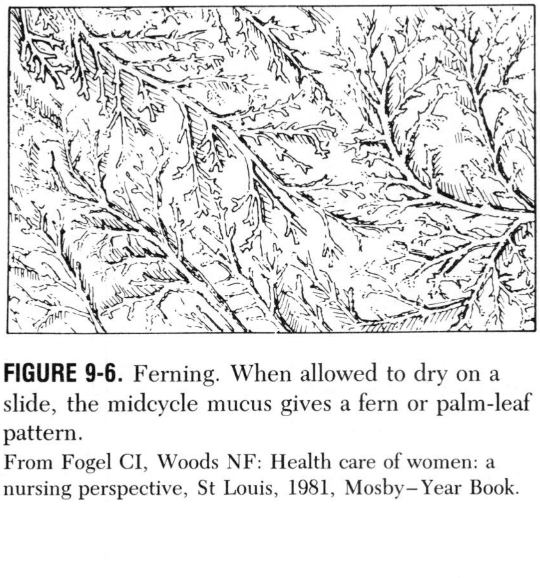

FIGURE 9-6. Ferning. When allowed to dry on a slide, the midcycle mucus gives a fern or palm-leaf pattern.
From Fogel CI, Woods NF: Health care of women: a nursing perspective, St Louis, 1981, Mosby–Year Book.

Procedure. This procedure is performed at midcycle to detect estrogen-induced ferning. It is then repeated approximately 7 days later to detect the progesterone inhibition of ferning. The patient is placed in the lithotomy position.

An unlubricated speculum is inserted into the vagina to expose the cervix. A cotton-tipped applicator is gently inserted into the cervical canal and rotated. The mucus that adheres to the cotton swab is spread on the clean glass slide and allowed to dry at room temperature. No staining is used. The dried spread of mucus is then examined under the low-power lens of a microscope for the presence of ferning (Figure 9-6).

The slides used for the mucus must be washed in distilled water, because the electrolytes in tap water may produce false ferning. Ferning may be inhibited if the cervix is traumatized during this procedure and blood mixes with the mucus.

This procedure is performed by a physician in approximately 15 minutes. The only discomfort associated with this study is the insertion of the speculum (as for a Pap smear).

Contraindications. None.

Nursing considerations

Nursing Diagnoses/Collaborative Problems

- Possible knowledge deficit related to test purpose, preparation, and procedure
- Possible anxiety related to unknown sensations of procedure
- Possible alteration in comfort related to test procedure
- Possible anxiety related to test results

Nursing Implications with Rationale

- Explain the procedure to the patient. Encourage the patient to ask questions. Many patients are poorly informed and worry needlessly about diagnostic studies.
- Many patients undergoing infertility studies are fearful that the test results may affect their fertility and sexuality. Provide emotional support.
- Keep the patient as comfortable as possible during the study. Ensure that draping is done effectively to prevent unnecessary exposure of the patient.
- Usually the patient is given the results immediately after the test. If not, tell her when to call the physician for the results.

Endometrial biopsy

Normal value: presence of a "secretory-type" endometrium 3 to 5 days before normal menses; no abnormal cells

Rationale. Performing an endometrial biopsy can determine whether ovulation has occurred. As discussed in the anatomy and physiology section, ovulation is followed by transformation of the ovarian follicle to a corpus luteum, which secretes the progesterone (Figure 9-3) responsible for endometrial buildup (secretory phase) in anticipation of nidation. A biopsy specimen taken 3 to 5 days before normal menses (days 21 to 25 of the cycle) should demonstrate a "secretory-type" endometrium on histologic examination if ovulation and corpus luteum formation have occurred. If not, only a preovulatory "proliferative-type" endometrium will be seen. This test also detects ovulation defects in addition to anovulation.

Occasionally an endometrial biopsy is performed to indicate estrogen's effect in patients with suspected ovarian dysfunction or absence. Similarly, adequate circulating progesterone levels can be determined by identifying secretory endometrium. Another major use of endometrial biopsy is to diagnose endometrial cancer. This study is also used to detect tuberculosis, polyps, or inflammatory conditions. Complications of this study include perforation of the uterus, uterine bleeding, and interference with early pregnancy. If lateral scrapings are used for hormone workup, the chances of interfering with pregnancy are minimal because most implantation occurs on the anterior or posterior surfaces.

Procedure. This study is performed on the nonfasting and unsedated patient in the physician's office. No anesthesia is required. The patient is placed in the lithotomy position, and a bimanual pelvic examination is performed to determine the position of the uterus. The cervix is exposed and cleaned. After a tenaculum is placed on the cervix for stabilization, a sound (metal probe) is passed into the uterine cavity to determine the size of the uterus. This prevents inadvertent perforation of the uterus during biopsy specimen removal. A suction tube—curet or an endometrial biopsy curet (Novak) is inserted into the uterus, and specimens are obtained from the anterior, posterior, and lateral walls. (Specimens are taken only from the lateral wall in infertility workups.) The specimens are placed in a solution containing 10% formalin solution and are sent to the pathologist for histologic examination. This study is performed by an obstetrician-gynecologist in approximately 10 to 30 minutes. Obtaining the biopsy tissue may cause the patient momentary discomfort (mild to severe menstrual-type cramping).

This procedure differs from a dilation and curettage (D and C) in that no cervical dilation is required. Also the curettage is much more extensive during a D and C. In effect, such curettage involves the taking of an endometrial biopsy specimen from the entire endometrium. (D and C usually requires general anesthesia with progressive cervical dilation before the curettage.) When an endometrial biopsy alone is performed to rule out endometrial cancer, it may easily miss the cancer. This is not true with a D and C. D and Cs are often therapeutic, in that endometrial polyps and other growths that may cause uterine bleeding can be removed.

Contraindications. Endometrial biopsy is contraindicated in:

1. Patients in whom the cervix fails to visualize because of previous cervical mutilation, senility, abnormal cervical position, or previous surgery
2. Patients with infections (such as trichomonal, monilial, or suspected gonococcal) of the cervix or vagina
3. Uncooperative patients

Nursing considerations

Nursing Diagnoses/Collaborative Problems

- Possible knowledge deficit related to test purpose, preparation, and procedure
- High risk for anxiety related to unknown sensations of procedure
- High risk for alteration in comfort related to test procedure
- Possible anxiety related to test results
- Potential complication: perforation of uterus
- Potential complication: uterine bleeding

Nursing Implications with Rationale

- Explain the procedure to the patient. Tell her that although momentary discomfort is associated with this study, analgesics are not needed. Encourage verbalization of the patient's fears. Provide emotional support.
- After the procedure assess the patient's vital signs at routine, regular intervals for the next 48 hours. Any temperature elevations (>100.4° F) should be reported to the physician, because this procedure may activate PID (pelvic inflammatory disease).
- Advise the patient to rest during the next 24 hours and to avoid heavy lifting to prevent uterine hemorrhage.
- After the procedure advise the patient to wear a pad because some vaginal bleeding is to be expected. Instruct the patient to call her physician if excessive bleeding (requiring more than one pad per hour) occurs.
- Inform the patient that douching and intercourse are not permitted for 72 hours after the biopsy specimen removal.
- Tell the patient how to obtain her test results. Generally the report is available within 72 hours.

Basal body temperature measurement

(BBT)

Normal value: a slight drop in basal body temperature followed by a sharp increase at time of ovulation

Rationale. Basal body temperature (BBT) measurement is a simple and inexpensive method of determining ovulation. Both the occurrence and the timing of ovulation can be determined by the taking of a daily rectal temperature reading throughout the menstrual cycle. The BBT remains at a relatively low level during the preovulatory estrogen phase of the cycle. Ovulation is heralded by a slight drop in the BBT (to its nadir) followed by a sharp increase of 0.5 to 0.7° F. Ovulation is thought to occur 12 hours before the sharp increase in temperature. Patients who wish to become pregnant should have intercourse during this time of ovulation, while those who wish to avoid pregnancy should abstain (the BBT method of birth control).

The temperature rise is maintained with slight variation until 1 to 2 days before menstruation. When the BBT measurements are charted, a "biphasic curve," which is indicative of progesterone production and ovulation, is produced (Figure 9-7, **A**). If both ovulation and fertilization have occurred, the temperature rise is maintained past the expected date of menses. A persistent elevation of BBT for 7 to 10 days after a missed period is suggestive of early pregnancy. This temperature elevation (caused by the thermogenic effect of progesterone) gradually falls after 2 weeks of pregnancy.

Patients whose temperatures remain low during the complete cycle are considered to have a monophasic curve (Figure 9-7, **B**), which indicates that ovulation has not occurred. For proper evaluation accurate temperature recordings should be kept over a period of at least three menstrual cycles. No complications are associated with this study. However, when BBT readings are obtained over long periods of time, the procedure may become a source of irritation to the patient or her husband or both.

Procedure. The first day of menses is considered the first day of the menstrual cycle. The duration of menses is recorded on the special chart as in Figure 9-7. Following the cessation of menses, the morning temperature is taken. The woman is instructed to keep a thermometer at the bedside and to take a daily rectal temperature reading before arising, smoking, drinking, eating, or moving about (that is, in a basal state). The measurement is taken with a special thermometer marked in tenths for a more accurate reading. The temperature reading should be taken at approximately the same time each day and charted on a graph for several months. If intercourse has occurred, a square should be placed around the recording, as in Figure 9-7.

Contraindications. This study is contraindicated in the uncooperative patient.

Nursing considerations

Nursing Diagnoses/Collaborative Problems

- Possible knowledge deficit related to test purpose, preparation, and procedure
- Possible anxiety related to test results

Nursing Implications with Rationale

- Explain the procedure to the patient. The temperature charts are confusing to many patients. Encourage the patient to ask questions.
- Let the patient practice reading the basal thermometer. Show her how it is "shaken down" after each reading. The thermometer should be kept at the bedside and shaken down the night before.
- Instruct the patient on how to record the temperature on a chart.
- Have the patient note other sources of temperature changes (for example, on upper respiratory tract infection).

Hormone assay for urinary pregnanediol

Normal value: increased excretion after ovulation to >1 mg/24 hours. Values vary according to week of pregnancy.

Rationale. Urinary pregnanediol is measured to evaluate progesterone production by the ova-

A

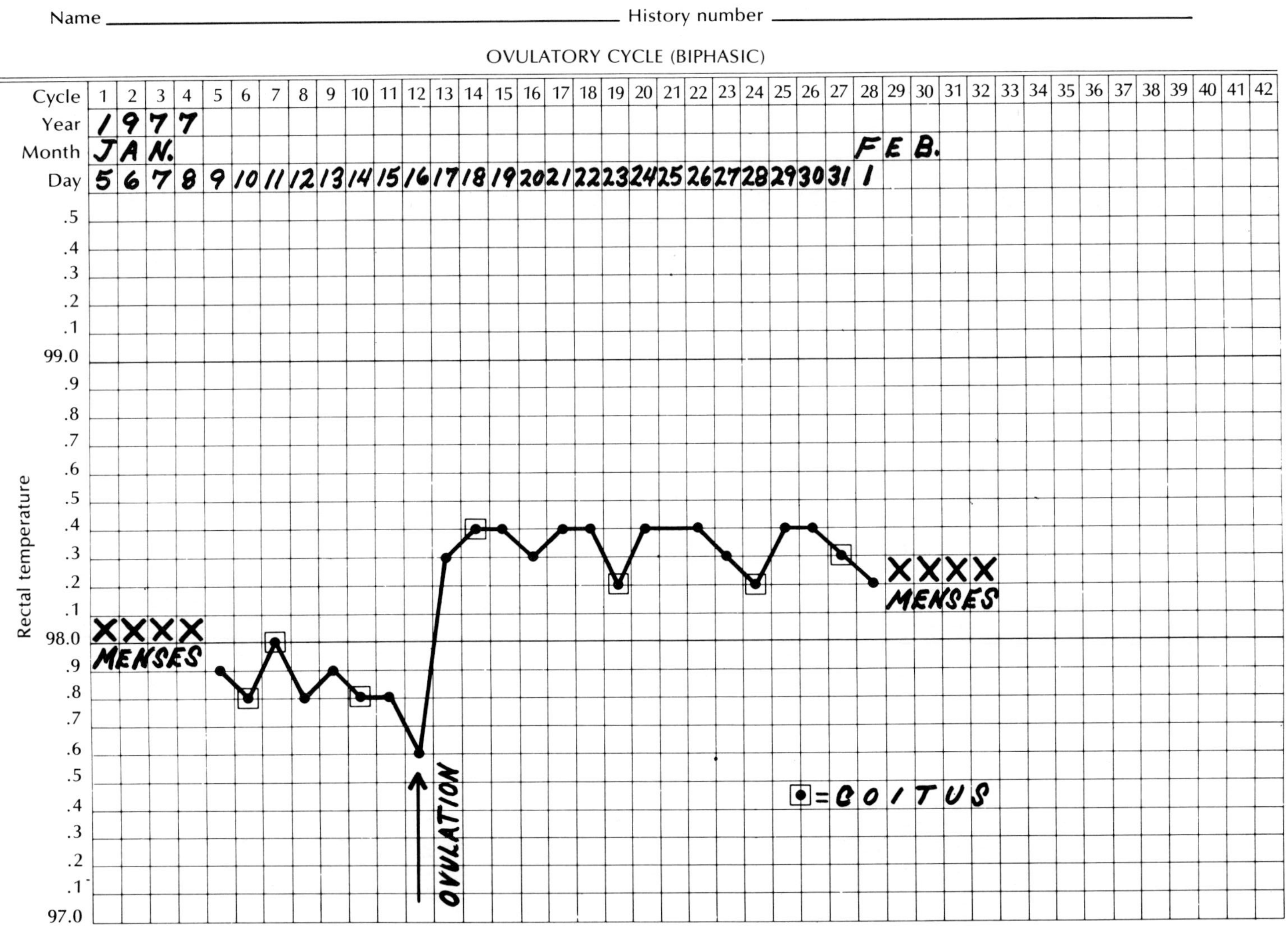

FIGURE 9-7. A, Basal body temperature (BBT) record shows drop and sharp rise at time of ovulation. Biphasic curve is indicative of ovulatory cycle.

From Jensen MD, Benson RC, Bobak IM: Maternity care: the nurse and the family, St Louis, 1977, Mosby–Year Book.

B

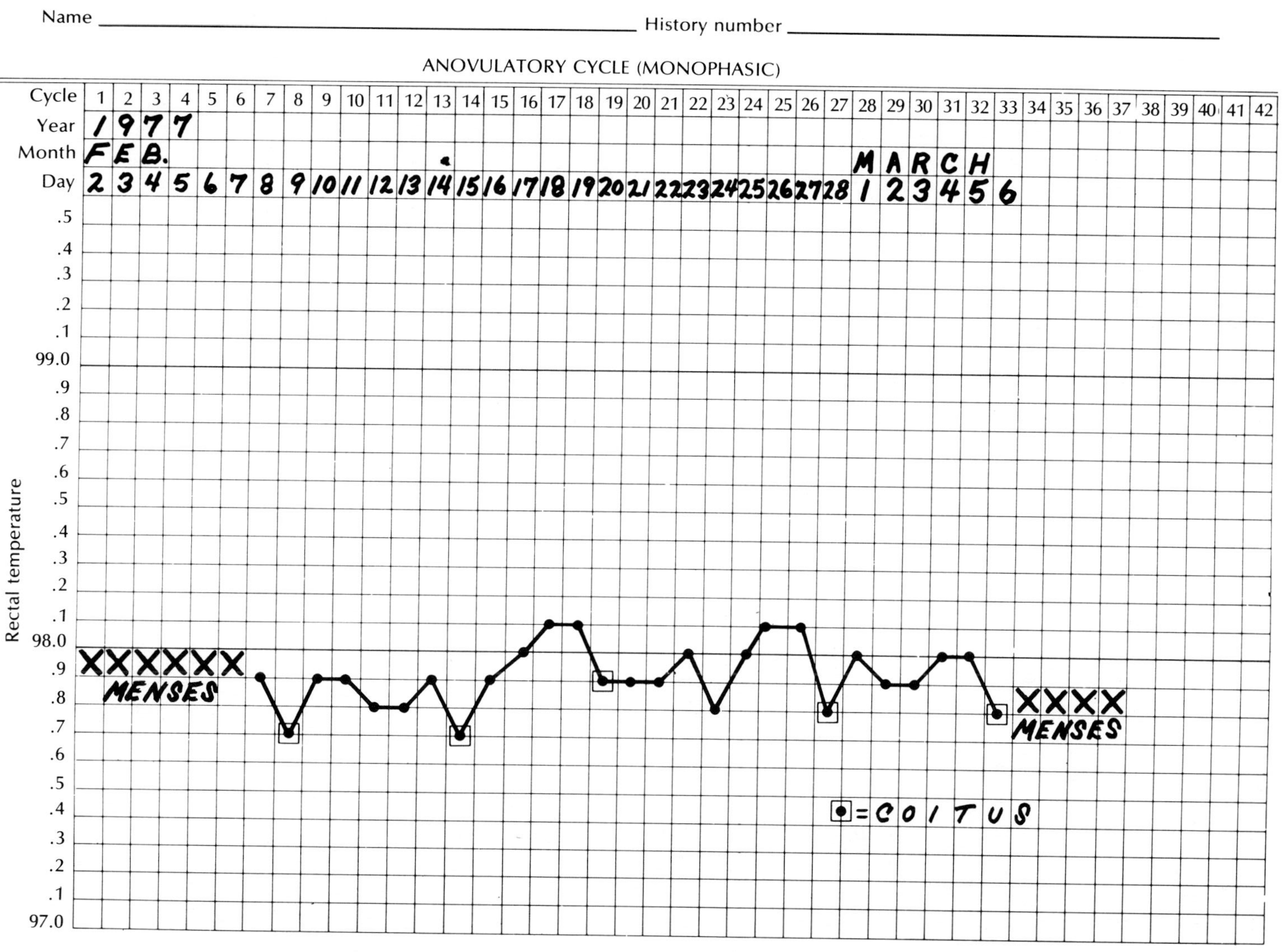

FIGURE 9-7, cont'd. B, BBT record shows monophasic (flat) curve indicative of anovulatory cycle.

ries and placenta. Now that serum progesterone levels are available (see p. 345), urinary levels are rarely performed. The main effect of progesterone is on the endometrium. It initiates the secretory phase in anticipation of implantation of a fertilized ovum. Normally progesterone is secreted by the ovarian corpus luteum following ovulation (Figure 9-3). Both serum progesterone levels and the urine concentration of progesterone metabolites (pregnanediol and others) are significantly increased during the latter half of an ovulatory cycle.

Pregnanediol is the most easily measured metabolite of progesterone. The urinary pregnanediol excretion increases after ovulation for approximately 10 days, to more than 1 mg/24 hours (compared with 0.4 ±0.1 mg/24 hours before ovulation). Since pregnanediol levels rise rapidly after ovulation, this study is useful in documenting whether ovulation has occurred and, if so, its exact time. During pregnancy, pregnanediol levels normally rise because of placental production of progesterone. Repeated assays can be used to monitor the status of the placenta. Increased levels may also be seen with luteal cysts of the ovary, arrhenoblastoma of the ovary, and hyperadrenocorticism. A decrease in pregnanediol levels may precede a spontaneous abortion. Decreased levels may also be associated with fetal death, toxemia of pregnancy, and amenorrhea.

Hormone assays for urinary pregnanediol are primarily used today to monitor progesterone supplementation in patients who have an inadequate luteal phase. Again, urinary assays are now being supplanted by plasma assays, which are quicker and more accurate.

Procedure. Progesterone determinations begin 4 to 6 days after a change in the biphasic curve (according to BBT measurements) when the patient is being followed for an inadequate luteal phase. A 24-hour urine specimen is collected in a standard specimen container and sent to the chemistry laboratory. During the entire collection, the specimen should be refrigerated. No foods or fluid restrictions are necessary during the collection period.

Contraindications. None.

Nursing considerations

Nursing Diagnoses/Collaborative Problems

See Urine studies, p. 3.

- Possible anxiety related to test results

Nursing Implications with Rationale

- Explain the procedure to the patient. See Chapter 7, pp. 230-231, Nursing implications for the creatinine clearance test (except for the first and last implications), for 24-hour urine collection. Keep the specimen refrigerated.
- Tell the patient when and how she can get the results of this urinary assay.

Sims-Huhner test

(postcoital test, postcoital cervical mucus test)

Normal values: cervical mucus adequate for sperm transmission, survival, and penetration; 6 to 20 active sperm per high-power field

Rationale. This study consists of a postcoital examination of the cervical mucus to measure the ability of the sperm to penetrate the mucus and maintain motility. This test evaluates the interaction between the sperm and the cervical mucus. It is also a measure of the quality of the cervical mucus. One can determine the effect of vaginal and cervical secretions on the activity of the sperm. Of course, this test is only performed after a previously performed semen analysis has been determined to be normal (see pp. 328-329).

This study is performed at the middle of the ovulatory cycle because at this time the secretions should be optimal for sperm penetration and survival. During ovulation, the quantity of cervical mucus is maximal whereas the viscosity is minimal, thus facilitating sperm penetration. The endocervical mucus sample is examined for color, viscosity, and tenacity (spinnbarkheit) (see Figure 9-5). The fresh specimen is then spread on a clean glass slide and examined for the presence of sperm. Estimates of the total number and the number of motile sperm per high-power field are reported. Normally 6 to 20 active sperm cells should be seen in each high-power field. If the sperm cells are present but not active, the cervical environment is unsuitable (for example, of abnormal pH) for their survival. After the specimen has dried on a glass slide, the mucus can be examined for arborization, or ferning (see Cervical mucus test and Figure 9-6). This study is invaluable in fertility examinations. It is not, however, a substitute for the semen analysis. If the results of the Sims-Huhner test are less than optimal, the test is usually repeated during the same or the next ovulatory cycle.

This analysis is also helpful in documenting cases of suspected rape by testing the vaginal and cervical secretions for sperm.

Procedure. During ovulation (as determined by BBT measurement) the woman is instructed to report to the physician for examination of her cervical mucus within 2 hours after coitus. (Some clinics suggest 4 to 8 hours.) Precoital lubrication and postcoital douching, bathing, or voiding are not permitted. This study should be performed after 3 days of abstinence. After intercourse the patient should rest in bed for 10 to 15 minutes to ensure cervical exposure to semen. After resting, the patient should wear a perineal pad until she is placed in the lithotomy position in the physician's office. The cervix is then exposed by an unlubricated speculum. The specimen is aspirated from the endocervix and delivered to the laboratory for analysis.

This procedure is performed by a physician in approximately 5 minutes. The specimen analysis is done in 15 minutes. The only discomfort associated with this study is the insertion of the speculum (as for a normal pelvic examination).

Contraindications. None.

Nursing considerations

Nursing Diagnoses/Collaborative Problems

See Cervical mucus test, p. 333.

Nursing Implications with Rationale

- Explain the procedure to the patient. Inform her that BBT recordings (see pp. 334-335) should be used to indicate ovulation. No vaginal lubrication, douching, or bathing is permitted until after the vaginal cervical examination because these factors alter the cervical mucus. After intercourse, the patient should rest in bed for 10 to 15 minutes and then wear a perineal pad and report to her physician within 2 hours.
- Encourage the patient to verbalize her feelings. Many patients are very anxious at this point in the fertility workup. They often fear that the results of this study will determine that they are infertile.
- Tell the patient how and when she may obtain the results.

Laparoscopy

(pelvic endoscopy)

Normal value: normal-appearing reproductive organs

Rationale. During a laparoscopy the abdominal organs can be visualized by inserting a fiberoptic scope through the abdominal wall and into the peritoneum. This scope is attached to a videocamera and the picture is projected on a television monitor. When the initial clinical evaluation is negative, this procedure is particularly helpful in diagnosing pelvic adhesions, ovarian tumors and cysts, and other tubal and uterine causes of infertility. Also endometriosis, ectopic pregnancy, ruptured ovarian cyst, and salpingitis can be detected during an evaluation for pelvic pain. Surgical procedures (e.g., cholecystectomy, hysterectomy, hernia repair, lysis of adhesions, oophorectomy) can be performed with the laparoscope. Laparoscopy is more informative than culdoscopy (see Supplemental information) in that a greater area of the abdominal cavity is able to be examined more carefully. Retroperitoneal organs (kidneys, ureters, pancreas, and colon) cannot be visualized well with this scope.

This procedure is relatively safe. However, the complication rate varies according to the laparoscopic operation. General anesthesia is required. While most patients are admitted after surgery, some laparoscopic procedures can be performed on outpatients. Acidosis may result from CO_2 insufflation of the abdominal cavity during the procedure.

Procedure. The routine preoperative procedure of the hospital is performed. The patient is kept NPO after midnight on the day of the procedure. In the morning, she empties her bladder and is premedicated before going to the operating room. After induction of anesthesia (general or regional) the patient is placed in a modified lithotomy position. Foley catheterization and temporary nasogastric aspiration are usually performed. For gynecologic purposes the uterus and ovaries can be better visualized by the insertion of a cannula into the cervix to permit manipulation of the uterus during laparoscopy. Other probes may also be introduced for manipulation of other abdominal organs.

After the abdominal skin is cleansed with povidone-iodine (Betadine), a blunt-tipped needle is inserted through a small incision in the periumbilical area into the peritoneal cavity. The peritoneal cavity is then filled with approximately 3 to 4 liters of carbon dioxide (pneumoperitoneum) to separate the abdominal wall from the intraabdominal viscera, thus enhancing visualization of pelvic and abdominal structures. After pneumoperitoneum has been established, a trocar within a cannula is introduced into the peritoneal cavity. The trocar is removed and the laparoscope (attached to the fiberoptic light source and videocamera) is inserted (Fig-

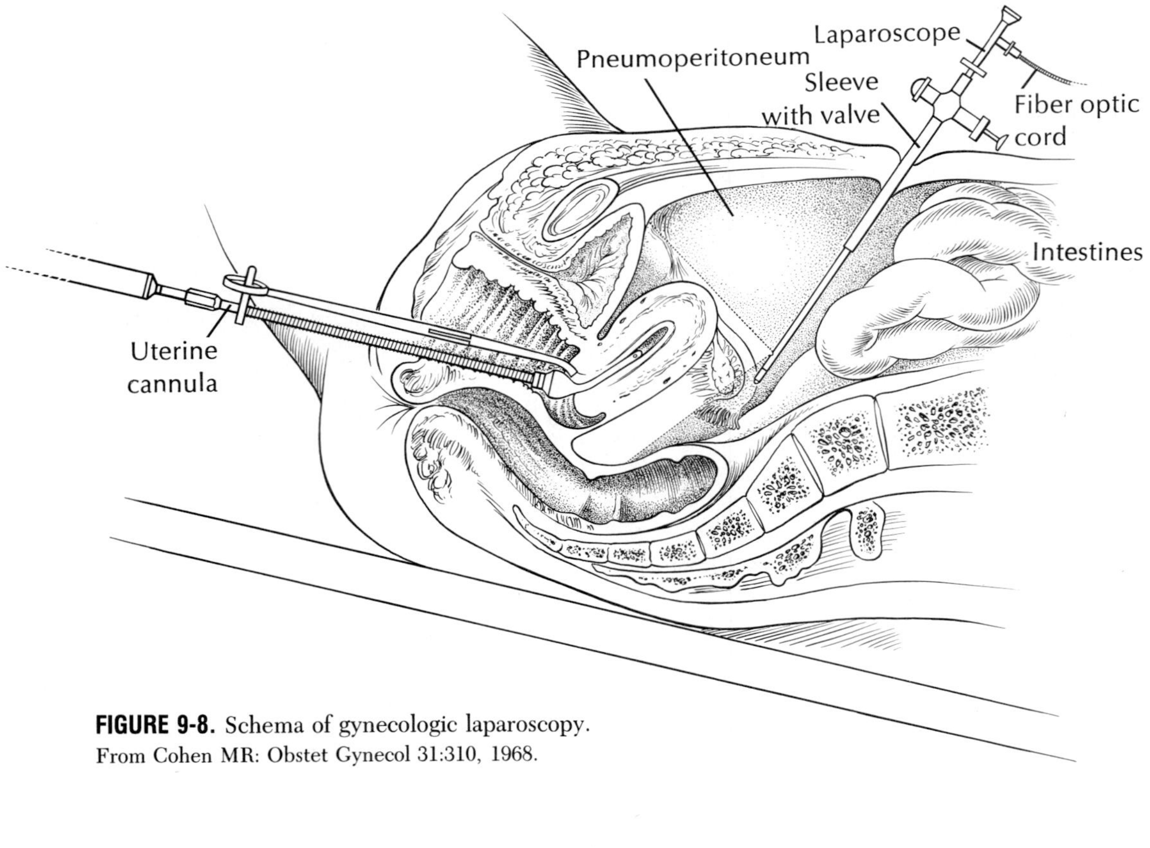

FIGURE 9-8. Schema of gynecologic laparoscopy.
From Cohen MR: Obstet Gynecol 31:310, 1968.

ure 9-8). The abdominal organs are then examined. After the desired procedure is completed, the laparoscope is removed and the CO_2 is allowed to escape. The incision is closed with a few skin stitches and covered with an adhesive bandage. After the procedure, most patients have mild incisional pain. Some patients may complain of referred pain in their shoulder caused by CO_2 insufflation pushing their diaphragms up.

Laparoscopy is performed by a surgeon in the operating room. The duration of this procedure varies according to the operation. The patient is usually discharged in 1-3 days.

Contraindications. This study is contraindicated in:

1. Patients with localized peritonitis because laparoscopy may spread the infection throughout the abdominal cavity
2. Patients who have had multiple operations, because adhesions may have formed between the viscera and the abdominal wall, and the chance of penetrating organs attached to the abdominal wall by the trocar is significant
3. Patients with suspected intraabdominal hemorrhage, since visualization through the scope will be obscured by the blood

Nursing considerations

Nursing Diagnoses/Collaborative Problems

See Endoscopic procedure, p. 7.

- Possible anxiety related to test results
- Potential complication: acidosis

Nursing Implications with Rationale

- Explain the procedure to the patient. Describe the preoperative and postoperative routines. Shave and prepare the abdomen. Some physicians order a Fleet's enema on the night before the study.
- Ensure that the written and informed consent form for this study is obtained by the physician.
- Laparoscopies are performed for various reasons. Ascertain the reason for this procedure. Allow the patient ample time to discuss her fears and verbalize her questions.
- If required, type and cross-match the patient's blood before the procedure.
- Keep the patient NPO after midnight. Food and fluid in the GI tract may result in pulmonary aspiration in the anesthetized patient.
- Be certain the patient voids before going to the operating room. It is very easy to penetrate a distended bladder if Foley catheterization is not to be done.
- After the procedure assess the patient frequently for signs of bleeding (increased pulse rate, decreased blood pressure); perforated viscus (abdominal tenderness, guarding, and decreased bowel sounds); and acidosis (increased respiration rate). Normally take vital signs every 15 minutes for four times, then every 30 minutes for four times, then every hour for four times, and then every 4 hours. Report any significant findings to the physician.
- If the patients report shoulder or subcostal discomfort (from pneumoperitoneum), assure them that this usually lasts only 24 hours. Minor analgesics usually relieve the discomfort.
- Many patients are fearful of the results of this study. If the results are not given immediately after the study, inform patients when they can obtain them. Provide patient support.

SUPPLEMENTAL INFORMATION

Culdoscopy

Normal value: normal-appearing reproductive organs

Rationale. The pelvic organs can be directly visualized by placing a culdoscope (a lighted instrument similar to a cystoscope) through a small incision in the posterior vaginal vault and into the perineal space between the rectum and the uterus (cul-de-sac of Douglas). This procedure affords direct visualization of the uterus, fallopian tubes, broad ligaments, uterosacral ligaments, rectal wall, and the sigmoid colon. This procedure is rarely performed because it is complicated and dangerous.

Culdoscopy is used in the evaluation of infertility because it can determine tubal abnormalities. It is also used in the detection of suspected ectopic pregnancy and in the study of unexplained pelvic pain or masses. Culdoscopy has fallen out of favor since the introduction of laparoscopy (see previous study). Laparoscopy has largely replaced culdoscopy because:

1. Laparoscopy affords superior visualization because of the CO_2 insufflation of the peritoneum.
2. A lower infection rate is associated with the abdominal approach used in laparoscopy.
3. Laparoscopy is more successful in visualizing the abdominal organs. Culdoscopic visualization often may be inadequate because of pelvic adhesions.

This procedure is accurate and relatively safe if it is performed by an experienced gynecologist. Possible complications include pelvic infection or hemorrhage and penetration of the rectum, bladder, or small intestines.

Procedure. The patient is prepared for culdoscopy in the same manner as for any type of vaginal surgery. The patient is kept NPO after midnight. This procedure is performed in the operating room with the patient in the knee-chest position. The head of the table is tilted downward to displace the bowel from the pelvis. Spinal or local anesthesia is used. A small incision is made in the posterior vaginal vault, and a culdoscope (light, tubular, lighted scope) is passed into the cul-de-sac (Figure 9-9). The pelvic and abdominal organs are then visualized and examined.

After the study the scope is removed. No sutures are used to close the incision in the vaginal cuff. No douching or intercourse is permitted until the healing is complete (usually 1 to 2 weeks). This procedure is performed by a physician in 1 hour. Patients are usually very un-

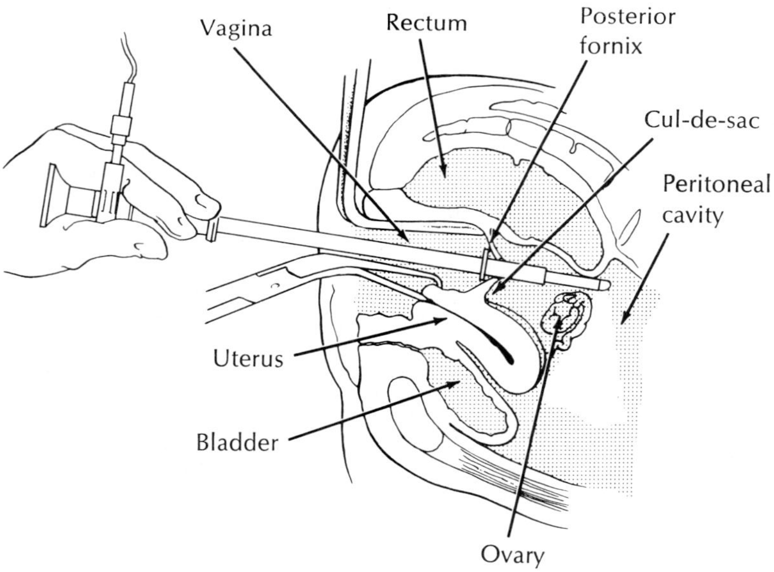

FIGURE 9-9. Culdoscopy. With patient in knee-chest position, culdoscope is inserted through posterior fornix of vagina into cul-de-sac of Douglas. Note that ovaries can be seen. From Cinkota E, Woods NF: Assessment of the reproductive and sexual systems. In Phipps WJ, Long BC, and Woods NF, editors: Medical-surgical nursing: concepts and clinical practice, St Louis, 1979, Mosby–Year Book.

comfortable from the required knee-chest position.

Contraindications. This study is contraindicated in patients who have:

1. An inability to assume the knee-chest position
2. Acute vulvar or vaginal infections
3. Acute peritonitis
4. Palpable masses in the cul-de-sac
5. Previous pelvic surgery causing an adhesion of the bowel to the cul-de-sac.

Nursing considerations

Nursing Diagnoses/Collaborative Problems

See Endoscopic procedures, p. 7.

- Possible anxiety related to test results

Nursing Implications with Rationale

- Explain the procedure to the patient. Describe the preoperative and postoperative routines. Minimize the stress associated with this study by providing factual information. A picture may be helpful.
- Encourage the patient to verbalize her questions or fears regarding this study. Provide emotional support.
- Ensure that the written and informed consent for this study is obtained by the physician before the study.
- Many patients are fearful of the results of this study. Arrange a time for the patient to call or to see her physician for the results.
- Inform the patient that douching or intercourse is not permitted until the vaginal septum has healed. This healing takes approximately 1 to 2 weeks. The patient may take sitz baths 4 days after the procedure. Mild oral analgesics may be ordered for discomfort.

Hysteroscopy

Normal value: normal endometrium

Rationale. A D & C is a blind scraping of endometrial tissue. Whether or not pathology is obtained is, in part, related to chance. However, with the use of hysteroscopy, the entire endometrial cavity can be visualized. Very rarely is endometrial pathology missed. Also endometrial cancers, hyperplasia, and polyps can be biopsied and removed. Endometrial ablation can be performed with the use of cautery or laser beam.

Complications of this study include perforation of the uterus, uterine bleeding, and interference with early pregnancy.

Procedure. The patient is placed in the lithotomy position. Under general or regional anesthesia, the hysteroscope is placed through the cervical os and into the endometrial cavity. Usually no cervical dilation is required. The entire endometrium is examined. Areas suspicious for cancer or hyperplasia can be sampled for biopsy. Polyps can be removed and the base ablated. The procedure takes only about 30 minutes and is not associated with any significant postoperative pain. This test is usually performed by a gynecologist.

Contraindications. Hysteroscopy is contraindicated in:

1. Patients in whom the cervix cannot be visualized because of previous cervical mutilation, senility, abnormal cervical position, or previous surgery
2. Patients with cervical or vaginal infections
3. Uncooperative patients.

Nursing Considerations

Nursing Diagnoses/Collaborative Problems

- Possible knowledge deficit related to test purpose, preparation, and procedure
- Possible anxiety related to unknown sensations of procedure
- Possible alteration in comfort related to test procedure
- Possible anxiety related to test results
- Potential complication: perforation of uterus
- Potential complication: uterine bleeding

Nursing Implications and Rationale

- See Endometrial biopsy, p. 334.

Antispermatozoal antibody test

(sperm agglutination and inhibition, sperm antibodies)

Normal value: negative

Rationale. The antispermatozoal antibody test is an infertility screening test used to detect the presence of sperm antibodies. Antibodies directed toward sperm antigens can result in diminished fertility. In addition to a semen specimen, serum of both partners should be studied for sperm antibodies, since a relationship may exist between spermatozoal antibodies in serum of women and unexplained infertility.

Antisperm antibodies may be found in men with blocked efferent ducts in the testes or in those who have had a vasectomy. Possibly the reabsorption of sperm from blocked ducts results in the formation of autoantibodies to sperm. Antisperm antibodies are also found in some women with unexplained infertility.

Procedure. Blood is collected from both partners in a red-top tube. A semen specimen should be collected after avoiding ejaculation for at least 3 days and brought to the laboratory in a plastic cup within 2 hours after collection. The most widely used serum-sperm bioassays are the *gelatin agglutination test* and the *sperm immobilization test*. Radioimmunoassays have also been developed to detect antibodies in serum and seminal fluid.

Contraindications. None.

Nursing considerations

Nursing Diagnoses/Collaborative Problems

- Possible knowledge deficit related to test purpose, preparation, and procedure
- Possible anxiety related to test results

Nursing Implications with Rationale

- Explain the procedure to the patient. Assess the venipuncture site for bleeding.
- Explain the sperm collection procedure. Be certain that the patient knows that a 3-day period of sexual abstinence is necessary.
- Give the male patient the proper container for the sperm collection. He may find the collection and delivery of the semen to the laboratory embarrassing. Do not add to his embarrassment. Be matter-of-fact about the specimen collection and delivery.
- If the specimen is to be obtained at home, be certain that the patient is told that it must be taken to the laboratory for testing within 2 hours after collection.
- Allow time for the patients to discuss any questions or fears regarding the results of this study. Instruct them when and how to obtain the test results. Abnormal results may have a devastating effect on a patient's sexuality.

Luteinizing hormone (LH) assay

Normal value:
- Men: 7-24 ImU/ml
- Women: 6-30 ImU/ml
  - Midcycle peak—over three times the baseline
  - Post menopause—>30 ImU/ml
- Children: up to 12 ImU/ml

Rationale. Luteinizing hormone (LH) is a gonadotropin secreted by the anterior pituitary gland. Luteinizing hormone, along with follicle stimulating hormone (FSH), is necessary for ovulation. The FSH is commonly measured with LH.

Performing an LH assay is an easy way to determine if ovulation has occurred. An LH surge in blood levels indicates ovulation has occurred. Under the influence of LH, the corpus luteum develops from the ruptured graafian follicle (see Figure 9-3). Daily samples of serum LH around the midcycle can detect the LH surge, believed to occur on the day of maximum fertility.

LH assays also determine whether a gonadal insufficiency is primary (problem with the ovary/testicle) or secondary (because of insufficient stimulation by the pituitary hormones, for example, LH). LH assays are used to study testicular dysfunction in men and to evaluate endocrine problems related to precocious puberty in children.

Procedure. LH assays can be performed using a home urine test, a 24-hour urine test, or a blood study. A red-top tube is used for the blood study. No fluid or food restrictions apply. The date of the last menstrual period should be indicated on the laboratory slip.

Contraindications. None.

Nursing considerations

Nursing Diagnoses/Collaborative Problems

See Urine studies, p. 3, or Blood studies, p. 2.

Nursing Implications with Rationale

- Explain the procedure to the patient. Make sure that patient understands that the peak period is the time of maximum fertility.
- Instruct the patient on how to perform the urine test and record the results.
- If a blood test is drawn, apply pressure to the venipuncture site and assess the site for bleeding.

Progesterone assay

Normal values:
Preovulation: 20-150 ng/dl
Midcycle: 300-2400 ng/dl
Pregnancy: >2400 ng/dl

Rationale. Determination of the progesterone level provides evidence to confirm ovulation and to evaluate the function of the corpus luteum. Plasma progesterone levels start to rise with the LH surge (see previous study) and continue to rise for approximately 6 to 10 days, and then fall. Normally, blood samples drawn at days 8 and 21 of the menstrual cycle will show a large increase in progesterone levels with normal ovulation and development of a corpus luteum. Progesterone levels are also very high in pregnancy. Repeated assays can be used to monitor the status of the placenta. Diminishing levels of progesterone in pregnancy can indicate fetal death, toxemia, or imminent spontaneous abortion. Certain adrenal or ovarian tumors may also produce elevated levels.

Urinary pregnanediol levels (see p. 335) are an indirect measurement of progesterone production. Serum progesterone levels can provide comparable information and are sometimes done in place of endometrial biopsy (see p. 333) to determine the phase of the menstrual cycle.

Procedure. A venous blood sample is obtained by peripheral venipuncture in a red-top tube. The laboratory request should include the date of the last menstrual period.

Contraindications. None.

Nursing considerations

Nursing Diagnoses/Collaborative Problems

See Blood studies, p. 2.

Nursing Implications with Rationale

- Explain the reason for progesterone testing to the patient. Assess the venipuncture site for bleeding.

CASE STUDY 2: ROUTINE PRENATAL EVALUATION

Mr. and Mrs. K., a 23-year-old black couple, were excited when Mrs. K's menstrual period was 3 weeks late. Mrs. K. was seen by her obstetrician, and her pregnancy was confirmed. The following routine laboratory tests were performed.

First prenatal visit Studies	Results
Urinalysis (see Chapter 7)	WNL
Urine culture (see Chapter 7)	Negative (normal: negative)
Complete blood count (CBC) and platelets (see Chapter 10)	WNL
Papanicolaou (Pap) smear	Negative (normal: negative)
Serologic test for syphilis	Negative (normal: negative)
Gonorrhea culture	Negative (normal: negative)
Toxoplasmosis antibody titer	1:100 (normal: 1:4 to 1:256 in general population)
Blood type and Rh factor (see Chapter 10)	B+

First prenatal visit—cont'd

Studies	Results
Rubella antibodies	1:20 (titer >1:10-1:20 indicates immunity)
Tuberculin skin test (see Chapter 5)	Negative (normal: negative)
Sickle cell test (see Chapter 10)	Negative (normal: negative)

28-week checkup

Studies	Results
Hematocrit (Hct) (see Chapter 10)	WNL
2-hour postprandial glucose (PPG) test (see Chapter 8)	WNL

36-week checkup

Studies	Results
Hct	WNL

The urinalysis was done primarily to detect sugar (glycosuria), which could have suggested diabetes, and to detect albumin (proteinuria), which could have suggested preeclampsia. The urine culture results did not detect urinary tract infection or renal problems. The normal CBC and platelets ruled out anemia (the most common nutritional complication of pregnancy), infectious processes, and alterations in the blood clotting ability. The sexually transmitted diseases of syphilis and gonorrhea were not detected. The level of the toxoplasmosis antibody titer did not indicate any problem for the mother or for the fetus. The blood typing and Rh factor determination studies were performed to detect a possible incompatibility disease. If the mother had been Rh negative, checking the father would have been necessary. Antibody titer levels would then have been followed throughout the pregnancy. The rubella antibody test assured Mrs. K. that she was protected from rubella. The Pap smear was normal and the tine test indicated tuberculosis was not suspected. The sickle cell test, which was done because the disease occurs more frequently in blacks, was negative. Her Hct was checked again at weeks 28 and 36. The 2-hour PPG test ruled out gestational diabetes.

The patient and her husband were happy that all the studies showed good results. Mrs. K. was seen by a certified nurse-midwife (CNM) monthly until week 28, biweekly from weeks 28 through 36, and weekly from week 36 until delivery. Her urine was checked at each visit for sugar and acetone, which may have indicated gestational diabetes, and protein, which would have indicated preeclampsia. She and her husband attended Lamaze classes. With the assistance of a CNM, Mrs. K. delivered a healthy 8-pound, 2-ounce baby boy 4 days after her estimated date of confinement (EDC).

DISCUSSION OF TESTS

Papanicolaou smear

(Pap smear, Pap test, cytologic test for cancer)

Normal value: no abnormal or atypical cells

Rationale. A Pap smear is taken to detect neoplastic cells in cervical and vaginal secretions. This test is based on the fact that normal and abnormal cervical and endometrial neoplastic cells are shed into the cervical and vaginal secretions. By examining these secretions microscopically, one can detect early cellular changes compatible with premalignant conditions or an outright malignant condition. The Pap smear is 95% accurate in detecting cervical carcinoma. Its accuracy in detection of endometrial carcinoma approaches 40%. There are several classifications designed to communicate the cytopathologic findings. One method is as follows:

- **Class 1:** Absence of atypical or abnormal cells (normal)
- **Class 2:** Atypical cells, but no evidence of malignancy (worrisome but most frequently caused by inflammation of the cervix)
- **Class 3:** Cytologic findings suggestive of but not conclusive concerning malignancy (should be evaluated more extensively)

Class 4: Cytologic findings strongly suggestive of malignancy (requires more extensive evaluation)
Class 5: Cytologic findings conclusive of malignancy (requires treatment)

Abnormal smears in classes 2 through 4 do not necessarily indicate that the patient has a malignancy. For these women, additional procedures, such as a D & C (see p. 334), or colposcopy with cervical biopsy (see pp. 371-372), are indicated.

Cervical intraepithelial neoplasia (CIN) is a simple designation of the spectrum of intraepithelial dysplasia, which usually occurs before invasive cervical cancer. In contrast to the previous classification, CIN reporting recognizes the continuum of cervical dysplasia and allows for some overlap. The subclasses of CIN are defined as follows:

CIN 1: mild and mild-to-moderate dysplasia
CIN 2: moderate and moderate-to-severe dysplasia
CIN 3: severe dysplasia and carcinoma in situ

Roughly CIN 1 includes classes 2 and 3, CIN 2 includes class 3, and CIN 3 comprises classes 4 and 5.

Most recently The Bethesda System (TBS) for reporting cervical/vaginal cytologic diagnoses was developed (1988) and revised (1991) by the National Cancer Institute. This system includes the following:

- Adequacy of specimen
  - Satisfactory for evaluation
  - Satisfactory for evaluation but limited by (specify disease)
  - Unsatisfactory for evaluation (specify reason)
- General categorization (optional)
  - Within normal limits
  - Benign cellular changes: see descriptive diagnosis
  - Epithelial cell abnormality: see descriptive diagnosis
- Descriptive diagnosis
  - Benign cellular changes
    - Infection
      - Trichomonas
      - Fungal organisms
      - Coccobacilli
      - Herpes simplex
      - Other
    - Reactive changes
      - Inflammation
      - Atrophy
      - Radiation
      - IUD
      - Other
  - Epithelial cell abnormalities
    - Squamous cell
      - Atypical squamous cells
      - Low-grade squamous intraepithelial lesion
      - High-grade squamous intraepithelial lesion
      - Squamous cell carcinoma
    - Glandular cell
      - Endometrial cells, cytologically benign
      - Atypical glandular cell
      - Endocervical adenocarcinoma
      - Endometrial adenocarcinoma
      - Extrauterine adenocarcinoma
      - Adenocarcinoma

A Pap smear may also be performed to follow some abnormalities (such as infertility). An abnormal maturation index is characteristic of estrogen-progesterone imbalance. These patients may even be taught to obtain their own Pap smears.

Pap smears should be part of the routine pelvic examination, which is usually performed once a year on women over 18 years old (or even earlier when the patient is sexually active). There are differences of opinion regarding the necessity for annual Pap smears. The American Cancer Society recommends that a Pap smear be taken annually for two negative examinations and then repeated once every 3 years until age 65 in asymptomatic women. More frequent testing may be indicated for patients with previously abnormal Pap smears, sexually transmitted diseases, those with a family history of cervical cancer, and those whose mothers had ingested diethylstilbestrol (DES) during their pregnancies. Usually a routine cervical culture for gonococcus is obtained during the Pap smear examination.

Procedure. The patient should refrain from douching and tub bathing for 24 to 48 hours before her Pap smear. She should not be menstruating. If abnormal bleeding is present, however, the Pap smear and examination should be performed because of the significant possibility that serious cervical or uterine lesions may be present. A common error is to delay Pap testing 2 to 3 months because of intermittent bleeding or continuous spotting.

The patient is placed in the lithotomy position. An examining light is positioned for visualization of the pelvic area. A nonlubricated vaginal speculum is inserted to expose the cervix. Material is collected from the cervical canal by rotating a moist, saline cotton swab or spatula within the cervical canal and in the squamocolumnar junction. The cells are immediately wiped across a clean glass slide and fixed either by immersing the slide in equal parts of 95% alcohol and ether or by using a commercial spray. Aqua Net hair spray is also an effective fixative. The secretions must be fixed before drying because drying distorts the cells and make interpretation difficult. The slide is labeled with the patient's name. The patient's name, age, and parity, the date of her last menstrual period, and the reason for the cytologic examination should be written on the request form.

No discomfort other than that of the insertion of the speculum is associated with this procedure. A Pap smear is obtained in about 10 minutes by a physician or a nurse.

The *Gravlee test* is a new screening test that differs from the Pap smear in that the cells are obtained by washing the uterine cavity with normal saline solution and then collecting the washed materials. The Gravlee jet washer is used for this procedure. The collected cells are then evaluated and classified as those obtained by the Pap smear.

Contraindications. The Pap smear is contraindicated in women who are presently having their routine, normal menses.

Nursing considerations

Nursing Diagnoses/Collaborative Problems

- Possible knowledge deficit related to test purpose, preparation, and procedure
- Possible anxiety related to unknown sensations of procedure
- Possible anxiety related to test results
- Possible alteration in comfort related to test procedures

Nursing Implications with Rationale

- Explain the procedure to the patient. Assure the patient that she will be appropriately draped to prevent unnecessary exposure.
- Determine if the patient has douched or tub bathed during the 24 hours before the Pap smear. Douching and tub baths may wash away cellular deposits, which are desired in the specimen.
- After the study inform the patient about how to obtain the test results. Usually the patient is notified by the office only if further evaluation is necessary. If the smears were abnormal, assure the patient that this does not necessarily mean that she has a malignancy. Many patients associate a suspicious test with malignancy and become very frightened. Provide emotional support.
- After the smear is obtained ensure that it is fixed immediately without being allowed to dry. Fixing causes rapid killing of the cells so that they look as much as possible as they did in situ. If the cells are allowed to die slowly and dry, they will not be able to be evaluated accurately.

Serologic test for syphilis

(STS, VDRL, RPR, FTA)

Normal value: negative, or nonreactive

Rationale. The serologic test for syphilis (STS) is a test used to detect antibodies to *Treponema* *pallidum,* the causative agent of syphilis. There are two groups of antibodies. The first is a nontreponemal antibody (reagin) directed against a lipoidal antigen that results from the *Treponema pallidum* infection. The second is an antibody directed against the *Treponema* organism itself. The nontreponemal antibody test is relatively nonspecific. These antibodies are most commonly detected by the Wassermann test or the Venereal Disease Research Laboratory (VDRL) test. A newer, more sensitive nontreponemal test is the rapid plasma reagin (RPR) test.

If the VDRL test or the RPR test is positive, the diagnosis may be confirmed by the *Treponema* test (such as fluorescent treponemal antibody absorption test [FTA-ABS]). This second test is much more specific.

The VDRL and RPR tests, by virtue of their testing for a nonspecific antibody, have a high false positive rate. Conditions such as mycoplasia, pneumonia, malaria, acute bacterial and viral infections, autoimmune diseases, and pregnancy can cause false positive results. VDRL tests become positive about 2 weeks after the patient's inoculation with *Treponema* and return to normal shortly after adequate treatment is given. The test is positive in nearly all primary and secondary stages of syphilis and in two thirds of patients with tertiary syphilis.

The FTA test, which tests for a much more specific antibody, is more accurate than the VDRL and RPR tests. False-positive and false-negative results are rare in all stages of the disease but can occur in patients with collagen vascular disease. The FTA test is required before the diagnosis of syphilis can be made with certainty. Positive results must be reported to the state health department.

Screening for syphilis is usually done during the first prenatal checkup for pregnant women. Syphilis, if untreated, may cause abortion, stillbirth, and premature labor. The effect on the fetus could be central nervous system damage, hearing loss, and possible death.

Syphilis can also be diagnosed by dark-field microscopic examination of scrapings from a primary syphilitic cancer.

Procedure. The VDRL, RPR, and FTA tests can be performed on a specimen of 7 ml of peripheral venous blood collected in a red-top tube. The test is performed in the clinical serologic lab. Some laboratories request that the specimen be taken before meals. For the VDRL and RPR tests the patient's serum is added to a synthetic lipoid antigen, and the mixture is observed for clumping (flocculation). The ingestion of alcohol may decrease the intensity of this reaction. For this reason, patients are instructed to abstain from drinking alcohol for 2 hours before having their blood sample taken.

For the FTA test the patient's serum is placed on a slide that contains dried *Treponema pallidum* organisms. Fluorescent antibodies against human globulin are added. After the slide is rinsed, it is observed for evidence of fluorescence. If fluorescence is present, the test is positive. If no fluorescence is seen, the test is negative and the patient does not have syphilis.

These tests are performed by a technician and are not associated with any patient discomfort except for the venipuncture. Hemolysis can affect the results.

Contraindications. The VDRL and RPR tests are contraindicated in any patient with a disease known to cause false positive results.

Nursing considerations

Nursing Diagnoses/Collaborative Problems

See Blood studies, p. 2.

- Possible anxiety related to test results

Nursing Implications with Rationale

- Explain the procedure to the patient. Obtain the blood as ordered. Assess the patient for other diseases that may cause false-positive results.
- If the test is positive, obtain a history of the patient's recent sexual contacts so that these persons may be evaluated for syphilis.
- If the test is positive, be sure the patient receives the appropriate antibiotic therapy.

Gonorrhea culture test

Normal value: no evidence of *Neisseria gonorrhoeae*

Rationale. Performing a culture for gonorrhea as part of the prenatal workup is often routine because gonorrhea is a widely spread, infectious disease that is frequently asymptomatic in a high-risk population. If the culture is positive, treatment during pregnancy can prevent possible fetal complications (such as ophthalmia neonatorum) and maternal complications. Rectal and orogastric cultures should be done on neonates of infected mothers.

Cultures for gonococcal infections are performed on men and women in whom gonorrhea may be suspected. If the culture is positive, sexual partners should be evaluated and treated. Cervical cultures are usually done in women; urethral cultures are done in men. Rectal and throat cultures are performed in persons who have engaged in anal and oral intercourse. Because rectal gonorrhea accompanies genital gonorrhea in a high percentage of women, rectal cultures may be recommended in all suspected cases of gonorrhea.

Procedure. Gram stains of smears or bacterial cultures should be taken before a patient begins antibiotic therapy. Bacterial cultures use a special media such as Thayer-Martin, designed for the cultivation of *Neisseria gonorrhoeae*.

Cervical culture. The female patient should refrain from douching and tub bathing before the cervical culture is performed. The patient is placed in the lithotomy position, and a nonlubricated vaginal speculum is inserted to expose the cervix. Cervical mucus is removed with a cotton ball held in ring forceps. Then a sterile cotton-tipped swab is inserted into the endocervical canal and moved from side to side.

Anal canal culture. An anal culture of the female or male is taken by inserting a sterile, cotton-tipped swab about 1 inch into the anal canal. If stool contaminates the swab, a repeat swab is taken.

Urethral culture. The urethral specimen should be obtained from the man before voiding. A culture is taken by inserting a sterile swab gently into the anterior urethra.

Oropharyngeal culture. This culture should be obtained in men and women who have engaged in oral intercourse. A throat culture is best obtained by depressing the patient's tongue with a wooden blade (tongue blade) and touching the posterior wall of the throat with a sterile cotton-tipped swab.

After the cultures are obtained, the swabs are placed in the Thayer-Martin medium and rolled from side to side. The swabs are then discarded. The culture bottle is labeled and sent to the microbiology laboratory.

Contraindications. Gonorrheal cultures are not done in women who are presently having their routine normal menses.

Nursing considerations

Nursing Diagnoses/Collaborative Problems

- Possible knowledge deficit related to test purpose, preparation, and procedure
- Possible anxiety related to test results
- Possible alteration in comfort related to test procedure

Nursing Implications with Rationale

- Explain the purpose and procedure to the patient. Use a matter-of-fact, nonjudgmental approach.
- Drape the patient appropriately during the procedure to prevent any unnecessary exposure.
- Obtain the specimens in a sterile manner. Sterile, disposable gloves should be worn. Handle all specimens as though they were capable of transmitting disease. Specimens should be transported to the laboratory as soon as possible after their collection (at least within 30 minutes).
- Obtain the specimens before initiating any antibiotic therapy. Antibiotics will alter the growth of the organisms in the culture medium.

- If culture results are positive, be aware that sexual partners should be evaluated and treated.

Toxoplasmosis antibody titer test

Normal values:
Titer <1:16 indicates no previous infection
Titer 1:16 to 1:256 generally prevalent in the general population
Titer >256 suggests a recent infection
Rising titers are of great significance

Rationale. Toxoplasmosis is a protozoan disease caused by *Toxoplasma gondii,* which is found in poorly cooked or raw meat and in the feces of cats. This disease is characterized by central nervous system lesions, which may lead to blindness, brain damage, and death. The condition may occur congenitally or postnatally. Because about one quarter to one half of the adult population are asymptomatically affected with toxoplasmosis, the Centers for Disease Control recommends that pregnant patients be serologically tested for this disease. The Sabin-Feldman dye tests or the indirect fluorescent antibody (IFA) tests are performed on a serologic specimen to detect toxoplasmosis antibody titers. A complement-fixation test will have a positive result in active disease.

The presence of antibodies before pregnancy probably assures protection against congenital toxoplasmosis in the child. Chronic toxoplasmosis (which a large percentage of adults have) will not cause spontaneous abortion or infection of the fetus. Fetal infection occurs only if the mother acquires toxoplasmosis after conception. Repeat testing of the pregnant patient with high or negative titers may be done before the twentieth week and before delivery to identify antibody converters and to determine appropriate therapy (such as therapeutic abortion at 20 weeks, treatment during the remainder of the pregnancy, or treatment of the newborn). Hydrocephaly, microcephaly, and chronic retinitis and convulsions are complications of congenital toxoplasmosis. Congenital toxoplasmosis is diagnosed when the Sabin-Feldman dye test (the oldest test for toxoplasmosis) or the indirect fluorescent antibody titer test levels are persistently elevated or a rising titer is found in the infant 2 to 3 months after birth. (This is because initially high titer activity may be caused by the transfer of antibodies from the mother to the infant.)

The patient with suspected toxoplasmosis may have studies done for infectious mononucleosis. However, unlike infectious mononucleosis, there is no elevated heterophil antibody activity test in toxoplasmosis.

Procedure. A peripheral venipuncture is performed, and approximately 5 ml of blood is sent to the laboratory for analysis. Some laboratories request that the lab slip indicate if the patient is pregnant or has been exposed to cats.

Contraindications. None.

Nursing considerations

Nursing Diagnoses/Collaborative Problems

See Blood studies, p. 2.

Nursing Implications with Rationale

- Explain the purpose of the test to the patient.
- Assess the venipuncture site for bleeding.

Rubella (German measles) antibody test

(hemagglutination inhibition, HAI, test)

Normal value: lack of susceptibility to rubella if HAI titer is >1:10 to 1:20 or if complement fixation test is positive

Rationale. Screening for rubella antibodies is done to determine immunity to rubella. These tests detect the presence of IgG and IgM antibodies of past and active infections and determine the susceptibility or immunity to the rubella virus, which is the causative agent for German measles. It is vitally important to identify exposure to rubella infection and susceptibility status in pregnant women because maternal infection in the first trimester of pregnancy is associated with congenital abnormalities, abortion, or stillbirth. All pregnant women should be screened for rubella during the first prenatal visit.

If the woman's titer is >1:10 to 1:20, she is not susceptible to rubella. If the mother's titer is ≤1:8, she has little or no immunity to rubella. She should be strongly advised to stay away from any small children, especially those with symptoms of an upper respiratory infection (prodromal symptoms of rubella). In addition, all hospital personnel associated with maternal and child care should be screened for rubella. Immunization is not done during pregnancy but should be done after delivery for nonimmune mothers.

A change in the HAI titer activity from the acute to the chronic phase in a patient with a rash is the most useful method of demonstrating a rise in antibody titer levels. With a rubella rash, diagnosis of rubella is confirmed by taking an acute sample (taken about 3 days after the onset of the rash) and a convalescent sample (taken around 3 weeks later). A four-fold increase in titer from the acute to the convalescent titer indicates that the rash was caused by rubella.

When pregnant women with an immunity to rubella (titer >1:10 to 1:20) are exposed to rubella, the HAI test should be repeated. A rise in antibody titer indicates that both the mother and the fetus have been infected by rubella. If the exposure occurred during the first trimester of pregnancy, the fetus is at risk for congenital heart defects, deafness, mental retardation, and cataracts.

Rubacell, Rubascan, or Rubazyme (enzyme-linked immunosorbent assay [ELISA]) tests, which detect immune status (IgG), can also be done. A positive result on any of these tests indicates that the woman is immune. She and the fetus are thus protected from rubella.

Procedure. A peripheral venous blood sample is obtained and sent to the laboratory for analysis.

Contraindications. None.

Nursing considerations

Nursing Diagnoses/Collaborative Problems

See Blood studies, p. 2.

Nursing Implications with Rationale

- Explain the purpose of the test to the patient.
- Apply pressure or a pressure dressing to the venipuncture site. Assess the site for bleeding.

SUPPLEMENTAL INFORMATION

Chlamydiae smears

Normal value: negative

Rationale. *Chlamydia trachomatis* is now isolated more frequently in clinics for sexually transmitted diseases than either gonorrhea or syphilis. This organism causes the eye disease trachoma, which is the most common form of preventable blindness. Chlamydia is the causative agent of lymphogranuloma venereum. *Chlamydia* can also cause salpingitis, urethritis, and epididymitis.

It is estimated that the incidence of chlamydial infections in infants is 28/1000 live births. This rate far exceeds that of herpes simplex and toxoplasmosis. Prenatal screening and treatment of pregnant women are beginning to be considered in some areas. This screening technique could prevent trachoma, ophthalmia neonatorum, inclusion conjunctivitis, chlamydial pneumonia, and genital tract infections (such as nonspecific urethritis).

Procedure. Cervical and urethral smears for women and men are obtained as described in the procedure for gonorrheal cultures (see p. 350). In men and women a gram stain of the smear showing polymorphonuclear leukocytes is diagnostic for chlamydial infections. *Chlamydia* can be isolated in culture. Direct fluorescent tests on a clinical skin lesion or pus can now be performed. Patients with positive smears should be treated with antibiotics. Sexual partners should be examined.

Contraindications. Smears for *Chlamydia* are not done in women who are presently having their routine menses.

Nursing Considerations

Nursing Diagnoses/Collaborative Problems

- Possible knowledge deficit related to test purpose, preparation, and procedure
- Possible anxiety related to test results
- Possible alteration in comfort related to test procedure

Nursing Implications with Rationale

- Same as for gonorrhea culture (see p. 350).

Herpes genitalis (Herpes virus type 2)

(herpes simplex virus type 2, HSV-2)

Normal value: not present

Rationale. Herpes virus type 2, or herpes genitalis, is a sexually transmitted viral infection of the urogenital tract. Because most infants become infected if they pass through a birth canal containing the virus, determining its presence before the time of delivery is necessary. A vaginal delivery is possible if no virus is present, and a cesarean section is needed if the virus is present. Viral testing can be performed on males or females to determine risk of sexual transmission.

This virus is one of the infections evaluated in the TORCH test (see next study).

Procedure. The cervical culture is obtained as described in the procedure for gonorrhea cultures (p. 350). The cervix is cultured weekly for the herpes virus beginning 4 to 8 weeks before the due date. Vaginal delivery is possible if the following criteria are met: the two most recent cultures are negative; the woman is not experiencing any symptoms; no lesions are visible on inspection of the vagina and vulva; and throughout her pregnancy, the woman has not had more than one positive culture during which she was symptom-free.

Serologic testing. ELISA is available to detect antibodies to herpes. The antibodies appear in the blood 4 to 6 weeks after infection.

Contraindications. None.

Nursing considerations

Nursing Diagnoses/Collaborative Problems

- Possible knowledge deficit related to test purpose, preparation, and procedure
- Possible anxiety related to unknown sensations of procedure
- Possible anxiety related to test results
- Possible alteration in comfort related to test procedure

Nursing Implications with Rationale

- Explain the procedure to the patient. Assure her that she will be appropriately draped to prevent unnecessary exposure.
- Allow ample time for the patient to verbalize her feelings. Many herpes victims experience anger, shame, and depression.
- After the study, inform the patient how to obtain the test results. Many patients are very anxious regarding the test results.

TORCH test

Normal value: negative

Rationale. The acronym TORCH (*t*oxoplasmosis, *o*ther, *r*ubella, *c*ytomegalovirus, *h*erpes) has been applied to infections with recognized detrimental effects on the fetus. The effects on the fetus may be direct or indirect (such as precipitating abortion or premature labor).

Toxoplasmosis (see p. 351). This infection can occur during early pregnancy and result in congenital infection. If this disease is recognized in early pregnancy by clinical evaluation or seroconversion, abortion is usually recommended because damage to the fetus is usually more severe than if acquired later in the pregnancy. If the infection occurs later in the pregnancy, treatment of the mother with triple sulfa drugs may reduce the fetal impact.

Other. Infections such as syphilis (see p. 348), varicella, and group B beta-hemolytic streptococcus are included in the *other* category. These infections are thought to be contracted by contact during birth.

Rubella, or German measles (see p. 351). Rubella may cause serious problems even as late as the fifth month of gestation. Abortion is usually recommended if the nonimmune pregnant mother develops clinical rubella or rubella antibodies because of the high rate of fetal involvement.

Cytomegalovirus. Cytomegalovirus is the most common of the congenital infections. Approximately 10% of infected newborns exhibit permanent damage, usually mental retardation and auditory damage. Fetal infection can cause microcephaly, hydrocephaly, cerebral palsy, mental retardation, or death. No specific therapy is known for this infection. If the diagnosis is established early by viral culture or serology, abortion may be an option.

Herpes simplex. The herpes simplex virus can be classified as either type I (primarily responsible for oral lesions) or type II (primarily responsible for genital lesions). Congenital infection, which is rare, has its greatest impact on the fetus in early pregnancy. Problems such as microcephaly, chorioretinitis, and mental retardation may result. Neonatal infection is much more common and is contracted during delivery by exposure to the virus in genital lesions. Disease in the newborn may be systematic (with a mortality of 90%) or localized (with a good prognosis). Treatment consists of performing a cesarean section if genital lesions are present at delivery (see p. 353).

Procedure. A venous or cord blood sample is obtained. See also separate studies.

Contraindications. None.

Nursing considerations

Nursing Diagnoses/Collaborative Problems

See Blood studies, p. 2.

- Possible anxiety related to test results

Nursing Implications with Rationale

- Explain the procedure to the patient and assess the venipuncture site for bleeding.
- Allow time for the patient to verbalize her feelings regarding these tests.

CASE STUDY 3: HIGH-RISK PREGNANCY

Mrs. P., a 22-year-old patient with a known history of juvenile diabetes mellitus, had been well regulated on insulin in the past few years. She had been trying to conceive. She went to her obstetrician 4 weeks after missing her expected menstrual period. Her physical examination results were essentially normal. Positive findings on the pelvic examination included mild uterine enlargement associated with softening and cyanosis of the cervix.

Studies	Results
Routine laboratory studies	Blood and urine tests WNL except: fasting blood sugar (FBS): 160 mg/dl (normal: 60-120 mg/dl) 2-hour postprandial glucose (2-hour PPG): 200 mg/dl (normal: 60-120 mg/dl)
Pap smear	Class I cytologic findings (normal)
Pregnancy test (latex agglutination)	Positive
Ultrasonography (at 24 weeks)	Biparietal diameter of the fetal skull 5 cm (baseline value)

The routine Pap smear did not indicate any neoplastic cells. The pregnancy test confirmed the clinical diagnosis of pregnancy with 80% accuracy. With close monitoring of her diabetes the patient was doing well at her thirty-sixth week of pregnancy. The following studies were then performed:

Studies	Results
Ultrasonography (at 36 weeks)	Normal placenta located high in fundus; biparietal diameter of the fetal skull 8.7 cm
Amniocentesis	L/S ratio: 3:1 (normal: >2:1) Creatinine level: 2.3 mg/dl (normal: ≥2 mg/dl) Cytologic findings: 30% of cells stained orange with Nile blue sulfate (normal: >20%)

Studies	Results
	Male child with no genetic or chromosomal abnormalities

In the patient's thirty-sixth week of pregnancy, ultrasonography indicated that fetal size was compatible with gestational age (by comparison of the ultrasonography value at 24 weeks with the value at 36 weeks) and that there were no abnormalities in placental location. Amniocentesis indicated fetal maturity compatible with life outside the womb.

In the patient's thirty-eighth week of pregnancy, spontaneous fetal movement ceased. The following studies were then performed:

Studies	Results
Serial 24-hour urine tests for estriol	12 mg/24 hours 11.2 mg/24 hours 10.0 mg/24 hours Abnormal, falling results (normal: >12 mg/24 hours)
Nonstress test	No accelerations with fetal movement (normal: heart rate acceleration with movement)
Contraction stress test	Positive: late decelerations of fetal heart rate (normal: negative)
X-ray pelvimetry	Birth canal size inadequate for vaginal delivery (normal: birth canal size adequate for vaginal delivery)
Amnioscopy	No meconium staining (normal: no meconium staining)

In the patient's thirty-eighth week of pregnancy, although amnioscopy ruled out fetal distress, the urine test for estriols and the contraction stress test (CST) indicated fetoplacental deterioration. X-ray pelvimetry implied cephalopelvic disproportion (CPD).

A cesarean section was performed, and a healthy 5-pound, 8-ounce boy was delivered. Both mother and child were discharged 1 week after delivery.

DISCUSSION OF TESTS

Pregnancy tests

Normal value: negative, unless patient is pregnant

Rationale. All pregnancy tests are based on the detection of human chorionic gonadotropin (HCG), which is secreted by the trophoblast after the ovum is fertilized. HCG appears in the blood and urine of pregnant women as early as 10 days after conception. Methods of pregnancy testing fall into the following four categories.

Biologic tests. Biologic (animal) tests have been used since the 1920s and are primarily of historical interest today. They are no longer used clinically. Urine from the patient is injected into an animal. If HCG is present, a specific response occurs in that animal, which varies according to the animal used. Each test is associated with an eponym. The Aschheim-Zondek test is based on corpus luteum formation in female mice; the Friedman test evaluates HCG-induced ovulation in female rabbits; the *Xenopus laevis* test is based on ova release in female South African toads; and the *Rana pipiens* frog test depends on sperm release in male toads. These tests all require the injection of urine from the patient into the animal. Biologic tests are 98% accurate 2 weeks after the first missed menstrual period. The disadvantage of these tests is that they require 48 hours to obtain a result. These tests have largely been replaced by less expensive, more accurate, and more rapidly performed immunologic tests.

Immunologic tests (agglutination inhibition test, AIT). These tests are performed by the use of commercially prepared reagents and can be completed within 2 minutes or 2 hours, depending on the method used. Immunologic tests are based on the reaction of HCG with antiserum to chorionic gonadotropin (rabbit anti-HCG). The tests can be performed with latex particles (slide test) or sheep erythrocytes (test tube assay).

In the slide test, one drop of urine and one drop of antiserum (against chorionic gonadotropin) are stirred together on a slide. Two drops of latex particles coated with the HCG are added and mixed completely for 2 minutes. If the woman is not pregnant, the urine contains no HCG to bind the HCG antibody and therefore the unaffected antibodies react with the HCG-coated latex particles and agglutinate (clump). This is a negative test. If the woman is pregnant, HCG in her urine neutralizes the antiserum. No HCG antibodies remain to agglutinate to the latex particles, and clumping does not occur. This is a positive test. These tests are frequently performed in a hospital's emergency department to detect if a woman is pregnant.

The test tube assay is similarly performed except that instead of HCG-coated latex particles, HCG-coated sheep red blood cells are used. This test requires 2 hours but is slightly more accurate and sensitive than the slide test. False-positive results may occur as often as 20% of the time.

Home pregnancy tests. Home pregnancy test kits are examples of urine- and agglutination-inhibition tests. Reliability of the test results is high if the test is done approximately 15 days after the last menstrual period (LMP) and if the urine specimen is clear, straw colored, and free of particles.

Radioimmunoassay (RIA). RIA is a highly sensitive and reliable blood test for the detection of the Beta subunit of HCG. In this test maternal serum HCG (unlabeled) and HCG that has been radioactively bound to antibody (labeled) compete for binding sites. The higher the concentration of HCG in the maternal serum, the greater the number of binding sites that are occupied by the unlabeled HCG. This study requires a blood sample (in a red-top tube), although it can also be performed on urine. In the past this test required 48 hours for completion; however, with newer techniques RIA can now be performed in 1 to 5 hours. This test is so sensitive that pregnancy can be diagnosed before the first missed menstrual period.

Radioreceptor assay (RRA). Radioreceptor assay for serum HCG is highly sensitive and accurate. It can be performed within 1 hour. The major advantage of this study is in its reliable diagnosis of early gestation in patients requesting an early termination of pregnancy and in cases in which infertile couples are anxious to confirm pregnancy. This study is 90% to 95% accurate 6 to 8 days after conception. Even the minute amounts of HCG secreted in an ectopic pregnancy can be measured with this study. This test is also useful in determining early spontaneous abortion in patients who desire to maintain the pregnancy. HCG production decreases when pregnancy is interrupted. Two minor disadvantages of this study are that the laboratory must be able to handle radioactive materials and it must be equipped with a Geiger counter. This test measures the ability of the blood sample to inhibit the binding of radiolabeled HCG to receptors.

False-negative tests most frequently result from performance of these different tests too early in the pregnancy, before there is a sufficient HCG level. Urine diluted by diuretic-induced excesses of excreted free water and laboratory technical errors are less common causes of false-negative results. False-positive results occur in some premenopausal or perimenopausal patients with gonadal hormone deficiencies caused by overproduction of pituitary gonadotropin, which can cause HCG-like positive reactions. Tranquilizers (especially promazine and its derivatives) may also produce false-positive results.

It is important to know that all of these pregnancy studies demonstrate the presence of HCG and do not necessarily indicate a normal pregnancy. Hydatidiform mole of the uterus and choriocarcinoma of the uterus, testes, or ovaries can produce HCG. Ectopic HCG production can occur with neoplasms of the GI tract. Because HCG is also produced by tumors, determination of HCG can be a valuable test for tumor activity. When HCG levels are elevated in these patients, tumor progression must be suspected. Decreasing HCG levels indicate effective antitumor treatment.

Procedure

Urine. Urine specimens should be collected in a standard container and taken to the laboratory. A first-voided morning specimen is preferred. Urine tests for pregnancy are usually recommended at least 2 weeks after the first missed menstrual period.

Blood. Blood samples are obtained according to the requirements of the specific test to be performed. Hemolysis of blood may interfere with test results.

Contraindications. None.

Nursing considerations

Nursing Diagnoses/Collaborative Problems

See Blood studies, p. 2, or Urine studies, p. 3.

- Possible anxiety related to test results

Nursing Implications with Rationale

- Explain the procedure to the patient. Encourage verbalization of the patient's fears. Many patients are very anxious in anticipation of the results. Inform the patient of how and when to obtain the test results.
- If urine specimens are required, give the patient the urine container on the evening before the test so that she can provide a first-voided morning specimen. This specimen generally contains the greatest concentration of HCG.
- If the patient is using a home pregnancy testing kit, be sure to emphasize that she should still have antepartal health examinations.
- If a blood sample is required, obtain this as indicated by the laboratory. Check the site afterward for bleeding.

Obstetric Ultrasonography

(obstetric echography, pregnant uterus ultrasonography)

Normal values: normal fetal and placental size and position

Rationale. Ultrasound evaluation of the obstetric patient has proven to be a harmless, noninvasive method of evaluating the female genital tract and fetus. In diagnostic ultrasound, harmless, high-frequency sound waves are emitted from a transducer and penetrate the structure (uterus, placenta, fetus, for example) to be studied. These sound waves are bounced back to a sensor within the transducer and, by electronic conversion, are arranged into a pictorial image of the desired organ. A realistic picture is reproduced on print paper or x-ray film.

Obstetric ultrasonography may be useful in:

1. Making an early diagnosis of normal pregnancy and abnormal pregnancy (such as tubal pregnancy and abdominal pregnancy). Pregnancy may be diagnosed as early as 5 weeks after the LMP. With the use of a probe placed vaginally, the embryo-fetal unit can be identified as early as 10 days after conception, and the fetal heartbeat can be observed as early as 6 to 7 weeks.
2. Identifying multiple pregnancies. Multiple pregnancies can be detected by 13 to 14 weeks' gestation by demonstrating the presence of more than one fetal head.
3. Differentiating a tumor (such as a hydatidiform mole) from a normal pregnancy.
4. Determining the age of the fetus by the diameter of its head. A single scan after 32 weeks is not completely reliable in determining fetal age (error: ±3 weeks). Ultrasound is more accurate if an earlier reference scan is available for comparison. At 36 weeks the biparietal diameter (BPD) of the fetal head should approximate 8.7 cm. Term pregnancy can usually be assured when the diameter is in excess of 9.8 cm.
5. Measuring the rate of fetal growth. Intrauterine growth retardation of the fetus can be indicated by sequential cephalometry. Growth retardation should be confirmed by estriol level determinations, nonstress testing, or contraction stress testing. Problems with twins can be detected by a disparity in BPDs in the

second trimester. Fetal death can be determined by sequential scans showing lack of growth, loss of fetal outline, and an increased number of echoes coming from within the fetal body.

6. Identifying placental abnormalities such as abruptio placentae (partial or complete premature separation of the placenta) and placenta previa (abnormally implanted placenta in the thin, lower part of the uterus).
7. Determining the position of the placenta. Ultrasound localization of the placenta is done before amniocentesis to avoid puncture of the placenta and before cesarean section so that the placenta can be avoided when the uterus is opened.
8. Making differential diagnoses of various uterine and ovarian enlargements (such as polyhydramnios, benign and malignant neoplasms, cysts, and abscesses). The ultrasound findings must be correlated with the clinical findings because malignancy, tuboovarian abscess, and endometriosis may appear similar.
9. Determining fetal position. This information is helpful when a normal vaginal delivery may not be possible because of the fetus's transverse or breech position.
10. Determining fetal maturity. A biophysical profile uses ultrasound to watch the fetus for 20 to 30 minutes. Lung movement, tonicity of arm movements and amniotic fluid volume are measured.

No known complications are associated with this study for the mother or the fetus. This study appears to be safe, even when used repeatedly. The patient is not exposed to any ionizing radiation.

A *general pelvic ultrasound* (or *gynecologic sonogram*) is performed in the nonpregnant female to examine the pelvic organs and surrounding tissues in men and women. Pelvic ultrasounds are used to evaluate delayed puberty, postmenopausal bleeding, pelvic masses, and uterine fibroids and to aid in the diagnosis of cysts and tumors affecting the pelvic organs.

Procedure. No fasting or sedation is required. The patient is given three to four glasses of water 1 hour before the study and is instructed *not* to void. The full bladder provides better transmission of the sound waves and better visualization of the uterus by pushing the uterus away from the symphysis and by pushing the bowel out of the pelvis. The patient is then taken to the ultrasound room (usually in the radiology department) and placed in the supine position on the examining table. The ultrasonographer (usually a radiologist) applies a greasy, conductive paste to the abdomen used to enhance sound transmission and reception. An abdominal transducer is then passed vertically and horizontally over the skin, and pictures are taken of the reflections (Figure 9-10). The duration of this study is approximately 20 minutes, and no discomfort is associated with it.

During the ultrasound examination, the fetal structures should be pointed out to the mother. Seeing the fetus during ultrasound may promote prenatal attachment.

The general pelvic ultrasound can be done transabdominally or transvaginally. With the *transvaginal approach*, a lubricated transducer is gently inserted into the vagina with the patient in a lithotomy position. A full bladder is not necessary.

Contraindications. This study is contraindicated in patients who have recently had GI contrast studies. The barium used in such studies creates severe distortion of the reflected sound waves. Also the results may be uninterpretable in patients with an air-filled bowel. Gas does not transmit the sound waves well.

Nursing considerations

Nursing Diagnoses/Collaborative Problems

See Ultrasound studies, p. 6.

Nursing Implications with Rationale

- Explain the procedure to the patient. Assure the patient that this study has no known del-

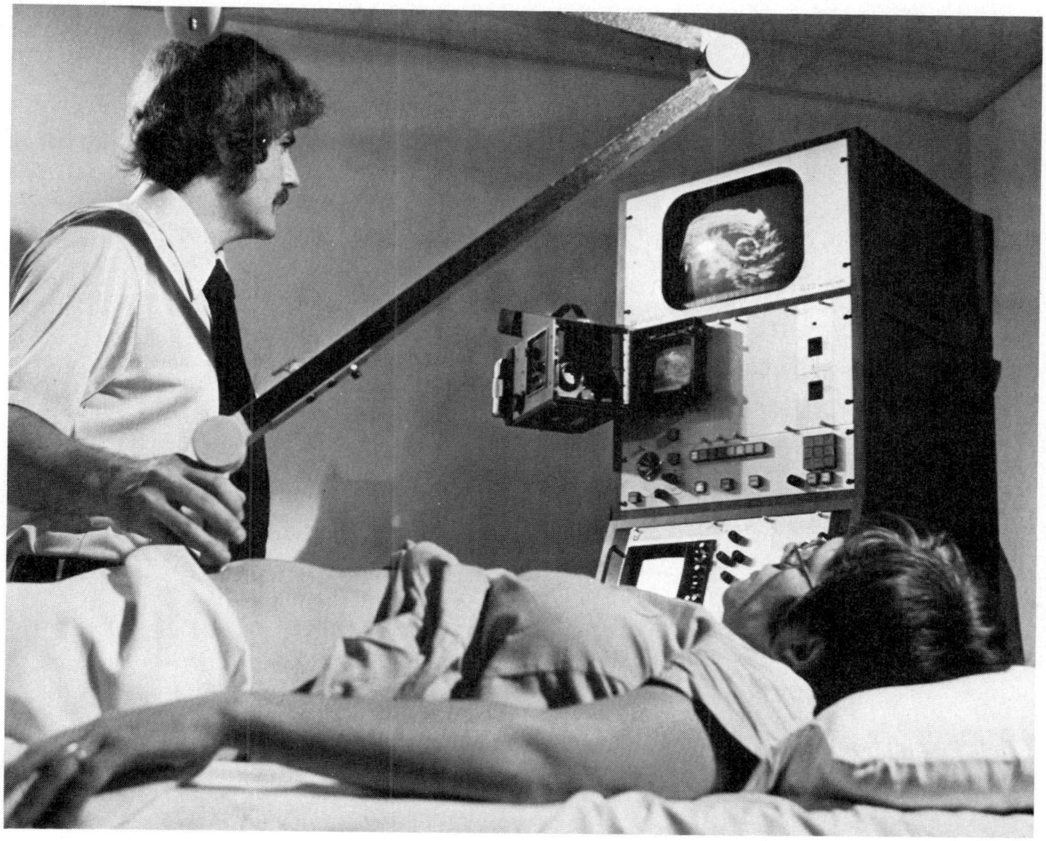

FIGURE 9-10. Ultrasonography is a safe, painless method of scanning mother's abdomen with high-frequency sound waves to follow fetal growth and development.
Courtesy March of Dimes.

eterious effect on maternal or fetal tissues even when it is repeated several times.

- Give the patient 3 or 4 glasses (200 to 350 ml) of water or other liquids 1 hour before the examination, and instruct her *not* to void until after ultrasonography is completed. This permits better transmission of the sound waves and enhances visualization of the uterus.
- Tell the patient that this study is not associated with any pain. The patient may have some discomfort because she will have a full bladder and the urge to void. Some patients may be uncomfortable lying on a hard x-ray table.
- Explain to the patient that a liberal amount of gel or lubricant will be applied to her skin to enhance the transmission and reception of the sound waves. The gel will feel cold.
- After the study remove the lubricant from the patient's skin and allow the patient an opportunity to void.

Amniocentesis

Normal values: dependent on the reason for the study

Rationale. Amniocentesis involves the placement of a needle through the patient's abdominal and uterine walls into the amniotic cavity to withdraw fluid for analysis (see Figure 9-11).

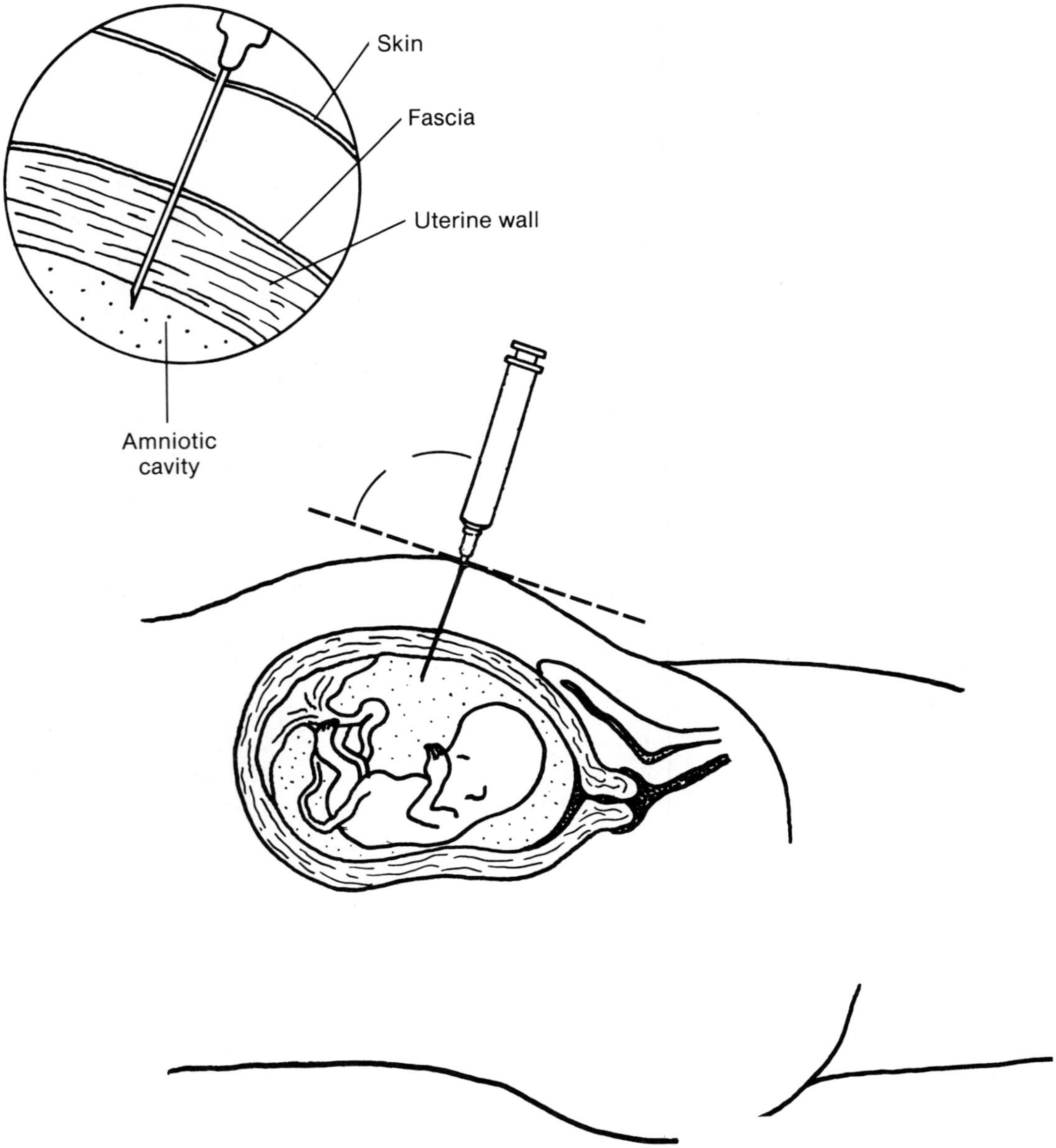

FIGURE 9-11. Amniocentesis. Ultrasound scanning is usually used to determine the placental site and to locate a pocket of amniotic fluid. The needle is then inserted. Three levels of resistance are felt as the needle penetrates the skin, fascia, and uterine wall. When the needle is placed within the uterine cavity, amniotic fluid is withdrawn.

Studying amniotic fluid is vitally important in assessing the following:

1. Fetal maturity status (in cases where early delivery is preferred).
2. Sex of the fetus. Sons of mothers who are known to be carriers of X-linked recessive traits would have a 50 : 50 chance of inheritance.
3. Genetic and chromosomal aberrations (such as hemophilia, Down's syndrome, and galactosemia).
4. Fetal status affected by Rh isoimmunization. Mothers with Rh isoimmunization have a series of amniocentesis procedures during the second half of pregnancy to assess the level of bilirubin pigment in the amniotic fluid. The quantity of bilirubin in the amniotic fluid is used to assess the severity of hemolytic anemia in Rh-sensitized pregnancy. The higher the amount of bilirubin, the lower the amount of fetal hemoglobin. Amniocentesis is usually initiated at 24 to 25 weeks. This allows assessment of the severity of the disease and the status of the fetus. Early delivery or blood transfusion may be indicated.
5. Hereditary metabolic disorders (such as cystic fibrosis).
6. Anatomic abnormalities such as neural tube closure defects (myelomeningocele, anecephaly, and spina bifida).
7. Fetal distress detected by meconium staining of the amniotic fluid. This is caused by relaxation of the anal sphincter.

Fetal maturity is determined by analysis of the amniotic fluid for the following:

1. Lecithin/sphingomyelin (L/S) ratio. The L/S ratio is a measure of fetal lung maturity, which is determined by measuring the phospholipids in amniotic fluid. Lecithin is the major constituent of surfactant (an important substance required for alveolar ventilation). If surfactant is insufficient, the alveoli collapse during expiration. This results in atelectasis and respiratory distress syndrome (RDS), which is a major cause of death in immature babies. In the immature fetal lung the sphingomyelin concentration in amniotic fluid is higher than the lecithin concentration. At 35 weeks' gestation, the concentration of lecithin rapidly increases, whereas sphingomyelin concentration decreases. An L/S ratio of $\geq 2:1$ ($3:1$ in diabetic mothers) is a highly reliable indication that the fetal lung, and therefore the fetus, is mature. In such a case, after birth the infant would be unlikely to develop RDS. Another phospholipid screening test for phosphatidyl glycerol is available and more accurate than the L/S ratio, especially in diabetic pregnant women. Phosphatidyl glycerol is the gold standard for determining fetal lung maturity. It appears at 36 weeks and increases until term.

The amount of surfactant in amniotic fluid can be evaluated by a quick, inexpensive, simple technique called the *shake test* (also called *foam stability* or *rapid surfactant test*). This test, which is used to assess fetal lung maturity, is based on the principle that surfactant should prolong the stability of an emulsifier. For this test a small amount of amniotic fluid is diluted with saline solution. Ninety-five percent ethyl alcohol is then added, and the mixture is shaken vigorously for about 30 seconds. The persistence of fine bubbles indicates the presence of surfactant. A dilutional table is used to determine the stage of lung maturity. The test result is positive when the fine bubbles (foam) are present. A positive test has a high accuracy for indicating pulmonary maturity. If no foam is seen, the test is negative and the risk for RDS is high. This test is now rarely performed because of the greater accuracy of phosphatidyl glycerol testing.

2. Creatinine concentration. Creatinine is excreted in the fetal urine and is used to assess fetal renal function and fetal muscle mass. The creatinine concentration rises sharply between the thirty-fourth and the thirty-sixth week of gestation. Values of ≥2 mg/dl of amniotic fluid usually correlate with a gestational age of at least 36 weeks and therefore indicate fetal maturity. The measurement of the creatinine concentration is much less reliable (60%) than is the L/S ratio (90%); however, when the two measurements are combined, their accuracy is greater than that of either test performed separately.
3. Bilirubin levels. The amount of bilirubin in amniotic fluid is a measure of liver maturity and should decrease near term in a normal fetus. When the optical density (OD) of bilirubinoid pigments in amniotic fluid at 450 nm is ≤0.01, the gestational age is greater than 38 weeks and the fetus is considered mature. Bilirubin level measurements are no longer routinely performed for determining fetal maturity because they are nonspecific (for example, bilirubin levels indicating maturity may be present earlier in an Rh-sensitized pregnancy).
4. Cytologic findings. The sebaceous glands of the fetus begin to function and to shed cells near term. As the fetus matures, the percentage of cells containing lipids increases. By staining amniotic fluid with Nile blue stain, lipid cells can be identified. When more than 20% of the fetal cells stain orange with 0.1% Nile blue sulfate, the gestational age is considered to be greater than 35 weeks. At this time the probable weight of the fetus is 2500 g. One advantage of this test is that it can be done without sophisticated laboratory equipment.

Genetic and chromosomal studies performed on cells aspirated within the amniotic fluid can indicate the sex of the fetus (important in sex-linked diseases such as hemophilia) or any of the described genetic and chromosomal aberrations. Increased levels of alpha-fetoproteins (AFP) in the amniotic fluid may indicate a neural crest abnormality, as listed earlier. Amniocentesis may be done on the premise that elective abortion may be performed if the fetus is severely defective.

Timing of the amniocentesis varies according to the clinical circumstances. With advanced maternal age and if chromosomal or genetic aberrations are suspected, the test should be done early enough (14 to 16 weeks) to easily allow safe abortion. This timing is essential because of the 3-week period necessary for cell growth to determine the results of the study. If knowledge of fetal maturity is sought, performing the study during or after the thirty-fifth week of gestation is best. Placental localization (by ultrasonography) should be done before amniocentesis to avoid the needle's passing into the placenta, possibly interrupting the placenta and inducing bleeding or abortion.

Amniocentesis with its probability of risk of less than 1% is considered a safe diagnostic procedure when family history or maternal age suggests a potential problem. The potential risks of amniocentesis for the fetus include miscarriage, fetal injury, subsequent leak of amniotic fluid, infection (amnionitis), abortion, and premature labor. Risks to the mother include hemorrhage, fetomaternal hemorrhage with possible maternal Rh isoimmunization, premature labor, amniotic fluid embolism, infection, abruptio placentae, and inadvertent damage to the bladder or intestines.

Procedure. Amniocentesis is usually performed on an outpatient basis under strict aseptic conditions. The bladder is emptied to minimize the chance of puncture after 20 weeks' gestational age. Before 20 weeks' gestation, the bladder is often kept full to support the uterus. Before the test the mother's blood pressure is taken and the fetal heart is auscultated. The placenta should be localized before the study (by ultrasound) to permit selection of a site that will

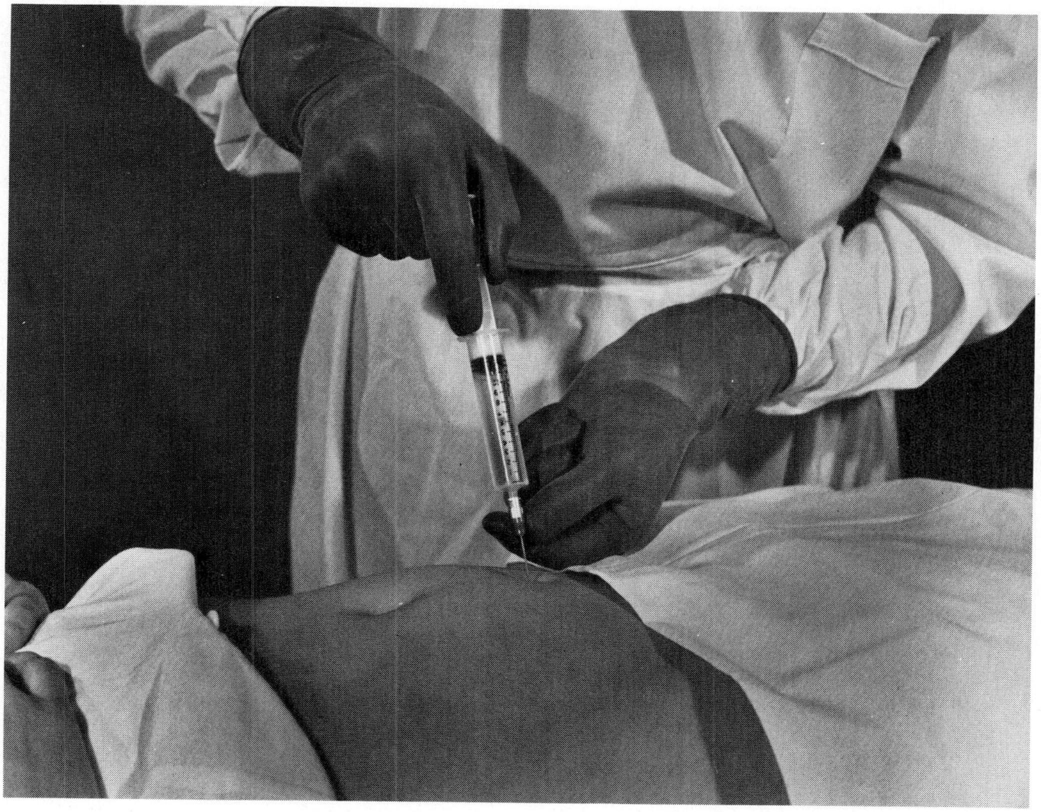

FIGURE 9-12. Transabdominal amniocentesis.
Courtesy March of Dimes.

avoid placental puncture. Ultrasonography also aids in identification of uterine abnormalities (such as bicornuate uterus) that may complicate the amniocentesis procedure.

The patient is then placed in a supine position, and the skin overlying the chosen site is prepared, draped, and locally anesthetized. (Some physicians do not use local anesthesia because the anesthetic would sting and two needles would be needed. Once the skin is pierced, the patient feels pressure, but not pain.)

A 22-gauge, 5-inch spinal needle with a stylet is inserted through the midabdominal wall and directed at an angle toward the middle of the uterine cavity. The stylet is then removed and a sterile plastic syringe is attached (Figure 9-12). After 10 to 15 ml of amniotic fluid is withdrawn, the needle is removed. This fluid volume is replaced by newly formed amniotic fluid within 3 to 4 hours after the procedure. The site is covered with an adhesive bandage. If the amniotic fluid is bloody, the physician must determine whether the blood is maternal or fetal in origin. Kleihauer-Böetke stain will stain fetal cells pink. Meconium in the fluid is usually associated with a compromised fetus.

The amniotic fluid is placed in a sterile, siliconized glass container and transported to a special chemistry laboratory for analysis. Sometimes the specimen may be sent by air mail to another commercial laboratory. The results are usually not available for at least 10 days.

After the procedure the mother's blood pressure is checked and the fetal heart tone is assessed. The patient should be instructed to report any fluid loss, bleeding, cramping, dizziness, or fever following this study.

Amniocentesis should be performed by an experienced obstetrician who is able to provide counseling and treatment based on the results of this study. The discomfort associated with this study is that of mild uterine cramping, which occurs when the needle contacts the uterus. Some women may complain of a "pulling" sensation as the amniotic fluid is withdrawn. Most women describe the injection of the local anesthetic as the major discomfort of the procedure. Many women are extremely anxious during this procedure. The duration of this procedure is approximately 20 to 30 minutes.

The maternal blood type should be determined (if unknown). Women who have Rh negative blood should receive RhoGAM because of the risk of immunization from the fetal blood, which can jeopardize the fetus.

Contraindications. This study is contraindicated in patients with:

1. Abruptio placentae
2. Placenta previa
3. A history of premature labor (before 34 weeks), unless the patient is receiving antilabor medication at this time
4. Incompetent cervix

Nursing considerations

Nursing Diagnoses/Collaborative Problems

- Possible knowledge deficit related to test purpose, preparation, and procedure
- Possible anxiety related to unknown sensations of procedure
- High risk for anxiety related to test results
- Possible alteration in comfort related to test procedure
- Potential complication: miscarriage
- Potential complication: infection
- Potential complication: premature labor
- Potential complication: fetomaternal hemorrhage

Nursing Implications with Rationale

- Explain the procedure to the patient. Assure the patient that precautions will be taken to minimize risk to both her and the fetus. Encourage the patient to verbalize her fears concerning this study. Most patients are very apprehensive. Relaxation techniques such as focusing and slow breathing can help relieve some maternal anxiety.
- Be certain that the physician has obtained a signed consent form from the husband and wife before the procedure.
- Assess the fetal heart rate (FHR) before and after the study to detect any ill effects related to the procedure. With detection of any ill effects, bed rest and fetal heart monitoring are prescribed. An immediate cesarean section may be performed if gestation is greater than 35 weeks and signs of fetal dizziness are evident.
- Tell the patient that the needle used in this procedure is long because it passes through layers of fat and muscle before reaching the uterus. Only a small portion of the needle passes into the uterus.
- If the woman feels dizzy or nauseated during the procedure, allow her to rest on her left side for several minutes before leaving the examining room.
- Instruct the patient to call her physician if she has any fluid loss or temperature elevation.
- Inform the patient about how she can obtain the results of this study from her physician. Be certain that the patient knows the results are not available for at least 3 weeks.

Estriol excretion studies

Normal values: rising urinary estriol values indicate normal fetal growth

Rationale

Twenty-four-hour urine studies. Serial 24-hour urine studies for estriol excretion provide an objective means of assessing placental function and fetal normality in high-risk pregnancies. Because there are better ways of determining placental function and fetal health, this test is rarely performed. Estriol (the type of estrogen present in blood and urine in the largest amounts) excretion increases around the eighth week of gestation and continues to rise until shortly before delivery. Because the fetal contribution to the estriol value is considerable, the measurement of excreted urinary estriol has become an important index of fetal well-being. Rising urinary values and those greater than 12 mg/24 hours indicate an adequately functioning fetoplacental unit. Decreasing values suggest fetoplacental deterioration (failing pregnancy, dysmaturity, preeclampsia/eclampsia, complicated diabetes mellitus, encephaly, fetal death) and require prompt reassessment of the pregnancy. If the estriol levels fall, early delivery of the fetus may be indicated.

Because urinary creatine excretion is relatively constant (0.7 to 1.5 mg/dl), its determination can be used to assess the adequacy of the 24-hour urine collection. A serially increasing estriol/creatinine ratio is a favorable sign in pregnancy.

Plasma estriol studies. Plasma estriol determinations are now used to evaluate the fetoplacental unit. (Urinary estriol excretion of 1 mg/24 hours is approximately equivalent to 0.6 to 0.8 ng/ml of unconjugated plasma estriol.) These studies can conveniently and rapidly (in 7 to 12 hours) assess the quantity of free estriol in the plasma by radioimmunoassay. The plasma collected by venipuncture is an accurate reflection of the current status of the placenta and fetus. The advantage of the plasma estriol determination is that it is more easily obtained than a 24-hour urine specimen. Another advantage is that glycosuria and maternal drugs (such as ampicillin and methenamine mandelate) do not affect plasma levels, as they do urine estriol levels.

Procedure. Serial studies are usually begun around 28 to 30 weeks of gestation and repeated at weekly intervals. The frequency of these estriol determinations can be increased as needed to evaluate a high-risk pregnancy. Collections may be done daily. Although the first collection is the baseline value, all collection results are compared with previous ones because decreasing values suggest fetal deterioration. Some physicians suggest using an average of three previous values as a control value.

Twenty-four–hour urine studies. A 24-hour urine specimen is collected using a preservative. The urine specimen must be refrigerated or kept on ice during the collection period. It is taken to the laboratory at the end of the collection period.

Plasma estriol studies. For plasma estriol studies a venipuncture is performed and 5 ml of venous blood is obtained in the manner specified by the laboratory. Some labs require a heparinized container.

Contraindications. Estriol excretion studies are contraindicated in patients receiving barbiturates or steroids because these drugs may alter estriol levels.

Nursing considerations

Nursing Diagnoses/Collaborative Problems

See Blood studies, p. 2, or Urine studies, p. 3.

- Possible anxiety related to test results

Nursing Implications with Rationale

- Explain the procedure to the patient. Allow ample time for the patient to verbalize her fears regarding the results of this study. Provide emotional support.
- See pp. 230-231, Nursing implications for the creatinine clearance test (except for the first and last implications), for 24-hour urine collection. Explain to the patient the importance of a complete collection. Every urine specimen must be included or the study must be started over. The specimen requires a preservative and must be kept on ice throughout the collection period.
- If the woman is going to collect the 24-hour urine specimen at home, give her the collection bottle (with the preservative) and instruct

her to keep the urine refrigerated. If one is available, supply the container (which is hat-like) to fit under the toilet seat. Collection and delivery to the laboratory may be inconvenient to the patient and her family.

- If serum estriol studies are needed, draw the blood according to the laboratory's procedure. Assess the site for bleeding afterward.
- Inform the patient of how and when to obtain the results of this study from her physician.

Contraction stress test

(CST, oxytocin challenge test, OCT)

Normal value: negative

Rationale. The contraction stress test (CST), frequently called the oxytocin challenge test (OCT), is a relatively noninvasive test of fetoplacental adequacy used in the assessment of high-risk pregnancy. For this study a temporary stress in the form of uterine contractions is applied to the fetus. The reaction of the fetus to the contractions is assessed by an external fetal heart monitor. Uterine contractions cause transient impediment of placental blood flow. If the placental reserve is adequate, the maternal-fetal oxygen transfer is not significantly compromised during the contractions and the FHR remains normal (a *negative* test). The fetoplacental unit can then be considered adequate for the next 7 days. If the placental reserve is inadequate, the fetus does not receive enough oxygen during the contraction. This results in intrauterine hypoxia and late deceleration of the FHR. The test is considered *positive* if there are consistent, persistent late decelerations of the FHR with two or more uterine contractions. False-positive results caused by uterine hyperstimulation can occur in 10% to 30% of patients. Thus positive test results warrant a complete review of other studies (such as amniocentesis) before the pregnancy is terminated by delivery.

Results are considered *equivocal* if there are inconsistent, late decelerations, and the test should be repeated 24 hours later. The concept of a "10-minute window"—a period of 10 minutes in which the criteria for either a positive or a negative test should be satisfied—has reduced the incidence of equivocal results. If an occasional late deceleration is followed by a 10-minute period of no decelerations during three contractions, the result is called a "negative window." The test is then negative rather than equivocal. A positive result can be ascertained from a 10-minute "positive window," in which there is a 10-minute time interval that meets the criteria of a positive test.

The test is considered *unsatisfactory* if the results cannot be interpreted (for example, because of hyperstimulation of the uterus or excessive movement of the mother), and it should be repeated.

Two advantages of the CST are that it can be done at any time and its results are available shortly afterward. Although this test can be performed reliably at 32 weeks of gestation, it usually is done after 34 weeks. CST can induce labor, and a fetus at 34 weeks is more likely to survive an unexpected induced delivery than a fetus at 32 weeks. Nonstress testing of the fetus (see next study) is the preferred test in almost every instance and can be performed more safely at 32 weeks and then followed 2 weeks later by CST if necessary. The CST may be performed weekly until delivery terminates pregnancy.

The CST can be used clinically in any high-risk pregnancy where fetal well-being is threatened. These include pregnancies marked by diabetes, hypertensive disease of pregnancy (eclampsia), intrauterine growth retardation, Rh-factor sensitization, history of stillbirth, postmaturity, or low estriol levels.

Procedure. The CST is safely performed on an outpatient basis in the labor and delivery unit, where qualified nurses and necessary equipment are accessible. If the CST is performed on an elective basis, the patient should be kept NPO in case labor occurs as a result of testing. Performance of the CST should not be delayed if the patient is not fasting and fetal distress is suspected. The test is performed by a nurse, with a physician available. After emptying her bladder, the patient is placed in the semi-Fowler position and tilted slightly to one side to avoid vena caval compression by the enlarged uterus. Her blood pressure is checked every 10 minutes to avoid hypotension, which may cause diminished placental blood flow and a false-positive test result. Blood pressure is then checked routinely every 15 minutes throughout the test. An external fetal monitor is placed over the abdomen to record the fetal heart tones, and an external tocodynamometer is attached to the abdomen at the fundal region to monitor uterine contractions. The output of the fetal heart tones and uterine contractions is recorded on a two-channel strip recorder. Baseline FHR and uterine activity are monitored for 15 to 20 minutes. If uterine contractions are detected during this pretest period, oxytocin is withheld and the response of the fetal heart tone to spontaneous uterine contractions is monitored.

If no spontaneous uterine contractions occur, oxytocin (Pitocin) is administered by intravenous infusion using a pump at 0.5 to 1.0 mU/minute. The rate of oxytocin infusion is increased every 20 minutes until the patient is having three "moderate-quality" contractions per 10-minute period. The FHR pattern is recorded.

The oxytocin infusion is then discontinued, while FHR monitoring is continued for another 30 minutes until the uterine activity has returned to its preoxytocin state. The body metabolizes oxytocin in approximately 20 to 25 minutes. The woman should be informed of the test results at this time.

A new noninvasive method of performing the CST is called the *breast stimulation* or *nipple stimulation technique*. Stimulation of the nipple causes nerve impulses to the hypothalamus that trigger the release of oxytocin into the mother's blood stream. This causes uterine contractions and may eliminate the need for the intravenous administration of oxytocin. Uterine contractions are usually satisfactory after 15 minutes of nipple stimulation (gentle twisting of the nipples). Advantages of this technique include ease of performing the test; shorter duration of the study; and elimination of the need to start, monitor, and stop intravenous infusions. If sufficient contractions do not result from nipple stimulation, the standard CST procedure is followed.

The discomfort associated with these procedures may consist of mild labor contractions. Usually breathing exercises are enough to control any discomfort. Analgesics are given if needed. The duration of this study is approximately 2 hours.

Contraindications. The CST is contraindicated in:

1. Multiple pregnancy, because the myometrium is under greater tension and is more likely to be stimulated to premature labor
2. Premature ruptured membrane, because labor may be stimulated by the CST
3. Placenta previa, because vaginal delivery may be induced, leading to life-threatening exsanguination from the mother and child
4. Abruptio placentae, because the placenta may separate from the uterus as a result of the oxytocin-induced uterine contractions
5. Previous hysterotomy, because the strong uterine contractions may cause uterine rupture
6. Previous vertical or classical cesarean section (for the same reasons as given previously); however, if necessary, the CST may be performed if it is carefully monitored and controlled
7. Pregnancies of less than 32 weeks, because early delivery may be induced before the development of adequate fetal maturity to sustain life outside the womb

Nursing considerations

Nursing Diagnoses/Collaborative Problems

- Possible knowledge deficit related to test purpose, preparation, and procedure
- High risk for anxiety related to unknown sensations of procedure

- Possible alteration in comfort related to test procedure
- High risk for anxiety related to test results
- Potential complication: premature labor

Nursing Implications with Rationale

- Explain the procedure to the patient. The necessity of the test usually raises realistic fears in the mother. Encourage verbalization and provide factual information. Provide emotional support for the patient.
- Practice breathing and relaxation exercises with the patient before the study. Administer analgesics during the study, if ordered. The need for narcotics must be carefully assessed, because these drugs may affect the FHR tracing.
- Monitor the patient's blood pressure and the FHR before, during, and after the study, as indicated. Record these signs and the oxytocin infusion rate every 15 minutes on the monitor strip.
- Administer the oxytocin by means of an infusion pump, because it can be more precisely controlled than manual methods. Discontinue the intravenous line after the study and apply an adhesive bandage to the site. Continue fetal monitoring for 30 minutes. Assess the intravenous site for bleeding.
- Many patients have this study repeated at weekly intervals until delivery. This regimen is tiring and produces anxiety for the parents, who require emotional support.

Nonstress test

(NST, fetal activity determination)

Normal value: "reactive" fetus (heart rate acceleration associated with fetal movement)

Rationale. The nonstress test (NST) is a noninvasive study in which FHR acceleration in response to fetal movement is monitored. This FHR acceleration reflects the integrity of the CNS and fetal well-being. Fetal activity may be spontaneous, induced by uterine contraction, or induced by external manipulation. Oxytocin stimulation is not used. Fetal response is characterized as "reactive" or "nonreactive." The NST indicates a reactive fetus (Figure 9-13), when, with fetal movement, two or more FHR accelerations are detected, each of which must be at least 15 beats/minute for 15 seconds or more within any 10-minute period. The test is 99% reliable in indicating fetal viability and negates the need for the CST (see previous study). If the test detects a nonreactive fetus (that is, no FHR acceleration with fetal movement) within forty minutes, the patient is then a candidate for the CST. A 40-minute period is used because this is the average duration of the sleep-wake cycle of the fetus. However, the cycle may vary considerably.

The NST is useful in screening high-risk pregnancies and in selecting those patients who may require the CST. An NST is now routinely performed before the CST to avoid the complications associated with oxytocin administration. No complications are associated with the NST.

Procedure. The NST is performed by a nurse in the physician's office or on a hospital ward. After emptying her bladder, the patient is placed in the Sim's position. An external fetal monitor is placed on the abdomen to record the FHR. The mother can indicate the occurrence of fetal movement by pressing a button on the fetal monitor whenever she feels the fetus move. FHR and fetal movement are concomitantly recorded on a two-channel strip graph. The fetal monitor is then observed for FHR accelerations associated with fetal movement. If the baby is quiet for 20 minutes, fetal activity is stimulated by external methods, such as rubbing the mother's abdomen, compressing the abdomen, ringing a bell near the abdomen, or placing a pan on the abdomen and banging on the pan.

This study should be performed after a recent meal, because the fetus frequently is more active when the maternal serum glucose level is increased. The duration of the study is ap-

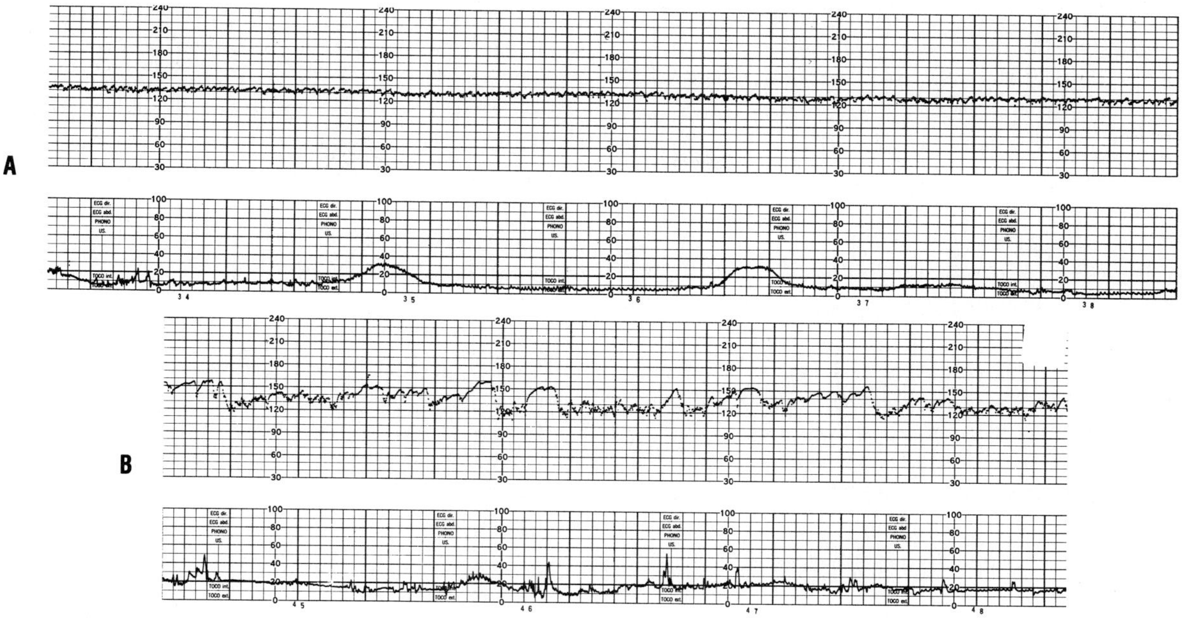

FIGURE 9-13. Nonstress test. **A,** Decreased variability caused by fetal sleep cycle. **B,** Reactive nonstress test 15 minutes later.
From Perez RH: Protocols for perinatal nursing practice, St Louis, 1981, Mosby–Year Book.

proximately 20 to 40 minutes. No discomfort is associated with the NST.

Contraindications. None.

Nursing considerations

Nursing Diagnoses/Collaborative Problems

- Possible knowledge deficit related to test purpose, preparation, and procedure
- Possible anxiety related to unknown sensations of procedure
- Possible anxiety related to test results

Nursing Implications with Rationale

- Explain the procedure to the patient. Assure the patient that no discomfort or adverse effects are associated with this study.
- Encourage verbalization of the patient's fears. The necessity for this study usually raises realistic fears in the expectant mother. Provide emotional support.
- If the patient is hungry, sending her to the cafeteria before initiating the NST may be helpful. Fetal activity is enhanced with a high maternal serum glucose level.

X-ray pelvimetry

(radiographic pelvimetry)

Normal value: transverse diameter of midpelvis >10.5 cm

Rationale. Although most abnormalities of the pelvis can be suspected by clinical measurement, x-ray pelvimetry is the most accurate means of determining adequacy of the pelvic bony structures for a normal vaginal delivery. By x-ray pelvimetry, one can compare the capacity of the pelvis with the size of the infant's head and discover any cephalopelvic disproportion (CPD).

X-ray pelvimetry is an outmoded procedure that is used only rarely in modern obstetrics because of the risks associated with radiation. However this study may be indicated in:

1. Patients suspected of having fetuses in abnormal positions (such as breech) when a vaginal delivery is anticipated
2. Patients who have had injury or disease of the bony pelvis or hips that may have caused pelvic distortion.

Other indications may include:

1. Patients with clinically abnormal pelvic measurements
2. Patients who have a debilitating illness complicating their pregnancy and a clinically small or unfavorable pelvis, because an elective cesarean section may then be recommended if a difficult or hazardous delivery is predicted
3. Patients who have a history of difficult delivery
4. Primiparas in early labor, with the fetus's head unengaged (to rule out CPD)
5. Patients admitted for trial labor to rule out a contracted pelvis
6. Patients having dysfunctional labor, especially when the physician is considering oxytocin administration.

Although measuring the pelvis clinically is less accurate than x-ray determination, it is adequate for most patients. Radiographic pelvimetry is only important late in pregnancy or during labor. If pelvimetry indicates a difficult or dangerous vaginal delivery, cesarean section is recommended. Cesarean section is now more frequently performed in cases where vaginal delivery is *clinically* suspected to be difficult. As a result, x-ray pelvimetry rarely affects the physician's decision concerning the type of delivery. In those rare situations in which vaginal delivery is attempted despite an anticipated difficult delivery, x-ray pelvimetry is performed more for legal purposes than for medical benefits.

Procedure. The patient is taken to the radiology department and dons a long x-ray gown. A lateral x-ray film is taken with the patient standing to detect the effect of gravity on engagement and to indicate the position of the fetal head when it reaches the lower level of the birth canal. The patient is then placed in the supine, lateral, and semirecumbent positions. During the x-ray exposure, the patient is asked to stop breathing. Generally the patient is instructed to hyperventilate and then stop breathing while the film is taken. The important measurements in determining pelvic adequacy are now more accurately made by the use of a pelvic CT scan. See p. 123.

No discomfort is associated with this study. A radiologic technician performs this study in approximately 15 minutes and a radiologist then interprets the results.

Contraindications. This study is contraindicated in early pregnancy because x-rays at this time may injure the fetus.

Nursing considerations

Nursing Diagnoses/Collaborative Problems

See X-ray studies, p. 5.

Nursing Implications with Rationale

- Explain the procedure to the patient. Encourage the patient to verbalize her feelings. She may suspect that she is undergoing this procedure because something may be wrong. Provide emotional support at this difficult time.
- Tell the patient that she must remove all clothing and don a long x-ray gown. Having the patient put on the gown before she leaves the nursing unit is a good idea.

Amnioscopy

Normal value: normal color of amniotic fluid; no meconium staining

Rationale. Amnioscopy allows direct transcervical visualization of the amniotic fluid to detect meconium staining of the fluid. Fetal hypoxia results in passage of meconium through the rectum of the fetus. This meconium, which can be detected through the intact membranes with a vaginal speculum, may indicate fetal distress or death. Meconium is also present in some normal pregnancies. Therefore, results must be evaluated within the overall clinical situation.

Amnioscopy is also used for fetal blood sampling. Fetal blood sampling for pH is described on p. 372.

The major risk associated with amnioscopy is inadvertent rupture of the membrane. A disadvantage of this study is that although the color of the fluid can be evaluated, no fluid is obtained for laboratory analysis.

Procedure. The patient is placed in the lithotomy position. The cervix is dilated 2 cm, and an endoscope (amnioscope) is introduced into the cervical canal. The color of the amniotic fluid is evaluated.

This study is performed by a physician in approximately 10 to 15 minutes. The patient will be uncomfortable during cervical dilation. After the study the patient may have vaginal discomfort and menstrual-type cramping.

Contraindications. This study is contraindicated in patients with:

1. Labor
2. Premature membrane rupture
3. Active cervical infection (such as gonorrhea).

Nursing considerations

Nursing Diagnoses/Collaborative Problems

- Possible knowledge deficit related to test purpose, preparation, and procedure
- Possible alteration in comfort related to procedure
- Possible anxiety related to unknown sensations of test
- Possible anxiety related to test results
- Potential complication: membrane rupture

Nursing Implications with Rationale

- Explain the procedure to the patient. Encourage verbalization of the patient's questions and fears. Provide emotional support.
- After the study assess the patient for rupture of the membranes and for uterine contractions.

SUPPLEMENTAL INFORMATION

Colposcopy

Normal value: normal vagina and cervix

Rationale. Colposcopy provides in situ macroscopic examination of the vagina and cervix with a colposcope, which is a microscope with a light source and a magnifying lens. With this procedure tiny areas of dysplasia, carcinoma in situ, and invasive cancer, which would be missed by the naked eye, can be visualized, and biopsy specimens can be removed. This study is performed on patients with abnormal vaginal epithelial patterns, cervical lesions, or suspicious Pap smear results and in those exposed to DES while in utero. Colposcopy may be a sufficient substitute for cone biopsy (removal and examination of a cone of tissue from the cervix) in evaluating the cause of abnormal cervical cytologic findings.

Realizing that colposcopy is useful only in identifying a suspicious lesion is important. Definitive diagnosis requires biopsy of the tissue. One of the major advantages of this procedure is that of directing the biopsy to the area most likely to be truly representative of the lesion. A biopsy performed without colposcopy may not necessarily be representative of the lesion's true pathologic condition, resulting in a significant risk of missing a serious lesion.

Procedure. The patient is placed in the lithotomy position, and a vaginal speculum is used to expose the vagina and cervix. After the cervix is sampled for cytologic findings, it is cleansed with a 3% acetic acid solution to remove excess mucus and cellular debris. The acetic acid also accentuates the difference between normal and abnormal epithelial tissues. The colposcope is then focused on the cervix (especially the squamocolumnar junction), which is then carefully examined. Usually the entire lesion can be outlined and the most atypical areas selected for biopsy specimen removal.

The patient will need to be hospitalized for diagnostic conization if:

1. Colposcopy and endocervical curettage do

not determine the problem or match the cytologic findings of the Pap smear within one grade.
2. The entire transformation zone is not seen.
3. The lesion extends up the cervical canal beyond the vision of colposcope.

The need for up to 90% of cone biopsies is eliminated by an experienced colposcopist. Endocervical curettage may routinely accompany colposcopy to detect unknown lesions in the endocervical canal.

Colposcopy is performed by a physician in approximately 5 to 10 minutes. Some patients complain of pressure pains from the vaginal speculum. Momentary discomfort may be felt when the biopsy specimens are obtained.

Contraindications. This test is contraindicated in uncooperative patients and in patients with heavy menstrual flow.

Nursing considerations

Nursing Diagnoses/Collaborative Problems

- Possible knowledge deficit related to test purpose, preparation, and procedure
- Possible alteration in comfort related to procedure
- Possible anxiety related to unknown sensations of test
- Possible anxiety related to test results

Nursing Implications with Rationale

- Explain the procedure to the patient. The very fact that this study is required arouses anxiety in most women. Encourage verbalization of the patient's fears and provide emotional support.
- Describe the sensations that the patient may feel during this study.
- After the study inform the patient she may have some vaginal bleeding if biopsy specimens were taken. Suggest she wear a sanitary pad.
- Inform the patient of when and how to obtain the results of this study (usually 2 to 3 days).

Fetal scalp blood pH

Normal values:
pH 7.25-7.35
O_2 saturation 30% to 50%
Po_2 18-22 mm Hg
Pco_2 40-50 mm Hg
Base excess 0 to −10 mEq/L

Rationale. Measurement of the pH of fetal scalp blood provides valuable information of fetal acid-base status. This screening test is useful clinically for diagnosing fetal distress.

Although the Po_2, Pco_2, and bicarbonate ion concentration can be measured on the fetal scalp blood sample, the pH is the most useful clinically. The pH normally ranges between 7.25 and 7.35 during labor. A mild decline of pH within the normal range is noted with contractions and as labor progresses.

Fetal hypoxia causes anaerobic glycolysis, resulting in excess production of lactic acid. This causes an increase in hydrogen ion concentration (acidosis) and a decrease in pH. Acidosis reflects the effect of hypoxia on cellular metabolism. A high correlation exists between low pH levels and low Apgar scores.

Procedure. Amnioscopy (see p. 370) is performed with the mother in the lithotomy position. Under sterile conditions the amnioscope is introduced into the vagina and the dilated cervix. The fetal scalp is cleansed with an antiseptic and dried with a sterile cotton ball. A small amount of petroleum jelly is applied to the fetal scalp to cause droplets of fetal blood to bead. After the skin on the scalp is pierced with a small metal blade, beaded droplets of blood are collected in long, heparinized capillary tubes. The tube is then sealed with wax and placed on ice to retard cellular respiration, which can alter the pH. The physician performing the procedure then applies firm pressure to the puncture site to retard bleeding. Scalp blood sampling can be repeated as necessary.

Complications of this procedure include continued bleeding from the puncture site, hematoma, ecchymosis, and infection. A blood sample may be obtained simultaneously from the mother to aid in interpretation of the fetal pH and to reduce the frequency of false-positive results.

Contraindications. See Amnioscopy, p. 371.

Nursing considerations

Nursing Diagnoses/Collaborative Problems

- Possible knowledge deficit related to test purpose, preparation, and procedure
- Possible alteration in comfort related to procedure
- High risk for anxiety related to unknown sensations of test
- High risk for anxiety related to test results
- Potential complication: fetal hemorrhage
- Potential complication: infection

Nursing Implications with Rationale

- See Amnioscopy, p. 371.
- After the delivery of the infant, assess the newborn and identify and document the puncture site(s).
- Cleanse the fetal scalp puncture site with an antiseptic solution. Then apply an antibiotic ointment.

Serum alpha-fetoprotein test

(AFP)

Normal values:
Adult: <40 ng/ml or <40 µg/L (SI units)
Child: (<1 yr): <30 ng/ml
Ranges are stratified by weeks of gestation and vary according to different laboratories.

Rationale. Serum alpha-fetoprotein (AFP) obstetric fraction levels are obtained to screen for neural tube defects (NTD) and Down's syndrome. AFP is a protein produced by the yolk sac and the fetal liver. Because serum AFP levels have detected myelomeningocele, anencephaly and Down's syndrome, widespread screening for serum AFP is now a routine aspect of prenatal care in the United States.

Serum AFP levels are very low in normal adults. AFP from fetal sources can be detected in the mother's blood after 10 weeks of gestation. Since peak levels occur between weeks 16 and 18, the AFP test is done at this time. When the serum AFP level is elevated, further evaluation (including a repeat serum AFP, ultrasound, and amniocentesis) must be done before an open NTD can be documented.

AFP is also an effective screening test for Down's syndrome when combined with HCG and unconjugated estriol serum levels. This combination of studies is known as AFP triple screen profile. The results are given as a risk for Down's syndrome, e.g., 1 out of 800. If the risk is greater than 1:190, ultrasound is performed to determine gestational age. If gestational age is correct and the patient is more than 15 weeks' pregnant, amniocentesis is offered. Imminent abortion, multiple pregnancy, and intrauterine fetal death also result in high AFP levels.

Increased AFP levels are also useful in the diagnosis of primary hepatocellular cancer because only *primary* liver tumors secrete AFP. AFP levels >500 ng/ml indicate primary liver cancer in approximately 97% of cases. Levels of AFP may also be elevated in patients with Hodgkin's disease, lymphoma, renal tumor, or a recurrent tumor. AFP levels are also useful in monitoring cancer treatment.

Procedure. Peripheral venipuncture is performed, and approximately 10 ml of blood is withdrawn. No food or fluid restrictions are necessary. For the AFP triple screen profile, maternal age, weight, and race; presence of diabetes; and gestational age must also be provided.

Contraindications. None.

Nursing considerations

Nursing Diagnoses/Collaborative Problems

See Blood studies, p. 2.

Nursing Implications with Rationale

- Explain the purpose of this test to the patient. Anticipate parental anxiety. Provide opportunities for verbalization of fears.

- After the procedure assess the venipuncture site for bleeding.
- If the AFP level is elevated, refer the patient for further testing. Explain the normal evaluation procedure.

Human placental lactogen study

(HPL)

Normal value: value should rise progressively during pregnancy

Rationale. Human placental lactogen (HPL), also called human chorionic somatomammotropin (HCS), is a hormone produced by the placenta that is used to evaluate placental functioning. HPL can be detected in the maternal serum as early as the fifth week of gestation. Levels gradually rise until week 36 of pregnancy and then tend to stabilize.

Values of <4 mg/dl are rarely found in the last 10 weeks of pregnancy. Low HPL levels may indicate fetal distress, threatened abortion, eclampsia, intrauterine growth retardation, and postmaturity.

HPL levels may be high in cases of maternal sickle cell disease, maternal liver disease, maternal diabetes mellitis, Rh sensitization, or multiple pregnancies.

Procedure. Peripheral venipuncture is performed and blood is collected in a red-top tube.

Contraindications. None.

Nursing considerations

Nursing Diagnoses/Collaborative Problems

See Blood studies, p. 2.

Nursing Implications with Rationale

- Explain the purpose and the procedure to the patient.
- After venipuncture is performed, assess the site for bleeding.

Fetoscopy

Normal values: no fetal distress

Rationale. Fetoscopy is an endoscopic procedure that allows direct visualization of the fetus via the insertion of a tiny telescope-like instrument through the abdominal wall and into the uterine cavity (see Figure 9-14). Direct visualization may lead to diagnosis of a severe malformation such as a neural tube defect (NTD). During the procedure, fetal blood samples for congenital blood disorders (hemophilia and sickle cell anemia, for example) can be drawn from a blood vessel in the umbilical cord for biochemical analysis. Fetal skin biopsies can also be done to detect primary skin disorders.

Fetoscopy is performed at approximately 18 weeks' gestation. At this time the vessels of the placental surface are of adequate size and the fetal parts are readily identifiable. A therapeutic abortion would not be as hazardous at this time as if done later in the pregnancy. Complications associated with fetoscopy include spontaneous abortion, preterm delivery, amniotic fluid leak, and intrauterine fetal death. Antibiotics may be given prophylatically after the test to prevent amnionitis.

Procedure. Before this procedure, the mother may be given meperidine (Demerol) because it crosses the placenta and quiets the fetus. This prevents excessive fetal movement, which makes the procedure more difficult. For this procedure the woman is placed in the supine position on an examining table. The abdominal wall is anesthetized with a local anesthetic. Ultrasonography is done to locate the fetus and the placenta. The endoscope is then inserted. Biopsies and blood samples may be obtained. This procedure is performed by a physician in 1 to 2 hours.

After the study, the mother and fetus are monitored for several hours for alterations in blood pressure and pulse, fetal heart rate abnormalities, uterine activity, vaginal bleeding, and loss of amniotic fluid. Rh negative mothers are given RhoGAM unless the fetal blood is found to be Rh negative. A repeat ultrasound is often performed the day following the procedure to confirm the adequacy of the amniotic fluid and fetal viability. The mother is advised to avoid strenuous activity for 1 to 2 weeks following the

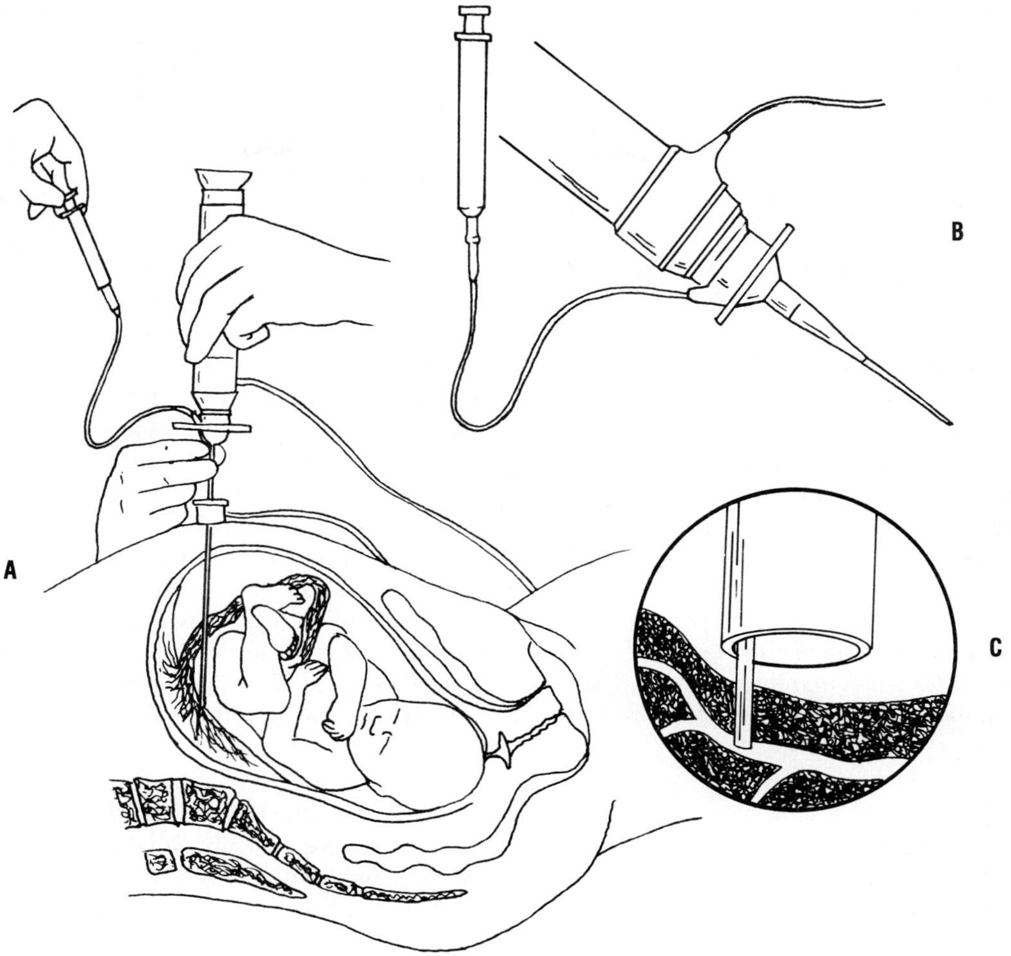

FIGURE 9-14. **A,** Schematic diagram of fetoscopy for fetal blood sampling. **B,** Detail of aspiration apparatus. **C,** Detail of needle puncturing fetal blood vessel.
From McCormack MK: Amniocentesis for detection of sickle cell anemia and the thalassemia disorders using recombinant DNA methodologies. In Filkins K and Russo JF, editors: Human prenatal diagnosis, New York, 1985, Marcel Dekker.

procedure and to report any pain, bleeding, amniotic fluid loss, or fever.

Contraindications. None.

Nursing considerations

Nursing Diagnoses/Collaborative Problems

- Possible knowledge deficit related to test purpose, preparation, and procedure
- Possible alteration in comfort related to procedure
- Possible anxiety related to unknown sensations of test
- Possible injury related to the effects of sedatives
- Potential complication: spontaneous abortion
- Potential complication: preterm delivery
- Potential complication: amniotic fluid leakage

- Potential complication: intrauterine fetal death

Nursing Implications with Rationale

- Explain the procedure to the patient. Assure the patient that precautions are taken to minimize risk to both her and the fetus. Encourage the patient to verbalize her fears concerning this study. Most patients are very apprehensive.
- Be certain that the physician has obtained a signed consent form before the procedure.
- Assess the fetal heart rate before and after the study to detect any ill effects related to the procedure. After the study, monitor the mother and fetus very carefully for alterations in blood pressure, pulse, fetal heart rate abnormalities, uterine activity, vaginal bleeding, and loss of amniotic fluid. If a woman is Rh negative and the fetus is Rh positive, make certain that she receives RhoGAM.
- Instruct the woman to report any pain, bleeding, amniotic fluid loss, or fever after the study.

Fetography

(amniography)

Fetography is a special x-ray technique that involves the instillation of contrast medium into the amniotic fluid. The contrast medium adheres to the fetal skin and produces a clear fetal silhouette on an x-ray film. Fetography, although not commonly performed, permits visualization of gross fetal structural abnormalities.

Chorionic villus sampling

(CVS)

Normal value: no genetic or biochemical disorders

Rationale. Chorionic villus sampling (CVS) (see Figure 9-15) is a relatively new procedure that can be performed between 8 to 12 weeks of pregnancy for the early detection of genetic and biochemical disorders. With the exception of diagnosing neural tube disorders, it is hoped that CVS will eventually replace amniocentesis for early prenatal diagnosis. Because CVS detects congenital defects early, first trimester therapeutic abortions can be done, if indicated and so desired.

For this study, a sample of chorionic villi is obtained for analysis. The villi in the chorion frondosum are present from 8 to 12 weeks and are believed to reflect fetal chromosome, enzyme, and DNA content. This permits a much earlier diagnosis of prenatal problems than amniocentesis (p. 359), which cannot be done before 14 to 16 weeks. Complications associated with CVS include accidental abortion, infection, bleeding, and limb reduction deformities.

Procedure. The client is placed in the lithotomy position. A cannula is inserted into the cervix and uterine cavity. Under ultrasonic guidance, the cannula is rotated to the site of the developing placenta. A syringe is attached and suction is applied to obtain several samples of villi. This procedure is performed by an obstetrician in approximately 5 minutes. Discomfort associated with this study is similar to that of a Pap smear.

After the procedure, some Rh negative mothers may receive RhoGAM. The clients are briefly monitored for signs of bleeding and discharged shortly after the procedure because no cervical dilation is required. Ultrasound is often performed in 2 to 4 days after the procedure to determine the continued viability of the fetus. Genetic determinations require 3 to 5 weeks to obtain results.

Contraindications. None.

Nursing considerations

Nursing Diagnoses/Collaborative Problems

- Possible knowledge deficit related to test purpose, preparation, and procedure
- Possible alteration in comfort related to procedure
- Possible anxiety related to unknown sensations of tests

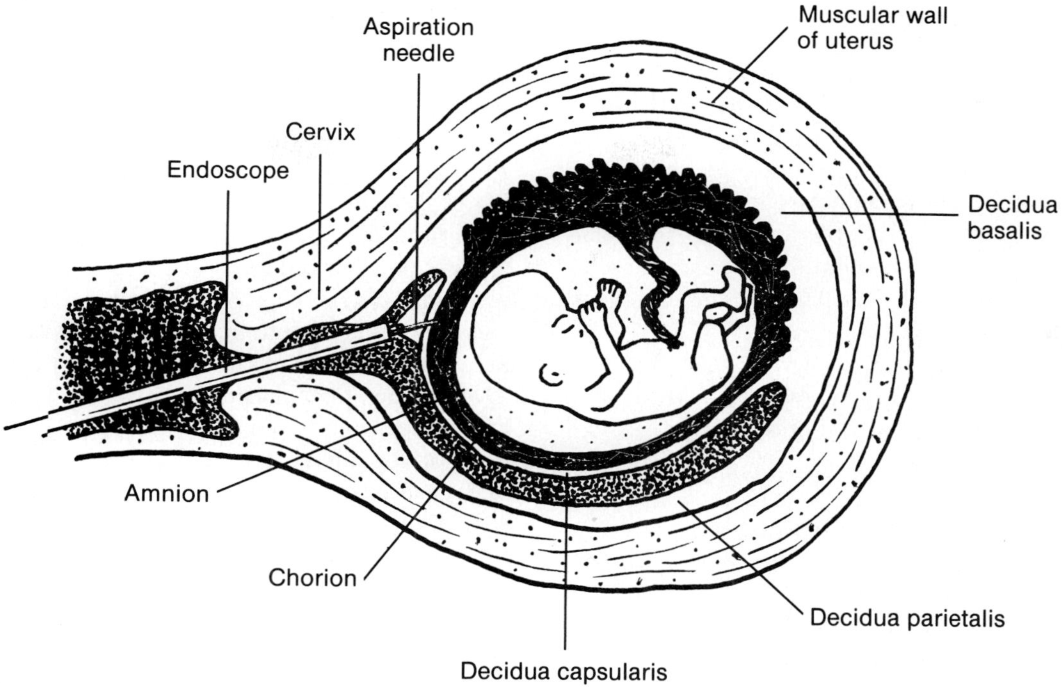

FIGURE 9-15. Chorionic villus sampling. Diagram of 8-week pregnancy showing endoscopic needle aspiration of extraplacental villi.
From Rodeck CH and Morsman JM: First semester chorion biopsy. In Ferguson-Smith MA, editor: Early prenatal diagnosis, Edinburgh, 1983, Longman Group, Ltd.

- Potential complication: abortion
- Potential complication: bleeding
- Potential complication: infection

Nursing Implications with Rationale

- Explain the procedure to the patient. Assure the patient that precautions are taken to minimize risk to both her and the fetus. Encourage the patient to verbalize her fears concerning this study. Most patients are very apprehensive.
- Be certain that the physician has obtained a signed consent before the procedure.
- After the study, administer RhoGAM if ordered to Rh negative mothers. It is given because of the risk of immunization from the fetal blood, which can jeopardize the fetus.
- After the study, carefully monitor the mother for signs of bleeding. Before discharging the patient, schedule her for ultrasound in 2 to 4 days to affirm the continued viability of the fetus.
- Inform the patient how she may obtain the results from her physician. Make sure she knows that the results are not available for at least 3 to 5 weeks.

CASE STUDY 4: ROUTINE WELL-BABY NEWBORN EVALUATION

After an 8-hour labor, Mrs. R. (age 26) delivered her first child—a 7-pound, 13-ounce, 21-inch boy. The baby's Apgar scores at 1 minute and 5 minutes after birth were both 9. Because the newborn cried seconds after birth, no special procedures were necessary other than the routine close observation, maintaining a clear airway, and supplying warmth. The umbilical cord was evaluated; it contained the normal two arteries and one vein. The infant's eyes received a prophylactic treatment for protection against ophthalmia neonatorum. A single dose (1 mg, 0.5 ml) of phytonadione solution (aquamephyton) was administered intramuscularly as a preventative measure against neonatal hemorrhagic disease.

Studies	Results
Phenylketonuria (PKU) test	Negative (normal: negative)
T_4 (see Chapter 8), TSH	Negative for hypothyroidism
Galactose-1-phosphate uridyl transferase test	21.2 U/g Hgb (normal: 18.5-28.5 U/g Hgb)
Hemoglobin and hematocrit	WNL for newborn
WBC	WNL for newborn

The healthy infant and his mother were discharged 3 days after birth. The PKU test was done on the day of discharge. A well-baby clinic appointment was scheduled before discharge.

DISCUSSION OF TESTS

Phenylketonuria test

(PKU test)

Normal values:
Blood: negative (<2 mg/dl) (Guthrie technique)
Urine: no green coloration
Possible critical value ≥4 mg/dl (Guthrie technique)

Rationale. PKU is an inherited disease characterized by deficiency of the enzyme phenylalanine hydroxylase, which converts phenylalanine to tyrosine. Phenylalanine is an essential amino acid necessary for growth. However, any excess must be degraded by conversion to tyrosine. An infant with PKU lacks the ability to make this necessary conversion. Hence, phenylalanine accumulates in the body and spills over into the urine. If the amount of phenylalanine is not restricted in babies with PKU, progressive mental retardation results. Dietary control must begin early to avoid brain damage; therefore, diagnosis must be made early.

Routine screening of newborn infants for PKU is now mandatory in most of the United States. It is important to note that the test is not valid until the newborn has ingested an ample amount (for 2 or 3 days) of the amino acid phenylalanine, which is a constituent of both human and cow's milk. The urine PKU test is normally done after 4 to 6 weeks of age. If the test is positive, a blood phenylalanine test should be performed.

Procedure. Blood is usually collected on the infant's discharge day from the hospital and analyzed for increased amounts of phenylalanine. For this procedure a few drops of blood obtained by a heel stick are placed on a filter paper for the *Guthrie test.* If the infant is discharged early or if there has been a feeding problem (such as vomiting), the test may be falsely negative. To prevent this, the test should be performed several days after the discharge.

Urine tests can also be used to detect PKU in infants who are at least 4 to 6 weeks of age. These tests are usually done at the baby's first checkup. For the *diaper test,* 10% ferric chloride is dropped on a freshly wet diaper. A green spot indicates probable PKU. Another test, the *Phenistix test,* is done by pressing a test stick against a wet diaper or dipping the stick in urine. A green color reaction indicates probable PKU.

PKU tests are usually performed by the nurse in less than 2 minutes. The amount of discomfort associated with the heel stick is slight.

Contraindications. None.

Nursing considerations

Nursing Diagnoses/Collaborative Problems

See Blood studies, p. 2, and Urine studies, p. 3.

Nursing Implications with Rationale

- Inform the mother about the purpose of the test and the method of performance.

- Assess the infant's feeding patterns before performing the PKU test. An inadequate amount of protein before performing the test can cause false-negative results.
- Note that urine tests for PKU are commonly done on the infant's first well-baby examination. This is vitally important if the infant was not checked for PKU while in the hospital. The infant must be at least 4 to 6 weeks old for appropriate screening with the urine test.
- If the results of the test are positive, inform the mother that dietary control must begin immediately to prevent brain damage. This is done by substituting Lofenalac for milk. Later, strained foods low in protein are added to the diet. Monitor the dietary treatment by blood and urine testing.
- Instruct women with PKU who wish to have children to begin a low phenylalanine diet before conception and continue it throughout the pregnancy. The risk of producing a mentally retarded infant is very high if the mother remains on a general diet.

Galactose-1-phosphate uridyl transferase test

(Gal-1-PUT test)

Normal value: 18.5-28.5 U/g hemoglobin

Rationale. Galactosemia is an inborn error of metabolism that causes a disorder of carbohydrate metabolism. This inherited disorder is characterized by lack of the enzyme galactose-1-phosphate uridyl transferase (Gal-1-PUT), which prevents the infant from converting galactose to glucose. This impairs normal glucose metabolism. The most common form of galactate is milk, which contains lactose.

Galactosemia is manifested by mental retardation, cataracts, jaundice, hepatomegaly, cirrhosis of the liver, and failure to thrive. Therapy consists of eliminating galactose from the diet. As with PKU, detection and treatment should begin in the first several weeks of life.

Procedure. Several screening tests may be used to detect galactosemia. The most popular are the Paigen assay (a bacterial inhibition test) and the Beutler fluorometric test. The Paigen assay measures elevated blood galactose (or galactose-6-phosphate) levels. Because this test depends on the presence of an elevated blood galactose level, milk feeding is necessary. The Beutler assay measures Gal-1-PUT activity and does not depend on milk feeding.

Both of these tests can be performed on filter paper blood spots. Approximately 1 ml of blood is obtained by a heel stick. The discomfort of this test to the infant is minimal.

Contraindications. None.

Nursing considerations

Nursing Diagnoses/Collaborative Problems

See Blood studies, p. 2.

Nursing Implications with Rationale

- Inform the mother about the purpose of this test and the method of obtaining the specimen.
- If the test results for galactosemia are positive, inform the mother that dietary therapy should begin at once. Foods containing galactose, especially milk, should be removed from the diet.

SUPPLEMENTAL INFORMATION

Barr body analysis

(sex chromatin body, chromatin-positive body, buccal smear for sex chromatin evaluation)

Normal value: depends on the sex of the child

Rationale. Barr body analysis studies may be performed when ambiguity of the newborn's genitalia makes it difficult to assign a sex to the infant. This test is also done to detect sex chromosomal abnormalities, such as Turner's syndrome and Klinefelter's syndrome.

The Barr body is a chromatin mass derived from one of the X chromosomes. The number of Barr bodies is one less than the total number of X chromosomes in the cell nucleus. Therefore, females (XX) normally contain one Barr body and are considered chromatin-positive. Normal males (XY) have no Barr bodies and are chromatin-negative. A female with Turner's syndrome (XO) would have no Barr body. These females are characterized by ovarian dysgenesis, have amenorrhea, and lack secondary sexual maturation. A male with Klinefelter's syndrome (XXY) would have one Barr body. Klinefelter's syndrome is the most common form of male hypogonadism, which is caused by a chromosomal abnormality that results in primary testicular failure. An XXX female would have two Barr bodies.

Procedure. Sex chromatin analysis can be performed from any cell in the body. The most easily obtained are those from the buccal mucosa, obtained by scraping the oral mucosa with a tongue depressor and smearing the cells onto a glass slide. Epithelial cells can also be obtained from a vaginal smear. After chemical fixation and staining, the cells are studied. Assessment of the results, together with the secondary sexual characteristics and genitalia of the patient, permit presumptive diagnosis of certain sex chromosome abnormalities. If necessary, the results can be confirmed by chromosome *karyotyping* (systematic arrangement of photographed chromosomes to demonstrate structure and number). See next study.

Buccal smear specimens may show false lowering of sex chromatin Barr bodies if specimens are taken during the first week of life or during adrenocorticosteroid or estrogen therapy. Poor slide preparation can also obscure the results.

The buccal smear is performed by a technician in approximately less than 5 minutes. The pathologist studies the slide smear. The discomfort associated with this test is minimal to none.

Contraindications. This test is contraindicated in patients with mouth lesions and bleeding abnormalities.

Nursing considerations

Nursing Diagnoses/Collaborative Problems

- Possible knowledge deficit related to test purpose, preparation, and procedure
- Possible anxiety related to unknown sensations of test
- Possible anxiety related to test results

Nursing Implications with Rationale

- Explain the procedure to the patient (or family).
- Allow plenty of time for verbalization of feelings. Much anxiety and emotion usually accompanies patients and families with potential or confirmed chromosomal abnormalities.

Chromosome karyotype

(blood chromosome analysis, chromosome studies, cytogenetics, karyotype)

Normal values:
Female: 44 autosomes + 2X chromosomes
Karyotype: 46,XX
Males: 44 autosomes + 1X, 1Y chromosomes
Karyotype: 46,XY

Rationale. This test is used to study an individual's chromosomal makeup. The term *karyotyping* refers to the arrangement of cell chromosomes in order from the largest to the smallest for the purpose of analyzing their number and structure. This test involves the determination of chromosome number and structure. Variations in either the number or structure can produce numerous abnormalities. A normal karyotype of chromosomes consists of a pattern of 22 pairs of autosomal chromosomes and a pair of sex chromosomes; XY for the male or XX for the female.

Chromosome karyotyping can be useful in evaluating the following clinical situations: congenital anomalies, mental retardation, growth retardation, delayed puberty, infertility, hypogonadism, primary amenorrhea, ambiguous genitalia, chronic myelogenous leukemia, neoplasm, recurrent miscarriage, prenatal diagnosis in situations of advanced maternal age, Turner's syndrome, Klinefelter's syndrome, Down's syndrome, and other suspected genetic disorders. The products of conception can also be studied to determine the cause of stillbirth or miscarriage.

Procedure. Specimens for chromosome analysis can be obtained from numerous sources. Leukocytes from a peripheral venipuncture are the most easily and most often used for this study. Bone marrow biopsies and surgical specimens can sometimes also be used as sources for analysis. During pregnancy, specimens can be collected by amniocentesis (see p. 359) and chorionic villus sampling (see p. 376). Fetal tissue or products of conception can also be studied to determine the reason for the loss of the pregnancy.

Contraindications. None.

Nursing considerations

Nursing Diagnoses/Collaborative Problems

- Possible knowledge deficit related to test purpose, preparation, and procedure
- Possible alteration in comfort related to test procedure
- Possible anxiety related to test results

Nursing Implications with Rationale

- Explain the procedure to the patient.
- Determine how the specimen will be collected. Many patients are fearful of the test results and require considerable emotional support.
- Aftercare depends on how the specimen was collected.
- If the test results showed an abnormality, encourage the patient to verbalize his or her feelings. Provide emotional support.
- Inform the patient that test results are generally not available for several months.

QUESTIONS AND ANSWERS

1. **QUESTION:** Your patient has not had a Pap smear in 5 years and asks you how often she should have this test done. What should you recommend?
   ANSWER: The American Cancer Society recommends that all asymptomatic women age 20 and over, and those under 20 who are sexually active, have a Pap test annually for two negative examinations and then one every 3 years until age 65. However, this recommendation is not supported by many gynecologists who recommend yearly Pap smears.
2. **QUESTION:** Your neighbor calls and asks for your advice. She has just been told that her Pap smear contains cells that "do not appear to be too good." What should you tell her?
   ANSWER: Explain to your neighbor that many possible causes exist for the type of cells reported as being "not too good." These include inflammation as well as benign and malignant tumors. Tell her that her physician will most probably recommend colposcopy or cervical cone biopsy. Briefly and optimistically describe both procedures. Provide support for your neighbor during this very anxious time.
3. **QUESTION:** Your patient has been trying unsuccessfully to get pregnant for 6 months. She says she would like to have a laparoscopy to elucidate the cause of her "infertility." How might she best be advised?
   ANSWER: The patient should be made to understand that to be considered for an infertility evaluation, she should have been trying to get pregnant for at least 1 year. Furthermore, she should be told that laparoscopy is not the first step of the evaluation. She should also be reminded that because nearly 40% of all cases of infertility are caused by a male factor, her husband should undergo concomitant evaluation.

   The patient should be advised to have coitus around the time of expected ovulation for another 6 months. If she still does not become pregnant she and her husband then should return for an infertility workup.
4. **QUESTION:** Your patient is scheduled to have hysterosalpingography. In your assessment of the patient you find that she has had a recent onset of a foul-smelling cervical discharge. Should the test be performed?
   ANSWER: No. The cervical discharge may be the result of an acute pelvic infection. Because this infection can be spread by hysterosalpingography, the test should be cancelled. The cervical discharge should be sent for a culture and sensitivity determination and also a fresh specimen should be

examined under a microscope for evidence of trichomoniasis or candidiasis. Treatment should be instituted pending these results.

5. **QUESTION:** While you are working on the night shift, a patient who is 36 weeks' pregnant calls and states that she had a CST that morning. She is now having vaginal bleeding and thinks her "water may have broken." How should you advise this patient?

   ANSWER: Labor may have been unexpectedly induced by the CST. Her condition certainly warrants a physical evaluation. Recommend that she call her physician immediately to arrange for such an examination.

6. **QUESTION:** Your pregnant patient has been instructed to collect a 24-hour urine specimen for estriol determination to evaluate fetal viability. Because she was out at a party during the evening, she voided once without collecting the urine. Should the specimen be sent for the analysis?

   ANSWER: No. The collection must be complete. An incomplete specimen may artificially lower the estriol value. Because a low estriol level is indicative of fetal distress, the consequences of an incomplete specimen analysis are grave. Therefore, the patient should be instructed to repeat the 24-hour urine collection.

BIBLIOGRAPHY

Bernsleen IM and others: Ultrasonographic estimation of fetal body composition for children of diabetic mothers, Invest Radiol 26(8):722-726, Aug 1991.

Brambati B, Oldrini A: CVS for first-trimester fetal diagnosis, Contemp OB/GYN 25:94, 1985.

Brent RL and others: Medical sonography: reproductive effects and risks, Teratology 44(2):123-146, Aug 1991.

Canfield RE and others: Biological markers on human pregnancy, Biomed Environ Sci 4(1-2):56-68, June 1991.

Cohen FL: Neural tube defects: epidemiology, detection, and prevention, J Obstet Gynecol Neonat Nurs 16(2):105, 1987.

Corey L, Spear PG: Infections with herpes simplex, N Engl J Med 314(11):686, 1986.

Daffos F, Capella-Pavlovsky M, Forestier F: Fetal blood sampling during pregnancy with use of a needle guided by ultrasound: a study of 606 consecutive cases, Am J Obstet Gynecol 153(6):655, 1985.

Deep R: Clinical evaluation of fetal status. In Scott JR and others, editors: Danforth's Obstetrics and Gynecology, ed 6, Philadelphia, 1990, JB Lippincott.

Elhose P: The "other" STDs: as dangerous as ever, RN 51(6):52-57, 1988.

Hogge JS, Hogge WA, and Golbus MS: Chorionic villus sampling, J Obstet Gynecol Neonat Nurs 15:24, 1986.

Hohlfeld RE and others: Cytomegalovirus fetal infection: prenatal diagnosis, Obstet Gynecol 78(4):6158, Oct 1991.

Hughes CL and others: Infertility. In Scott JR and others, editors: Danforth's Obstetrics and Gynecology, ed 6, Philadelphia, 1990, JB Lippincott.

Jaffe SB and others: The basic infertility investigation, Fertil Steril 56(4):599-613, Oct 1991.

Kochenour NK: Normal pregnancy and prenatal care. In Scott JR and others, editors: Danforth's Obstetrics and Gynecology, ed 6, Philadelphia, 1990, JB Lippincott.

Marrero MA. Unexplained infertility, Curr Opin Obstet Gynecol 3(2):211-218, April 1991.

Marshall C: The nipple stimulation contraction stress test, J Obstet Gynecol Neonat Nurs 15:459, 1986.

Mayberry LJ and Inturrisi-Levy M: Use of breast stimulation for contraction stress test, J Obstet Gynecol Neonat Nurs 16(2):121, 1987.

Millard S: Emotional responses to infertility: understanding patients' needs, AORN J 54(2):301-305, Aug 1991.

Reed KL: Ultrasound in obstetrics. In Scott JR and others, editors: Danforth's Obstetrics and Gynecology, ed 6, Philadelphia, 1990, JB Lippincott.

Spellacy WN: Diabetes mellitus and pregnancy. In Scott JR and others, editors: Danforth's Obstetrics and Gynecology, ed 6, Philadelphia, 1990, JB Lippincott.

Zeitune M and others: Screening for Down's syndrome in older women based on maternal serum alpha-fetoprotein levels and age: preliminary results, Prenatal Diagnosis 11(6):393-398, June 1991.

Zilianti M and others: Transperineal sonography in second trimester to term pregnancy and early labor, J Ultrasound Med 10(9):481-485, Sept 1991.

Chapter 10

DIAGNOSTIC STUDIES USED IN THE ASSESSMENT OF THE
HEMATOLOGIC SYSTEM

ANATOMY AND PHYSIOLOGY

The hematologic system is responsible for the production of red blood cells (RBCs), white blood cells (WBCs), and platelets and for the function of hemostasis (that is, the ability of the blood to clot following vascular injury). The bone marrow within the central bones (such as the ilium, sternum, and the proximal long bones) is the site of blood cell production (hematopoiesis). The primary function of the RBCs is to transport oxygen from the lungs to the tissues. WBCs are primarily a defense against infection, foreign particles, and foreign tissues. Blood clotting (coagulation) is the primary function of the platelets.

Red blood cells (erythrocytes)

Pluripotent stem cells, which exist in the bone marrow, are capable of differentiating into the RBC line or the WBC line. In differentiation toward RBC production, a proerythroblast is formed. With further cell division and differentiation, the proerythroblast becomes a normoblast. As the cell matures, it accumulates hemoglobin and gradually loses its nucleus. These cells are called reticulocytes and are deposited into the circulating blood. They further differentiate into mature RBCs (erythrocytes). This process is stimulated by many factors (such as hypoxia, catecholamines and growth hormone); however, the major stimulating factor is erythropoietin, a hormone produced primarily by the kidney.

Packed within each RBC are molecules of hemoglobin that permit the transport and exchange of O_2 and CO_2. Four polypeptide chains (two alpha and two beta) make up the normal hemoglobin protein called hemoglobin A_1. Hemoglobin A_2, a normal variant, is composed of two alpha and two delta chains. Hemoglobin F is the main hemoglobin component in the fetus and infant and consists of two alpha and two gamma chains. Hemoglobin F is capable of transporting oxygen even when very little oxygen is available. Hemoglobinopathies (such as sickle cell disease, hemoglobin C disease, and thalassemias) are a result of genetically induced abnormalities in the normal alpha and beta polypeptide hemoglobin chains.

Iron is the major inorganic component of hemoglobin and is essential for hemoglobin synthesis. When the patient is iron-deficient, hemoglobin synthesis is markedly diminished, resulting in small (microcytic), pale (hypochromic) RBCs.

The primary role of the RBC is the transportation of oxygen from the lungs to the tissues. Carbon dioxide is transported in the opposite direction. Normally the RBCs exist in the peripheral blood for about 120 days. Toward the end of the RBC's life, the cell membrane becomes less pliable and the aged RBC is then hemolyzed and extracted from the circulation by the spleen. Abnormal RBCs have a shorter life span and are extracted earlier. Intravascular RBC trauma (such as that caused by artificial heart valves or peripheral vascular atherosclerotic plaques) also shortens the RBC's life. An enlarged spleen (such as that caused by portal hypertension or leukemias) may inappropriately destroy and remove normal RBCs from the circulation.

With RBC destruction, the heme molecule of hemoglobin is broken down and metabolized into bilirubin. Bilirubin is then handled and excreted by the normal liver into bile. Liver disease, bile duct obstruction, or increased hemolysis can all result in hyperbilirubinemia and jaundice (see Figure 4-2).

White blood cells (leukocytes)

The major function of the WBCs is to fight infection and react against foreign bodies or tissues. Five types of WBCs can easily be identified on a routine blood smear. These cells, in order of frequency, include neutrophils, lymphocytes, monocytes, eosinophils, and basophils. All of these WBCs arise from the same pluripotent stem cell within the bone marrow as the RBC does. Beyond this origin, however, each cell line differentiates separately. The mature white cell is then deposited into the circulating blood.

Polymorphonuclear (PMN) *neutrophils* are produced in 7 to 14 days and exist in the circulation for only 6 hours. The primary function of the neutrophil is phagocytosis (killing and digestion of bacterial microorganisms). Acute bacterial infections and trauma stimulate neutrophil production, resulting in an increased WBC count. Often when neutrophil production is stimulated, early immature forms of neutrophils enter the circulation. These immature forms are called *band* or *stab cells.* This process, called a "shift to the left" in WBC production, is indicative of an ongoing acute bacterial infection.

Lymphocytes are divided into two types: T cells and B cells. T cells are primarily involved with cellular-type immune reactions, whereas B cells participate in humoral immunity (antibody production). The primary function of the lymphocytes is fighting chronic bacterial infection and acute viral infections.

Monocytes are phagocytic cells capable of fighting bacteria in a way very similar to that of the neutrophil. However, they can be produced more rapidly and can spend a longer time in the circulation than the neutrophils.

Basophils, and especially *eosinophils,* are involved in the allergic reaction. Parasitic infestations also are capable of stimulating the production of these cells.

Platelets (thrombocytes)

Platelets are formed in the bone marrow, the lungs, and to some extent, the spleen. Platelets play a vital role in hemostasis (stopping blood flow) and blood clotting. The pluripotent stem cell differentiates into a megakaryocyte. When this cell fragmentizes, platelets are formed and discharged into the circulation.

Physiologic hemostasis is an ongoing response to vascular injury to avoid excessive loss of blood. The entire process involves platelet aggregation around the site of the injury, thereby creating an early and temporary plug over the injury site. In the presence of the platelets and thromboplastin, a serial activation of clotting factors occurs that results in fibrin production. The fibrin strengthens the platelet plug into a fibrin clot. Vascular repair is followed by a dissolution of the fibrin clot. This lysis of the clot is accomplished by the fibrinolytic (or plasmin) system (Figure 10-1).

Abnormalities in any part of this normal physiologic process can result in bleeding tendencies or in hypercoagulable states. The balance of hemostasis and fibrinolysis must be constantly intact, otherwise bleeding tendencies or hypercoagulation results.

Hemostasis

Hemostasis (Figure 10-1) is a multiphasic process that involves:

1. Platelet aggregation and plugging of the hole in the injured vessel
2. Fibrin formation to strengthen the platelet plug
3. Vessel repair and lysis of the fibrin clot (fibrinolysis).

Platelet aggregation, although quickly initiated, offers only transient interruption of active blood loss. The platelet aggregate (red clot) must be strengthened and supported by fibrin strands (white clot). Fibrin is the result of a process in which the clotting factors are sequentially activated by chemical enzymes. Two mechanisms are capable of producing fibrin. The first is the intrinsic system, which includes activation of factors XII, XI, IX, and VIII. Injury of the vessel surface is the stimulus for this system. Tissue damage, on the other hand, is capable of stimulating the extrinsic system of clot formation, which includes factors VII and III. Both the intrinsic and extrinsic systems activate the common pathway, which involves activation of factors X, V, II, and I (fibrinogen). Fibrin is the final result.

Fibrinolysis, through the action of plasmin (an activated form of plasminogen), is necessary to police and appropriately restrict the clotting system by dissolving fibrin clots after vascular repair.

CASE STUDY 1: SICKLE CELL ANEMIA

Bobby J. was a 10-year-old black boy who developed a sudden attack of abdominal, chest, and diffuse joint pain while playing ice hockey. Both his father and mother had a history of sickle cell disease in their families. The results of physical examination were negative except for conjunctival pallor.

Studies	Results
Complete blood count (CBC)	
RBC count	3.8 million/mm^3 (normal: 3.8-5.5 million/mm^3)
Hemoglobin (Hgb) concentration	9.4 g/dl (normal: 11-16 g/dl)
Hematocrit (Hct)	28% (normal: 31%-43%)
Mean corpuscular volume (MCV)	83 μ^3 (normal: 80-95 μ^3)
Mean corpuscular hemoglobin (MCH)	28 pg (normal: 27-31 pg)
Mean corpuscular hemoglobin concentration (MCHC)	34 g/dl (normal: 32-36 g/dl)
WBC and differential counts	
Total WBC	6,500/mm^3 (normal: 5,000-10,000/mm^3)
Neutrophils	60% (normal: 55%-70%)
Lymphocytes	29% (normal: 20%-40%)
Monocytes	8% (normal: 2%-8%)
Eosinophils	2% (normal: 1%-4%)

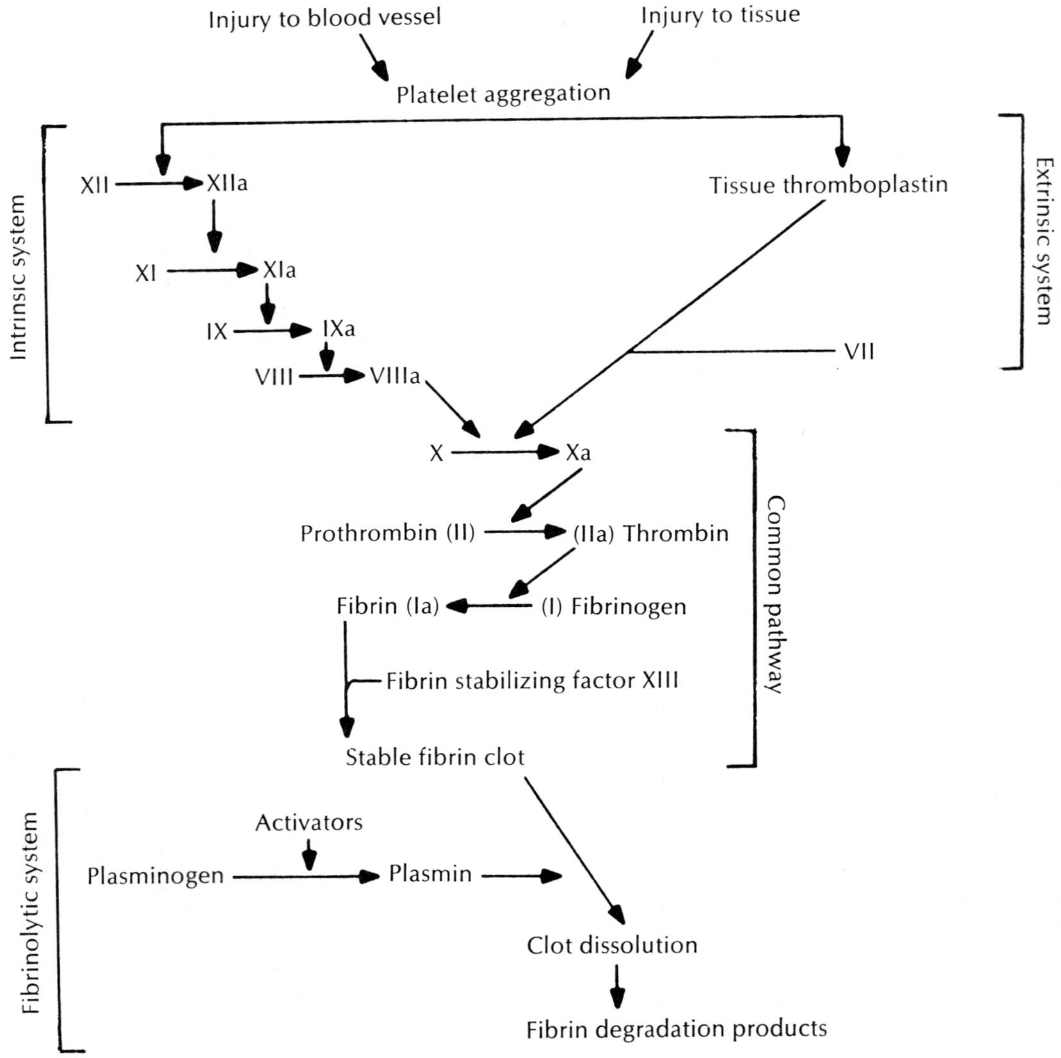

FIGURE 10-1. Process of hemostasis and fibrinolysis. Injury to blood vessel surface or tissue initiates platelet aggregation. Intrinsic or extrinsic system is activated and then activates common pathway of fibrin formation. Finally, fibrin is physiologically dissolved by fibrinolytic system.

Studies	Results
Basophils	1% (normal: 0.5%-1%)
Peripheral blood smear	Sickled forms of RBCs (normal: normocytic normochromic RBCs)
Reticulocyte count	4% (normal: 0.5%-2%)
Iron level	125 μg/dl (normal: 60-190 μg/dl)
Total iron-binding capacity (TIBC)	328 μg/dl (normal: 250-420 μg/dl)
Ferritin level	150 ng/ml (normal: 12-300 ng/ml)
Serum haptoglobin level	74 mg/dl (normal: 100-150 mg/dl)
Bone marrow aspiration	Erythroid hyperplasia M:E ratio (ratio of myeloid cells to erythroid cells): 2:1 (normal: 3:1)
Hemoglobin electrophoresis	
Hgb F	20% (normal: <1%)
Hgb A_2	3% (normal: approximately 2%)
Hgb S	77% (normal: 0)
Hgb A_1	0 (normal: 95%-98%)
Sickle cell test	Positive (normal: negative)
Coombs' test direct	Negative (normal: negative)
Blood type	O+

Bobby's doctor clinically suspected that the child had sickle cell anemia. The CBC indicated that Bobby had a normochromic, normocytic anemia. The increased reticulocyte count and erythroplasia seen on bone marrow aspiration indicated that his marrow was attempting to compensate for the anemia. His iron level and iron-binding capacity were normal, as expected, and these values eliminated the possibility of iron deficiency as a cause of the anemia. His decreased serum haptoglobin level indicated that hemolysis was occurring. A negative Coombs' test eliminated an autoimmune cause of the hemolysis. The peripheral blood smear, sickle cell test, and hemoglobin electrophoresis confirmed the diagnosis of sickle cell anemia.

Bobby was treated for his sickle cell crisis and released from the hospital. He had many future sickle cell crises and frequently required transfusion of O+ blood. He died at the age of 18 from pneumonia.

DISCUSSION OF TESTS

Complete blood count and differential count

(CBC and diff, hemogram)

Rationale. The CBC and differential count are a series of tests of the peripheral blood that provide a tremendous amount of information about the hematologic system and many other organ systems. They are inexpensively, easily, and rapidly performed as a screening test on almost every patient that enters the hospital. Each test included in the series is discussed below.

Red blood cell count

Normal values:
- Adult/elderly
  - Men: 4.7-6.1 million/mm^3
  - Women: 4.2-5.4 million/mm^3
- Infants and children: 3.8-5.5 million/mm^3
- Newborn: 4.8-7.1 million/mm^3

This is a count of the number of the circulating RBCs in 1 mm^3 of peripheral venous blood. Normal values vary according to sex and age. When the value is decreased by more than 10% of the expected normal value, the patient is said to be anemic. There are many causes for low RBC values. These include:

1. Hemorrhage (as in gastrointestinal bleeding or trauma)
2. Hemolysis (as in glucose-6-phosphate dehydrogenase deficiency, spherocytosis, or secondary splenomegaly)
3. Dietary deficiency (as of iron or vitamin B_{12})
4. Genetic aberrations (as in sickle cell anemia or thalassemia)
5. Drug ingestion (as of chloramphenicol, hydantoins, or quinidine)

6. Marrow failure (as in fibrosis, leukemia, or antineoplastic chemotherapy)
7. Chronic illness (as in tumor or sepsis)
8. Other organ failure (as in renal disease).

RBC counts greater than normal can be physiologically induced as a result of the body's requirements for greater oxygen-carrying capacity (such as at high altitudes). Diseases that produce chronic anoxia (such as congenital heart disease) also provoke this physiologic increase in RBCs. Polycythemia vera is a neoplastic condition involving uncontrolled production of RBCs.

Hemoglobin (Hgb) concentration

Normal values:
- Male: 14-18 g/dl or 8.7-11.2 mmol/L (SI units)
- Female: 12-16 g/dl or 7.4-9.9 mmol/L (pregnancy, >11 g/dl)
- Elderly: values are slightly decreased
- Child: 11-16 g/dl
- Infant: 10-15 g/dl
- Newborn: 14-24 g/dl

Possible critical values <5.0 g/dl

This is a measure of the total amount of hemoglobin in the peripheral blood. Hemoglobin serves as a vehicle for oxygen and carbon dioxide transport. As with RBC counts, normal values vary according to sex and age. The clinical implications of this test closely parallel the RBC count (see above for implications of high and low values). In addition, however, changes in plasma volume are more accurately reflected by hemoglobin concentrations. Dilutional overhydration decreases the concentration, whereas dehydration tends to cause an artificially high value. Slight decreases in the values of hemoglobin and hematocrit during pregnancy reflect the expanded blood volume. The number of cells is actually increased during pregnancy.

Hematocrit (Hct), packed red cell volume, or packed cell volume (PCV)

Normal values:
- Male: 42%-52%
- Female: 37%-47% (pregnancy, >33%)
- Elderly: values may be slightly decreased
- Child: 31%-43%
- Infant: 30%-40%
- Newborn: 44%-64%

Possible critical values <15%

This is a measure of the percentage of the total blood volume made up by RBCs. It, therefore, closely reflects the hemoglobin and RBC values. The hematocrit in percentage points is usually about three times the hemoglobin concentration in grams per deciliter when the RBCs are of normal size and contain normal amounts of hemoglobin. Normal values also vary according to sex and age. Abnormal values indicate the same pathologic states as abnormal RBC counts and hemoglobin concentrations do (see previous mention).

Mean corpuscular volume (MCV)

Normal values:
- Adults and children: 80-95 μ^3
- Newborns: 96-108 μ^3

This is a measure of the average volume, or size, of a single red blood cell and is therefore useful in classifying anemias. It is derived by dividing the hematocrit by the total RBC. Normal values vary according to age and sex. When the MCV value is increased, the RBC is said to be abnormally large, or "macrocytic" (see RBC size, p. 392). This is most frequently seen in megaloblastic anemias (such as vitamin B_{12} or folic acid deficiency). When the MCV value is decreased, the RBC is said to be abnormally small, or "microcytic" (see RBC size, p. 392). This is associated with iron deficiency anemia or thalassemia.

Mean corpuscular hemoglobin (MCH)

Normal values:
- Adults and children: 27-31 pg
- Newborns: 32-34 pg

This is a measure of the average amount of hemoglobin within an RBC. It is derived by dividing the total hemoglobin concentration by the number of RBCs. Because macrocytic cells generally have more hemoglobin and microcytic cells generally have less hemoglobin, the causes for these values closely resemble those for the MCV value.

Mean corpuscular hemoglobin concentration (MCHC)

Normal values:
- Adults and children: 32-36 g/dl (or 32%-36%)
- Newborns: 32-33 g/dl (or 32%-33%)

The MCHC is a measure of the average concentration or the percentage of hemoglobin within a single RBC. It is derived by dividing the total hemoglobin concentration by the hematocrit. When values are decreased, the cell has a deficiency of hemoglobin and is said to be "hypochromic" (frequently seen in iron deficiency anemia and thalassemia) (see RBC color, p. 392).

When one investigates the causes of an anemia, it is helpful to categorize the anemia according to the RBC indexes (MCV, MCH, MCHC) as follows in Table 10-1.

Red cell distribution width (RDW)

Normal values: 11.0-14.5%

The RDW is an indication of variation in the RBC size. It is calculated by machine using the MCV and RBC values. Variation of the width of the RBC may be helpful in classifying certain types of anemia. The RDW is essentially an indicator of the degree of anisocytosis, a blood condition characterized by RBCs of variable and abnormal size.

White blood cell count

Normal values:
- Total WBCs
  - Adults and children over 2 years old: 5,000-10,000/mm^3
  - Children 2 years old and younger: 6,200-17,000/mm^3
  - Newborns: 9,000-30,000/mm^3
- Differential count
  - Neutrophils: 55%-70%
  - Lymphocytes: 20%-40%
  - Monocytes: 2%-8%
  - Eosinophils: 1%-4%
  - Basophils: 0.5%-1%

Possible critical values: WBCs <2,500 or >30,000/mm^3

The WBC count has two components. One is a count of the total number of WBCs (leukocytes) in 1 mm^3 of peripheral venous blood. The other component, the differential count, measures the percentage of each type of leukocyte present in the same specimen. An increase in

TABLE 10-1. Categorization of Anemia According to the RBC Indexes

Normocytic.*, Normochromic Anemia†

- Iron deficiency (detected early)
- Chronic illness (such as sepsis or tumor)
- Acute blood loss
- Aplastic anemia (such as chloramphenicol toxicosis)
- Acquired hemolytic anemias (such as from a prosthetic cardiac valve)

Microcytic.‡, Hypochromic Anemia§

- Iron deficiency (detected late)
- Thalassemia
- Lead poisoning

Microcytic, Normochromic Anemia

- Renal disease (because of the loss of erythropoietin)

Macrocytic.||, Normochromic Anemia||

- Vitamin B_{12} or folic acid deficiency
- Hydantoin ingestion
- Chemotherapy

*Normocytic: normal RBC size.
†Normochromic: normal color (normal hemoglobin content).
‡Microcytic: smaller than normal RBC size.
§Hypochromic: less than normal color (decreased hemoglobin content).
||Macrocytic: larger than normal RBC size.

the percentage of one type means a decrease in the percentage of another type. *Granulocytes* include the neutrophils, eosinophils, and basophils and make up about 65% of the total number of leukocytes. *Agranulocytes,* which include the lymphocytes and monocytes, comprise the remaining 35% of the leukocytes. These leukocyte types can be identified easily by their morphology on a peripheral blood smear. The total leukocyte count has a wide range of normal values, but many diseases can induce abnormal values. An increased total WBC count (leukocytosis) usually indicates infection or leukemic neoplasia. Trauma or stress, either emotional or physical, can increase the WBC count. Leukopenia (that is, a decreased WBC count) occurs in many forms of bone marrow failure (such as after antineoplastic therapy or in agranulocytosis), overwhelming infections, dietary deficiency, and autoimmune diseases.

In the body's defense against microbial invasion, the neutrophils (because of their ability of phagocytosis) are the most important leukocyte. These cells are called *stab* or *band cells* in their immature stage of development. Mature neutrophils are often referred to as "segs," for segmented neutrophils, or "polys," for polymorphonuclear neutrophils (PMNs). (See anatomy and physiology section of this chapter [p. 383] for a brief discussion of neutrophils, lymphocytes, monocytes, basophils, and eosinophils.) Elevation of any one type of leukocyte may indicate a specific disease. Therefore, the differential categorization can be very valuable in the diagnosis and treatment of disease processes (see Table 10-2).

Serial CBCs and differential counts have both diagnostic and prognostic value. For example, a persistent increase in WBC count may indicate a worsening of an ongoing infectious process (such as appendicitis). A dramatic decrease in WBC count may delay chemotherapy.

Procedure. A peripheral venipuncture using at least a 20-gauge needle is performed, and 5 to 7 ml of blood is obtained in an EDTA-containing (lavender top) tube. Capillary blood sticks of the finger may be performed for some of these individual tests. The blood tube is tilted up and down several times to ensure adequate mixture of EDTA (an anticoagulant) with the blood. The specimen is then sent to the hematology laboratory for analysis.

Most modern clinical hospital laboratories have a machine that automatically measures the WBC, RBC, Hgb, MCV, and MCHC and calculates the Hct and MCH values. With some reliability a machine can provide a WBC differential. The differential count may be performed by a technician who examines a cubic millimeter of a blood smear under a microscope. Each type of WBC is counted, and the percentages are recorded. The only discomfort associated with this study is that of the peripheral venipuncture. A laboratory technician or nurse draws the blood.

Contraindications. None.

Nursing considerations

Nursing Diagnoses/Collaborative Problems

See Blood studies, p. 2.

Nursing Implications with Rationale

- Explain the procedure to the patient. If serial determinations are necessary, explain the rationale.
- Obtain the specimen and immediately transfer the blood to the appropriate container. Thoroughly mix the blood with the anticoagulant by tilting the blood specimen.
- Apply pressure or a pressure dressing to the venipuncture site. Assess the site for bleeding.

Peripheral blood smear

Normal values: normal quantity of RBCs, WBCs, and platelets; normal size, shape, and color of RBCs; normal white cell differential count

Rationale. When adequately prepared and examined microscopically by an experienced physician, a smear of the peripheral blood is the

TABLE 10-2. Causes for Abnormalities in the WBC Differential Count

Type of WBC	Elevated	Decreased
Neutrophils	*Neutrophilia* Physical or emotional stress Acute suppurative infection Myelocytic leukemia Trauma Cushing's syndrome Inflammatory disorders (such as rheumatic fever, thyroiditis, rheumatoid arthritis) Metabolic disorders (such as ketoacidosis, gout, eclampsia)	*Neutropenia* Aplastic anemia Dietary deficiency Overwhelming bacterial infection (especially in the elderly) Viral infections (such as hepatitis, influenza, measles) Radiation therapy Addison's disease Drug therapy: myelotoxic drugs (as in chemotherapy)
Lymphocytes	*Lymphocytosis* Chronic bacterial infection Viral infection (such as mumps, rubella) Lymphocytic leukemia Multiple myeloma Infectious mononucleosis Radiation Infectious hepatitis	*Lymphocytopenia* Leukemia Sepsis Immune deficiency diseases Lupus erythematosus Acquired immunodeficiency syndrome Drug therapy: adrenal corticosteroids, antineoplastics Radiation therapy
Monocytes	*Monocytosis* Chronic inflammatory disorders Viral infections (such as infectious mononucleosis) Tuberculosis Chronic ulcerative colitis	*Monocytopenia* Drug therapy: prednisone
Eosinophils	*Eosinophilia* Parasitic infections Allergic reactions Eczema Leukemia Autoimmune diseases	*Eosinopenia* Increased adrenal steroid production
Basophils	*Basophilia* Myeloproliferative disease (such as myelofibrosis, polycythemia rubra vera) Leukemia	*Basopenia* Acute allergic reactions Hyperthyroidism Stress reactions

most informative of all hematologic tests. All three hematologic cell lines (red cells, white cells, and platelets) can be examined.

Microscopic examination of the RBCs can reveal variation in red cell size (anisocytosis), shape (poikilocytosis), color, or intracellular content. Classification of RBCs according to these variables is most helpful in identifying the causes of anemia.

- *RBC size*
  - Microcytes (small RBC)
    - Iron deficiency
    - Hereditary spherocytosis
    - Thalassemia
  - Macrocytes (larger size)
    - Vitamin B_{12} or folic acid deficiency
    - Reticulocytosis secondary to increased erythropoiesis (RBC production)
    - Occasional liver disorder
    - Postsplenectomy anemia
- *RBC shape*
  - Spherocytes (small and round)
    - Hereditary spherocytosis
    - Acquired immunohemolytic anemia
  - Elliptocytes (crescent or sickled)
    - Hereditary elliptocytosis
    - Sickle cell anemia
  - Leptocytes, or "target cells" (thin and with less hemoglobin)
    - Hemoglobinopathies
    - Thalassemia
  - Spicule cell
    - Uremia
    - Liver disease
    - Bleeding ulcer
- *RBC color*
  - Hypochromic (pale)
    - Iron deficiency
    - Thalassemia
    - Cardiac disease
  - Hyperchromasia (more colored)
    - Concentrated hemoglobin usually caused by dehydration
- *RBC intracellular structure*
  - Nucleus (because the maturation process of the RBC results in the loss of the nucleus, nucleated RBCs [normoblasts] seen in the peripheral smear indicate increased RBC production)
    - "Normal" for infant's blood
    - Physiologic response to RBC deficiency (as in hemolytic anemias, sickle cell crisis, transfusion reaction, and erythroblastosis fetalis)
    - Physiologic response to hypoxemia (as in congenital heart disease and congestive heart failure)
    - Marrow-occupying neoplasm or fibrotic tissue (as in myeloma and leukemia)
  - Basophilic stippling (refers to bodies enclosed or included in the cells)
    - Lead poisoning
    - Reticulocytosis (see next study)
  - Howell-Jolly bodies (small, round remnants of nuclear material)
    - Postsplenectomy
    - Hemolytic anemia
    - Megaloblastic anemia
  - Heinz bodies (small, irregular particles of hemoglobin)
    - Drug-induced RBC injury
    - Hemoglobinopathies
    - Hemolytic anemia

The WBCs are examined for total quantity, differential count, and degree of maturity. An increased number of immature WBCs may indicate leukemia. A decreased WBC count indicates marrow failure caused by drugs, chronic disease, neoplasia, or fibrosis.

Finally, an experienced cell examiner can estimate platelet number (see p. 409) on a peripheral blood smear.

No complications are associated with this study. It is only as uncomfortable as the required finger stick. The smear takes only a few minutes to prepare for examination.

Procedure. In the hematology department a finger stick is usually performed. The finger is prepared with alcohol. A drop of blood is spread on a slide, and a second slide is used to smear the drop across the first slide. The slide is then colored with a polychromatic stain (usually Wright's or Giemsa). The stained slide is then examined under the microscope. The slide is prepared by a technician and best examined by an experienced physician. The only discomfort associated with the study is that of the finger stick.

Contraindications. None.

Nursing Considerations

Nursing Diagnoses/Collaborative Problems

See Blood studies, p. 2.

Nursing Implications with Rationale

- Explain the procedure to the patient.
- Prepare the finger appropriately with alcohol, and perform the finger stick. Many laboratories prefer to have the patient sent to the hematology department for the finger stick.

Reticulocyte count

Normal values:
Adults/elderly/children: 0.5%-2% of total erythrocytes
Infants: 0.5%-3.1% of total erythrocytes
Newborns: 2.5%-6.5% of total erythrocytes
Reticulocyte index: 1

Rationale. The reticulocyte count is a test for determining bone marrow function. It is useful in determining the cause of anemia. A reticulocyte is an immature RBC that can be readily identified under the microscope by the staining of a peripheral blood smear with a supravital stain. The reticulocyte count represents a direct measurement of RBC production by the bone marrow. Increased reticulocyte counts are expected as physiologic compensation in patients who are anemic. A normal or low reticulocyte count in an anemic patient indicates that the marrow production of RBCs is inadequate and perhaps is the cause of the anemia (as in aplastic anemia, iron deficiency, and vitamin B_{12} deficiency).

An elevated reticulocyte count found in patients with a normal hemogram indicates increased RBC production (compensated hemolysis or acute hemorrhage). To detect if the increased reticulocyte count is reflective of adequate erythropoiesis in anemic patients with a decreased hematocrit, one can determine the reticulocyte index:

Reticulocyte index =

$$\text{Reticulocyte count (\%)} \times \frac{\text{Patient's hematocrit}}{\text{Normal hematocrit}}$$

The reticulocyte index in a patient who has a good marrow response to the anemia should be 1. If it is below 1, even though the reticulocyte count is elevated in the anemic patient, the bone marrow response is inadequate in its ability to compensate (as in iron deficiency or vitamin B_{12} deficiency). No complications are associated with this study.

Procedure. Blood is obtained for a CBC (see p. 390) and sent to the hematology lab. A technician applies a supravital stain to a peripheral blood smear and examines the slide under a microscope. Young RBCs (reticulocytes) exhibit a network of purple strands. The reticulocytes are counted and their percentage of the total RBCs is determined.

Contraindications. None.

Nursing considerations

Nursing Diagnoses/Collaborative Problems

See Blood studies, p. 2.

Nursing Implications with Rationale

- See CBC, p. 390.

Iron level and total iron-binding capacity test

(Fe and TIBC)

Normal values:
Iron: 60-190 μg/dl or 13-31 μmol/L (SI units)
TIBC: 250-420 μg/dl or 45-73 μmol/L (SI units)
Transferrin saturation: 30%-40%

Rationale. Abnormal levels of iron and total iron-binding capacity are characteristic of many diseases, including iron deficiency anemia. Most of the iron in the body is found in the hemoglobin of the RBCs. Iron, supplied by the diet, is absorbed in the small intestine and transported to the plasma. There the iron is bound to a globulin protein called *transferrin* and carried to the bone marrow for incorporation into hemoglobin. The serum iron determination is a measurement of the quantity of iron bound to transferrin. The TIBC is a direct, quantitative measurement of transferrin. The percentage of saturation is calculated by dividing the serum iron level by the TIBC.

$$\text{Transferrin saturation (in \%)} = \frac{\text{Serum iron level}}{\text{TIBC}} \times 100\%$$

The normal value for transferrin saturation is between 30% and 40%. Calculation of transferrin saturation is helpful in determining the cause of abnormal iron and TIBC levels.

Iron deficiency anemia has many causes, including:

1. Insufficient iron intake
2. Inadequate gut absorption
3. Increased requirements (as in growing children)
4. Loss of blood (as in menstruation, bleeding peptic ulcer, or colon neoplasm).

Iron deficiency results in a decreased production of hemoglobin available for RBC synthesis. The RBCs that are present have reduced hemoglobin concentration and appear small and pale (microcytic, hypochromic). A decreased serum iron level, an elevated TIBC and a low transferrin saturation value are characteristic of iron deficiency anemia. A decrease in the MCV and MCHC indexes is also found (see pp. 388-390).

Chronic illnesses (such as infections, neoplasia, nephrosis, and cirrhosis) are characterized by a low serum iron level, a decreased iron-binding capacity, and a normal transferrin saturation. Pregnancy is marked by high levels of protein, including transferrin. Because iron requirements are high, it is not unusual to find low serum iron levels, high TIBC, and a low percentage of transferrin saturation in late pregnancy.

Increased intake or absorption of iron (as in hemochromatosis) leads to elevated iron levels. In such cases the TIBC is unchanged, and as a result, the percentage of transferrin saturation is very high. Excess iron is usually deposited in the brain, liver, and heart and causes severe dysfunction of these organs.

Because serum iron levels may vary significantly during the day, the blood specimen should be obtained in the morning, especially when the results are used to monitor iron replacement therapy. The patient should refrain from eating for about 12 hours to avoid artificially high iron measurements caused by eating food with a high iron content. Blood transfusions also markedly raise the iron level (although the increase is only transient), and should be avoided before serum iron level determinations.

TIBC, on the other hand, varies minimally according to intake. The TIBC is more of a reflection of liver function (transferrin is produced by the liver) and nutrition (protein intake) than of iron metabolism. Often TIBC values are used to monitor the course of patients receiving hyperalimentation.

Chloramphenicol, estrogens, alcohol, and oral contraceptives cause high serum iron values. Allopurinol, anabolic steroids, and aspirin will decrease serum values.

Procedure. The patient should be kept fasting except for water for at least 12 hours before the study. Approximately 7 ml of peripheral venous blood is obtained in a red-top tube. Some laboratories require the use of iron-free needles and iron-free plastic containers for the blood collection. The specimens should always be obtained using a 20-gauge or larger needle. Smaller needles may traumatize the RBC during collection, resulting in hemolysis. With hemolysis the iron usually contained in the RBC pours out into the serum and causes artificially high iron levels. The serum is transported to the chemistry laboratory for analysis.

Contraindications. Contraindications for this study include:

1. Recent transfusions
2. Recent ingestion of a meal containing a high iron content

3. Hemolytic diseases that may be associated with an artificially high iron content.

Nursing considerations

Nursing Diagnoses/Collaborative Problems

See Blood studies, p. 2.

Nursing Implications with Rationale

- Explain the procedure to the patient. Keep the patient fasting except for water for 12 hours before the blood test.
- Assess the patient for a history of blood transfusions and recent meals high in iron content.
- Perform a peripheral venipuncture, using a needle size of at least 20-gauge. Blood is usually drawn in the morning.
- After the venipuncture has been performed, apply pressure or a pressure dressing to the site. Assess the site for bleeding.

Serum ferritin test

Normal values:
Men: 12-300 ng/ml or 12-300 μg/L (SI units)
Women: 10-150 ng/ml or
10-150 μg/L (SI units)

Rationale. The serum ferritin study is a good indicator of available iron stores. Ferritin, the major iron-storage protein, is normally present in the serum in concentrations directly related to iron storage. In healthy people, 1 ng/ml of serum ferritin corresponds to approximately 8 mg of stored iron. Ferritin levels in adult men and postmenopausal women are generally significantly higher than in younger adult females. Decreases are associated with iron deficiency anemia (see previous study) and are also seen in severe protein depletion. Increased levels are a sign of iron excess (as seen in hemochromatosis, hemosiderosis, megaloblastic anemia, hemolytic anemia, and alcohol/inflammatory liver disorders). A limitation of the study is that ferritin levels can also be elevated in conditions not reflecting iron stores (such as in acute inflammatory diseases, infections, metastatic cancer, leukemias, and lymphomas).

When combined with the serum iron and TIBC (see previous study), this test is useful in differentiating and classifying anemias. For example, in iron deficiency anemia, the ferritin, iron, and saturation levels are low, while the TIBC and transferrin levels are high. Ferritin levels are normal or high in thalassemia.

Procedure. A peripheral venous blood sample is collected in a red-top tube.

Contraindications. See Iron level and TIBC (previous study).

Nursing considerations

Nursing Diagnoses/Collaborative Problems

See Blood studies, p. 2.

Nursing Implications with Rationale

- Explain the procedure to the patient.
- Perform a peripheral venipuncture and obtain the needed blood sample. Apply pressure to the site and assess the site for bleeding.

Serum haptoglobin test

Normal values:
Newborn: 5-48 mg/dl
Adult:
Male 26-185 mg/dl
Female 40-175 mg/dl
Possible critical value: <40 mg/dl in adults

Rationale. The serum haptoglobin test is used to detect intravascular destruction (hemolysis) of RBCs. Haptoglobins are glycoproteins that are produced by the liver. These haptoglobins are powerful, free hemoglobin–binding proteins. In hemolytic anemias associated with intravascular destruction of RBCs (for example, hemoglobinopathies and autoimmune and mechanical destruction of RBCs [as from artificial heart valves]), the released hemoglobin is quickly bound to haptoglobin and the new complex is quickly catabolized by the liver. This causes a precipitous drop in the amount of free haptoglobin in the serum that cannot be quickly compensated for by normal liver production. As a consequence, the patient demonstrates a transient reduced level of haptoglobin in the serum.

Haptoglobins are also decreased in patients with primary liver disease unassociated with hemolytic anemias. This is because the diseased liver is unable to produce these glycoproteins.

Elevated haptoglobin concentrations are found in many inflammatory diseases and can therefore be used as a nonspecific test of disease in much the same way as a sedimentation rate test (see p. 444). Anabolic steroids increase haptoglobin levels. Birth control pills and tamoxifen decrease serum haptoglobin. No complications are associated with this blood study.

Procedure. A peripheral venous blood sample is obtained from the nonfasting patient and placed in a red-top tube (containing no anticoagulant). The blood is then sent to the chemistry laboratory for analysis.

Contraindications. None.

Nursing considerations

Nursing Diagnoses/Collaborative Problems

See Blood studies, p. 2.

Nursing Implications with Rationale

- Explain the procedure to the patient.
- Assess the patient for signs of ongoing infection that could falsely elevate the results. Notify the physician of any significant findings.
- Perform a peripheral venipuncture and obtain the needed blood sample. Apply a pressure dressing to the site and assess the site for bleeding.

Bone marrow examination

(bone marrow biopsy, bone marrow aspiration)

Normal values: active erythroid cell, myeloid cell, and megakaryocyte (platelet) production

Rationale. By examination of a bone marrow specimen, the hematologist can fully evaluate hematopoiesis. Examination of the bone marrow reveals the number, size, and shape of the RBCs, WBCs, and megakaryocytes (platelet precursors) as these cells evolve through various stages of development in the bone marrow. Samples of the bone marrow can be obtained by either aspiration or surgical removal. Microscopic examination includes estimation of cellularity, determination of the presence of fibrotic tissue or neoplasms (both primary and metastatic), and estimation of iron storage.

For the estimation of cellularity, the specimen is examined and the relative quantity of each cell type is determined. This is more accurately performed on a biopsy specimen than on an aspirate because the aspirate may not be truly representative of the entire marrow. Leukemias or leukemoid reactions are suspected when increased numbers of leukocyte precursors are present. Physiologic marrow compensation for infection is also recognized by an increased number of leukocyte precursors. Decreased numbers of marrow leukocyte precursors occur in patients with myelofibrosis, old age, metastatic neoplasia, or agranulocytosis and following radiation therapy or chemotherapy.

Increased numbers of marrow RBC precursors occur with polycythemia vera or as physiologic compensation to hemorrhagic or hemolytic anemias. Decreased numbers of marrow RBC precursors occur with erythroid hypoplasia following chemotherapy or radiation therapy, administration of other toxic drugs, or marrow replacement by fibrotic tissue or neoplasms.

Increased numbers of platelet precursors (megakaryocytes) are seen in the marrow of patients following acute hemorrhage or some forms of chronic myeloid leukemia. This increase may also be compensatory in patients with secondary hypersplenism associated with portal hypertension or other conditions. Decreased megakaryocytes occur in patients who have had radiation therapy or chemotherapy and in patients with neoplastic or fibrotic marrow infiltrative diseases. Patients with aplastic anemia also have decreased megakaryocytes.

Lymphocyte precursors are increased in infections (such as mononucleosis), lymphocytic leukemia, and lymphoma. Plasma cells (plasmocytes) are increased in patients with multiple myelomas, Hodgkin's disease, hypersensitivity states, rheumatic fever, and other chronic inflammatory diseases.

Estimation of cellularity can also be expressed as a ratio of myeloid (WBC) to erythroid (RBC) cells. The normal M:E ratio is about 3:1. The M:E ratio is greater than normal in those diseases mentioned previously in which increased leukocyte precursors are present or in which there is a decrease in erythroid precursors. The M:E ratio is below normal when either leukocyte precursors are decreased or erythroid precursors are increased. A more detailed listing of diseases affecting the M:E ratio can be found in most hematology textbooks.

Drug-induced or idiopathic myelofibrosis can be detected by examination of the bone marrow. With the use of special stains, iron stores can be estimated by the marrow biopsy. Although fibrosis or neoplasia can occasionally be detected in aspiration studies, biopsy is the best method. Leukemias, multiple myelomas, and polycythemia vera can easily be detected in biopsy specimens. Similarly, diffusely metastatic tumors (as of the breast, kidney, and lung) can be seen with metastases to the bone marrow.

The rare complications associated with marrow biopsies or aspiration studies include severe bleeding (especially if the patient has a coagulopathy), infection (especially if the patient is leukopenic), and puncture of the heart or great vessels when the test is performed on the sternum.

Procedure. Bone marrow aspiration is performed on the sternum (see Figure 11-1, p. 421), iliac crest, anterior or posterior iliac spines, and proximal tibia (in children). The removal of specimens for bone marrow biopsy is done on the iliac spines or wherever tumor is suspected. Bone marrow aspiration is usually performed at the patient's bedside using local anesthesia. The preferred site is the posterior iliac crest with the patient placed prone or on his or her side. The area overlying the bone is prepared and draped in a sterile manner. The overlying skin and soft tissue, along with the periosteum of the bone, is infiltrated with lidocaine (Xylocaine). If *aspiration* is to be done, a large-bore (14-gauge) needle containing a stylus is slowly advanced through the soft tissues and into the outer table of the bone. Once inside the marrow, the stylus is removed and a syringe is attached. One half to 2 ml of bone marrow is aspirated, smeared on slides, and allowed to dry. The slides are then sprayed with a preservative and taken to the pathology laboratory. There some of the slides are stained with Wright's stain and others with a supravital stain.

If bone marrow *biopsy* is to be performed, the skin and soft tissues overlying the bone are incised and a core biopsy instrument is screwed into the bone. The biopsy specimen is obtained and sent to the pathology laboratory for analysis.

Aspiration is performed by a trained nurse or a physician. Bone marrow biopsy specimen removal is performed only by a physician. The duration of the study is approximately 10 to 20 minutes. After the needle or core biopsy instrument is removed, pressure is applied to the site and a sterile dressing is supplied. The patient usually feels pain during lidocaine infiltration and pressure when the syringe plunger is pulled back for aspiration. The patient may have some apprehension when pressure is applied to the bone for outer table puncture during biopsy specimen removal or aspiration.

Contraindications. This study is contraindicated in uncooperative patients.

Nursing considerations

Nursing Diagnoses/Collaborative Problems

- Possible knowledge deficit related to test purpose, preparation, and procedure
- Possible anxiety related to unknown sensations of procedure
- Possible anxiety related to test results
- Possible alteration in comfort related to test procedure
- Potential complication: hemorrhage

- Potential complication: infection
- Potential complication: perforation

Nursing Implications with Rationale

- Explain the procedure to the patient. Describe the purpose of the study. Encourage the patient to verbalize fears because many patients are anxious concerning this study. Provide emotional support.
- Be sure that the physician has obtained the signed and informed consent forms before the study.
- Assess the coagulation studies performed on the patient before the study. Report any evidence of coagulopathy to the physician.
- Obtain an order for sedatives if the patient appears extremely apprehensive before the study.
- Assist the physician or nurse in obtaining the specimen. During the study remind the patient to remain very still. If the patient moves, the needle could accidentally puncture a vital organ.
- Label the slides appropriately, with the patient's name, date, and room number.
- After the needle is removed, apply pressure to arrest the scant amount of bleeding from the puncture site. Pressure usually stops any bleeding from the biopsy or aspiration site. Apply an adhesive bandage. Ice packs may be used to help control bleeding. Uncontrolled hemorrhage can lead to hematoma formation, which can be very uncomfortable.
- Observe the puncture site for bleeding. Tenderness and erythema may indicate infection and should be reported to the physician.
- After the study assess the patient for signs of shock (increased pulse rate, decreased blood pressure) and pain. Normally, bed rest is prescribed for 30 to 60 minutes after the study. After that time, allow the patient to resume normal activity.
- Some patients complain of tenderness at the puncture site for several days after the study. Administer mild analgesics as ordered.

Hemoglobin electrophoresis

Normal values
  Adult/elderly:
    Hgb A_1: 95%-98%
    Hgb A_2: 2%-3%
    Hgb F: 0.8%-2%
    Hgb S: 0
    Hgb C: 0
  Children: Hgb F
    Newborn: 50%-80%
    6 months: 8%
    >6 months: 1%-2%

Rationale. The hemoglobin electrophoresis is a test that enables abnormal forms of hemoglobin (that is, hemoglobinopathies) to be detected. Although many different hemoglobin variations have been described, the more common types are A_1, A_2, F, S, and C. Each major hemoglobin type is charged to varying degrees. When placed in an electromagnetic field, the hemoglobin variants migrate at different rates and therefore spread apart from each other. One is able to quantitate each band as a percentage of the total hemoglobin.

Hgb A_1 constitutes the major component of hemoglobin in the normal RBC. Hgb A_2 is only a minor component (2% to 3%) of the normal hemoglobin total. Hgb F is the major hemoglobin in the fetus, yet exists in only minimal quantities in the normal adult. Levels of Hgb F greater than 2% in patients over the age of 3 years are considered abnormal. Hgb F is able to transport oxygen when only small amounts of oxygen are available (as in fetal life). In patients requiring compensation for prolonged chronic hypoxia (as in congenital cardiac abnormalities), Hgb F may be found in increased levels to assist in the transport of the available oxygen.

Hgb S is an abnormal form of hemoglobin that is associated with sickle cell anemia, which occurs predominantly in African-Americans. Hgb S is a relatively insoluble variant. When little oxygen is available, it assumes a crescent (sickletype) shape that greatly distorts the RBC morphology. Vascular sludging is a consequence of the localized sickling and may lead to organ infarction.

Hgb C is another hemoglobin variant that exists in African-Americans. RBCs containing Hgb C have a decreased life span and are more readily lysed than normal RBCs. Mild hemolytic anemia may result.

The hemoglobin contents of the common hemoglobinopathies as determined by electrophoresis are as follows:

Sickle cell disease (homozygous SS)
- Hgb S: 80%-100%
- Hgb A_1: 0
- Hgb A_2: 2%-3%
- Hgb F: <2%

Sickle cell trait (heterozygous SA)
- Hgb S: 20%-40%
- Hgb A_1: 60%-80%
- Hgb A_2: 2%-3%
- Hgb F: 2%

Hemoglobin C disease (homozygous)
- Hgb C: 90%-100%
- Hgb A_1: 0
- Hgb A_2: 2%-3%
- Hgb F: 2%

Hemoglobin H disease
- Hgb A_1: 65%-90%
- Hgb A_2: 2%-3%
- Hgb H: 5%-30%

Thalassemia major (homozygous)
- Hgb A_1: 5%-20%
- Hgb A_2: 2%-3%
- Hgb F: 65%-100%

Thalassemia minor (heterozygous)
- Hgb A_1: 50%-85%
- Hgb A_2: 4%-6%
- Hgb F: 1-3%

No complications are associated with hemoglobin electrophoresis. This test is no more uncomfortable than a peripheral venipuncture. Because not all clinical laboratories are equipped to perform this test, frequently the blood must be sent to a commercial lab, often requiring days for the results to be received. The test itself takes only between 2 and 36 hours to be performed, depending on the method used.

Procedure. A lavender-top tube, or any EDTA-containing tube, is filled with 7 ml of peripheral venous blood and sent to the hematology lab as soon as possible. There, a small quantity is placed on a starch gel or cellulose acetate medium. Electrophoresis ensues within an electromagnetic field, and the hemoglobin variants are separated out and quantified by spectrophotometry.

Contraindications. Patients who have received a blood transfusion within the previous 12 weeks should not have hemoglobin electrophorersis. The donor's blood can, if normal, mask and dilute an abnormal hemoglobin variation that may exist in the recipient.

Nursing considerations

Nursing Diagnoses/Collaborative Problem

See Blood studies, p. 2.

Nursing Implications with Rationale

- Explain the procedure to the patient.
- Assess the patient to make sure that he or she has not had any recent blood transfusions, which could alter the test results.
- Perform a peripheral venipuncture and obtain the blood specimen. Apply pressure or a pressure dressing to the venipuncture site. Assess the site for bleeding.
- Transport the blood specimen to the laboratory as soon as possible to avoid hemoglobin dilution, which could alter the results.

Sickle cell test

(sickle cell preparation, Sickledex, Hgb S test)

Normal value: no sickle cells

Rationale. Both sickle cell disease (homozygous for Hgb S) and sickle cell trait (heterozygous for Hgb S) can be detected by this study. Sickle cell anemia is caused by Hgb S, which is an abnormal form of hemoglobin. When Hgb S becomes deoxygenated, it tends to band in a way that causes the RBC to assume a sickle shape. These sickled RBCs cannot pass freely through the capillaries, resulting in plugging of the microvascular tree. This may compromise the blood supply to various organs. Hgb S is found in 8% to 10% of the black population.

The routine peripheral blood smear of patients with sickle cell disease does not contain sickled RBCs unless hypoxemia is present. In the sickle cell test, a deoxygenating agent is added to the patient's blood. If 25% or more of the patient's hemoglobin is of the S variation, the cells assume the crescent (sickle) shape and the test is positive. If there is no sickling, the test is negative. A negative test indicates that the patient has no or very little Hgb S. Other, less common hemoglobin variants can also cause sickling.

This test is only a screening test, and its sensitivity varies according to the method used by the laboratory. The definitive diagnosis is made by hemoglobin electrophoresis (see previous study), where Hgb S can be identified and quantified.

Any transfusions within 3 to 4 months before the sickle cell test can cause false-negative results because the donor's normal hemoglobin may dilute out the recipient's abnormal Hgb S. Some drugs (especially the phenothiazines) may cause false negative results. No complications are associated with this study.

Procedure. Approximately 7 ml of peripheral venous blood is obtained, placed in a lavender-top vacutainer, and transported to the hematology laboratory. In the laboratory a technician mixes a small quantity of blood with a bisulfite solution and then examines a peripheral blood smear for crescent-shaped RBCs. The sickling procedure takes less than 30 minutes. The only discomfort associated with this study is the venipuncture.

Contraindications. The sickle cell test is contraindicated in patients who have received blood transfusions within 3 months before the time of the test.

Nursing considerations

Nursing Diagnosis/Collaborative Problems

See Blood studies, p. 2.

Nursing Implications with Rationale

- Explain the procedure to the patient. Assess the patient for recent transfusions of blood.
- Perform the venipuncture and send the blood to the laboratory. Assess the venipuncture site for bleeding.
- If the test is positive, be aware that the family should be offered genetic counseling. A patient with one recessive gene (heterozygous) is said to have sickle cell *trait*. A patient with two recessive genes (homozygous) has sickle cell *anemia*.
- Inform patients with sickle cell anemia that they should avoid situations in which hypoxia may occur (such as strenuous exercise, air travel in unpressurized aircraft, and travel to high-altitude regions).

Direct Coombs' test

(direct antiglobin test)

Normal value: negative, no agglutination

Rationale. The direct Coombs' test is used to detect autoantibodies against RBCs, which can cause cellular damage. Many diseases (such as erythroblastosis fetalis, lymphomas, lupus erythematosus, mycoplasmal infection, and infectious mononucleosis) along with drugs (such as alpha-methyldopa, levodopa, penicillin, cephalosporins, sulfonamides, acetaminophen, quinidine, aspirin, and many other drugs) are associated with the production of these autoantibodies. These antibodies result in hemolytic anemia. Frequently, the production of these autoantibodies against RBCs is not associated with any disease, and the resulting hemolytic anemia is therefore called *idiopathic*.

This test is performed by mixing the patient's RBCs, which are suspected of being covered with autoantibodies against RBCs, with Coombs' serum. Coombs' serum is a solution containing antibodies against human antibodies. If the RBCs are coated with the patient's autoantibodies against RBCs, the Coombs' antibodies react with those antibodies on the RBC and cause agglutination (clumping) of the RBCs. The greater the quantity of antibodies against RBCs present, the more clumping occurs. This test is read as positive with clumping on a scale of trace to +4. If the RBCs are not coated with the patient's autoantibodies against RBCs (immunoglobulins), agglutination does not occur. This is a negative test.

When a transfusion with incompatible blood is given, the Coombs' test can detect the antibodies coating the transfused RBCs. The Coombs' test is therefore very helpful in evaluating suspected transfusion reactions. No complications are associated with this study.

Procedure. No food or drink restrictions are associated with this test. Coombs' serum is produced by injecting human serum antibodies into a rabbit, which then makes antibodies to the human serum antibodies. The rabbit's serum contains antibodies against human serum (Coombs' serum). The patient's blood is collected in a red-top vacutainer and transported to the blood bank. (Venous blood from the umbilical cord is used to detect the presence of antibodies in the newborn.) The patient's RBCs are mixed with the Coombs' serum. Agglutination indicates a positive test, and the patient is said to have an autogenous production of antibodies against RBCs that causes RBC hemolysis. No agglutination indicates a negative study.

Contraindications. None.

Nursing considerations

Nursing Diagnoses/Collaborative Problems

See Blood studies, p. 2.

Nursing Implications with Rationale

- Explain the procedure to the patient.
- Obtain the blood specimen as ordered. Be certain that the blood specimen is correctly labeled with a stamped name plate sticker.
- Transport the blood to the laboratory as soon as possible.

Indirect Coombs' test

(blood antibody screening, indirect antiglobulin test)

Normal value: negative

Rationale. The indirect Coombs' study detects the presence of circulating antibodies against RBCs. The major purpose of this test is to determine if the patient has serum antibodies (other than major ABO system) to RBCs that he or she is about to receive by blood transfusions. Therefore, this test is the "screening" portion of the "type and screen" routinely performed for blood compatibility testing (cross-matching).

In this test a small amount of the recipient's serum is added to the donor's RBCs. Then Coombs' serum is added to the mixture. Visible agglutination indicates that the recipient has antibodies to the donor's RBCs. Thus clumping, or agglutination, occurs when the antibodies against human serum in the Coombs' serum react with the recipient's antibodies, which have coated the donor's RBCs. If the recipient has no antibodies against the donor's RBCs, agglutination does not occur. Transfusion should then proceed safely and without any cross-reaction.

Circulating antibodies against RBCs may also occur in a pregnant woman who is Rh negative and is carrying an Rh positive fetus.

Procedure. Seven milliliters of peripheral venous blood is obtained from the proposed recipient in a red-top vacutainer (without an anticoagulant) and transported to the blood bank. The proposed recipient's serum is mixed with the donor's RBCs, and Coombs' serum is subsequently added. Agglutination, or clumping, indicates a positive test. The degree of agglutination is an indication of the quantity of antibodies against RBCs present in the recipient's serum. Positive results vary from trace to +4. No agglutination indicates a negative result. No food or drink restrictions are associated with this test.

Contraindications. None.

Nursing considerations

Nursing Diagnoses/Collaborative Problems

See Blood studies, p. 2.

Nursing Implications with Rationale

- See Direct Coombs' test (preceding study).

Blood typing

Rationale. By blood typing, ABO and Rh antigens can be detected in the blood of prospective blood donors and potential blood recipients. This test is also used to determine the blood type of expectant mothers and newborns. Human blood is grouped according to the presence or absence of these antigens. The two major antigens, A and B, form the basis of the ABO system (group A RBCs contain A antigens; group B RBCs contain B antigens; group AB RBCs have both A and B antigens; group O RBCs have neither A nor B antigens) (Table 10-3). The presence or absence of Rh antigens on the RBCs determines the classification of Rh positive or Rh negative.

All pregnant patients should have a blood typing and Rh factor determination. If the pregnant patient's blood is Rh negative or type O (the most common type of ABO disease), the husband's blood should also be typed. If his blood is Rh positive, the woman's blood should be examined for the presence of Rh antibodies (by the indirect Coombs' test, see previous study). If the initial screening is negative (no antibodies to Rh found), the test is repeated at weeks 30 and 36 of pregnancy. If these tests are also negative, no risk is involved to the fetus. If the Coombs' test is positive, the fetus may have been affected. That is, the mother is making antibodies to the Rh positive RBCs of the fetus causing hemolysis. The severity of the hemolytic anemia is then evaluated by the quantity of bilirubin in the amniotic fluid (see Amniocentesis, p. 359). ABO and Rh typing is also performed during pregnancy to advise the mother whether or not she is a candidate for RhoGAM (Rh immunoglobulin) after the delivery.

Blood transfusions are actually transplantations of tissue (blood) from one person to another. It is important that the recipient does not have antibodies to the donor's RBCs and that the donor does not have antibodies to the recipient's RBCs. If either of these conditions exists, there is a hypersensitivity reaction, which can vary in severity from mild fever to anaphylaxis with severe intravascular hemolysis. Although typing for the major ABO and Rh antigens does not guarantee that a reaction will not occur, it does greatly reduce the possibility of such a reaction.

Many potential minor antigens are not routinely detected during blood typing. If allowed to go unrecognized, these minor antigens can also initiate a blood transfusion reaction. Therefore, blood is not only typed but also cross-matched to identify compatability with the minor antigens. Cross-matching consists of mixing the recipient's serum with the donor's RBCs in saline solution followed by the addition of Coombs' serum (indirect Coombs' test, see preceding study).

Procedure. Usually 14 ml of peripheral venous blood is obtained in two red-top vacutainers and sent to the blood bank. The RBCs are diluted and suspended in saline solution divided into many quanta. Antisera A, B, and Rh_O are each added to a quantum and mixed. The blood is typed by RBC agglutination in one or more of the antisera.

TABLE 10-3. Blood Typing

Blood type	Antigen	Antibody
Group A	A	B
Group B	B	A
Group AB (universal receiver)	A, B	None
Group O (universal donor)	None	A, B

Agglutination In	Blood Type
A only	A−
B only	B−
A and B only	AB−
A and Rh_O only	A+
B and Rh_O only	B+
A, B, and Rh_O	AB+
None	O−
Rh_O only	O+

Next, cross-matching is performed by placement of a small quantum of the patient's serum and a quantum of the proposed donor's blood in saline solution. The solution is assessed for agglutination. The indirect Coombs' test (see preceding study) is then performed. If no agglutination occurs, the blood can be given safely with a minimal chance of an in vivo blood reaction. The type and cross-match is done in the blood bank in approximately 45 minutes.

Contraindications. Cross-matching is not performed when the patient requires immediate transfusion and the risk of the blood reaction is outweighed by the urgent need of a blood transfusion (as in ongoing acute hemorrhage). In these situations, type-specific (ABO and Rh) matched blood can be given. In those very rare situations when the transfusion cannot be delayed for even the few minutes required for blood typing, type O− blood is given. Type O− blood contains no major antigens; therefore, the chances of blood reaction are fewer when it is given to a patient with an unknown blood type.

Nursing considerations

Nursing Diagnoses/Collaborative Problems

See Blood studies, p. 2.

Nursing Implications with Rationale

- Explain the procedure to the patient. Assess the patient for a previous allergic reaction to transfused blood products.
- Draw the blood as indicated. Label the blood tubes appropriately with a stamped nameplate sticker. Label the blood request slips appropriately and deliver the blood to the blood bank.
- Before administering the blood, do the following:
  - Check the patient's identification band.
  - Check the patient's blood type as determined by the blood bank.
  - Compare the blood type of the donor's unit to the patient's type and be certain they match. Two professional nurses must verify this and sign a blood transfusion sheet indicating that the proper blood was given to the proper patient.
  - Aseptically, start an intravenous (IV) line with saline solution. The needle must be at least 20-gauge to avoid hemolysis of the RBCs. (The IV line should be taped securely to avoid infiltration.) The IV line is always started with saline solution, because dextrose (which is hypertonic) may cause hemolysis or clumping of the donor RBCs.
  - Administer the first 50 ml of the donor's blood over a 30-minute period, and observe the patient for signs of cross match reaction (such as fever, back pain, urticaria, tachycardia, or wheezing). If no reaction is suspected, you can increase the rate of infusion, unless this is contraindicated (as in congestive heart failure).
  - Provide the blood bank with a fresh blood sample if further transfusions are required 48 hours after the first one.
- If you suspect a blood reaction, do the following:
  - Immediately stop the blood infusion and infuse the normal saline solution. Assess the vital signs and notify the physician.
  - Obtain blood for a direct Coombs' test, a serum haptoglobin test, free hemoglobin, and retyping of the patient's blood (two red-top tubes and one lavender-top tube are needed). Obtain a urine specimen for hemoglobinuria.
  - Administer an antihistamine or steroid preparation if ordered by the physician.
  - Do not administer any more blood until the cause of the reaction is determined. Do

not discard the blood bag and tubing. Return them to the laboratory for further analysis.

SUPPLEMENTAL INFORMATION

Red blood cell survival study

(RBC survival study, splenic sequestration study)

Normal values:
Half-life of RBC = 26-30 days
Spleen/liver ratio = 1:1
Spleen/pericardium ratio <2:1

Rationale. In patients who have hemolytic anemia the RBCs are destroyed and normally sequestered in the spleen. As a result of this ongoing RBC destruction, the RBC life span will be significantly reduced. This reduction in RBC survival indicates that active hemolysis is occurring and is the cause of the patient's anemia.

Hemolysis can be identified by determination of the catabolic products of hemoglobin (which are increased) or by measuring the level of circulating haptoglobin—the transport protein that binds hemoglobin (which is decreased). With this test, the nuclear determination of RBC life span can provide a semiquantitative measurement of the degree of hemolysis. This quantitation can be best performed by determining the half-life of the RBC within the circulation. This portion of the test is performed by extracting some of the patient's RBCs, labeling them with chromium-51 (^{51}Cr), and reinjecting them into the patient. Subsequent blood levels of ^{51}Cr indicate the half-life of the labeled RBCs. Decreased RBC survival is seen in patients with hemolysis, hemorrhage, and abnormally increased erythropoiesis.

The second portion of the test is the imaging of the spleen, liver, and pericardium. In patients who have hemolytic anemia associated with abnormal splenic sequestration, the spleen/liver ratio is in excess of 1:1. However, this abnormally high ratio can occur in patients who have splenomegaly caused by a disease other than hemolytic anemia. Therefore, spleen/pericardium ratios are performed; those greater than 2:1 indicate abnormal splenic sequestration of hemolyzed RBCs. A normal spleen/pericardium ratio with an increased spleen/liver ratio indicates splenomegaly.

This second portion of the splenic sequestration study is also helpful in determining which patients with hemolytic anemia will benefit from splenectomy. Patients who have increased splenic sequestration can be expected to improve greatly as a result of splenectomy. Splenic sequestration is eliminated, and RBC blood cell survival is prolonged.

Procedure. Usually a hematocrit, WBC count, platelet count, and reticulocyte count are performed before this test. Then, approximately 20 ml of blood is withdrawn from the patient and the RBCs are labeled with ^{51}Cr. The RBCs are immediately reinjected into the patient. On the first day of testing, 10 ml of blood is withdrawn by peripheral venipuncture in a red-top tube. The RBCs are quantitated for ^{51}Cr counts per minute. Nuclear imaging of the spleen, liver, and pericardium is carried out. This process is repeated 3 times a week for about 3 weeks. The peripheral venous blood ^{51}Cr counts are plotted on a graph and a half-life is determined. The spleen/liver and spleen/pericardium ratios and nuclear counts are determined.

This test takes place over a 2- to 3-week period. The results are available on the day after the test is completed. The study is performed by a nuclear medicine technologist or by a physician. There is no pain or discomfort associated with this test other than the frequent venipuncture. The patient must also lie still during the nuclear imaging portion of the test.

Contraindications. This test is contraindicated in patients who are pregnant because of the risk of fetal damage.

Nursing considerations

Nursing Diagnoses/Collaborative Problems

See Blood studies, p. 2, and Nuclear scan, p. 5.

Nursing Implications with Rationale

- Explain the procedure to the patient.

- Assure the patient that he or she will not be exposed to large amounts of radioactivity since only tracer doses of the isotope are used. No precautions need to be taken against radioactive exposure.
- Tell the patient that no special preparation or sedation is required.
- Notify the nuclear medicine technologist or physician if blood transfusion or hemorrhage has occurred shortly before or during the test.
- After the test, assess the venipuncture site for bleeding and apply a pressure dressing.

Glucose-6-phosphate dehydrogenase

(G-6-PD)

Normal values: 8-18.6 U/g hemoglobin or negative (screening test)

Rationale. The G-6-PD test is used to determine if hemolytic anemia is caused by lack of G-6-PD (an enzyme normally present in the RBC). Decreased levels of this enzyme are associated with G-6-PD deficiency, which is a sex-linked, recessive trait carried on the X chromosome. Affected males inherit this abnormal gene from their mothers, who are usually asymptomatic. Hemolytic episodes in these individuals may be triggered by drugs (such as sulfonamides, nitrofurantoin, phenacetin, antipyretics, and primaquine), infections, or acidotic states. Because there are two common types of G-6-PD deficiencies (Mediterranean and Type A), some drugs cause hemolysis in only one or the other type. Certain foods, such as fava beans, are not tolerated by patients with the Mediterranean type of G-6-PD found in whites and Asians. Type A is found in the black population.

Levels of G-6-PD may be increased in patients with pernicious anemia, myocardial infarction, hepatic coma, hyperthyroidism, chronic blood loss, and other megaloblastic anemias.

Procedure. No food or fluid restrictions are associated with this test. Venipuncture is performed according to the laboratory guidelines.

Contraindications. None.

Nursing considerations

Nursing Diagnoses/Collaborative Problems

See Blood studies, p. 2.

Nursing Implications with Rationale

- Explain the procedure to the patient
- Obtain the blood specimen as ordered. Assess the venipuncture site for bleeding.
- If the test indicates that a lack of G-6-PD exists, give the patient a list of drugs (see Rationale) that can precipitate hemolysis. Fava beans should not be eaten by patients with the Mediterranean variant of this disease. Teaching the patient to read the labels on any over-the-counter drugs for the presence of products (such as aspirin and phenacetin) that may cause hemolytic anemia is also very important.

CASE STUDY 2: HEMOPHILIA

Kenny D. was a 10-year-old boy who fell and lacerated his lower leg while climbing a fence. In the emergency department, no signs of neurovascular damage were detected and the wound was closed. One hour later, the dressings were saturated with blood. The patient was then taken to the operating room, where the wound was explored. No arterial lacerations were seen. There was a diffuse oozing of blood from the wound's edges. In a review of the patient's bleeding history, it was found that he seemed to have a tendency to bleed larger quantities and for a greater duration than normal.

Studies	Results
Routine laboratory studies	WNL
Prothrombin time (PT)	Patient/control: 11 sec/12 sec; 85% (normal: 11-12.5 sec or 85%-100%)
Activated partial thromboplastin time (APTT)	62 sec (normal: 30-40 sec)
Platelet count	200,000/mm^3 (normal: 150,000-400,000/mm^3)
Ivy bleeding time	8.5 min (normal: 1-9 min)
Blood clot retraction test	WNL

Studies	Results
Factor VIII concentration	10% of normal concentration (absolute normal varies according to the laboratory performing the test)
DIC screening test	No evidence of DIC (normal: negative)

The abnormal APTT result indicated a defect in the intrinsic system or common pathway of clot formation (see p. 386). The extrinsic pathway of clot formation was found to be adequate because of the normal PT results. The normal bleeding time, platelet count, and blood clot retraction test eliminated insufficient platelet quantity or function as a cause of the coagulopathy. The factor VIII concentration was well below normal and was found to be the cause of the failure to clot. Hemophilia was diagnosed and the patient was given factor VIII concentration. All obvious bleeding ceased and the leg wound healed.

After discharge the patient returned to the hospital at regular intervals for factor VIII concentration (such as cryoprecipitate). He had no further bleeding difficulties.

DISCUSSION OF TESTS

Prothrombin time test

(pro-time, PT test)

Normal values: 11-12.5 seconds; 85%-100%
 Full anticoagulant therapy: 1½-2 times control value; 20%-30%
Possible critical values: >20 seconds
 Full anticoagulant therapy: >3 times control value

Rationale. The prothrombin time study is used to evaluate the adequacy of the extrinsic system and common pathway in the clotting mechanism. The PT measures the clotting ability of factors I (fibrinogen), II (prothrombin), V, VII, and X. When these clotting factors (especially factors V and VII) are deficient, prothrombin time (PT) is prolonged. Many diseases and drugs are associated with decreased levels of these factors. These include:

1. Hepatocellular liver disease (such as cirrhosis, hepatitis, Reye's syndrome, and neoplastic invasive processes). Factors II, V, VII, IX, and X and fibrinogen are produced in the liver. With severe hepatocellular dysfunction, this synthesis does not occur, and serum concentration of these factors are decreased. Even a small decrease in factor VII results in marked prolongation of the PT.
2. Obstructive biliary disease (such as bile duct obstruction secondary to tumor or stones or intrahepatic cholestasis secondary to sepsis or drugs). As a result of the biliary obstruction, the bile necessary for fat absorption fails to enter the gut and fat malabsorption results. Vitamins A, D, E, and K are fat-soluble and are not absorbed with fat malabsorption. Because the synthesis of factors II, VII, IX, and X is dependent on vitamin K, these factors will not be adequately produced and serum concentrations fall. Factor VII is the first to decrease and results in prolongation of PT.

   Parenchymal liver disease can be differentiated from obstructive biliary disease by determination of the patient's response to parenteral vitamin K administration. If the PT returns to normal after 3 days of vitamin K administration (10 mg, intramuscularly, twice a day), it is safe to assume that the patient has obstructive biliary disease that is causing vitamin K malabsorption. If, on the other hand, PT does not return to normal with the vitamin K injections, it can be assumed that severe hepatocellular disease exists and that the liver cells are incapable of synthesizing the clotting factors no matter how much vitamin K is available.
3. Coumarin ingestion. The coumarin derivatives, dicumarol and warfarin (Coumadin, Panwarfin) are used to prevent coag-

ulation in patients with thromboembolic disease (such as pulmonary embolism, thrombophlebitis, and arterial embolism). These drugs interfere with the production of vitamin K–dependent clotting factors, which results in a prolongation of PT (as described above). The adequacy of coumarin therapy can be monitored by following the patient's PT. Appropriate coumarin therapy should prolong PT by 1½-2 times the control value (or 20% to 30% of the normal value if percentages are used).

Coumarin derivatives are slow-acting, but their action may persist for 7 to 14 days after discontinuation of the drug. The action of a coumarin drug can be fairly rapidly reversed (in 12 to 24 hours) by the parenteral administration of vitamin K (phytonadione) given very slowly.

The action of the coumarin drugs can be enhanced by drugs such as aspirin, quinidine, sulfa, and indomethacin. Barbiturates, chloral hydrate, and oral contraceptives may decrease the effects of coumarin drugs.

4. Disseminated intravascular coagulation (DIC). Several clotting factors are used up by this uncontrolled form of coagulation, and none are left for normal necessary hemostasis.
5. Excessive bleeding. The clotting factors are lost during the bleeding. While replacement with banked blood replenishes the RBCs, the clotting factors are not replaced. The PT is therefore prolonged.

PT test results are usually given in seconds along with a control value. The control value usually varies somewhat from day to day because the reagents used may vary. The patient's PT should be about equal to the control value. Some laboratories report PT values as percentages of normal activity, as the patient's results are compared with a curve representing normal clotting time. Normally, the patient's PT is 85% to 100%. A patient receiving anticoagulants should be within a therapeutic range of 20% to 30%.

In order to have uniform PT results for physicians in different parts of the country and the world, the World Health Organization has recommended that PT results now include the use of the *international normalized ratio* (INR) value. The reported INR results are independent of the reagents or methods used since the standard method of keeping PT ratios of 1½ to 2 times the control value in certain clinical indications would be converted to a figure that takes the sensitivity of the thromboplastin used as reagent and the type of instrument into account. These international sensitivity indexes are different for various thromboplastins and according to whether mechanical or photo-optical methods and instruments are used. Many hospitals are now reporting PT times in both absolute numbers and in INR numbers.

Many drugs prolong the PT by enhancing the effect of oral anticoagulants. They include aspirin, acetaminophen in high doses, anabolic steroids, many antibiotics, large amounts of alcohol, and heparin.

Procedure. Peripheral venipuncture is performed, and one or two blue-top tubes (containing sodium citrate) are filled with blood. The tubes must be filled to capacity, otherwise the PT results may be artificially prolonged because of the extra citrate in the tube. The blood samples should be transported on ice to the laboratory as soon as possible to avoid deterioration of factors. In the lab tissue thromboplastin is added, thereby circumventing the intrinsic system of clotting. The time required for clotting is then noted.

Contraindications. None.

Nursing considerations

Nursing Diagnoses/Collaborative Problems

See Blood studies, p. 2.

Nursing Implications with Rationale

- Explain the procedure to the patient. Tell him or her that you are drawing blood to assess how quickly the blood clots. Be sure to fill completely the blue-top tubes with blood.

Deliver the blood specimen to the laboratory immediately after venipuncture.

- If the patient is receiving warfarin, the PT specimen should be drawn before the patient is given the daily dose of warfarin. The daily dose may be increased, decreased, or kept the same, depending on the PT test results for that day. Maintain a flow chart indicating the PT test results, control value, and dose of anticoagulant.
- Check the site for bleeding after the venipuncture; apply pressure to the site until the bleeding stops. Remember, the bleeding time will be prolonged if the patient is taking warfarin or if the patient has any coagulopathies.
- If the PT is markedly prolonged, evaluate the patient for bleeding tendencies (that is, check for blood in the urine and all excretia and assess the patient for bruises, petechiae, and low back pain).
- If severe bleeding occurs, the anticoagulant effect of warfarin can be reversed by the slow parenteral administration of vitamin K (phytonadione).
- Because of drug interactions, instruct the patient not to take any medication unless it is specifically ordered by the physician.

Partial thromboplastin time (activated) test

(PTT, APTT)

Normal values:
APTT: 30-40 seconds
PTT: 60-70 seconds
Patients receiving anticoagulant therapy:
1.5-2.5 times control value in seconds
Possible critical values:
APTT: >70 seconds
PTT: >100 seconds

Rationale. The partial thromboplastin time (PTT) test is used to assess the intrinsic system and the common pathway of clot formation. It evaluates factors I, II, V, VIII, IX, X, XI, and XII. When any of these factors exists in inadequate quantities (as in hemophilia A and B or consumptive coagulopathy), the PTT is prolonged. Because factors II, IX, and X are vitamin K–dependent factors produced in the liver, hepatocellular disease or biliary obstruction can reduce their concentration and thus prolong the PTT. Von Willebrand's disease, hemophilia, and DIC are also associated with prolongation of PTT.

Heparin has been found to inactivate prothrombin (factor II) to prevent the formation of thromboplastin and, to a lesser degree, factors VIII and IX. These actions prolong the intrinsic clotting pathway for about 4 to 6 hours after each dose of heparin. Therefore, heparin is capable of providing therapeutic anticoagulation. The appropriate dose of heparin can be monitored by the PTT. PTT test results are given in seconds along with a control value. The control value may vary slightly from day to day because of the reagents used. Recently, activators have been added to the PTT test reagents to shorten normal clotting time and provide a narrow normal range. This shortened time is called the activated partial thromboplastin time (APTT). The normal APTT is 30 to 40 seconds. Desired ranges for therapeutic anticoagulation are 1½ to 2½ times normal (for example, 70 seconds). The APTT specimen should be drawn 30 to 60 minutes before the patient's next heparin dose is given. If the APTT is less than 50 seconds, the patient is not receiving therapeutic anticoagulation and needs more heparin. An APTT of greater than 100 seconds indicates that too much heparin is being given. The risk of serious spontaneous bleeding exists when the APTT is this high. The effects of heparin can be reversed immediately by the administration of 1 mg of protamine sulfate for every 100 units of the heparin dose.

Heparin's effect (unlike that of warfarin) is immediate. This drug is often given during cardiac and vascular surgery to prevent intravascular clotting during clamping of the vessels. When a thromboembolic episode (such as pulmonary embolism, arterial embolism, or thrombophlebitis) occurs, immediate and complete anticoagulation is best achieved by heparin administration. Often small doses of heparin

(5,000 units subcutaneously every 12 hours) are administered to prevent thromboembolism in high-risk patients. This dose alters the PTT very little, and the risk of spontaneous bleeding is minimal.

Procedure. Peripheral venipuncture is performed, and one or two blue-top tubes (containing sodium citrate) are filled with blood. The blue-top tubes must be filled to capacity, otherwise the PTT value may be incorrect because of the extra citrate within the tube. The blood samples are usually transported on ice to the laboratory as soon as possible.

PTT levels are now being determined from finger stick specimens using a machine similar to a glucometer. This is generally done in the critical care units. Nurses vary the heparin dose based on sliding-scale heparin orders.

Contraindications. None.

Nursing considerations

Nursing Diagnoses/Collaborative Problems

See Blood studies, p. 2.

Nursing Implications with Rationale

- Explain to the patient that blood is drawn to assess how quickly it clots.
- Usually the PTT specimen is drawn daily 30 minutes to 1 hour before one of the heparin administrations. The heparin dosage may be altered depending on the results. Maintain a flow chart indicating the PTT test results, control values, and dosage of anticoagulants.
- Be sure that the blue-top tubes of blood are completely full.
- Check the site for bleeding after the venipuncture. Apply pressure to the site until the bleeding stops. Remember, if the patient is receiving anticoagulants or has coagulopathies, bleeding time will be increased.
- Deliver the blood specimen to the laboratory immediately.
- Assess the patient to detect possible bleeding (that is, check for blood in the urine and all excretia and assess the patient for bruises, petechiae, and low back pain).
- If severe bleeding occurs, the anticoagulant effect of heparin can be reversed by parenteral administration of protamine sulfate.

Platelet count

(thrombocyte count)

Normal values:
Adult/elderly: 150,000-400,000/mm^3 or 150 to 400 × 10^9/L (SI units)
Premature infant: 100,000-300,000/mm^3
Newborn: 150,000-300,000/mm^3
Infant: 200,000-475,000/mm^3
Child: 150,000-400,000/mm^3
Possible critical values: <50,000 or >1 million/mm^3

Rationale. The platelet count is an actual count of the number of platelets (thrombocytes) per cubic milliliter of blood. Platelet activity is essential to blood clotting (see p. 384 for a review of platelet function). Because platelets can clump together, automated counting is subject to at least a 10% to 15% error. Counts between 150,000 and 400,000/mm^3 are considered normal. Counts below 100,000/mm^3 are considered to constitute thrombocytopenia; thrombocytosis is said to exist when counts are >400,000/mm^3. Vascular thrombosis with organ infarction is the major complication of thrombocytosis. Paradoxical hemorrhage may occur with thrombocytopenia.

Spontaneous bleeding is a serious danger when platelet counts fall below 15,000/mm^3. With counts above 40,000/mm^3, spontaneous bleeding rarely occurs. However, prolonged bleeding from trauma or surgery may occur at this level.

Causes of thrombocytopenia (decreased number of platelets) include:

1. Reduced production (secondary to bone marrow failure or infiltration)
2. Sequestration (secondary to hypersplenism)
3. Accelerated destruction of platelets (secondary to antibodies, infections, prosthetic heart valves)

4. Consumption (secondary to disseminated intravascular coagulation)
5. Platelet loss from hemorrhage requiring massive blood transfusion of platelet-poor products
6. Hereditary thrombocytopenia, Wiscott-Aldrich syndrome, Fanconi's syndrome, and other less common syndromes
7. Idiopathic autoimmune disorders, e.g., idiopathic thrombocytopenic purpura
8. Extracorporeal circulation damage to platelets, which are then sequestered
9. Uremia. Patients with chronic renal failure have platelets reduced in quantity and in function.

Thrombocytosis (increased number of platelets) may occur as a compensatory response to severe hemorrhage. Other conditions associated with thrombocytosis include polycythemia vera, leukemia, rheumatoid arthritis, inflammatory bowel disease, postsplenectomy syndromes, and various malignant disorders.

No complications are associated with this procedure other than ongoing bleeding from the venipuncture site in patients with thrombocytopenia.

Procedure. Five to seven milliliters of peripheral venous blood is obtained in a lavender-top tube and sent to the hematology laboratory. A small quantity of blood is then analyzed by an automatic counter simultaneously with the CBC.

Contraindications. None.

Nursing considerations

Nursing Diagnoses/Collaborative Problems

See Blood studies, p. 2.

Nursing Implications with Rationale

- See CBC, p. 390.

Bleeding time test

(Ivy bleeding time)

Normal values: 1-9 minutes.
Possible critical value: >12 minutes

Rationale. This test is used to evaluate the vascular and platelet factors associated with hemostasis (see p. 385 for a review of hemostasis). When injury occurs, the first hemostatic response is a spastic contraction of any lacerated microvessels. Next, platelets adhere to the wall of the vessel at the area of laceration in an attempt to plug the hole. Failure of either of these processes results in a prolonged bleeding time.

For this study a small standard incision is made in the forearm, and the time required for the bleeding to stop is recorded. This is called the bleeding time. Normal values vary according to the method used. The method most commonly used today is the Ivy bleeding time test.

Prolonged values occur in the following:

1. Patients with decreased platelet counts (see p. 409)
2. Patients who have prolonged prothrombin time (see p. 406)
3. Patients with DIC
4. Uremic patients, because platelets are reduced in number and function
5. Coumadin overdose
6. Increased capillary fragility secondary to collagen vascular disease, Cushing's disease, or Henoch-Schönlein syndrome
7. Ingestion of antiinflammatory drugs (such as aspirin or indomethacin).

Because this test requires only a small incision, it is rare to have a complication such as laceration of the nerve, tendon, artery, or vein. Infections do not occur if appropriate skin preparation and aftercare are given.

Procedure. The bleeding time test is usually performed at the patient's bedside. The skin of the inner part of the forearm is cleansed with alcohol or povidone-iodine (Betadine). A blood pressure cuff (tourniquet) is placed on the arm above the elbow, inflated to 40 mm Hg, and maintained at this pressure during the study. A small laceration is then made 3 mm deep into the skin, and the time is recorded. Bleeding ensues and the blood is blotted clean at 30-second intervals. When no new bleeding occurs, the time is again recorded. The time interval (from the beginning to the end of bleeding) is calculated and called the bleeding time. The blood pressure cuff is then removed and an adhesive bandage is applied to the patient's arm.

If the bleeding persists for more than 10 minutes, the test is stopped and a pressure dressing is applied. If the patient has a factor deficiency, the bleeding time may be normal, but subsequent oozing of blood from the test site may be seen 20 minutes after the original bleeding has stopped. Pressure should be applied to the wound. A minor amount of discomfort occurs with this test because of the skin laceration.

Contraindications. This test is contraindicated in the following:

1. Patients with known low platelet counts
2. Patients who are unable to cooperate
3. Patients who cannot have a blood pressure cuff placed on the arm (e.g., those with cellulitis)
4. Patients with a history of keloid formation
5. Patients with senile skin changes
6. Patients who have had a mastectomy. (Avoid the arm on that side.)

Nursing considerations

Nursing Diagnoses/Collaborative Problems

- Possible knowledge deficit related to the purpose, preparation, and procedure
- Possible alteration in comfort related to the test purpose
- Potential complication: bleeding

Nursing Implications with Rationale

- Explain the procedure to the patient. Assess the patient for aspirin ingestion or other nonsteroidal antiinflammatory agents, such as ibuprofen (Motrin), during the week preceding the test. These medications prolong bleeding time.
- If the patient is taking any anticoagulants, indicate this with the test results.
- Assist as needed in performing this test.
- Apply a dressing to the patient's forearm after the study. Assess the arm for subsequent bleeding. Apply a pressure dressing if oozing of blood is noted.

Whole blood clot retraction test

Normal values:
50%-100% clot retraction in 1-2 hours
Complete retraction within 24 hours

Rationale. The clot retraction test is used to determine if bleeding disorders may be caused by thrombocytopenia (decreased platelet count). Platelets (see discussion of anatomy and physiology, p. 384) play a vital role in hemostasis and blood clotting. This test measures the role and degree of blood clot retraction. The clot should contract to one half its original size within 1 to 2 hours. The retraction should be nearly complete in 4 hours and definitely completed within 24 hours.

If thrombocytopenia exists, the clot retraction is slower and the clot formation stays soft and watery. If fibrinolysins are present, no clot retraction occurs. This test is only reliable if the hematocrit and fibrinogen (factor I) concentration (Table 10-4) are within normal limits.

TABLE 10-4. Minimum Concentration of Coagulation Factors Required for Adequate Fibrin Production

Factor	Minimum hemostatic level (mg/dl)	Blood components*
I	60-100	C, FFP, FWB
II	10-15	P, WB, FFP, FWB
V	5-10	FFP, FWB
VII	5-20	P, WB, FFP, FWB
VIII	30	C, FFP, VIII
IX	30	FFP, FWB
X	8-10	P, WB, FFP, FWB
XI	25	P, WB, FFP, FWB

*Blood components capable of providing specific factor: *C*, cryoprecipitate; *FFP*, fresh frozen plasma; *FWB*, fresh whole blood (<24 hours old); *P*, unfrozen banked plasma; *WB*, banked whole blood; *VIII*, factor VIII concentrate.

In addition to thrombocytopenia, poor whole blood retraction occurs in patients with thrombasthenia (abnormal platelets), anemia, and Waldenström's macroglobulinemia.

Procedure. No food or fluid restrictions are associated with this test. Approximately 5 to 7 ml of venous blood is collected in a red-top tube. Clot retraction is then timed and evaluated.

Contraindications. None

Nursing considerations

Nursing Diagnoses/Collaborative Problems

See Blood studies, p. 2.

Nursing Implications with Rationale

- Explain the procedure to the patient. Carefully draw the blood sample. Avoid excessive probing during the venipuncture if a coagulation disorder is suspected. After drawing the blood, apply pressure to the venipuncture site and observe the site for bleeding.
- Handle the specimen carefully to avoid hemolysis.
- If the specimen is to be evaluated on the floor, ensure that it is accurately timed and carefully evaluated for contraction.

Coagulating factors concentration test

Normal values: 50%-200% of "normal"

Rationale. The coagulating factors concentration test measures the concentration of a specific coagulating factor in the blood. Testing is available to measure the quantity of factors I, II, V, VII, VIII, IX, X, XI, and XII. For example, fibrinogen (factor I) is essential to the blood clotting mechanism because it is converted to fibrin by the action of thrombin during the coagulation process (see Figure 10-1). Measurement of factor I is often referred to as a *quantitative fibrinogen*. When these factors exist in concentrations below their "minimum hemostatic level," clotting time is prolonged. These minimal hemostatic levels vary according to the factor involved (Table 10-4). Common medical conditions associated with decreased factor concentrations are listed in Table 10-5. It is important to identify the exact factor or factors involved in the coagulating defect so that appropriate blood component replacement can be administered (Table 10-4).

TABLE 10-5. Conditions that May Result in Coagulation Factor Deficiency

Condition	Factor diminished
Liver disease	I, II, V, VII, IX, X, XI
Disseminated intravascular coagulation	I, V, VIII
Fibrinolysis	I, V, VIII
Congenital deficiency	I, II, V, VII, VIII, IX, X, XI, XII
Heparin administration	II
Warfarin ingestion	II, VII, IX, X, XI
Autoimmune disease	VIII

Procedure. Peripheral venous blood is obtained and placed in a blue-top vacutainer. The blood is then sent to the hematology laboratory for bioassay of the desired coagulation factor. In most hospitals the specimen is sent to a commercial laboratory for analysis. The test results usually require 1 to 7 days to be reported, depending on whether the specimen has to be sent to a commercial laboratory or whether the test can be done in the hospital.

Contraindications. None.

Nursing considerations

Nursing Diagnoses/Collaborative Problems

See Blood studies, p. 2.

Nursing Implications with Rationale

- See PT test, pp. 406-408, and PTT test, pp. 406-408.

Disseminated intravascular coagulation screening

(DIC screening)

Normal value: no evidence of DIC

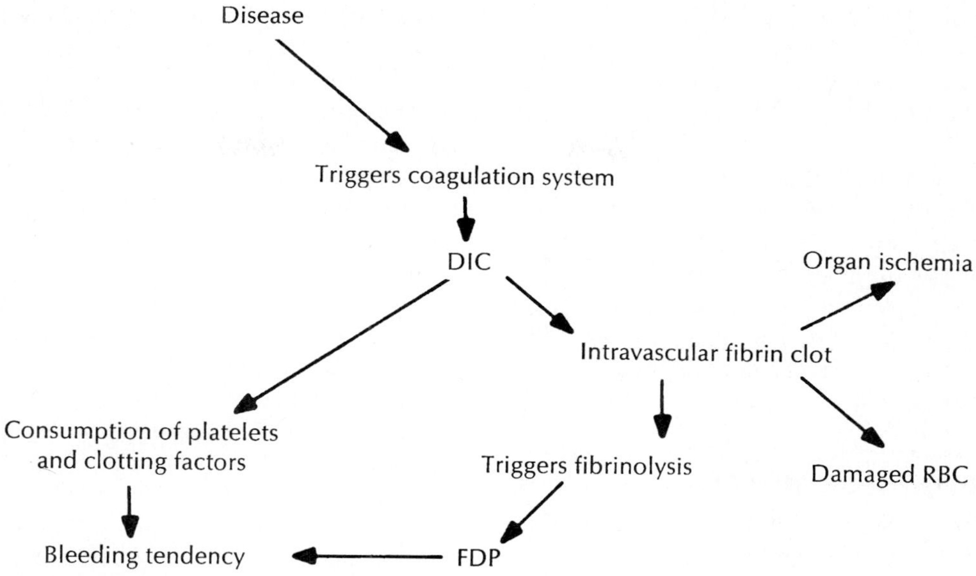

FIGURE 10-2. Illustration of pathophysiology of disseminated intravascular coagulation, which may result in bleeding tendency, organ ischemia, and hemolytic anemia.

Rationale. This group of tests is used to detect DIC. Many pathologic conditions instigate or are associated with DIC. The more common ones include bacterial septicemia, amniotic fluid embolism, retention of a dead fetus, malignant neoplasia, liver cirrhosis, postextracorporeal heart bypass, extensive trauma, and transfusion reactions.

In DIC the entire clotting mechanism is triggered inappropriately. This results in significant systemic or localized intravascular formation of fibrin clots. Consequences of this futile clotting are intravascular sludging and excessive bleeding caused by consumption of the platelets and clotting factors that have been used in intravascular clotting. The fibrinolytic system is also activated to break down the fibrin involved in the intravascular coagulation. This results in fibrin degradation products (FDPs), which by themselves act as anticoagulants. These FDPs only serve to enhance the bleeding tendency.

Organ injury can occur as a result of the intravascular clots, which cause microvascular occlusion in various organs. This may cause serious anoxic injury in organs affected. Also, RBCs passing through partly plugged vessels are injured and subsequently hemolyzed. The result may be ongoing hemolytic anemia. Figure 10-2 provides a summary of DIC pathophysiology

TABLE 10-6. Disseminated Intravascular Coagulation Screening Tests

Test	Positive result
Bleeding time	Prolonged
Platelet count	Decreased
Prothrombin time	Prolonged
Activated partial thromboplastin time	Prolonged
Fibrinogen (factor I concentration)	Decreased
Fibrin degradation products	Present
RBC smear	Damaged RBCs and decreased number of platelets
Euglobulin lysis time	Normal or prolonged

and effects. Heparin is sometimes used to treat DIC because it inhibits the ongoing futile thrombin formation. This decreases the use of clotting factors and platelets, and bleeding ceases.

When a patient with a bleeding tendency is suspected to have DIC, a series of readily performed laboratory tests should be done (Table 10-6). With these tests, the hematologist can make the appropriate diagnosis confidently. All of these tests have been discussed earlier in this chapter except for the euglobulin lysis time test and fibrin degradation products test, which are presented below.

SUPPLEMENTAL INFORMATION

Euglobulin lysis time test

(fibrinolysis/euglobulin lysis time test)

Normal values: 90 minutes to 6 hours
Possible critical value: <1 hour, indicating excessive fibrinolytic activity (danger of bleeding)

Rationale. The euglobulin lysis test is used to evaluate systemic fibrinolysis. As discussed in the Anatomy and physiology section (p. 385) the fibrinolytic system normally breaks down small fibrin deposits. When this system is abnormally overactive (as in primary fibrinolysis) any fibrin clot that is formed will be dissolved immediately, thereby resulting in a bleeding tendency. This system is only minimally overactive in patients with secondary fibrinolysis (e.g., DIC, pulmonary surgery, and various liver diseases).

The euglobulin lysis time is a measure of the activity of this fibrinolytic system. Fibrin formed in the euglobulin fraction of plasma is normally very rapidly dissolved by plasmin (fibrinolysin). The time measured from clot formation to clot lysis is referred to as the euglobulin lysis time. In primary fibrinolysis (caused by streptokinase administration, cancer of the prostate, shock, and other conditions) the euglobulin lysis time is rapid (short). In DIC, the euglobulin lysis time is usually normal. However, if all of the plasmin has been consumed, the time may be prolonged. This is one of the best tests used to differentiate primary fibrinolysis from DIC. This differentiation is important in considering appropriate therapy for the patient with bleeding tendencies. Epsilon aminocaproic acid may be required to treat primary fibrinolysis; heparin may be indicated for DIC.

This test also may be used to monitor streptokinase or urokinase therapy used to dissolve clots in deep-vein thrombophlebitis.

Procedure. A peripheral venipuncture is performed and 4.5 ml of blood is collected in a chilled oxalate-containing tube and taken to the hematology laboratory. A clot is formed and a solution is added that causes clot lysis. A timer is started and the specimen is observed for lysis. The time required to complete clot lysis is called the euglobulin lysis time. This test is performed in most clinical hematology laboratories. The results can be reported in less than 6 hours.

Contraindications. None.

Nursing considerations

Nursing Diagnoses/Collaborative Problems

See Blood studies, p. 2.

Nursing Implications with Rationale

- See PT test, pp. 406-408, and PTT test, pp. 408-409.

Fibrin degradation products test

(fibrin split products, FSP, fibrinogen degradation products)

Normal values: <10 μg/ml or dilution <1 : 20
Possible critical value: >40 μg/ml

Rationale. The measurement of FDPs provides a direct indication of the activity of the fibrinolytic system. When plasma acts to dissolve fibrin clots, fibrinogen and FDPs (X, D, E, and Y) are formed. These degradation products, which have their own anticoagulant effect, can be measured. When they are present in large amounts, they indicate increased fibrinolysis as occurs in DIC and primary fibrinolytic disorders.

Procedure. Peripheral venous blood is collected in a blue-top tube and taken on ice to the hematology laboratory. The specimen is mixed with a serum containing antifibrinogen degradation fragments A and E, which have been absorbed onto latex particles. If the patient's blood contains the degradation fragments, agglutination occurs. If no degradation fragments are present in the patient's blood, no agglutination occurs. Degradation product levels greater than 10 μg/ml indicate increased fibrinolysis (DIC or primary fibrinolysis).

Contraindications. None.

Nursing considerations

Nursing Diagnoses/Collaborative Problems

See Blood studies, p. 2.

Nursing Implications with Rationale

- See PTT test, pp. 408-409.

Folic acid test

(folate)

Normal values: 5-20 μg/ml, or
14-34 mmol/L (SI units)

Rationale. Folic acid, one of the B vitamins, is necessary for normal function of RBCs and WBCs and for the adequate synthesis of certain purines and pyrimidines, which are precursors for DNA. Like vitamin B_{12} (see Schilling test), folate is dependent on normal function of the intestinal mucosa.

The folic acid test is done to evaluate hemolytic disorders and to detect folic acid–deficient anemia (where the RBCs are abnormally large, causing a megaloblastic anemia). These RBCs have a shortened life span and impaired oxygen-carrying capacity.

The main causes for deficiency of folic acid include poor diet, malabsorption syndrome, pregnancy, and certain anticonvulsive drugs. Decreased folic acid levels are seen in patients with folic acid anemia (megaloblastic anemia), hemolytic anemia, malnutrition, malabsorption syndrome, malignancy, liver disease, sprue, and celiac disease. Some drugs (such as anticonvulsants, antimalarials, alcohol, aminopterin, and methotrexate) are folic acid antagonists and interfere with nucleic acid synthesis. Elevated levels of folic acid may be seen in patients with pernicious anemia. This test may be done in conjunction with vitamin B_{12} levels (see Schilling test).

Procedure. No fasting is usually required before this test; however, patients should not consume alcoholic beverages before the test. Seven to 10 ml of blood is collected in a red-top tube and sent to the laboratory.

Contraindications. None.

Nursing considerations

Nursing Diagnoses/Collaborative Problems

See Blood studies, p. 2.

Nursing Implications with Rationale

- Prevent hemolysis of the blood sample.
- Assess the venipuncture site for bleeding and hematoma formation.

Urinary porphyrins and porphobilinogens

Normal values:
Porphyrins: 50-300 mg/24 hours
Porphobilinogens: 1.5-2 mg/24 hours or negative

Rationale. Porphyrias are hereditary metabolic disorders of heme synthesis, which is needed for the formation of hemoglobin. Abnormalities of porphyrin metabolism may be genetic, drug, or lead induced. Normally insignificant amounts of porphyrins are excreted in the urine. In certain disease states (such as abnormal porphyrin metabolism, liver disease, lead poisoning, and pellagra) there is an increased level of porphyrins in the urine. Disorders in porphyrin metabolism also cause porphobilinogen. This test is a quantitative analysis of urinary porphyrins and their precursors (such as porphobilinogen [PBG]). If porphyrins are determined to be present in the urine, the urine may be colored amber red or burgundy. The urine may turn dark after standing in the light.

Procedure. A 24-hour urine specimen is collected in a light-resistant specimen bottle with a preservative to prevent degradation of the light-sensitive porphyrin. Porphobilinogens are usually elevated with the porphyrin test or in a single, fresh voided, random urine specimen. The specimen should be protected from light and taken immediately to the laboratory for analysis.

Contraindications. None.

Nursing considerations

Nursing Diagnoses/Collaborative Problems

See Urine studies, p. 2.

Nursing Implications with Rationale

- Explain the procedure to the patient and assist the patient as needed with the urine collection.
- Permit the patient food and fluids during the 24-hour urine collection.

Delta-aminolevulinic acid test

(ΔALA, aminolevulinic acid, ALA)

Normal values: 1-7 mg/24 hours, or 11.1-57.2 μmol/24 hr (SI units)
Possible critical value: >20 mg/24 hr

Rationale. Delta-aminolevulinic acid (ΔALA), the basic precursor for the porphyrins (see previous study), is an enzyme needed for the normal conversion to porphobilinogen during heme synthesis. Impaired conversion, which causes abnormal RBC formation, occurs in lead intoxication and in porphyrias. These conditions cause the urine levels of ALA to rise before other chemical or hematologic changes.

Urine levels of ALA are obtained to screen for lead poisoning and to aid in the diagnosis of certain kinds of genetic deficiencies of porphyrin metabolism (see porphyrias). Elevated levels may also be seen in patients with hepatitis and hepatic carcinoma.

Healthy people usually do not have ALA present in their urine. However, increased values may be seen in patients taking some medications (such as penicillin, barbiturates, and griseofulvin).

Procedure. A 24-hour urine specimen is collected in a light-resistant container containing a preservative. The specimen is kept on ice or refrigerated during the entire collection.

Contraindications. None.

Nursing considerations

Nursing Diagnoses/Collaborative Problems

See Urine studies, p. 3.

Nursing Implications with Rationale

- Explain the procedure to the patient. Ensure that the specimen is collected using a preservative in a light-resistant container and placed on ice to prevent degradation of ALA.
- Ensure that the 24-hour urine specimen is collected as described in the Nursing implications of the creatinine clearance test, all but the first and last implications (see pp. 230-231).
- If the patient has a Foley catheter in place, protect the drainage bag with a dark plastic bag to prevent light exposure.
- Indicate on the lab slip any medications that the patient is currently taking. Some medications (such as penicillin, barbiturates, and griseofulvin) may cause false-positive results.
- Because the chronic ingestion of lead eventually causes anemia, vomiting, stupor, or convulsions, the source of lead (such as paint) should be found and removed. Refer the child and his or her family to a community health nurse for follow-up in the community setting.

QUESTIONS AND ANSWERS

1. **QUESTION:** Your male patient who has a long history of peptic ulcer disease has been found to have a hematocrit of 24% (normal: 52%) on routine laboratory testing. His reticulocyte count is 1.5% (within normal range). Does this reticulocyte count represent adequate marrow response in light of this patient's low hematocrit?

   ANSWER: No. Although the reticulocyte count is "normal" for a patient with a "normal" hematocrit, it is probably low when one considers the fact that the appropriate marrow response in this anemic patient should raise the reticulocyte count well above normal. This is more accurately demonstrated by a determination of the reticulocyte index, which should be 1 or higher in all patients despite the hematocrit level.

Reticulocyte index =

$$\text{Reticulocyte count} \times \frac{\text{Patient's hematocrit}}{\text{Normal hematocrit}}$$

In this case:

$$\text{Reticulocyte index} = 1.5 \times \frac{24}{52} = 0.69$$

This represents an inadequate marrow response most probably caused by iron deficiency resulting from the chronic blood loss. The anemia therefore is caused by a combination of chronic blood loss and inadequate marrow response.

2. **QUESTION:** Your 72-year-old patient is suspected of having acute appendicitis. The WBC count is 3,800. Can an infectious process like appendicitis still be considered a possibility without the normally suspected leukocytosis?

   ANSWER: Yes. Although the expected normal response to infection is elevation of the WBC count, this may not occur in the geriatric and pediatric population. Leukopenia may actually occur in response to sepsis in these two groups of patients.

3. **QUESTION:** Your patient has been receiving IV heparin therapy (6,000 units) every 4 hours. A PTT specimen is drawn at 4 P.M. (1 hour before the next heparin dose). The results indicate that the PTT is greater than 100 seconds. At 5 P.M. bleeding develops from the patient's gums while she is eating her dinner. Shortly thereafter, she voids grossly bloody urine. Epistaxis (nosebleed) follows. What should you do for this patient?

   ANSWER:

   a. Place the patient in bed in the supine position. She may become hypovolemic and hypotensive from the blood loss. Monitor her vital signs every 15 minutes.

   b. Instruct the patient to pinch her nasal alae closed to try to stop the epistaxis.

   c. Notify the physician, who will probably want to order protamine sulfate as an antidote to the heparin. One milligram of protamine sulfate equilibrates 100 units of heparin. The physician needs to know when the last dose of heparin was given because after 2 hours 50% of the heparin will have been metabolized and after 4 hours almost all of the heparin will have metabolized. By knowing when the last dose of heparin was given, the physician can calculate how much heparin is present in the blood and can match the amount of heparin with the appropriate amount of protamine sulfate.

4. **QUESTION:** A male construction worker is brought to the emergency room with a severe laceration of the leg. He is bleeding profusely and in shock. After pressure is applied to the bleeding site, blood is obtained for a CBC and cross match. Then, IV access is obtained with several large-bore IV needles, and vigorous fluid replacement is begun. The hemoglobin concentration and hematocrit results return at 14 g/dl and 52% respectively. Can these values be correct in light of the apparent severe hemorrhage?

   ANSWER: Yes, because of the time at which the blood was drawn. One of the major physiologic responses to hemorrhage is complete conservation of all free body water. This, combined with vigorous IV fluid therapy, tends to dilute the RBC count and result in the decrease in hemoglobin associated with the hemorrhagic state. However, these physiologic responses take time to occur. This patient's CBC specimen was drawn before these physiologic responses became effective and before IV fluids were administered. Therefore, there was no time for dilution of the RBC count and hemoglobin to occur. A repeat CBC performed 4 to 8 hours later will probably more accurately reflect the severity of the patient's bleeding.

5. **QUESTION:** Your 2-year-old (12 kg) patient is admitted for lower gastrointestinal bleeding. The patient's hemoglobin concentration is 7.8 g/dl. How much blood is required to transfuse the patient to a hemoglobin concentration of 10 g/dl? How much blood would be required to transfuse an adult patient (70 kg) to the same hemoglobin concentration?

   ANSWER: In general, a useful guide to blood replacement in infants and children is to consider that 10 ml/kg of whole blood or 5 ml/kg of packed cells will raise the hemoglobin 1 g/dl. Therefore, the 12 kg child requires 264 ml of whole blood or 132 ml of packed cells to raise the hemoglobin concentration from 7.8 to 10 g/dl.

In adults 1 unit of packed cells or whole blood can be expected to raise the hemoglobin concentration 1 g/dl. Therefore, slightly more than 2 units of packed cells or whole blood is required to raise the adult's hemoglobin concentration from 7.8 to 10 g/dl.

6. **QUESTION:** During blood administration, your patient suddenly suffers fever, chills, flushing of the face, shortness of breath, tachycardia, and pain along the vein into which the blood is being transfused. What should you do for the patient and what laboratory studies should be performed to elucidate the cause of the acute problem?

   ANSWER: Your patient is most probably having a transfusion reaction. For the appropriate steps to management and diagnosis you should:

   a. Stop the transfusion and run saline solution through the IV line.
   b. Record the patient's vital signs and notify the physician immediately.
   c. Administer an antihistamine, steroids, or both (such as diphenhydramine, 50 mg intramuscularly; hydrocortisone sodium succinate, 100 mg intravenously; or both) as ordered. Epinephrine, administered subcutaneously, may also be indicated.
   d. Return the blood pack and tubing to the blood bank along with a completed transfusion reaction report.
   e. Obtain 20 ml of peripheral venous blood in one lavender-top and two red-top tubes and send them to the blood bank for testing (see below).
   f. Collect a urine specimen immediately and again 24 hours after the transfusion.
   g. Do not administer any more blood until the cause of the reaction is established. The following tests are helpful in determining the cause of the reaction:
      (1) Repeated blood typing of the patient's blood and the donor pack
      (2) Repeated cross-matching
      (3) Direct and indirect Coombs' tests
      (4) Free hemoglobin, haptoglobin, and bilirubin level determinations (which indicate hemolysis)
      (5) Serum hemoglobin level determination
      (6) Urine tests for free hemoglobin and bilirubin
      (7) Culture and sensitivity study of donor's packed cells to detect bacterial contamination.

7. **QUESTION:** A patient is being transferred to the intensive care unit after surgery following a severe motor vehicle accident. In receiving the patient, you are told that the patient has required 23 units of blood. As is appropriate, to replace clotting factors that are not present in banked blood, one pack of fresh frozen plasma has been given for every 5 units of blood. In the ensuing hours you notice that the patient seems to be oozing blood from all wound and venipuncture sites. You also detect cutaneous petechia. What would be helpful in elucidating the cause of this patient's bleeding tendency?

   ANSWER: A common problem with multiple transfusions is dilution of the patient's platelets. Banked blood contains very few functioning platelets, and no platelets are contained in fresh frozen plasma. A low platelet count and a normal PT and PTT would document the cause of this patient's bleeding tendency. The patient would need platelet transfusions to correct the bleeding.

BIBLIOGRAPHY

Andresen S, Bukowski R: Disseminated intravascular coagulation. In Rakel RE, editor: Conn's current therapy, Philadelphia, 1991, WB Saunders.

Bagby GC: Leukopenia. In Wyngaarden JB and others, editors: Cecil textbook of medicine, ed 19, Philadelphia, 1992, WB Saunders.

Bagby GC: Leukocytosis and leukemoid reaction. In Wyngaarden JB and others, editors: Cecil textbook of medicine, ed 19, Philadelphia, 1992, WB Saunders.

Bunn HF: Pathophysiology of the anemias. In Wilson J and others, editors: Harrison's principles of internal medicine, ed 12, New York, 1991, McGraw-Hill.

Gabrilove JL and Gordon MS: Neutropenia. In Rakel RE, editor: Conn's current therapy, Philadelphia, 1991, WB Saunders.

Handin RI: Disorders of coagulation and thrombosis. In Wilson J and others, editors: Harrison's principles of internal medicine, ed 12, New York, 1991, McGraw-Hill.

Handlin RI: Anticoagulant, fibrinolytic, and antiplatelet disorders. In Wilson J and others, editors: Harrison's principles of internal medicine, ed 12, New York, 1991, McGraw-Hill.

Koepke JA: Practical laboratory hematology, New York, 1991, Churchill Livingstone.

Lindenbaum J: An approach to the anemias. In Wyngaarden JB and others, editors: Cecil textbook of medicine, ed 19, Philadelphia, 1992, WB Saunders.

Martinelli AM: Sickle cell disease: etiology, symptoms, and patient care, AORN J 53(3):716-724, March 1991.

Menitove JE: Blood transfusion. In Wyngaarden JB and others, editors: Cecil textbook of medicine, ed 19, Philadelphia, 1992, WB Saunders.

Nathan DG: Introduction to hematologic diseases. In Wyngaarden JB and others, editors: Cecil textbook of medicine, ed 19, Philadelphia, 1992, WB Saunders.

Sears DA: Iron deficiency. In Rakel RE, editor: Conn's current therapy, Philadelphia, 1991, WB Saunders.

Tsevat J and others: Neonatal screening for sickle cell disease: a cost effectiveness analysis, J Pediatrics 118(4, pt 1):546-554, April 1991.

Williams WJ and others: Hematology, ed 4, New York, 1990, McGraw-Hill.

Chapter 11

DIAGNOSTIC STUDIES USED IN THE ASSESSMENT OF THE

SKELETAL SYSTEM

ANATOMY AND PHYSIOLOGY

The skeletal system (Figure 11-1) consists of a framework of bones whose main purpose is to support the tissues of the body, protect delicate internal organs, and facilitate movement. Bones also serve as a reservoir for calcium, magnesium, phosphorus, sodium, and other ions necessary for a variety of homeostatic functions. Hematopoiesis, which is the production of blood cells (see Chapter 10), is another important function of the bone.

Bones are classified according to shape.

Long bones. Long bones are found in the extremities. Examples include the bones of the upper and lower arm (humerus, ulna); and bones of the thigh and leg (femur, tibia, and fibula); and bones of the fingers and toes (phalanges). They are called long bones because their length is greater than their breadth.

Short bones. Examples of these are the wrist and ankle bones (carpals and tarsals).

Flat bones. These bones have a large surface area and provide protection for soft body parts. Examples are the frontal and parietal bones of the cranium, the ribs, the sternum, the scapulae, the ilium, and the pubis.

Irregular bones. These are bones of various shapes and compositions, which include the bones of the spinal column (such as the vertebrae, sacrum, coccyx) and certain skull bones (such as the mandible).

Histologically, bones are composed of cancellous (spongy) and compact (dense) bone. Red marrow, which produces blood cells, occupies the spaces of cancellous bone. Compact bone is strong and dense with many networks of interconnecting canals called haversian systems. A haversian canal runs centrally through each system, parallel to the bone's long axis, and contains one or two blood vessels, which supply most of the bone's blood. Bones have an intergenerative membrane called the marrow cavity. Yellow marrow is present in the shafts of the long bones and extends into the haversian system. Yellow marrow is composed of adipose cells and can change to red marrow if necessary to produce blood cells.

A typical long bone consists of the following structures: periosteum, diaphysis, epiphyses, articular cartilage, medullary (or marrow) cavity, and endosteum (Figure 11-2).

Periosteum. The periosteum is the dense,

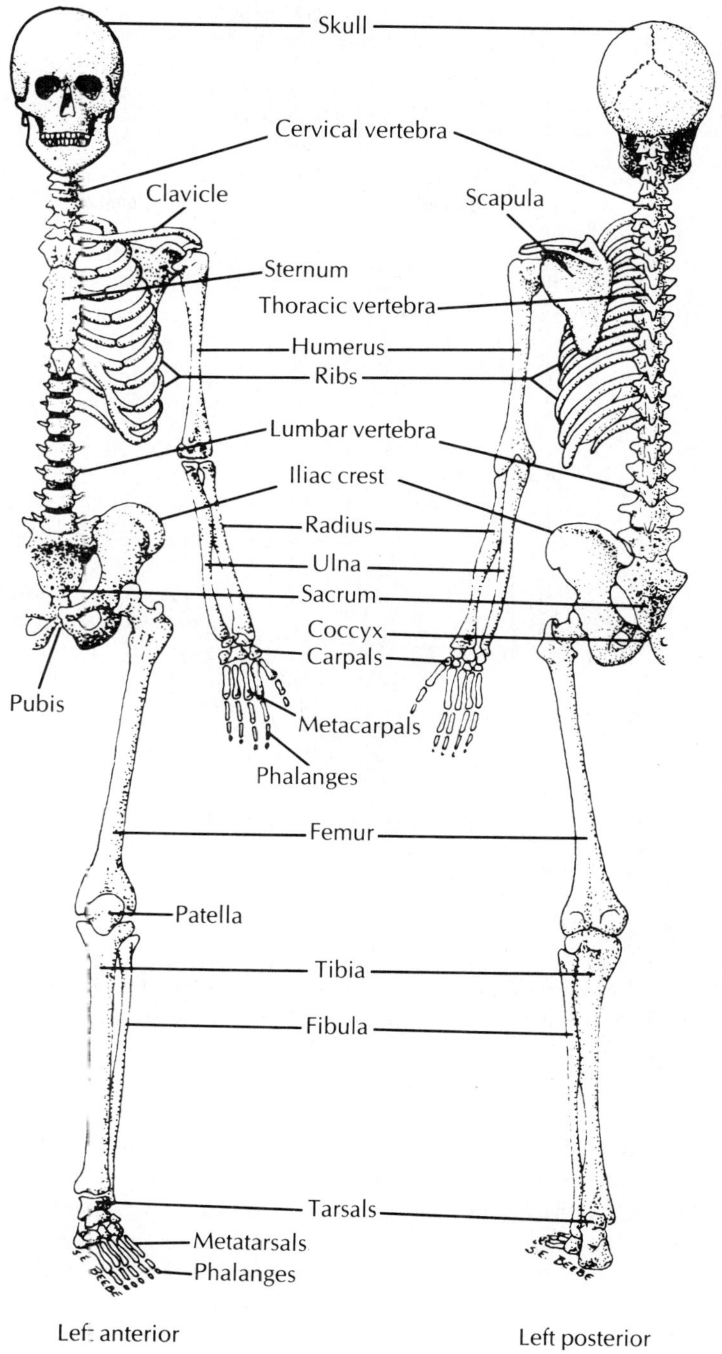

FIGURE 11-1. Musculoskeletal system.

From Tucker SM and others: Patient care standards, ed 3, St Louis, 1984, Mosby–Year Book.

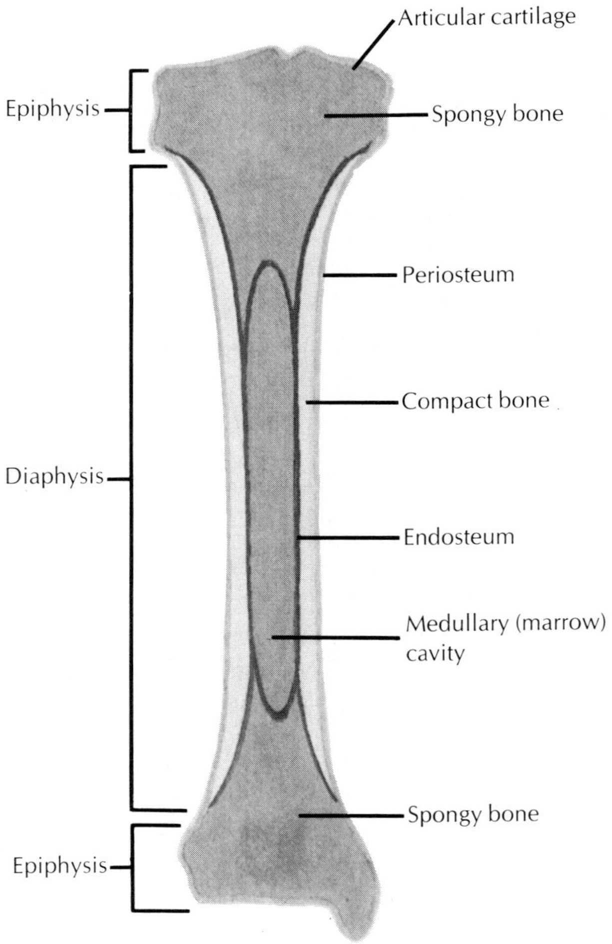

FIGURE 11-2. Structure of a long bone as seen in longitudinal section.
From Anthony CP and Thibodeau GA: Textbook of anatomy and physiology, ed 10, St Louis, 1979, Mosby–Year Book.

white, fibrous membrane that covers the bone except at the joint surface where the articular cartilage forms a covering. Periosteum contains many blood vessels and numerous osteoblasts, which are bone-forming cells. In children the periosteum produces new bone easily. Because the periosteum regenerates slowly in adults, fractures heal more slowly than in children.

Diaphysis. The diaphysis is the main shaft-like portion of the bone.

Epiphyses. These cancellous portions are ends of the bone. Note their bulbous shape at the end of the bone.

Articular cartilage. This cartilage covers the articular or joint surface of the epiphyses. The resiliency of this material cushions the bone.

Medullary (marrow) cavity. This cavity is tubelike and contains marrow.

Endosteum. The endosteum is the membrane that lines the medullary cavity. In long bones the cancellous portions (epiphyses) are found in the ends of the bones. Short bones, flat

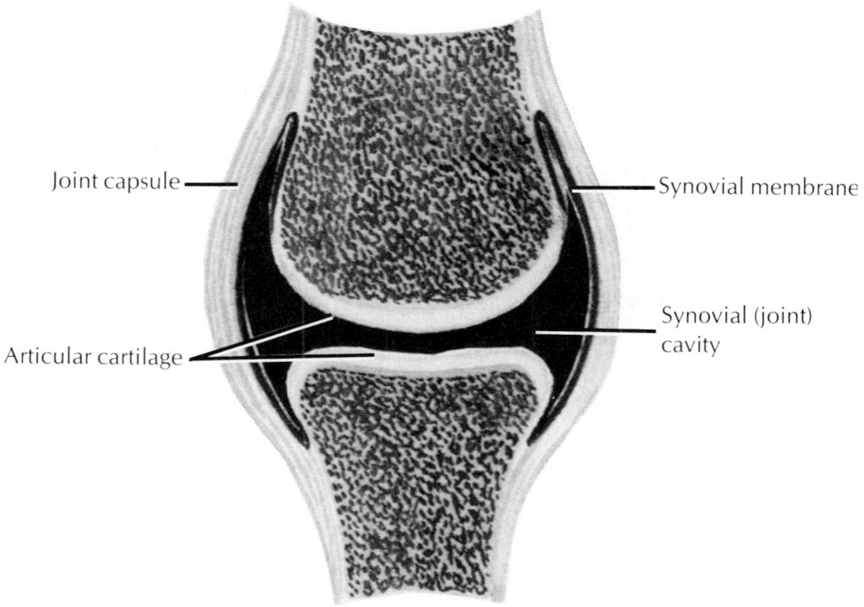

FIGURE 11-3. Structure of a diarthrotic joint.
From Anthony CP and Thibodeau GA: Textbook of anatomy and physiology, ed 10, St Louis, 1979, Mosby–Year Book.

bones, and irregular bones all have an inner portion of cancellous bone covered by an outside portion of compact bone.

Although the size and shape of the 208 bones in the human body vary greatly, bones are all subject to the same disease processes. Fractures, infections (osteomyelitis), tumors (osteogenic sarcoma), congenital defects (ranging from complete absence to extra limbs), demineralization (osteoporosis and osteomalacia), and acquired diseases (such as hyperparathyroidism and vitamin D insufficiency or deficiency) may involve and affect any of these bones.

A *joint* exists at the connection of two or more bones. Joints (articulations) hold the bones firmly to each other and permit movement between them. The three kinds of joints are classified according to their characteristic structural features. The *fibrous joints* are those in which the articular surface of two bones are connected by fibrous connective tissue that binds them closely and tightly. They allow only minute motion and provide stability when tight union is necessary (as in the sutures' joining of the skull's cranial bones). Cartilaginous joints are those in which cartilage joins one bone to another. They allow limited movement, as between the vertebrae. The majority of the body's articulations are *synovial* (or *diarthrodial*) *joints*, which provide free movement between two bones.

To achieve mobility, diarthrodial joints are of a complex structure (Figure 11-3). Each synovial joint contains a small space or *joint cavity* (synovial cavity) between the articulating surfaces of the bones that comprise the joint. The joint capsule completely encases the epiphyses and binds them to each other. Because no tissue grows between the articulating surfaces of the bones, the bones are free to move against one another. For this reason synovial joints are freely movable joints. The joint capsule is lined with a *synovial membrane,* which is a moist, slippery membrane that binds the inner surface of the joint capsule. The synovial membrane attaches to the margins of the articular cartilage and secretes synovial fluid, which lubricates and nourishes the inner joint surfaces. The *articular cartilage* is the hyaline cartilage that covers and cushions the articulating ends of the bones.

Ligaments are strong cords of dense, white, fibrous connective tissue that are present in some synovial joints to provide internal stability. Menisci are small pieces of dense cartilage that may be interposed between the articulating surfaces of two joints. The meniscus of the knee is most clinically significant, as it is most frequently injured in athletics.

The synovial membrane may become inflamed, granular, and eventually destroyed by ongoing arthritis. Common forms of arthritis include degenerative, which usually occurs in older age; rheumatoid, which can occur at any age; or infectious, which occurs as a result of direct bacterial contact. Similarly, the components of a joint can be involved in tumors, such as synovial cell sarcomas. Since the joints are supported by a series of fibrous ligaments, they can become partially or completely torn (minor or major sprains) when stressed.

CASE STUDY 1: KNEE INJURY

M.R., a 15-year-old gymnast, has noted increasing knee pain. This has become progressively worse during the last several months of intensive training for a state-wide gymnastic meet. Her physical examination indicated swelling in and around the left knee. She had some decreased range of motion and a clicking sound on flexion of the knee. The knee was otherwise stable.

Studies	Results
Routine laboratory values	WNL
Long bone (femur, fibula, and tibia) X-ray	No fracture
Arthrocentesis	
Appearance	Bloody (normal: clear and straw colored)
Mucin clot	Good (normal: good)
Fibrin clot	Small (normal: none)
WBC	<200 WBC/mm^3 (normal: <200 WBC/mm^3)
Neutrophils	<25% (WNL)
Glucose	100 mg/dl (normal: within 10 mg/dl of serum glucose level)
Arthrography	Small tear in medial meniscus of left knee
Arthroscopy	Tear in posterior aspect of medial meniscus

The x-ray studies of the long bones eliminated any possibility of fracture. Arthrocentesis indicated a bloody effusion, which was probably a result of trauma. The fibrin clot was further evidence of bleeding within the joint. Arthrography indicated a tear of the medial meniscus of the knee, a common injury for gymnasts. Arthroscopy corroborated that finding. Transarthroscopic medial meniscectomy was performed. Her postoperative course was uneventful.

DISCUSSION OF TESTS

X-ray examinations of the long bones

Normal values: no evidence of fracture, tumor, infection, or congenital abnormalities

Rationale. X-ray examinations of the long bones are usually taken when the patient complains about a particular body area. Fractures (Figure 11-4) or tumors are readily detected by x-ray studies. In patients who have a severe or chronic infection overlying a bone, an x-ray film may detect an infection involving that bone (osteomyelitis). X-ray studies of the long bones are also capable of detecting joint destruction (Figure 11-5) and bone spurring as a result of persistent arthritis. Growth patterns can be followed by a serial x-ray study of a long bone (usually of the wrist and hands). Healing of a fracture can also be documented and followed.

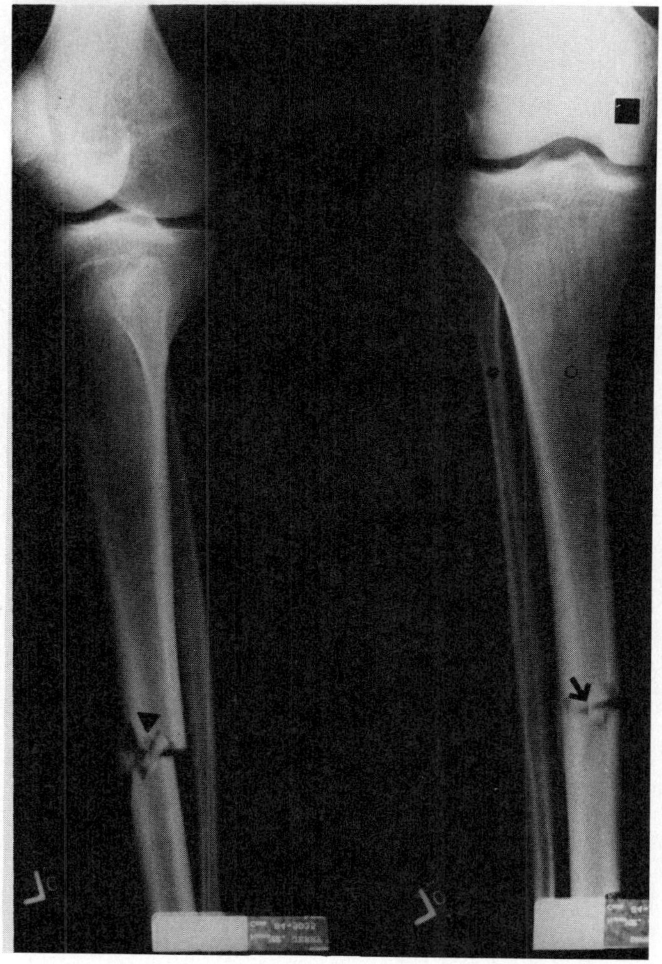

FIGURE 11-4. X-ray film of tibia and fibula. Left side of photograph is lateral view of tibia and fibula. Solid pointer indicates fracture. Right side of photograph indicates the same patient with a posterior-anterior view. Solid square indicates distal femur. Solid circle indicates fibula. Circle outline indicates tibia. Arrow indicates anterior-posterior view of tibia fracture.

X-ray films of the joints may reveal an abnormal collection of fluid in or around the joint.

Procedure. No fasting or sedation is required before x-ray examination of the long bones. The patient is asked to place the involved extremity in several positions; an x-ray picture is taken in each one. No discomfort or complications are associated with this test. This test is routinely performed in the radiology department by an x-ray technician in several minutes.

Contraindications. None.

Nursing considerations

Nursing Diagnoses/Collaborative Problems

See X-ray studies, p. 5.

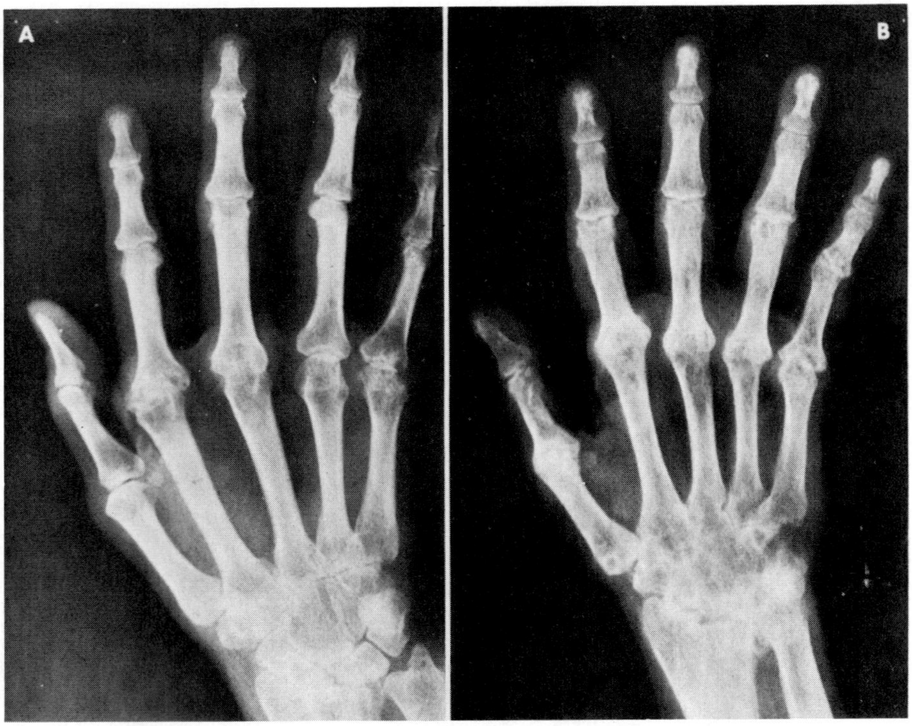

FIGURE 11-5. Roentgenograms of rheumatoid arthritis in the hand and wrist. **A,** Moderate changes ranging from atrophic bone areas and narrowed cartilage spaces to subluxation of second and third metacarpophalangeal joints. **B,** More advanced case with severe destructive changes, including multiple subluxations in the digits and ankyloses in the carpus.

From Brashear HR and Raney RB: Shands' handbook of orthopaedic surgery, ed 9, St Louis, 1978, Mosby–Year Book.

Nursing Implications with Rationale

- Explain the procedure to the patient. Carefully handle any injured parts of the body.
- Explain to the patient that holding the extremity still while the x-ray film is being taken is important. This can sometimes be difficult, especially when the patient has severe pain associated with a recent injury.
- Shield the patient's testes, ovaries, or pregnant abdomen during the procedure to avoid exposure from scatter radiation.
- Although no pain is associated with these x-ray examinations, many patients (especially those with arthritis) are extremely uncomfortable lying on a hard x-ray table.
- Young children requiring x-ray examinations are usually frightened by the large equipment and by the fear of being isolated from their parents. Check the radiology department's policy on allowing parents (protected with lead shielding) to accompany the child during the procedure.

Arthrocentesis with synovial fluid analysis

(synovial fluid analysis, joint aspiration)

Normal values: synovial fluid is clear and straw-colored with few white blood cells, no crystals, and a good mucin clot. Chemical test values (such as glucose determination) should approximate those found in the bloodstream

Rationale. Arthrocentesis is performed by inserting a sterile needle into a joint space (most commonly the knee) to obtain a specimen of synovial fluid for analysis. Synovial fluid (see Anatomy and physiology) is a liquid found in small amounts in the joints. The joint aspiration (withdrawal of the fluid) may be obtained from the knee, shoulder, hip, elbow, wrist, or ankle.

Arthrocentesis is performed for many different reasons, such as to establish the diagnosis of infection, crystal-induced arthritis, synovitis, or neoplasms involving the joint. This procedure is also done to identify the cause of joint effusion, to follow the progression of joint disease, and to inject antiinflammatory medications (most commonly corticosteroids) into a joint area.

A culture of the sample of synovial fluid is taken; the sample is also examined microscopically and chemically. Normal joint fluid is clear, straw-colored, and quite viscous because of hyaluronic acid. Viscosity is reduced in patients with an inflammatory type of arthritis. Viscosity can be grossly evaluated by forcing synovial fluid from a syringe. Fluid of high viscosity forms a "string" several inches long, in contrast to fluid of low viscosity, which drips like water. The mucin clot test correlates with the viscosity. The test is performed by adding acetic acid to joint fluid. The formation of a tight, ropy clot indicates qualitatively good mucin and the presence of adequate molecules of intact hyaluronic acid. Mucin clot is poor in quality and quantity in inflammatory joint diseases, such as rheumatoid arthritis. Synovial fluid should not form a fibrin clot because normal joint fluid does not contain fibrinogen. The fluid will clot only if blood entered the joint during the aspiration or in the presence of an inflammatory effusion.

The synovial fluid glucose value is usually within 10 ml/dl of the serum glucose value. For proper interpretation the synovial fluid glucose and the serum glucose samples should be drawn simultaneously after the patient has fasted for 6 hours. Synovial fluid glucose level falls with increasing inflammation. In septic arthritis the synovial fluid glucose value may be less than 50% of the serum glucose value. A low synovial glucose level may also be seen in patients with rheumatoid arthritis.

Cell counts should also be done on the synovial fluid. Normally the joint fluid contains less than 200 WBC/mm^3. A very high percentage of neutrophils (over 75%) is found in most cases of untreated acute bacterial infectious arthritis.

Acid-fast stains for tubercle bacilli are also performed on the synovial fluid. Bacterial and fungal cultures are obtained when these diseases are suspected. Gonococci are a major cause of joint infection. Previous antibiotic therapy reduces the chance of diagnosis by culture. Synovial fluid is also examined under polarized light for the presence of crystals. This enables a differential diagnosis to be made between gout and pseudogout.

Synovial fluid can also be analyzed for complement levels. The complement level may be decreased in patients with systemic lupus erythematosus or rheumatoid arthritis. Decreased joint complement levels may be caused by consumption of complement by antigen-autoantibody complexes in the joint cavity.

Complications of arthrocentesis include joint infection and hemorrhage into the joint area.

Procedure. For arthrocentesis the hospitalized patient may be asked to fast from midnight before the test. However, this study is often done either on an emergency basis or in a physician's office. If the patient does not fast, some of the chemical evaluations (such as glucose) may be altered from food. If glucose testing of the synovial fluid will not be performed, the patient need not restrict food intake before the test.

This procedure may also be performed at the patient's bedside. The patient lies on his or her back with the knee to be examined fully extended. The knee is then locally anesthetized to minimize pain. The area is meticulously cleansed since this procedure is done under strict sterile technique. A needle is then inserted through the skin and into the joint space. Fluid is obtained for analysis. Sometimes the joint area may be wrapped with an elastic bandage to compress free fluid into a certain area, enhancing the maximal collection of fluid.

If a corticosteroid is to be injected, a syringe containing the steroid preparation is attached to the needle and injected. The needle is then removed. Pressure or a pressure dressing is applied to the site. Sometimes a peripheral venous blood sample is taken after the study to compare chemical tests on the blood with chemical studies on the synovial fluid.

A physician performs this procedure in approximately 10 minutes. The only discomfort is that associated with injection of the local anesthetic.

Contraindications. This study is contraindicated in patients with skin or wound infections in the area of the needle puncture because of the risk of sepsis.

Nursing considerations

Nursing Diagnoses/Collaborative Problems

- Possible knowledge deficit related to test purpose, preparation and procedure
- Possible anxiety related to unknown sensations of the procedure
- Possible alteration in comfort related to test procedure
- Potential complication: hemorrhage
- Potential complication: joint infection

Nursing Implications with Rationale

- Explain the procedure to the patient. Ensure that the written and informed consent for this procedure is obtained.
- Before the study keep the patient NPO from midnight. This is done to prevent alterations of the chemical determinations (such as glucose) that may be performed with the study.
- After the study assess the joint for any pain, fever, or swelling, which may indicate infection. Apply ice to decrease pain and swelling. Keep a pressure dressing on the joint.
- After the study the patient will usually resume his or her usual activity. However, inform the patient that strenuous use of the joint should be avoided for the next several days.
- After the study check that the patient's normal diet is resumed.
- Send the specimen to the laboratory immediately after the procedure is completed. Collect all specimens in the appropriate containers. Add anticoagulants as indicated by the laboratory.

Arthrography

(arthrogram)

Normal values: normal bursae, menisci, ligaments, and articular cartilage of the joint

Rationale. Arthrography affords radiographic visualization of a joint after the injection of a radiopaque substance or air (or both) into the joint cavity to outline the soft tissue structures not normally seen on routine x-ray films. Bones with the meniscus, cartilage, and ligaments are clearly visualized with this procedure. Joint derangement and synovial cysts are also diagnosed with arthrography.

Arthrography is usually done on the knee and shoulder joints; however, it can also be done on other joints (such as the ankle, hip, wrists, or temporomandibular). This procedure is usually performed on patients with persistent, unexplained knee or shoulder pain. Arthography is done much less frequently now that arthroscopy and MRI scanning are available. These latter two studies are much more accurate in determining the extent of injury or disease involving the major joints.

Complications of this procedure may include infection at the puncture site or an allergic reaction to the contrast medium.

Procedure. No fasting or sedation is required for this procedure. The procedure is done under local anesthetic using sterile technique. The patient is placed in the supine position on an examining table. The skin overlying the desired joint is aseptically cleansed and anesthetized. The needle is then inserted into the joint space and fluid is aspirated to prevent dilution of the contrast agent and diminishment of the quality of the x-ray films. With the needle still in place, the aspirating syringe is removed and a syringe containing dye is replaced. The contrast agent or agents are then injected. The needle is removed, and the joint is manipulated to afford distribution of the contrast material. (The patient may be asked to walk a couple of steps or to pass the joint through a range-of-motion exercise.) X-ray films are then taken with the joint held in various positions.

A physician usually performs this procedure in approximately 30 minutes. The patient may feel pressure or a tingling sensation as the contrast medium is injected.

Contraindications. Arthrography is contraindicated in the pregnant patient and in patients with active arthritis, joint infection, or allergy to radiopaque material.

Nursing considerations

Nursing Diagnoses/Collaborative Problems

See X-ray studies, p. 5.

Nursing Implications with Rationale

- Explain the procedure to the patient. Obtain the written and informed consent forms for this procedure.
- Before the study ascertain whether the patient is allergic to iodine dye.
- After the study inform the patient that the joint is usually rested for at least 12 hours. Apply an elastic bandage to the involved joint and leave it in place for several days.
- If swelling occurs after the test, apply ice to the joint. Administer a mild analgesic, such as aspirin or acetaminophen (Tylenol), if the patient has minor discomfort. Report any increase in pain or swelling to the physician.
- Inform the patient that crepitant noises in the joint may be heard after the test. These symptoms are normal and usually disappear in 1 to 2 days. The noise is a result of the air that was injected into the joint during the procedure.

Arthroscopy

Normal values: normal ligaments, menisci, and articular surfaces of the joints

Rationale. Arthroscopy is an endoscopic procedure that allows examination of the interior of a joint with a specially designed endoscope. Endoscopy is a highly accurate test because it allows direct visualization of the anatomic site. Although this technique can visualize many joints of the body, it is most commonly used to evaluate the knee for meniscus cartilage or ligament tears. It is also used in the differential diagnosis of acute and chronic disorders of the knee. Physicians can now perform corrective surgery on the knee through the endoscope. Arthroscopy, thus, provides a safe, convenient alternative to open surgery (arthrotomy). Arthroscopy is also used to monitor the progression of disease and the effectiveness of therapy. Visual findings may be recorded by attaching a camera to the arthroscope. Arthroscopy is commonly done on knee, shoulder, and wrist joints.

Complications are rare with this procedure, but may include infection, hemarthrosis, swelling, thrombophlebitis, joint injury, and synovial rupture.

Procedure. For this study the patient must be kept NPO after midnight on the day of the procedure. This procedure is commonly performed with the patient under spinal or general anesthesia, especially when knee surgery is anticipated.

Before knee arthroscopy hair in the area 6 inches above and below the joint is removed by shaving or by a depilatory creme. The patient is placed on his or her back on an operating table. The patient's leg is then carefully, surgically scrubbed, elevated, and wrapped with an elastic bandage from the toes to the lower thigh to drain as much blood from the leg as possible. A tourniquet is then placed on the patient's leg. If a tourniquet is not used, a fluid solution may be instilled into the patient's knee immediately before insertion of the arthroscope to distend the knee and help reduce bleeding.

The foot of the table is then lowered so that the patient's knee is approximately at a 45° angle. The elastic bandage is opened. A small incision is made in the skin of the knee. The arthroscope (a lightened instrument) is then inserted in and out of the joint space to visualize the inside of the knee joint. Although the entire joint can be viewed from one puncture site, making additional punctures for better visualization is often necessary. After the area is examined, biopsy or appropriate surgery can be performed and the arthroscope is removed. The joint is then irrigated clean. Pressure is applied to the knee to remove the irrigating solution. After a few stitches are placed into the skin, a pressure dressing is applied over the incision site.

This procedure is performed in an operating room by an orthopedic surgeon. The total examining time is approximately 15 to 30 minutes. There is moderate joint pain postoperatively.

Contraindications. Arthroscopy is contraindicated in patients with ankylosis because it is almost impossible to maneuver the instrument into a joint stiffened by adhesions. This procedure is also contraindicated in patients with local skin or wound infections because of the risk of sepsis.

Nursing considerations

Nursing Diagnoses/Collaborative Problems

See Endoscopy procedures, p. 6–7.

- Potential complication: infection
- Potential complication: hemarthrosis
- Potential complication: thrombophlebitis
- Potential complication: joint injury
- Potential complication: synovial rupture

Nursing Implications with Rationale

- Explain this procedure to the patient. Follow the routine preoperative procedure. Keep the patient NPO after midnight on the day of the study.
- Ensure that the physician has obtained the written consent form.
- Before the procedure many orthopedic surgeons recommend that the patient learn the appropriate crutch gait. Check the surgeon and inform the patient. (Crutches should be used after arthroscopy until he or she can walk without limping.)
- After the procedure take the vital signs frequently according to hospital routine. Assess the neurovascular status of the affected leg by checking pulses, color, temperature, and sensation. Observe the patient for signs of infection, which include fever, swelling, increased pain, and redness or drainage at the incision site. After the procedure administer a mild analgesic, such as aspirin or acetaminophen (Tylenol), if needed.
- After the study instruct the patient to elevate the knee when sitting and to avoid twisting the knee.
- After the procedure the patient can usually walk with crutches. However, this depends on the extent of the procedure and the physician's protocol. Do not allow excessive use of the joint for several days. The patient should be taught isometric quadriceps exercises and be instructed to perform them per the physician's protocol.
- After the study examine the incision site for bleeding; apply ice to reduce pain and swelling.
- Check that the patient resumes a normal diet after the study.
- Tell the patient that the sutures will be removed in approximately 7 days.

SUPPLEMENTAL INFORMATION

Uric acid test

Normal values:
Serum:
Adult: male, 2.1-8.5 mg/dl, or
0.15-0.48 mmol/L (SI units)
female, 2.0-6.6 mg/dl, or
0.09-0.36 mmol/L (SI units)
Elderly: values may be slightly increased
Child: 2.5-5.5 mg/dl, or 0.12-0.32 mmol/L
Newborn: 2.0-6.2 mg/dl
Possible critical values: >12 mg/dl
Urine: 250-750 mg/24 hour

Rationale. Uric acid is a nitrogenous compound that is a product of purine (DNA building block) catabolism. It is excreted in a large degree by the kidney and to a smaller degree by the intestinal tract. When the uric acid levels are elevated (hyperuricemia), the patient may have gout. Causes of hyperuricemia can be overproduction or decreased excretion of uric acid (such as kidney failure). Overproduction of uric acid may occur in patients who have a catabolic enzyme deficiency that through feedback mechanisms stimulates purine metabolism. In patients with cancer the purine and DNA turnover is great, again causing high levels of uric acid. Other causes of hyperuricemia may include alcoholism, hyperlipoproteinemia, diabetes mellitus, renal failure, stress, lead poisoning, and dehydration caused by diuretic therapy. Ketoacids (as occur in diabetic or alcoholic ketoacidosis) may compete with uric acid for tubular excretion and can cause decreased uric acid excretion. Many causes of hyperuricemia production go undefined and are therefore labeled as *idiopathic.* Drugs such as diuretics, salicylates, nicotinic acid, levodopa, and diazoxide can cause hyperuricemia. A diet high in purines can cause high uric acid and precipitate a gouty attack.

Increased serum levels may be clinically associated with gout, arthritis, soft tissue deposits of uric acid (tophi), and uric acid kidney stones. Decreased uric acid levels are not associated with any clinical symptoms and are usually the result of poor liver function.

Routine performance of multiphasic blood analysis studies have permitted the early detection of increased levels of uric acid in patients who have no symptoms of gout. This allows the physician to treat the disease at an early stage; however, this is controversial because many physicians do not treat asymptomatic hyperuricemia. Uric acid levels can also be evaluated by a 24-hour urine specimen study.

Procedure. This test is usually included in any multiphasic automated systems analysis of the blood. Some hospitals require that the patient be fasting. Usually for these multiphasic analysis studies, two red-top tubes of blood are obtained from a peripheral vein.

Urine studies require the collection of a 24-hour urine specimen.

Contraindications. None.

Nursing considerations

Nursing Diagnoses/Collaborative Problems

See Blood studies, p. 2, and Urine studies, p. 3.

Nursing Implications with Rationale

- Explain the procedure to the patient. Follow the hospital requirements regarding fasting. Prevent hemolysis of the blood sample.
- After the blood study examine the venipuncture site for bleeding and hematoma formation.
- Check the information on 24-hour urine specimens described on p. 231 of creatinine clearance tests (see all but the first and last nursing implications).
- If the uric acid levels are high, instruct the patient to avoid foods high in purine, such as liver, kidney, heart, brain, sweet breads, sardines, anchovies, and mince meat. Foods that contain a moderate amount of purine nitrogens include poultry, fish, asparagus, mushrooms, peas, and spinach.
- Instruct patients with elevated uric acid levels to decrease their alcohol intake because alcohol causes renal retention of urate.

QUESTIONS AND ANSWERS

1. **QUESTION:** Mr. and Mrs. P. brought their crying 3-year-old daughter into the emergency room because she fell off a seesaw and landed on her shoulder. Because of the child's complaints of pain in the clavicle area, a fractured clavicle was the suspected diagnosis. The child was extremely frightened by the thought of an x-ray examination, and Mrs. P. insisted on accompanying her daughter during the procedure. What is the appropriate intervention in this situation?

   ANSWER: Because of exposure from scattered radiation during the x-ray procedure, you should first find out if Mrs. P is pregnant. If Mrs. P is not currently menstruating, you should suggest that Mr. P don a lead apron and accompany his daughter during this procedure.

2. **QUESTION:** Your 17-year-old male patient is scheduled for a knee arthroscopy in the morning. When you go into his room to shave the knee 6 inches above and below the joint, you note that the knee is red and swollen. Should the arthroscopy be canceled?

   ANSWER: Notify the physician. The procedure may be canceled because of the possibility of infection in the knee, which is a contraindication to arthroscopy because of the possibility of sepsis.

3. **QUESTION:** Your 62-year-old female patient has had an arthrocentesis of her right knee and an injection of steroids 2 days ago. She now complains of pain in the right knee, which she describes as worse than the initial symptoms. What is the appropriate nursing intervention?

   ANSWER: Having severe pain 48 hours after arthrocentesis is unusual. However, with the injection of steroids a temporary chemical arthritis frequently occurs. This often lasts from 1 to 3 days. The patient should be reassured of this possibility, and the physician should be contacted to prescribe an appropriate pain medication.

4. **QUESTION:** Your 55-year-old male patient was admitted to the hospital with complaints of a high temperature of unknown etiology. Initial orders called for blood, urine, and sputum cultures. During your nursing history, you detected that the patient had an arthrogram 3 days ago because of complaints of unexplained shoulder pain. What is the appropriate intervention?

   ANSWER: Septic arthritis is a known complication of arthrography. Notify the physician of the patient's recent arthrogram. The physician will probably order an arthrocentesis to identify the causative agent. The infection is then treated with the appropriate antibiotic.

5. **QUESTION:** Your 5-year-old patient fell during play therapy and injured his right arm. You notify the physician who requests an x-ray examination of both arms. Why should both arms be included in the x-ray examination?

   ANSWER: Fracture lines of the long bones in children are often difficult to distinguish from normal growth lines in x-ray film. If the suspicious line is seen in the x-ray film of both arms, one can be confident that a fracture did not occur. However, if the suspicious line is unilateral, a fracture is strongly suspected.

BIBLIOGRAPHY

Arnett FC: Rheumatoid arthritis. In Wyngaarden JB and others, editors: Cecil textbook of medicine, ed 19, Philadelphia, 1992, WB Saunders.

Bellamy N, Buchanan W: Clinical evaluation in rheumatic diseases. In McCarty DJ: Arthritis and allied conditions: a textbook of rheumatology, ed 11, Philadelphia, 1989, Lea and Febiger.

Baum J, Morris Z: Laboratory findings in rheumatoid arthritis. In McCarty DJ, editor: Arthritis and allied conditions: a textbook of rheumatology, ed 11, Philadelphia, 1989, Lea and Febiger.

Brandt KD, Kovalov-St. John K: Osteomyelitis. In Wilson J and others, editors: Harrison's principles of internal medicine, ed 12, New York, 1991, McGraw-Hill.

Cush JJ, Lipsky PE: Approaches to articular and musculoskeletal disorders. In Wilson J and others, editors: Harrison's principles of internal medicine, ed 12, New York, 1991, McGraw-Hill.

Fries JF: Approach to the patient with musculoskeletal disease. In Wyngaarden JB and others, editors: Cecil textbook of medicine, ed 19, Philadelphia, 1992, WB Saunders.

Halpern BC: Common sport injuries. In Rakel RE, editor: Conn's current therapy, Philadelphia, 1991, WB Saunders.

Jenkins DB: Hollinshead's functional anatomy of the limbs and back, ed 6, Philadelphia, 1991, WB Saunders.

Krane SM, Holic MF: Metabolic bone disease. In Wilson J and others, editors: Harrison's principles of internal medicine, ed 12, New York, 1991, McGraw-Hill.

Lance NJ, Ellman MH: Rheumatoid arthritis. In Rakel RE, editor: Conn's current therapy, Philadelphia, 1991, WB Saunders.

Macfarlane DG and others: Comparison of clinical, radionuclide, and radiographic features of osteoarthritis of the hands, Ann Rheum Dis 50(9):623-626, Sept 1991.

Malawista SE: Lyme disease. In McCarty DJ: Arthritis and allied conditions: a textbook of rheumatology, ed 11, Philadelphia, 1989, Lea and Febiger.

Marino C and others: Osteoarthritis and rheumatoid arthritis in elderly patients: differentiation and treatment, Postgrad Med 90(5):237-243, Oct 1991.

Maskowitz RW: Clinical and laboratory findings in osteoarthritis. In McCarty DJ: Arthritis and allied conditions: a textbook of rheumatology, ed 11, Philadelphia, 1989, Lea and Febiger.

McCarty DJ: Arthritis and allied conditions: a textbook of rheumatology, ed 11, Philadelphia, 1989, Lea and Febiger.

Neustadt DN and Neustadt N: Osteoarthritis. In Rakel RE, editor: Conn's current therapy, Philadelphia, 1991, WB Saunders.

Stalberg E: The value to the clinical neurologist of electromyography in the 1990s, Clin Exp Neurol 27:1-28, 1990.

Stoller DW and Genant HK: Magnetic resonance imaging of the joints. In McCarty DJ, editor: Arthritis and allied conditions: a textbook of rheumatology, ed 11, Philadelphia, 1989, Lea and Febiger.

Chapter 12

DIAGNOSTIC STUDIES USED IN THE ASSESSMENT OF DISEASES OF THE IMMUNE SYSTEM

Serologic tests are essentially studies used to diagnose and monitor diseases of the immune system. Often, these diseases are associated with antibodies directed against the connective tissue of the body. Therefore, these diseases are called connective tissue or collagen-vascular diseases. They are also often referred to as rheumatic diseases because musculoskeletal pain is a frequent manifestation. They all seem to be associated with production of an antibody that is directed against some component of the body. The various diseases within this group can be identified by performing several serologic tests and identifying the pattern most consistent with the disease suspected.

Systemic lupus erythematosus (SLE) and rheumatoid arthritis are the more common types of rheumatologic/immunologic diseases and are therefore discussed in the case studies. Many other diseases exist that are marked by the presence of antibodies that may cause false-positive serologic tests. These must be eliminated by other appropriate diagnostic testing.

Rheumatology deals with the study of joints and periarticular structures. Immunology studies the process involved in the recognition and protection of the body from foreign noxious elements. The immunologic system includes immunologic cells such as T and B lymphocytes, plasma cells, and other white blood cells (WBCs). Noncellular components, such as antibodies and the complement enzymatic system, are vitally important in the immunologic response. There are many variations of normal immunologic processes. Descriptions of these are beyond the scope of this text.

CASE STUDY 1: SYSTEMIC LUPUS ERYTHEMATOSUS

Mrs. R.D., 24 years old, had been complaining of multiple joint and muscular pains with some stiffness in the morning. She had also noted some hair loss and had complained of an increased skin sensitivity to light. Her physical examination showed slight erythema around the cheek bones and some swelling in the joints of her hands.

Studies	**Results**
Routine laboratory	WNL, except for a mild anemia
Urinalysis (see Chapter 7)	Profuse proteinuria and cellular casts
Lupus erythematosus (LE) cell prep	LE cells present (normal value: no LE cells present)
Antinuclear antibody	Positive, titer of 1:256
Sedimentation rate (normal value: negative)	75 mm/hour (normal: up to 20 mm/hour)
Immunoglobulin electrophoresis	IgG 1910 mg/dl (normal: 565-1,765 mg/dl)
	IgA 450 mg/dl (normal: 85-385 mg/dl)
	IgM 475 mg/dl (normal: 55-375 mg/dl)
Total complement assay	22 hemolytic U/ml (normal: 41-90 hemolytic U/ml)
Anti-DNA antibody test	High titer (normal: low titer or none)

The positive antinuclear antibody, LE cell prep, and positive anti-DNA antibody test strongly supported the diagnosis of SLE. She also had a facial rash suggestive of SLE. The elevated sedimentation rate indicated a systemic inflammatory process. The immunoelectrophoresis was compatible with either rheumatoid arthritis or SLE. However, a decreased complement assay is commonly associated with SLE. The abnormal urinalysis indicated that the kidneys were also involved with the disease process. The patient was treated with steroids and did quite well for 7 years. Unfortunately, her renal function deteriorated, and she required chronic renal dialysis.

DISCUSSION OF TESTS

Lupus erythematosus cell prep

(lupus erythematosus test)

Normal value: no LE cells seen

Rationale. The LE cell prep is a serologic test used in the diagnosis of SLE. Of the patients with active SLE, 70% to 80% have a positive LE prep. Patients with SLE have antibodies against the constituents of nuclei within the patient's own cells. LE preps are usually performed by traumatizing WBCs to expose nuclear material. This material is then incubated with the patient's serum, and the WBCs (neutrophils) in the serum phagocytize the nuclear material. This complex looks like a round amorphous mass. When stained with Wright's stain, the phagocytized amorphous mass appears as blue-staining bodies in the cytoplasm of the white cell. These cells are called LE cells.

The test is not only used to diagnose SLE but is also used to monitor its treatment. No LE cells should be seen several weeks after successful treatment for SLE. Sometimes positive LE cell preps persist despite successful treatment. Some feel that the severity of SLE is related to the number of LE cells present.

Certain drugs may cause false-positive LE cell preps; the most commonly used are dilantin, isoniazid, procainamide, and hydralazine. Steroids may tend to suppress LE cell production in patients with SLE. Because no LE cells may appear on a prep one day and many on the succeeding day, most physicians order LE preps daily for 3 days. In normal patients no LE cells are present. The anti-DNA antibody test (see p. 438) may be more specific in detecting SLE and other connective tissue diseases.

Procedure. Seven milliliters of blood are drawn into a red-top tube via a venipuncture. WBCs are traumatized to damage the nuclei, which are converted to hematoxylin bodies. They are then incubated with the patient's serum. The combination is placed on a slide, stained with Wright's stain, and examined by the pathologist for the presence of LE cells. This study is no more uncomfortable than a simple venipuncture. No pretechnique preparation is required. No complications to the study exist.

Contraindications. None.

Nursing considerations

Nursing Diagnoses/Collaborative Problems

See Blood studies, p. 2.

Nursing Implications with Rationale

- Describe the study to the patient.
- Ensure that the patient is not taking any of the drugs known to interfere with the test.
- Check the venipuncture site for bleeding because patients with autoimmune diseases may have prolonged bleeding times.
- Because a patient with SLE has immunologic disorders, he or she is at risk for infection. Be sure the patient understands the signs of infection that may occur at the venipuncture site. Instruct the patient to notify the physician if any of these signs are recognized.

Antinuclear antibody test

(ANA)

Normal value: no antinuclear antibodies (ANA) detected in a titer of greater than a dilution of 1:32

Rationale. Many abnormal antibodies exist in patients with autoimmune diseases. ANA is a protein antibody that reacts against cellular nuclear material. The ANA is quite sensitive in detecting SLE; positive results occur in approximately 95% of the patients with this disease. However, many other disorders, such as Sjögren's syndrome, rheumatoid arthritis, cirrhosis, and myositis, can cause false-positive ANA tests. As a result, the ANA is quite sensitive but not very specific. When a patient has a positive LE prep and a positive ANA test, SLE is strongly suspected. Oftentimes the ANA is used as a screening test for patients with SLE. If the ANA is negative, chances are that the patient does not have SLE. Unlike LE prep, ANA titer is not affected by steroids, and decreasing titers indicate true clinical remission of the disease.

The test is usually performed by combining the patient's serum with nuclear material derived from rat's liver or other such tissues. Fluorescein-labeled antihuman serum is then mixed with the patient's serum and the nuclear material of the rat's liver. The preparation is then examined under an ultraviolet microscope for fluorescent ANAs. The patient's serum is serially diluted, and the antinuclear test is carried out with each dilution. The most dilute serum in which the ANA are detected is called the titer. The test is considered positive if ANAs are found in a titer greater than a dilution of 1:32.

Procedure. Seven milliliters of blood are obtained by venipuncture and placed in a red-top tube. The patient's serum is then incubated with the traumatized rat's liver tissue to obtain the antinuclear immune complex. This is then incubated with fluorescein-labeled antihuman serum, which tags any immune complex with fluorescein. It is examined under an ultraviolet microscope. As stated before, the serum is serially diluted for titer quantitation. The pattern of nuclear fluorescence is also documented by the pathologist examining the specimen, since it is considered to be equally important in determining whether the patient has SLE or other autoimmune diseases. No complications are associated with this test. Like LE prep, many drugs and other diseases may cause false-positive ANA tests.

Contraindications. None.

Nursing considerations

Nursing Diagnoses/Collaborative Problems

See Blood studies, p. 2.

Nursing Implications with Rationale

- See LE prep (previous study).

Immunoglobulin electrophoresis

(gammaglobulin electrophoresis)

Normal values:
IgG: 565-1765 mg/dl
IgA: 85-385 mg/dl
IgM: 55-375 mg/dl
IgD and IgE: minimal

Rationale. Antibodies are also called gamma globulins or immunoglobulins. There are many classes of immunoglobulins. IgG comprises about 75% of the serum immunoglobulins; therefore, it constitutes the majority of antibodies. IgA constitutes about 15% of the immunoglobulins and is present primarily in the secretions of the gastrointestinal tract, saliva, and tears. IgM is an immunoglobulin primarily responsible for ABO blood grouping and rheumatoid factor. IgE is an immunoglobulin that often mediates an allergic response; it is used to detect allergic diseases. IgD constitutes the smallest portion of the immunoglobulins and is rarely evaluated. Patients with autoimmune disorders often have an increased quantity of immunoglobulins, which can be seen as an increased gamma globulin spike on the electrophoresis strip. This study is also used to diagnose multiple myeloma, macroglobulinemia, and hypergammaglobulinemias or hypogammaglobulinemias. Disorders such as hepatitis and cirrhosis are also associated with abnormalities seen on immunoglobulin profile. There are no complications associated with this test.

Procedure. Seven milliliters of blood are obtained by venipuncture and placed in a red-top tube. The serum is placed on a slide containing agar gel, and an electric current is passed through the gel. The immunoglobulins then separate according to the quantity and difference in electric charges. Specific antisera are placed alongside the slide to identify the specific type of immunoglobulin. In some laboratories the patient is asked to refrain from eating 12 hours before the blood sample is obtained. Drugs, such as those described in the LE prep study, can affect the quantity of immunoglobulins.

Contraindications. None.

Nursing considerations

Nursing Diagnoses/Collaborative Problems

See Blood studies, p. 2.

Nursing Implications with Rationale

- See LE prep (p. 435).

Complement assay

Normal values:
Total complement: 41-90 hemolytic U
C_3: 70-176 mg/dl
C_4: 16-45 mg/dl

Rationale. Serum complements comprise a group of globulin proteins that act as enzymes. These enzymes facilitate the immunologic and inflammatory response. Complement increases vascular permeability, thereby allowing antibodies and WBCs to be delivered to the area of inflammation. Complement also acts to increase chemotaxis (pulling of WBCs to the area of infection), phagocytosis, and immune adherence of the antibody to antigen. These processes are vitally important in the inflammatory response.

Serum complement levels are important in the detection of autoimmune diseases, such as lupus erythematosus and serum sickness. In these types of illnesses, the complement assays are decreased secondary to consumption of the complement created by the development of the "autoimmune complexes" (that is, antibody-antigen complexes). Normal complement levels are between 41 and 90 hemolytic units. Two particular components (C_3 and C_4) are often assayed along with the total complement level. C_3 and C_4 are more accurate in detecting the previously described diseases and in following the course of the disease.

Procedure. Seven milliliters of blood are obtained by venipuncture and placed in a red-top tube. It is mixed with antibody-coated sheep red blood cells (RBCs). When complement is present in normal quantities, 50% of the RBCs are lysed. No pretechnique preparation is needed. There are no complications associated with this test.

Contraindications. None.

Nursing considerations

Nursing Diagnoses/Collaborative Problems

See Blood studies, p. 2

Nursing Implications with Rationale

- See LE prep (p. 435).

Anti-DNA antibody test

(antibody to double-stranded DNA, anti-double-stranded DNA, anti-ds-DNA, DNA antibody, native double-stranded DNA)

Normal values: Low levels of antibody or none (units depend upon laboratory and methodology)

Rationale. The anti-ds-DNA test is done to confirm the diagnosis of SLE (systemic lupus erythematosus). This antibody is found in approximately 40% to 80% of patients with SLE and rarely in other diseases. High titers are characteristic of SLE; low titers may be found in other rheumatic diseases and also in patients with chronic hepatitis, infectious mononucleosis, and biliary cirrhosis. The anti-DNA titer may decrease with successful therapy but may increase with an exacerbation of SLE, and especially with the onset of glomerulonephritis.

Procedure. Peripheral venipuncture is performed and one red-top tube of blood is collected.

Contraindications. None.

Nursing considerations

Nursing Diagnosis/Collaborative Problems

See Blood studies p. 2.

Nursing Implications with Rationale

- After the venipuncture is obtained, assess the site for bleeding.

CASE STUDY 2: RHEUMATOID ARTHRITIS

Mrs. J.D., 46 years old, had been complaining of bilateral knee and hand pain for 2 years that had become progressively worse. She had also noted subcutaneous nodules about the elbow and knees. Her physical examination showed some ulnar deviation of the digits and swelling of the metacarpal phalangeal and proximal interphalangeal joints. There were also signs of acute inflammation and some instability of both knees. The condition of the right knee was worse than that of the left.

Studies	Results
Routine laboratory studies	WNL, except for mild anemia
Rheumatoid factor	Titer 1:320 (normal value: none)
C-reactive protein	4 mg/dl (normal value: <0.8 mg/dl)
HLA-B27 antigen	Negative
X-ray examination of the knee (see Chapter 11)	Marked destruction of both knees with joint narrowing
Synovial fluid analysis (see Chapter 11)	
Appearance	Turbid (normal value: clear)
Fibrin clot	Large (normal value: none)
Mucin clot	Fair to poor (normal value: good)
WBCs	8,000/mm^3 (normal values: <200)
Polymorphonuclear lymphocytes	80% (normal values: <25%)
Glucose level	60% (normal value: within 10 mg/dl of serum glucose)

The presenting symptoms of the patient were physical findings compatible with rheumatoid arthritis. The x-ray films of the knee joint confirmed the significant joint destruction. Her rheumatoid factor and C-reactive protein were markedly positive. Synovial fluid analysis corroborated the findings of rheumatoid arthritis. The HLA antigen was negative, thereby eliminating ankylosing spondylitis or Reiter's syndrome. The patient was given an aggressive antiarthritic regimen and aggressive physical therapy. She improved markedly and was able to enjoy a relatively normal life.

DISCUSSION OF TESTS

Rheumatoid factor test

Normal value: negative (<60 U/ml by nephelometric testing)

Rationale. The rheumatoid factor test is useful in the diagnosis of rheumatoid arthritis. Other diseases, such as SLE, Sjögren's syndrome, scleroderma, and myositis, may cause a positive rheumatoid factor test. Rheumatoid factor is also occasionally seen in tuberculosis, chronic hepatitis, infectious mononucleosis, and subacute bacterial endocarditis. Drugs such as methyldopa are associated with positive rheumatoid factor titers. The elderly often have false-positive results.

Rheumatoid arthritis is a chronic inflammatory disease that affects most joints, especially the metacarpal phalangeal joint, the proximal interphalangeal joints, and the wrists, although any synovial joint may be involved. In this disease abnormal IgG antibodies produced by lymphocytes in the synovial membranes act as antigens. These antigens react with IgG and IgM antibodies to produce immune complexes. These immune complexes can activate the complement system and other inflammatory systems to cause joint damage. It is the reactive IgM molecule that is the rheumatoid factor. Tissues other than the joints, including blood vessels, lungs, nerves, and heart, may also be involved in rheumatoid arthritis.

Tests for rheumatoid factor are directed toward identification of the IgM antibodies. Eighty percent of the patients with rheumatoid arthritis have positive rheumatoid factor titers. To be considered positive the rheumatoid factor must be found in a dilution of greater than 1:80. When rheumatoid factor is found in titers <1:80, diseases such as SLE, scleroderma, and other autoimmune diseases should be considered. Although the normal value is no rheumatoid factor identifiable at low titers, a small number of normal patients have rheumatoid factor present at a very low titer. When the nephelometric testing procedure is used, the normal value is considered to be less than 60 U/ml. No complications are associated with this test.

Procedure. Seven milliliters of blood are obtained by venipuncture and placed in a red-top tube. Although there are many ways of detecting the rheumatoid factor, the sheep cell agglutination test or the latex fixation test is commonly performed to detect the rheumatoid factor. In the sheep cell agglutination test, rabbit IgG is placed on the sheep RBCs. When this is mixed with the patient's serum (which has been serially diluted), visual agglutination occurs if any rheumatoid factor is present. In the latex fixation test, human IgG is placed on a synthetic latex particle and mixed with the patient's serum. Visual agglutination is then detected. No specific preparation is required. As mentioned previously, the study may be done by the nephelometric procedure. This study is as uncomfortable as a normal venipuncture.

Contraindications. None.

Nursing considerations

Nursing Diagnoses/Collaborative Problems

See Blood studies, p. 2.

Nursing Implications with Rationale

- See LE prep (p. 435).

C-reactive protein test

(CRP)

Normal values: <0.8 mg/dl

Rationale. C-reactive protein (CRP) is a nonspecific acute-phase reactant used to diagnose infectious disease and inflammatory disorders, such as acute rheumatic fever and rheumatoid arthritis. CRP is a more sensitive and rapidly responding indicator than the erythrocyte sedimentation rate (ESR, see p. 444). In an acute inflammatory change, CRP shows an earlier, more intense increase than ESR. With recovery, the disappearance of CRP precedes the return of the ESR to normal. The CRP also disappears when the inflammatory process is suppressed by salicylates or steroids.

This test is also useful in the evaluation of patients with an acute myocardial infarction (MI). The level of CRP correlates with peak CK-MB levels, but CRP peaks occur 1 to 3 days later. Failure of CRP to return to normal may indicate damage to the heart tissue. Levels are not elevated in patients with angina.

CRP may also be used postoperatively to detect wound infections. CRP levels increase within 4 to 6 hours after surgery and generally begin to decrease after the third postoperative day. Failure of the levels to fall is an indicator of complications such as infection or pulmonary infarction.

High levels of CRP are also seen in patients with many other problems, including kidney or marrow transplant rejection, malignant diseases, bacterial and viral infections, Crohn's disease, Reiter's syndrome, vasculitis syndromes, and lupus erythematosus.

Procedure. Peripheral venipuncture is performed and one red-top tube is collected. Fasting is not usually required.

Contraindications. None.

Nursing considerations

Nursing Diagnosis/Collaborative Problems

See Blood studies, p. 2.

Nursing Implications with Rationale

- After the study assess the venipuncture site for bleeding.

HLA-B27 antigen

Normal value: negative

Rationale. The human leukocyte antigens (HLA) are the major histocompatibility antigens important in tissue recognition. These antigens are under direct genetic control and share a locus on the chromosome. Some HLA antigens are derived from the father and some from the mother. These antigens are not only used in tissue transplantation, but also for paternity testing and for assessing other diseases. Many HLA antigens exist, but the one with the most clinical relevance is HLA-B27. This antigen is found commonly in patients with ankylosing spondylitis and Reiter's syndrome. HLA-B27 is used to detect and confirm these diagnoses. HLA-B27 is found in 5% to 7% of normal patients, but about 80% to 90% of patients with ankylosing spondylitis or Reiter's syndrome have HLA-B27. Other HLA associations include B47 (congenital adrenal hyperplasia), B35 (subacute thyroiditis), and DR2 (Goodpasture's syndrome).

Procedure. While HLA testing can be done on just about any human cell, RBCs are most easily accessible. A venous sample of at least 10 ml is obtained in a heparinized solution. Lymphocytes from the patient are then extracted and incubated with anti–HLA-B27 cytotoxic antibody. If the patient has HLA-B27 antigen, a complex is formed on the cell surface. Serum complement is then added to the mixture, thereby killing the lymphocyte and recognizing the titer of HLA-B27. No prestudy preparations exist. The test is as uncomfortable as a venipuncture.

Contraindications. None.

Nursing considerations

Nursing Diagnoses/Collaborative Problems

See Blood studies, p. 2.

Nursing Implications with Rationale

- Be sure the patient understands the test.
- Instruct the technician to be gentle with the patient while performing the venipuncture. Some patients have painful joints, and extending the arm completely for venipuncture is difficult.
- Assess the venipuncture site for bleeding or hematoma formation.

CASE STUDY 3: AIDS

Steve Z., a 30-year-old homosexual, complained of unexplained weight loss, chronic diarrhea, and respiratory congestion over the past 6 months. Physical examination was performed, and no evidence of Kaposi's sarcoma was noted. The following studies were performed:

Studies	Results
CBC (see Chapter 10)	
Hemoglobin	12 g/dl (normal: 14-18 g/dl)
Hematocrit	36% (normal: 42%-52%)
Bronchoscopy (see Chapter 5)	*Pneumocystis carinii* pneumonia (PCP)
Stool culture	*Cryptosporidium muris*
AIDS serology	
ELISA	Positive
Western blot	Positive

The bronchoscopic detection of *Pneumocystis carinii* pneumonia (PCP) confirmed the suspected diagnosis of acquired immunodeficiency syndrome (AIDS). PCP is an opportunistic infection occurring only in immunocompromised patients and is the most common infection in persons with AIDS. The diarrhea was caused by *Cryptosporidium muris,* an enteric pathogen, which occurs frequently with AIDS and can be identified on a stool culture. The AIDS serology tests supported the diagnoses.

The patient was initially hospitalized for a short time for the treatment of PCP. Several months later after he was discharged, he developed Kaposi's sarcoma. He eventually developed psychoneurologic problems and died 18 months after the diagnosis.

DISCUSSION OF TESTS

AIDS serology

(acquired immunodeficiency serology, AIDS screen, HIV antibody, Western blot test for HIV and antibody, enzyme-linked immunosorbent assay [ELISA])

Normal value: no evidence of HIV antigen or antibodies

Rationale. Tests used to detect the antibody to human immunodeficiency virus (HIV), which is the virus that causes AIDS, were first licensed by the FDA in 1985 for the screening of blood and plasma donors. HIV is also known as human T-lymphotrophic virus, type III (HTLV-III) or the lymphadenopathy-associated virus (LAV). Since 1985, millions of HIV antibody tests have been performed in blood banks, plasma collection centers, counseling centers, and clinical facilities for screening. Those at high risk for AIDS include sexually active homosexuals and bisexual men with multiple partners, intravenous drug abusers, persons receiving blood products containing HIV, and infants exposed to the virus during gestation. Accurate test results require attention to both the intrinsic quality of the tests and the technical performance of the technician performing the test.

Because of the medical and social significance of a positive test for HIV antibody, test results must be accurate and their interpretation correct. Therefore, the Public Health Service has emphasized that an individual can be said to have serologic evidence of HIV infection only after an enzyme immunoassay (EIA) screening test is repeatedly positive (i.e., two out of three times), and another test such as Western blot or immunofluorescence assay validates the results. The Western blot also measures IgG antibodies to HIV. However, in this test, several HIV proteins are used as the antigens.

The enzyme-linked immunosorbent assay (ELISA) test for antibodies to HIV in serum or plasma is the most widely used serologic test for AIDS. It is important to note that ELISA detects *antibodies* to HIV. Since it does not detect viral antigens, it cannot detect infection in its earliest stage before antibodies are formed. ELISA is used for clinical diagnosis, screening blood and blood products, and testing individuals who believe they may be infected with AIDS.

The sensitivity (probability that the test results will be reactive if the specimen is a true positive) of the ELISA test is approximately 99% for blood from persons infected for 4 to 12 weeks or more. The probability of a false-negative test is remote except during the first few weeks after infection, before detectable antibodies appear.

The specificity (probability that test results will be nonreactive if the specimen is a true negative) of the ELISA test is approximately 99% when repeatedly reactive tests are considered. To further increase the specificity of serologic tests, a supplemental test, most often the *Western blot,* is done to validate repeatedly reactive ELISA results. Sensitivity of the blot test is comparable to or greater than a repeatedly reactive ELISA. The testing sequence of a repeatedly reactive ELISA and a positive Western blot test is highly predictive of HIV infection.

Procedure. Many states have requirements for preserving confidentiality of results. Informed patient consent is also required.

No food or drink restrictions are necessary. Peripheral venipuncture is performed and blood is collected in a red-top tube. If the ELISA results are repeatedly reactive (test positively twice consecutively), the Western blot test is performed on the same blood sample. If the ELISA results have been repeatedly reactive and the Western blot is equivocal, a second serum specimen should be collected and tested in 2 to 4 months.

Contraindications. None.

Nursing considerations

Nursing Diagnoses/Collaborative Problems

See Blood studies, p. 2.

- High risk for anxiety related to test results
- Possible knowledge deficit related to spread of disease

Nursing Implications with Rationale

- Explain the purpose of the test to the patient, and follow hospital guidelines concerning confidentiality and informed consent.
- After the venipuncture, assess the site for bleeding and apply pressure as indicated.
- Most patients are extremely anxious regarding the need for the test. Be nonjudgmental and allow the patients ample time to express their feelings.
- Follow the institution's policy regarding test results. Results are not given over the telephone. With a positive result, patients may lose their jobs and not be able to get insurance.
- If the test results are positive, explain to the patient that this implies exposure to and probably the presence of the virus in the body. It does not mean the patient has AIDS. Not all patients with positive antibodies acquire the disease.
- Assess the patient for symptoms of AIDS, which include fever, fatigue, weight loss, anorexia, diarrhea, swollen neck glands and night sweats.
- Observe universal blood and body precautions when dealing with patients at risk for AIDS. Gloves should be worn for handling blood products. Cuts on the hands can serve as sites for entry of the virus.
- Encourage patients with AIDS to identify their sexual contacts so they can be informed and tested. Make sure the patient knows that unprotected sexual contact puts sexual partners at high risk for contracting the AIDS virus.

CASE STUDY 4: LYME DISEASE

Mr. J.W., 38 years old, had a 3-week history of fatigue and lethargy with intermittent complaints of headache, fever, chills, myalgia, and arthralgia. According to the history, the patient's symptoms began shortly after a camping vacation. The patient recalled a bug bite and rash on his thigh immediately after the trip. The following studies were ordered:

Studies	Results
Lyme disease test	Elevated IgM antibody titers against *Borrelia burgdorferi* (normal value: low)

Studies	Results
Erythrocyte sedimentation rate (ESR)	30 mm/hr (normal value: ≤15 mm/hr)
Serum aspartate aminotransferase (AST) (see p. 13)	32 U/L (normal value: 8-20 U/L)
Hemoglobin (see p. 388)	12 g/dl (normal value: 14-18 g/dl)
Hematocrit (see p. 388)	36% (normal value: 42-52%)
Rheumatoid factor (see p. 439)	negative (normal value: negative)
Antinuclear antibodies (see p. 436)	negative (normal value: negative)

Based upon the patient's history of camping in the woods and an insect bite and rash on the thigh, Lyme disease was suspected. Early in the course of this disease the specific IgM antibodies against *Borrelia burgdorferi* are the most helpful test in diagnosing Lyme disease. An elevated erythrocyte sedimentation rate, increased AST levels, and mild anemia are frequently seen early in this disease. Rheumatoid factor and antinuclear antibodies are usually absent.

The therapeutic goal for Lyme disease is to eradicate the causative organism. Lyme disease, like other spirochetal disease, is most responsive to antibodies early in its course. This patient was placed on oral doxycycline, 100 mg b.i.d., for 21 days. The symptoms resolved completely, and he had no further problems.

DISCUSSION OF TESTS

Lyme disease test

Normal values: Negative (low titers of IgM and IgG antibodies)

Rationale. Lyme disease was first recognized in Lyme, Connecticut, in 1975. The disease usually begins during the summer months with a skin lesion called erythema chronicum migrans (ECM), which occurs at the site of a bite by *Ixodes dammini* (in the Northeast and Midwest) or *I. pacificus* (in the West) or a related tick. Ticks are the best documented vectors of the spirochete *(Borrelia burgdorferi),* which is the causative agent for Lyme disease.

Weeks to months after the insect bite, some patients develop meningoencephalitis, cranial or peripheral neuropathies, myocarditis, atrioventricular nodal block, or arthritis. The last manifestation is joint involvement, which often occurs intermittently in a few large joints for several years.

Currently, ELISA is the best diagnostic test for Lyme disease and determines titers of specific IgM and specific IgG antibodies to the *I dammini* spirochete. Levels of specific IgM antibody peak during the third to sixth week after disease onset and then gradually decline.

Titers of specific IgG antibodies are generally low during the first several weeks of illness, become maximal months later during arthritis, and often remain elevated for years. Early in the illness, the diagnosis can usually be determined from the gross appearance of ECM and known exposure to an endemic area. These patients do not require antibody determination. However, in the absence of ECM lesions, Lyme disease can be confused with a number of viral infections. In these patients, a single titer of specific IgM antibody may suggest the correct diagnosis. Acute and convalescent sera can be tested to be certain. Later in the illness, determination of specific IgG antibodies can separate Lyme disease from aseptic meningitis or unexplained cranial or peripheral nerve palsies.

Procedure. No food or fluid restrictions are needed. Peripheral venipuncture is performed to collect a venous blood sample.

Contraindications. None.

Nursing considerations

Nursing Diagnoses/Collaborative Problems

See Blood studies, p. 2.

- Possible anxiety related to test results.

Nursing Implications with Rationale

- Explain the purpose of the test to the patient. Since Lyme disease is a relatively new disease, many people have never heard of it and have questions and concerns.

- After the venipuncture is performed, assess the site for bleeding.

Erythrocyte sedimentation rate test

(ESR, sed rate test)

Normal values: (Westergren method)
Men: up to 15 mm/hour
Women: up to 20 mm/hour
Children: up to 10 mm/hour
Newborn: 0-2 mm/hour

Rationale. The ESR test is a nonspecific test used to detect inflammatory, neoplastic, infectious, and necrotic processes. Since the sed rate test is a nonspecific test, it is not diagnostic for any specific organ disease or injury. The test is performed by measurement of the distance (in millimeters) that RBCs descend (or settle) in normal saline in 1 hour. Because the conditions mentioned above increase the protein content of plasma, RBCs have a tendency to stack up on one another, thereby increasing their weight and causing them to descend faster. Therefore, the sed rate is increased.

The test can be used to detect disease that is otherwise not suspected. Many physicians use the ESR test in this way for routine patient evaluations. Other physicians regard this test as so nonspecific that it is useless as a routine study. The ESR test can occasionally be helpful in differentiating disease entities or complaints (for example, in the patient with chest pain, the sed rate is increased with myocardial infarction but normal with angina).

ESR is a fairly reliable indicator of the course of the disease and can therefore be used to monitor disease therapy. In general, as the disease (e.g., lupus erythematosus) worsens the ESR increases, and as the disease improves the ESR decreases. Decreased values may be seen in patients with congestive heart failure, sickle cell anemia, hypofibrinogenemia, and polycythemia vera. Dextran, fat emulsions, and vitamin A fictitiously increase the sed rate. Steroids decrease the sed rate.

Procedure. Peripheral venous blood is obtained and placed in an oxalate or editate (EDTA) anticoagulated tube (lavender-top, as used for CBC). The blood is immediately taken to the hematology laboratory, where the sed rate is measured. If the specimen is allowed to stand before the test is done, the ESR may be retarded, thereby causing artificially low results. Therefore, the study should be performed within 3 hours after the specimen has been obtained. The only discomfort associated with this test is the venipuncture.

Contraindications. None.

Nursing considerations

Nursing Diagnoses/Collaborative Problems

See Blood studies, p. 2.

Nursing Implications with Rationale

- Explain the procedure to the patient.
- Perform the venipuncture as indicated. Apply pressure or a pressure dressing to the venipuncture site, and assess the site for bleeding.

CASE STUDY 5: CHRONIC FATIGUE SYNDROME

Ms. A.M., 35 years old, complained of persistent, debilitating fatigue for over 4 months with no history of similar symptoms. Her history and physical examination noted the following: mild fever, enlarged cervical and axillary lymph nodes, muscle weakness, generalized weakness, insomnia, and complaints of confusion and inability to concentrate. A thorough evaluation was done to exclude conditions with similar symptoms.

Studies	Results
CBC and differential count (see p. 387)	WNL
Electrolytes (see p. 475)	WNL
Glucose (see p. 310)	80 mg/dl (normal value: 70-105 mg/dl)
Creatinine (see p. 229)	0.8 mg/dl (normal values: 0.5-1.1 mg/dl)

Studies	Results
BUN (see p. 229)	13 mg/dl (normal value: 10-20 mg/dl)
Calcium (see p. 291)	9.4 mg/dl (normal value: 9.0-10.5 mg/dl)
Phosporus (see p. 294)	3.8 mg/dl (normal value: 3.0-4.5 mg/dl)
Bilirubin (total) (see p. 94)	0.8 mg/dl (normal value: 0.1-1.0 mg/dl)
Alkaline phosphatase (see p. 96)	64 ImU/ml (normal value: 30-85 ImU/ml)
ALT (see p. 96)	22 IU/L (normal values: 5-35 IU/L)
AST (see p. 96)	8 U/L (normal value: 8-20 U/L)
Creatine phosphokinase (CPK) (see p. 12)	29 U/ml (normal value: 10-55 U/ml)
Aldolase	4.9 U/dl (normal value: 3-8.2 U/dl)
Urinalysis (see p. 224)	WNL
Chest x-ray	normal
ESR (see p. 444)	15 mm/hour (normal value: ≤20 mm/hour)
ANA (see p. 436)	none (normal value: none)
Thyroid stimulating hormone (see p. 286)	8 μU/ml (normal value: 2-10 μU/ml)
HIV (see p. 441)	negative (normal value: negative)
PPD (tuberculin test)	negative (normal value: negative)
Lyme disease test	negative (normal value: negative)

All test results in the recommended evaluation were normal. If any test results had been abnormal, the physician would have had to search for other conditions that could have caused such a result. Based upon the history, physical, and lab test evaluation, chronic fatigue syndrome was diagnosed. The patient eventually had to quit her job because of her overwhelming fatigue and numerous symptoms. After 2½ years, she was able to resume working on a part-time basis.

SUPPLEMENTAL INFORMATION

Serum aldolase test

Normal values:
- Adult: 3.0-8.2 Sibley-Lehninger U/dl or 22-59 mU at 37° C (SI units)
- Child: approximately 2 times the adult values
- Newborn: approximately 4 times the adult values

Rationale. Serum aldolase is very similar to the enzymes serum aspartate aminotransferase (AST) and creatine phosphokinase (CPK). Aldolase is an enzyme that is used in the glycolytic breakdown of glucose. Like AST and CPK, aldolase exists throughout the body in most tissues. This test is most useful in indicating muscular cellular destruction or hepatocellular destruction. The serum aldolase level is very high in muscular dystrophies, dermatomyositis, and polymyositis. Levels are also increased in patients with gangrenous processes, muscular trauma, and muscular infectious diseases (such as trichinosis). Elevated levels are also noted in hepatitis, obstructive jaundice, and cirrhosis or metastatic tumor of the liver. Central nervous system (CNS) tumors and granulocytic leukemias also are associated with increased levels of serum aldolase.

Neurologic diseases causing weakness can be differentiated from muscular causes of weakness with this test. Normal values are seen in the neurologic diseases such as poliomyelitis, myasthenia gravis, and multiple sclerosis. Elevated aldolase levels are seen in primary muscular disorders. No complications are associated with this test.

Procedure. Seven milliliters of blood are obtained in a red-top tube from a fasting patient via venipuncture. The blood is then taken to the laboratory where it is analyzed for levels of aldolase.

Contraindications. None.

Nursing considerations

Nursing Diagnoses/Collaborative Problems

See Blood studies, p. 2.

Nursing Implications with Rationale

- See AST (p. 96).

Febrile/cold agglutinins test

Normal values:
Febrile (warm) agglutinins: no agglutination in titers ≤1:80
Cold agglutinins: no agglutination in titers ≤1:16

Rationale. Febrile agglutinins tests are serologic studies used to diagnose infectious diseases such as salmonellosis, rickettsial diseases, brucellosis, and tularemia. Agglutination at titers greater than 1:80 are considered positive. Appropriate antibiotic treatment toward the infectious agent is associated with a drop in the titer activity of febrile agglutinins.

Cold agglutinins occur in patients who are infected by other agents, most notably *Mycoplasma pneumoniae.* The febrile and cold agglutinins are antibodies that cause RBCs to aggregate at high or low temperatures, respectively. Normally, agglutination may occur in concentrated serum (below 1:32 dilution). Agglutination occurring at titers greater than 1:16 for cold agglutinins and 1:80 for febrile agglutinins are considered abnormal and diagnostic of the infectious agent they represent.

Other diseases causing abnormal cold agglutinins at elevated titer levels include many viral illnesses, infectious mononucleosis, multiple myeloma, scleroderma, cirrhosis, staphylococcemia and thymic tumors.

Procedure. Seven milliliters of blood are obtained by venipuncture in a red-top tube. For cold agglutinins, the red-top tube is previously warmed to above 37° C. For febrile agglutinins, the red-top tube is cooled. The specimen is then immediately taken to the laboratory so that no hemolysis occurs. Under no circumstances should the cold agglutinin specimen be refrigerated or the febrile agglutinin specimen heated.

Once in the laboratory the cold agglutinin specimen is chilled, and the specimen is evaluated for agglutination. The febrile agglutinin specimen is heated and inspected for agglutination. Serial dilutions are carried out to detect the titer of agglutination. No pretesting preparation is required. The test is as uncomfortable as a venipuncture.

Contraindications. None.

Nursing considerations

Nursing Diagnoses/Collaborative Problems

See Blood studies, p. 2.

Nursing Implications with Rationale

- Be sure that the specimen is taken to the laboratory as soon as possible. Avoid the refrigeration of the cold agglutinin specimen or the warming of the febrile agglutinin specimen. Be sure the patient has not been exposed to marked abnormalities in temperature that may affect the respective agglutination testing.

Mononucleosis spot test

(mononuclear heterophil test or heterophil antibody test, Monospot test)

Normal values: negative (<1:28 titer)

Rationale. The mononucleosis test is performed to aid in the diagnosis of infectious mononucleosis, a disease caused by the *Epstein-Barr virus.* Usually young adults are affected. The clinical presentation is that of fever, pharyngitis, lymphadenopathy, and splenomegaly. About 2 weeks after the onset of the disease, a large proportion of patients is found to have IgM antibodies in their serum that react against warm RBCs. When these antibodies are present in serial dilutions of greater than 1:56, infectious mononucleosis can be strongly considered. However, false positives exist. Occasionally patients with lymphoma or SLE may also have this antibody. Patients with Burkitt's lymphoma, leukemia, and some gastrointestinal cancers also have false-positive tests. Burkitt's lymphoma is strongly associated with the Epstein-Barr virus, the agent causing infectious mononucleosis. Narcotic addicts are also known to have high titer values of infectious mononuclear heterophil antibodies. No complications are associated with this test.

Procedure. Several heterophil agglutination tests are available, but the most commonly performed is the spot test for infectious mononucleosis (Monospot test). (Heterophil antibodies produced by humans react with the RBCs of another species.) The test is performed by diluting the patient's serum on one side of a slide by mixing it with guinea pig kidney antigen (containing only Forssman antigen). On the other side of the slide the patient's serum is mixed with beef RBCs (containing only infectious mononuclear antigen). Horse RBCs are then applied to each side. These RBCs contain Forssman and infectious mononuclear antigens. Agglutination of the beef cell indicates the presence of the infectious mononuclear heterophil antibody-antigen complexes and thereby confirms the diagnosis of infectious mononucleosis.

The serum is obtained by withdrawing 7 ml of blood into a red-top tube via venipuncture. The specimen is then taken to the laboratory where the mono spot test is carried out on the patient's serum. The results are available within an hour. No pretest preparations are required.

Contraindications. None.

Nursing considerations

Nursing Diagnoses/Collaborative Problems

See Blood studies, p. 2.

Nursing Implications with Rationale

- Observe the venipuncture site for signs of ecchymosis.

Epstein-Barr virus titer

Normal values:

Titers $\leq$1:10 nondiagnostic

1:10 to 1:60 indicates infection at some undetermined time.

1:320 or greater suggests active infection

4-fold increase in titer in paired sera drawn 10 to 14 days apart is usually indicative of an acute infection

Rationale. Epstein-Barr Virus (EBV) is the most common agent associated with infectious mononucleosis syndrome, seen most commonly in children, adolescents, and young adults. Clinical features include those of acute fatigue, fever, sore throat, and lymphadenopathy. Laboratory findings of lymphocytosis, atypical lymphocytes, and the development of transient serum heterophil antibodies (see previous study) are found in patients with *acute* EBV infection. After recovery from primary EBV infection, a life-long, latent EBV carrier status is established. Most patients with infectious mononucleosis recover uneventfully and return to normal activity within 4 to 6 weeks. In the last several years, specific immunologic tests to identify EBV activity indicate that latent EBV can reactivate and become associated with a constellation of chronic signs and symptoms resembling infectious mononucleosis.

Clinical manifestations of *chronic* EBV syndrome are variable with nonspecific symptoms such as profound fatigue, pharyngitis, myalgias, arthralgias, low-grade fever, headache, paresthesias, and loss of abstract thinking. The routine laboratory workup is of no diagnostic value. There are occasionally atypical lymphocytes, but the heterophil tests are almost always negative. Diagnosis is best established by demonstrating immunologic evidence of antibodies to the Diffuse (D) and Restricted (R) components of early antigen (EA) complex and/or by the absence of Epstein-Barr nuclear antigen (EBNA) measured 6 months after primary EBV infection, when it should be present.

EBV antibody titers are tests indicating the body's response to EBV antigens, complex substances produced by the EBV virus during various phases of replication. Although laboratories performing these tests present the results in slightly different units, the titers are recorded in four parts:

VCA (viral capsid antigen)
EAD (early antigen diffuse component)
EAR (early antigen restricted component)
EBNA (Epstein-Barr nuclear antigen)

The interpretation of EBV antibody tests is based on the following assumptions.

1. Once the person becomes infected with EBV, the anti-VCA antibodies appear first.
2. Anti-EA EAD antibodies appear next or are present with anti-VCA antibodies early in the course of illness. An anti-EA antibody titer greater than 80 in a patient 2 years after acute infectious mononucleosis indicates chronic Epstein-Barr virus syndrome.
3. As the patient recovers, anti-VCA and anti-EA antibodies decrease; and anti-EBNA antibodies appear. Anti-EBNA persists for life and reflects a past infection.
4. After the patient is well, anti-VCA and anti-EBNA are always present but at lower ranges. Occasionally, anti-EA may also be present after recovery.

Procedure. Peripheral venipuncture is performed and approximately 5 to 10 ml of blood is collected in a red-top tube. The day of illness onset should be recorded on the lab slip. Acute serum samples should be obtained as soon as possible after the onset of illness. A second specimen should be obtained 14 to 21 days later.

Contraindications. None.

Nursing considerations

Diagnoses/Collaborative Problems

See Blood studies, p. 2.

Nursing Implications with Rationale

- Observe the venipuncture site for signs of bleeding.
- Be sure that patients with infectious mononucleosis are taught the basic points of self-care, which include the following: resting in bed during febrile periods; taking analgesics (such as aspirin) for general discomfort and fever; and gargling with warm water and using throat lozenges to relieve sore throat.

Antimitochondrial antibody and antismooth muscle antibody test

Normal values:
No antimitochondrial antibodies at titers >1:5
No antismooth muscle antibodies at titers >1:20

Rationale. The antimitochondrial antibody and antismooth muscle antibody tests are used primarily to diagnose primary biliary cirrhosis and chronic hepatitis, respectively. They are also used to distinguish between surgical and nonsurgical obstructive jaundice. Surgical or obstructive jaundice on the basis of extrahepatic biliary duct obstruction is not associated with marked elevations of these antibodies. Normally the serum does not contain antimitochondrial antibodies at a titer >1 : 5, nor does it contain antismooth muscle antibodies at a titer of >1 : 20.

Antimitochondrial antibodies (AMA) appear in most patients with primary biliary cirrhosis. These patients also have markedly elevated liver enzymes and a normal cholangiogram. Their liver biopsy is compatible with primary liver cirrhosis.

Antismooth muscle antibodies (ASMA) are only present in approximately 30% of patients with primary biliary cirrhosis. However, the majority of patients with chronic hepatitis have antismooth muscle antibodies. False-positive antismooth muscle antibodies may be caused by infectious mononucleosis, acute hepatitis, or hepatomas.

Procedure. Seven milliliters of venous blood are withdrawn and placed in a red-top tube. For antismooth muscle antibodies the patient's serum is exposed to cut sections of smooth muscle. Fluorescent-labeled antibodies are then added and combine with antibody-antigen immune complexes. This binding can be quantitated with an ultraviolet microscope. Antimitochondrial antibodies can be incubated with renal tubules, gastric mucosa, or other organs to which antimitochondrial antibodies are known to react.

Contraindications. None.

Nursing considerations

Nursing Diagnoses/Collaborative Problems

See Blood studies, p. 2.

Nursing Implications with Rationale

- Be sure to check the venipuncture site for ongoing bleeding. Oftentimes jaundice patients may have coagulopathies associated with vitamin K deficiency.
- Avoid contact with the needles used to withdraw the blood, since the patient may have chronic hepatitis. Follow Universal Precautions for this and all blood tests.

Serum protein electrophoresis

Normal values:
Total protein: 6.6-7.9 g/dl
Albumin: 3.3-4.5 g/dl
$Alpha_1$ globulin: 0.1-0.4 g/dl
$Alpha_2$ globulin: 0.5-1.0 g/dl
Beta globulin: 0.7-1.2 g/dl
Gamma globulin: 0.5-1.6 g/dl

Rationale. Total serum protein is a combination of albumin and globulins. Albumin is the smaller molecule, which is most important in maintaining the oncotic pressure of plasma (that is, the pressure that keeps water in the bloodstream). Albumin also acts as a carrier protein for some drugs. Larger molecules called globulins are subclassified into four categories. $Alpha_1$ globulins include alpha antitrypsin and thyroid-binding globulin. $Alpha_2$ globulins include serum haptoglobins, ceruloplasmin, prothrombin, and cholinesterase. $Beta_1$ globulins include lipoproteins, transferrin, plasminogen, and complement proteins. $Beta_2$ globulins include fibrinogen. Gamma globulins are the immune proteins (see p. 437).

Serum protein electrophoresis is a process whereby the various components of a total protein can be separated and quantified according to their electrical charge. Several well-established electrophoretic patterns (variations of concentrations of the protein components) can be associated with specific disease entities. While there are no diseases marked by increased albumin levels, decreased albumin levels have many potential causes: (1) acute and chronic inflammation (e.g., rheumatic diseases); (2) granulomatosis, bacterial, or viral infections; (3) inflammatory bowel diseases; (4) decreased albumin synthesis from liver disease or malnutrition; (5) increased body loss of albumin from nephrotic syndrome, severe burns, peritonitis, or ascites; and (6) increased metabolism from thyrotoxicosis or Cushing's syndrome.

$Alpha_1$ globulin is increased in acute infections and neoplastic diseases. $Alpha_2$ globulin is increased as a compensatory mechanism in the nephrotic syndrome or in many chronic inflammatory or malignant disorders.

Beta globulin is increased in hyperlipoproteinemias or monoclonal gammopathies.

Gamma globulins are increased in polyclonal gammopathies, chronic liver diseases, autoimmune diseases, and chronic infections. Many drugs (such as aspirin, bicarbonates, chlorpromazine, corticosteroids, isoniazid, neomycin, phenacemide, salicylates, sulfonamides, estrogen, testosterone, and tolbutamide) can markedly affect protein component concentrations. One must be aware of the medication history before interpreting any specific electrophoretic pattern.

Procedure. Seven milliliters of peripheral venous blood are drawn into a red-top tube and taken to the chemistry laboratory. The serum is placed on a pH adjusted gel strip to which an electrical current is applied. Each protein component then migrates to a certain point, depending on its electrical charge. The final migration pattern is recognized as either normal or as one associated with a specific disease. No specific preparation is associated with the test. The test is as uncomfortable as any blood test.

Contraindications. None.

Nursing considerations

Nursing Diagnoses/Collaborative Problems

See Blood studies, p. 2.

Nursing Implications with Rationale

- Describe the test to the patient.
- Obtain a medication history to determine if the patient is taking any drug that may affect the results.
- If the patient is suspected of having an immune globulin abnormality, be sure to take extra precautions to prevent infection.

Cryoglobulin test

Normal value: no cryoglobulins detected

Rationale. Cryoglobulins are abnormal globulin protein complexes that precipitate at low temperatures and redissolve with rewarming. These proteins exist in the blood of patients with myeloma, macroglobulinemia, chronic leukemia, connective tissue diseases, mononucleosis, hepatitis, and infective endocarditis.

Serum levels >5 mm are associated with myeloma, macroglobulinemia, and leukemia. Globulin levels between 1 and 5 mm are associated with rheumatoid arthritis. Cryoglobulin levels >1 mm/ml can be associated with SLE, rheumatoid arthritis, infectious mononucleosis, viral hepatitis, cirrhosis, endocarditis, and glomerulonephritis. The cryoglobulin test detects levels of cryoglobulin that may be associated with specific disease entities.

Cryoglobulins can precipitate within the blood vessels of the fingers when exposed to cold temperatures. This precipitation causes sludging of blood within those vessels. The patient often has symptoms of Raynaud's disease (pain, cyanosis, and coldness of the fingers).

Procedure. Ten milliliters of blood are drawn from a peripheral vein into a red-top tube prewarmed to body temperature. The sample is taken to the chemistry laboratory where it is refrigerated for 72 hours. After that time the specimen is evaluated for precipitation. If precipitation is identified, the tube is then rewarmed and the specimen examined for dissolution of that precipitation. If precipitation of the refrigerated specimen is identified and dissolved upon rewarming, cryoglobulins are present. An 8-hour fast may be required to minimize turbidity of serum caused by the ingestion of a recent meal. Turbidity may make the detection of precipitation rather difficult.

Contraindications. None.

Nursing considerations

Nursing Diagnoses/Collaborative Problems

See Blood studies, p. 2.

Nursing Implications with Rationale

- Instruct the patient to fast for 8 hours before obtaining the specimen if indicated by the laboratory.
- If cryoglobulins are found to be present, warn the patient to avoid cold temperatures to minimize Raynaud's symptoms.
- Patients who have cryoglobulins may have diseases that are associated with coagulation defects. Observe the venipuncture site for possible hematoma.

Legionnaire's disease antibody test

(Legionella pneumophilia)

Normal value:

<4-fold change in titer between acute and convalescent sample

No *Legionella pneumophilia* seen on direct fluorescent antibody examination.

Rationale. This test is used to detect antibodies to *Legionella pneumophilia* to support the diagnosis of legionnaire's disease. Since there are more than 20 different species of *Legionella*, testing for multiple serogroups may be necessary since tests are species-specific. A 4-fold rise in titer >1:128 from acute to convalescent phase provides evidence of recent infection. A single titer equal to or greater than 1:256 provides evidence of infection at an undetermined time.

Procedure. Legionnaire's disease can be tested by either a blood test or by a direct fluorescent antibody (FA) microscopic examination of a specimen smear. The blood test is an easily performed venipuncture with the collection of one red-top tube of blood. A convalescent sample should be drawn 2 to 3 weeks after the acute sample.

Organisms may also be cultured on special media from pleural fluid, lung biopsies, bronchial washings, transtracheal or bronchial aspirates, or other body fluids. Direct immunofluorescent antibody staining may demonstrate the organism in sputum, lung tissue, or pleural fluid within 2 to 3 days after the onset of clinical disease. This direct FA method is more specific in comparison to the blood test.

Contraindications. None.

Nursing considerations

Nursing Diagnosis/Collaborative Problems

- Possible knowledge deficit related to test purpose, preparation, and procedure.
- Possible anxiety related to test results.

Nursing Implications with Rationale

- Explain the method of testing to the patient.
- Encourage the patient to verbalize his or her concerns regarding the possible diagnosis of Legionnaire's disease.

QUESTIONS AND ANSWERS

1. **QUESTION:** The physician has requested a rheumatoid factor test on your young female patient. She is terribly frightened that the doctor suspects rheumatoid arthritis and that she will soon be paralyzed by incapacity and joint pain. What is the appropriate nursing intervention?
   ANSWER: Remind the patient that many diseases are associated with a positive rheumatoid factor. Some of these diseases are self-limiting, viral symptoms. The rheumatoid factor is merely a part of an immunologic workup to document a pattern associated with the disease that may explain her complaints. Also, assist her in verbalizing her fears and frustrations concerning this workup.
2. **QUESTION:** Your patient has an antimitochondrial antibody and antismooth muscle antibody test performed. Several hours later you notice an enlarged hematoma around the venipuncture site. What might be the cause of that hematoma, and what should the appropriate nursing intervention be?
   ANSWER: The antimitochondrial antibody and antismooth muscle antibody test were performed to diagnose and distinguish forms of liver disease. These liver diseases are often associated with inadequate levels of coagulation factors. Your patient most probably has a coagulopathy and does not have the normal capability to form a clot at the venipuncture site. You should:
   a. Ensure that the hematoma has not caused compression of the arterial supply to the hand. Check the pulses.
   b. Ensure that there is no compression on the nerves of the hand. Check for muscular capability and pin prick sensation.
   c. Elevate the arm.
   d. Place cold compresses over the hematoma site.
   e. Notify the physician to document and determine the cause of the coagulopathy more accurately.
3. **QUESTION:** Your 65-year-old female patient is admitted to the hospital. On taking a history, you find that the patient has a cardiac arrhythmia for which she is taking procainamide. She is admitted now for a workup for generalized aches and pain. An LE prep has been performed and is positive. How should this be interpreted?
   ANSWER: Many diseases can cause LE cells to be present in the blood of a patient. The results do not necessarily mean that the patient has SLE. Also, many drugs including procainamide can cause such a phenomenon. Interpretation of the laboratory test results should be made in light of the patient's drug ingestion. The physician should be reminded that the patient has been taking procainamide, which may be the cause of the abnormal LE cell prep.

BIBLIOGRAPHY

Bradley WG, Fries T: Neuromuscular testing. In Kelley WN and others, editors: Textbook of rheumatology, ed 3, Philadelphia, 1989, WB Saunders.

Carson D: Rheumatoid factor. In Kelley WN and others, editors: Textbook of rheumatology, ed 3, Philadelphia, 1989, WB Saunders.

Cooper MD, Lawton AR: Primary immune deficiency diseases. In Wilson J and others, editors: Harrison's principles of internal medicine, ed 12, New York, 1991, McGraw-Hill.

Croft JE, Grodzicki RL, Steere AC: Antibody response to Lyme disease evaluation of diagnostic tests, J Infect Dis 149(5):789-795, 1984.

Densen P: Complement. In Mandell G and others, editors: Principles and practices of infectious diseases, ed 3, New York, 1990, Churchill Livingstone.

Dominquez A and others: Inclusion of laboratory test results in the surveillance of infectious diseases, Int J Epidemiol 20(1):290-292, March 1991.

Fauci AS, Lane HC: The acquired immunodeficiency syndrome (AIDS). In Wilson J and others, editors: Harrison's principles of internal medicine, ed 12, New York, 1991, McGraw-Hill.

Fries JF: Assessment of the patient with rheumatic diseases. In Kelley WN and others, editors: Textbook of rheumatology, ed 3, Philadelphia, 1989, WB Saunders.

Hahn JF: Systemic lupus erythematosus. In Wilson J and others, editors: Harrison's principles of internal medicine, ed 12, New York, McGraw-Hill.

Holmes GP and others: Chronic fatigue syndrome: a working case definition, Ann Intern Med 108(3):387-389, 1988.

Katz W: Diagnosis and management of rheumatic disease. Philadelphia, 1988, JB Lippincott.

Kieff ED: Infectious mononucleosis (Epstein-Barr virus infection). In Wyngaarden JB and others, editors: Cecil textbook of medicine, ed 19, Philadelphia, 1992, WB Saunders.

Kristoferitsch W: Neurological manifestation of Lyme borreliosis, Infection 19(4):268-272, July-Aug 1991.

Lavoie PE: Lyme disease. In Rakel RE, editor: Conn's current therapy, Philadelphia, 1991, WB Saunders.

Lipski PE: Rheumatoid arthritis. In Wilson J and others, editors: Harrison's principles of internal medicine, ed 12, New York, 1991, McGraw-Hill.

Malawista SE: Lyme disease. In Wyngaarden JB and others, editors: Cecil textbook of medicine, ed 19, Philadelphia, 1992, WB Saunders.

Metcalf RW: Arthroscopy. In Kelley WN and others, editors: Textbook of rheumatology, ed 3, Philadelphia, 1989, WB Saunders.

Miller SM, Cate TR: Management of HIV infection. In Rakel RE, editor: Conn's current therapy, Philadelphia, 1991, WB Saunders.

Milton JD and others: Immune responsiveness in chronic fatigue syndrome, Postgrad Med J 67(788):532-537, June 1991.

Reichlin M: Antinuclear antibodies. In Kelley WN and others, editors: Textbook of rheumatology, ed 3, Philadelphia, 1989, WB Saunders.

Ruddy S. Complement. In Kelley WN and others, editors: Textbook of rheumatology, ed 3, Philadelphia, 1989, WB Saunders.

Schleupner CJ: Detection of HIV-1 infection. In Mandell G and others, editors: Principles and practices of infectious deseases, ed 3, New York, 1990, Churchill Livingstone.

Stanek G: Laboratory and seroepidemiology of Lyme borreliosis, Infection 19(4):263-267, July-Aug 1991.

Sumaya CV: Infectious mononucleosis. In Rakel RE, editor: Conn's current therapy, Philadelphia, 1991, WB Saunders.

Tavris DE: Criteria for chronic fatigue syndrome, Penn Med 94(7):34, July 1991.

Willis D: Lyme disease, J Neurosci Nurs 23(4):211-217, Aug 1991.

Chapter 13

DIAGNOSTIC STUDIES USED IN THE ASSESSMENT OF CANCER

The following studies are commonly performed on the cancer patient to detect primary and metastatic tumors. The test results assist in more accurate staging of the tumor. When performed at appropriately timed intervals during the course of anticancer treatment, these studies can determine whether the tumor is becoming smaller (regressing) or getting larger (progressing). Metastasis is a form of progression.

Because the lymph nodes, bone, brain, liver, and lungs are organs commonly involved with metastatic cancer, staging diagnostic studies are directed toward the evaluation of these organs. Certain tumors are more commonly known to involve certain organs in their pattern of metastasis. These organs are evaluated during the diagnostic staging studies. If the staging studies indicate tumor progression, the physician may elect to change or reinstitute anticancer therapy. If, on the other hand, the staging studies indicate tumor regression, the present anticancer therapy would be continued. Therefore, accurate patient preparation and accurate test results are vitally important because they may significantly affect the clinical course of the patient.

CASE STUDY 1: BREAST CANCER

Mrs. M.W. was a 48-year-old woman with an asymptomatic lump in her breast. Her physical examination indicated a 2 cm lump in the upper outer quadrant of her left breast.

Studies	Results
Routine laboratory studies	WNL
Thermography	Hot spot in the upper outer quadrant of the left breast
Mammography	Poorly defined density in the upper outer quadrant of the left breast with microcalcifications strongly suspicious for cancer
Carcinoembryonic antigen (CEA) test (Chapter 3)	5.8 units (normal: <2 ng/ml)

Studies	Results
Computed tomography (CT) scan of liver (see CT of abdomen, Chapter 4)	No evidence of metastatic tumor
Liver/spleen scan (see Chapter 4)	No evidence of metastatic tumor
Bone scan	Mild arthritis in the lumbosacral (LS) spine
Estrogen receptor assay	2 fmol/mg (normal: ≤3 fmol/mg)
Progesterone receptor assay	4 fmol/mg (normal: ≤5 fmol/mg)
CT scan of the brain (see Chapter 6)	No metastasis
LS spinal x-ray examination (see Chapter 6)	Arthritis

The thermography indicated that the lump was warmer than the surrounding breast tissue. This finding is compatible with fibrocystic disease, infection, or tumor. Mammography, however, was quite specific for cancer. Other possibilities include cystic breast disease and benign tumors (such as fibroneuroma). The CEA level was mildly elevated, which is compatible with breast cancer. Other abnormalities, however, can mildly and transiently elevate the CEA level (see p. 74). CT scans of the liver and brain, a liver-spleen scan, and a bone scan were performed to detect metastasis of breast cancer. No metastasis was seen. The bone scan did "light up" in the lumbosacral (LS) spine area; however, this is compatible with arthritis. The LS spinal x-ray examination also showed arthritis, not bone destruction by tumor.

Mrs. M.W. underwent a breast biopsy, which indicated cancer. The tumor estrogen and progesterone receptor assays were negative, indicating a more aggressive tumor. After the alternatives to primary treatment for breast cancer were explained, she chose lumpectomy, axillary lymph node dissection, and primary radiation with preservation of her breast. She received chemotherapy for 6 months. Yearly chest x-ray examinations, bone scans, liver scans, CEA tests, and mammograms have all been negative, indicating no evidence of recurrent tumor.

DISCUSSION OF TESTS

Thermography

(mammothermography)

Normal value: Avascular pattern with even distribution of temperature patterns

Rationale. Thermography is a technique by which differences in heat energy emanating from the skin of the breast are photographed using an infrared camera. The result is a pictorial representation of the breast. Fibrocystic disease, infection, and tumor are all associated with increased blood supply to the affected area. This increased blood supply causes an increase of temperature in the suspicious area, and heat is emitted. That heat is detected by an infrared camera and is easily located on a pictorial representation.

Normal tissues and benign tumors are represented as shades of gray. The hot spots are demonstrated as black areas. Cysts are occasionally represented as cold spots or white areas. This test is moderately sensitive in detecting breast cancer. Because other abnormalities (such as fibrocystic disease and infection) may be misread as positive, the test is considered to be relatively nonspecific; that is, a great number of abnormalities may cause false-positive test results. Since not all breast cancers show up as hot spots, a significant number of false-negative test results occur. The overall accuracy of thermography, therefore, is far inferior to that of mammography (see the following study). However, because thermography can be done easily and inexpensively, it is considered a good screening tool in the attempt to diagnose breast cancer in its early stage. It can also be used to assess clients with joint disease, especially rheumatoid arthritis. With the development of low dose mammography, thermography is rarely used today.

Essentially no complications arise as a result of having thermography performed. The test is able to detect breast cancer, infection, fibrocystic disease, and benign tumors. The normal thermogram demonstrates an avascular pattern with even distribution of temperature ranges. Although small variations in temperature distribution indicated by variant shades of gray may exist, there is not a predominant area of increased heat emanation in the normal thermogram.

Procedure. The patient is taken to the radiology department, instructed to disrobe from the waist up, and asked to don an x-ray gown with the opening in the front. She is then taken to the thermography room and asked to wait approximately 10 minutes. This wait allows greater heat emanation from any abnormal areas in the breast. The patient is seated with her arms held up in the air. A thermoscope is placed over a small area of breast skin to determine normal breast temperatures. The infrared scanning unit is then adjusted to establish a baseline normal temperature. The unit is placed in a position to scan both breasts from the frontal and lateral views. The duration of this study is approximately 20 minutes, and no discomfort is associated with it. Mammothermography is usually performed by a technician and interpreted by a radiologist. No fasting or sedation is required.

Contraindications. The test is contraindicated in patients who:

1. Are in the premenstrual stage and have severe engorgement of their breast
2. Have recently been exposed to excessive sunlight causing a sunburn
3. Have recently had a breast infection.

These conditions can cause false-positive results.

Nursing considerations

Nursing Diagnoses/Collaborative Problems

- Possible knowledge deficit related to test purpose, preparation, and procedure
- Possible anxiety related to unknown sensations of procedure
- Possible anxiety related to test results

Nursing Implications with Rationale

- Explain the test completely to the patient and answer any questions that she may have.
- Question the patient regarding recent exposure to excessive sunlight, which can cause false-positive test results.
- Find out if the patient has applied any ointment or powder to her breast the day of the test, since these cause false-positive results if not removed before the study.
- Obtain a menstrual history. Be sure that the patient is in the postmenstrual stage. Thermography is not performed if the woman is pregnant, immediately premenstrual, or menstruating because the vascularity of the breasts increases at these times.
- This may be a time of high anxiety for the patient. Encourage her to express any concerns about breast cancer. If the results are positive, explain the other tests that are necessary to confirm the diagnosis.
- It may be reasonable to take this opportunity to instruct the patient in breast self-examination.

Mammography

Normal value: negative; no tumor shadow present

Rationale. Mammography is an x-ray examination of the breast. Careful interpretation of these x-ray films by a skilled radiologist can:

1. Detect nonpalpable breast cancers, especially in patients with large, pendulous breasts
2. Detect cancer 1 to 2 years before it may have become clinically palpable, thus providing an excellent opportunity for cure
3. Provide a reliable means of following patients at high risk for breast cancer

Although mammography is not a substitute for a biopsy, it is reliable and accurate when interpreted by a skilled radiologist. Radiographic signs of breast cancer include fine, calcific stippling, a localized area of increased radiodensity (nodule) with poorly defined margins (Figure

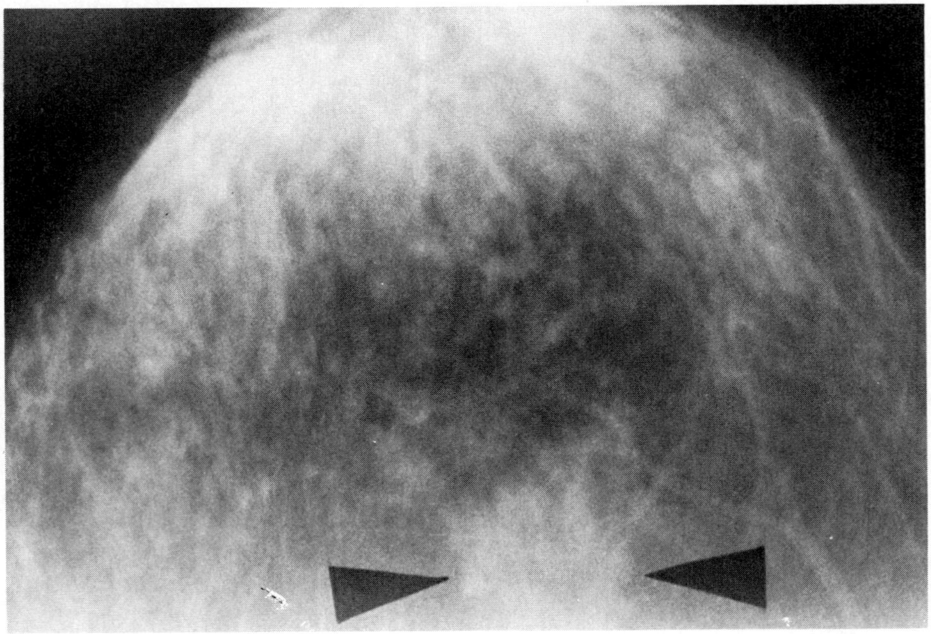

FIGURE 13-1. Mammogram. Craniocaudal view of breast. Pointers indicate typical breast cancer. Note poorly defined margins.

13-1), an area of edema surrounding a nodule, or thickening of the skin adjacent to a nodule.

Mammography cannot replace complete and careful physical examination, yet it frequently can substantiate questionable findings (Figure 13-2) or detect unrecognized lesions. There is some controversy concerning the role of mammography in the routine evaluation of patients. Because an x-ray study of the breast can induce cancer, there has been some resistance to the routine performance of mammography. However, with recent advances in technique, as little as 0.4 rad of radiation is delivered per examination. With this minimal exposure, the chance of radiation-induced cancer is minimal. Thus, in light of the fact that more early and easily curable breast cancers are being detected by routine mammography, few physicians now dispute the importance of mammography in certain groups of patients who are at risk for breast cancer. At present the American Cancer Society recommends that a baseline mammogram be taken when a woman is between 35 and 40 years old. Mammograms should be done at least every other year between ages 40 and 50. Women over 50 years old should have mammography yearly. Women who have had a breast cancer resected for cure should have mammography of the opposite breast performed yearly regardless of age.

Procedure. The nonfasting, unsedated patient is taken to the radiology department and placed in front of the mammographic x-ray machine (Figure 13-3). One breast is placed on an x-ray plate, and the x-ray cone is brought down on top of the breast to compress it gently between the broadened cone and the plate. An x-ray film is taken. This is called the craniocaudal view. Next, the x-ray plate is turned perpendicular to the floor and placed laterally on the outer as-

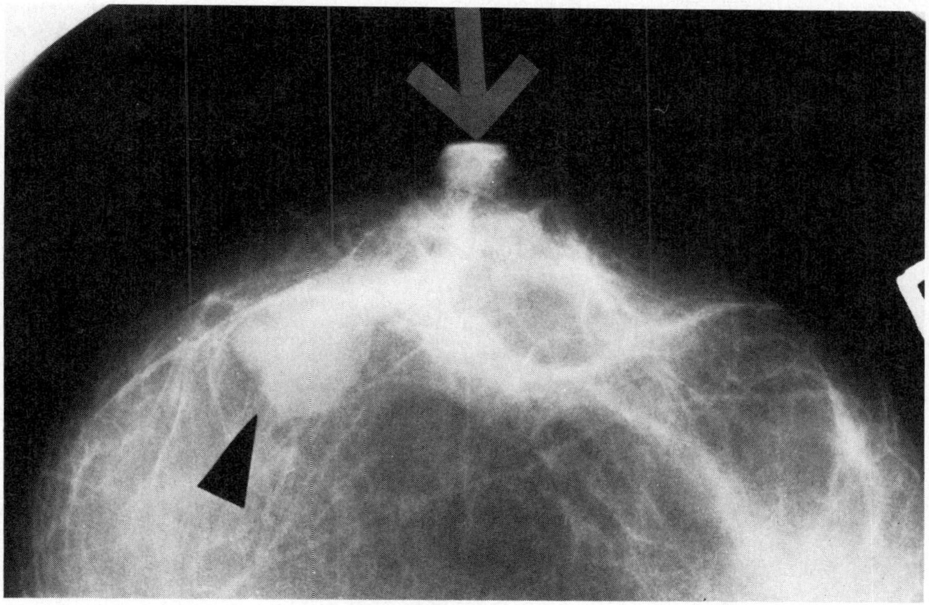

FIGURE 13-2. Mammogram. Craniocaudal view of breast. Pointer indicates typical benign fibroadenoma with well-circumscribed margin. Arrow indicates nipple. Note large cyst under breast.

pect of the breast. The broadened cone is brought in medially, and it again gently compresses the breast. This creates the lateral view. Oblique views are also performed. It is important to note that mammography can be falsely negative as often as 15% of the time.

Xeromammography provides the same information as mammography and has equal risks. The final picture is a positive print rather than the normal x-ray film's negative picture. The form of mammography used depends on the preference of the radiologist who must interpret the mammogram.

Discomfort associated with mammography varies. Some women report pain caused by the pressure, which is required to flatten the breast tissue on the x-ray plate. Mammography is performed by a radiologic technician in approximately 10 minutes. The x-ray films are viewed and interpreted by a skilled radiologist.

Contraindications. None (if the guidelines for the procedure are followed), with the exception of pregnancy.

Nursing considerations

Nursing Diagnoses/Collaborative Problems

See X-ray studies, p. 5.

Nursing Implications with Rationale

- Explain the procedure to the patient. Inform the patient of the recent advances in mammography and of the minimal risk associated with this study.
- Some patients may be embarrassed by this procedure. Allow them to verbalize their feelings.
- Patients are often very anxious regarding breast mammography. Provide emotional support.
- Tell the patient how and when she can get the

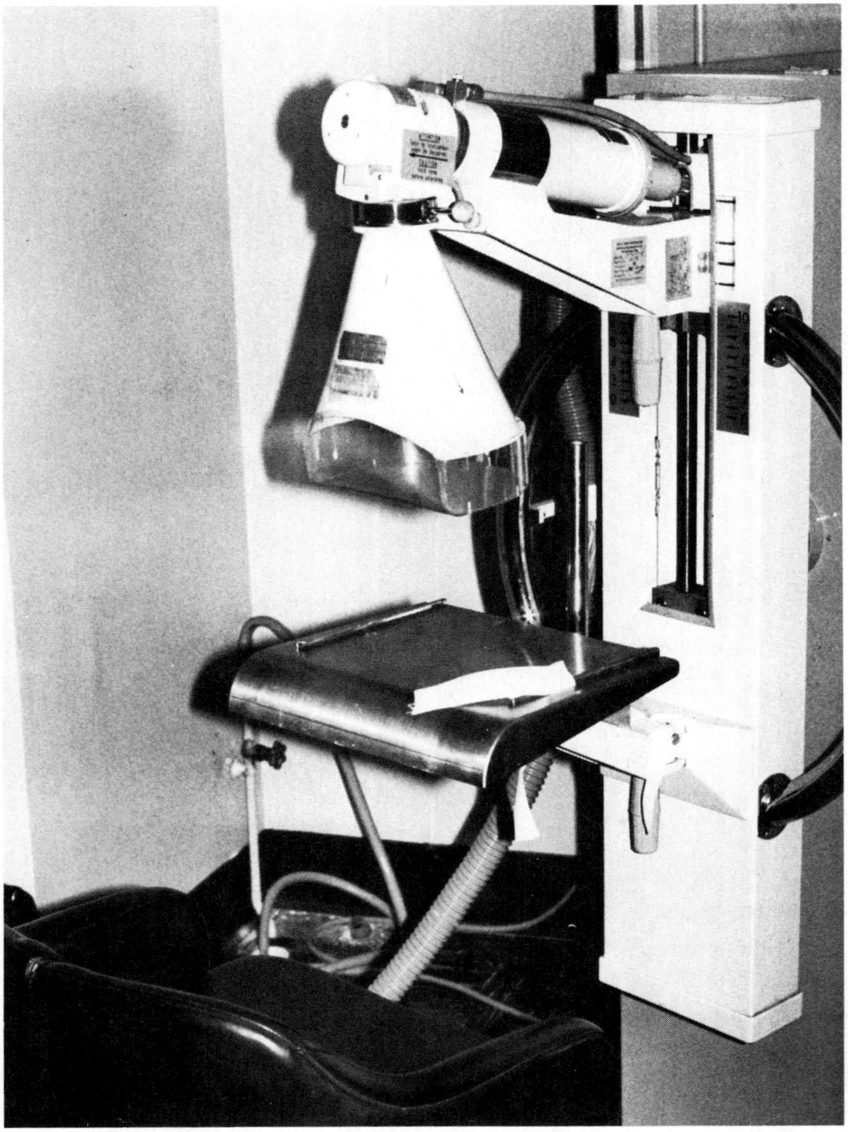

FIGURE 13-3. X-ray machine used in mammography.

results of this study. Usually the results are available 1 day after the test.

- Instruct the patient to perform a breast self-examination after each menstrual period. Teach this procedure if necessary.

Bone scan

Normal value: no evidence of abnormality

Rationale. Bone scanning is a test that permits examination of the skeleton by a scanning cam-

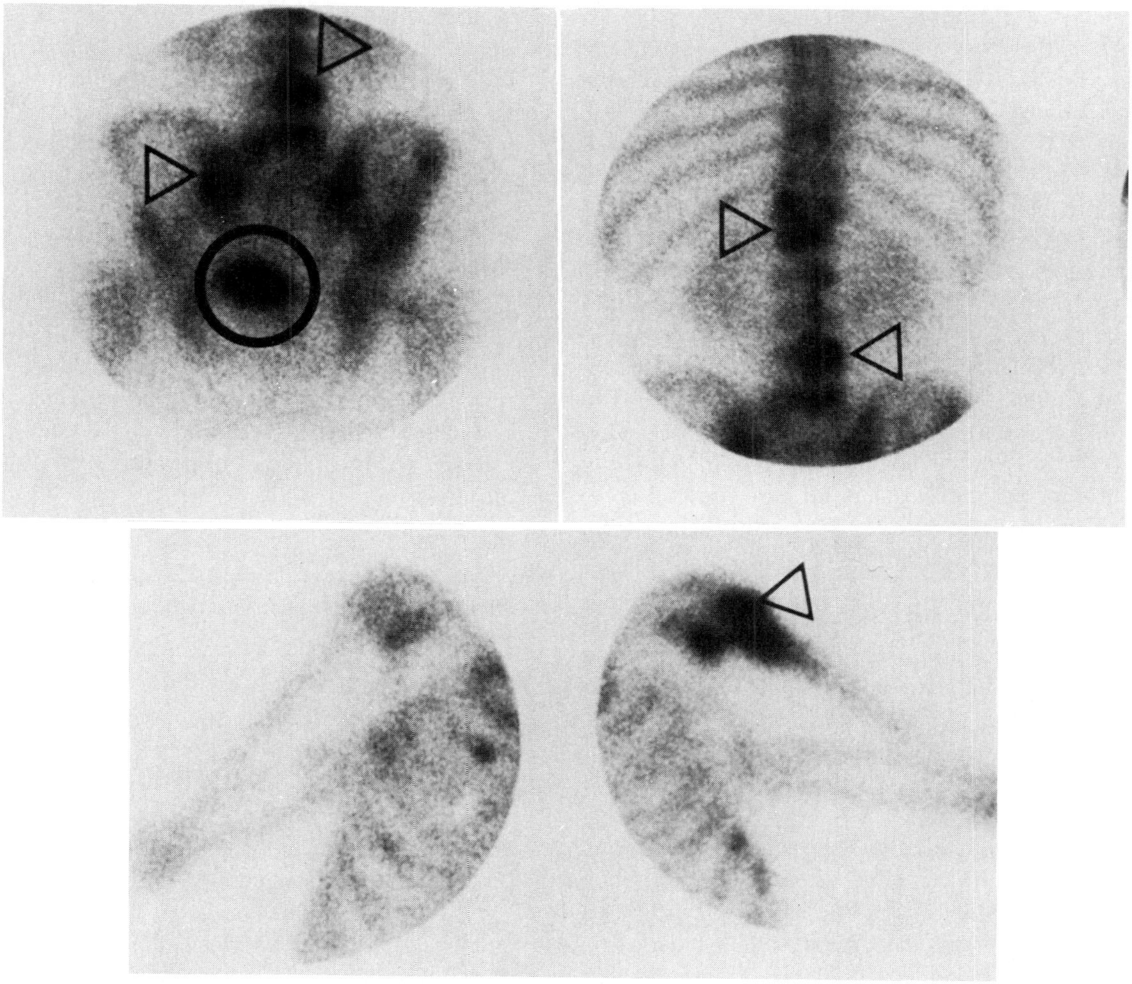

A B C

FIGURE 13-4. **A,** Abnormal bone scan demonstrating tumor metastasis to the vertebrae of L1 and L4. **B,** Abnormal bone scan demonstrating tumor metastasis in L4 and right sacroiliac joints (pointer outline). The bladder *(circled)* normally contains radionuclide tracer. **C,** Abnormal bone scan demonstrating increased uptake of radionuclide in the left humerus because of metastatic tumor in this area.

era after the intravenous injection of a radioactive material. The degree of radionuclide uptake is related to the metabolism of the bone. Normally a uniform concentration should be seen throughout the bones of the body. An increased uptake of isotope is abnormal and may represent tumor (Figure 13-4), arthritis, fracture, or degenerative disorders. These areas of concentrated nucleotide uptake are often called "hot spots" and are detectable months before an ordinary x-ray film can reveal a lesion.

Bone scan can detect primary and metastatic tumor. All malignancies capable of metastasis may reach the bone, especially those of the prostate, breast, lung, kidney, urinary bladder, and thyroid. Bone scanning may be repeated to detect the response of the body to radiation or chemotherapy.

Bone scanning also provides valuable information in the evaluation of patients with trauma or those with unexplained pain. Detection of hot spots can incriminate the bone or periosteal pathology as a source of the pain. Bone scanning is especially important in areas where fractures are not immediately seen on x-ray film, especially in the spine, ribs, face, and small bones of the extremities. With routine x-ray examinations the radiologist may not be able to detect secondary changes produced by healing before 10 to 14 days after trauma. In contrast, many fracture sites become abnormal 3 days after the trauma on bone scans. A fracture site that is revealed on an x-ray film but not on a bone scan at least 7 days after the trauma usually represents an old, healed injury.

Bone scanning is also valuable in the evaluation of patients with osteomyelitis. Routine x-ray examination changes usually do not appear before 10 to 14 days after the onset of the disease. However, bone scan abnormalities are evident days or weeks before detection on x-ray film.

The major disadvantage of bone scanning is that it is nonspecific. Many conditions (such as fractures, osteomyelitis, osteoarthritis, area bone necrosis, renal osteodystrophy, and Paget's disease) produce similar abnormal scans. No complications are associated with bone scanning.

Procedure. No fasting or sedation is required before bone scanning. For this test the patient receives an intravenous injection of an isotope (such as sodium pertechnetate ^{99m}Tc) in a vein in the arm. The patient is then encouraged to drink several glasses of water between the injection of the radioisotope and the actual scanning to facilitate renal clearance of the circulating tracer not picked up by the bone. The waiting period before scanning is approximately 1 to 3 hours. The patient is then instructed to urinate and is subsequently positioned on a scanning table in the radiology department. A scanning machine moves back and forth over the patient's body and detects radiation emitted by the skeleton. This information is then translated into x-ray film, thus showing a two-dimensional view of the skeleton. Many x-ray pictures are taken; the patient may have to be repositioned several times during the test.

The only discomfort associated with this study is that of the injection of the radioisotope. This test is performed by a physician or a nuclear medicine technician in 30 to 60 minutes. Sedatives may be given if a patient has difficulty remaining still during the scanning period.

Contraindications. This study is contraindicated in patients who are either pregnant or lactating.

Nursing considerations

Nursing Diagnoses/Collaborative Problems

See Nuclear scanning, p. 5.

Nursing Implications with Rationale

- Explain the procedure and assure the patient that the dose of radiation received is less than the amount he or she would receive from regular diagnostic x-rays.
- Tell the patient that the injected radionuclide will not affect the family, visitors, or other hospital staff members. The radioactive substance is usually excreted via the urine in 6 to 24 hours.
- Inform the patient that during the scanning the patient is not exposed to any radiation. The scanning machine detects the radiation emitted *from* the patient, as opposed to a regular x-ray machine where radiation is emitted from the machine to the body. Therefore, even though the patient may be scanned for 1 hour, the amount of exposure does not cause radiation effects, as an exposure of this length to an x-ray machine would. Tell the patient that the scanning machine makes a clicking sound as it detects radioactivity.
- Before the test instruct the patient to remove jewelry or any metal objects that may obscure x-ray visualization of the bones.

- After the patient receives the intravenous injection of the radioisotope, give him or her the exact time at which scanning will be done. The patient's activities are not restricted during this waiting period. However, encourage the patient to drink several glasses of water to facilitate renal clearance of the circulating radioisotope not picked up by the bone. The patient should void before scanning because a full bladder will mask the pelvic bones.
- Check the injection site of the radioisotope for redness or swelling. If a hematoma forms, apply warm soaks to the area to relieve pain.

Estrogen receptor assay

(ERA, ER, estradiol receptor)

Normal values:
Negative; ≤10 fmol/mg of protein
Positive; >10 fmol/mg

Rationale. Estrogen receptor (ER) assays are useful in the prognosis and treatment of breast carcinoma. They are used to determine whether a tumor is likely to respond to endocrine medical therapy or to removal of the ovaries or adrenal gland. Hormone receptor assays should be done on all primary or recurrent breast carcinomas. Levels tend to be higher in postmenopausal than in premenopausal women. In general, ER+ tumors have a better prognosis than ER− tumors.

Slightly more than half of patients with breast carcinoma who are ER+ respond to endocrine therapy (such as tamoxifen, estrogens, androgens, oophorectomy, or adrenalectomy). The response is greater when progesterone receptors (see next study) are also positive. Patients whose breast cancers lack these hormone receptors (ER−) have a much lower chance of tumor response to hormone therapy and may not be candidates for this form of therapy.

Specimens are collected during surgery according to the protocol of the pathologist. One gram of tissue is required. Tissue specimens are usually unfixed and frozen immediately after surgical removal. Hormones should be discontinued before breast biopsy. Antiestrogen preparations (e.g. Tamoxifen [Nolvadex]) during the past 2 months may cause false-negative estrogen receptor assays. Exogenous hormones that are taken for contraceptive purposes or menopausal estrogens may produce lower receptor values.

Procedure. Before biopsy, a gynecologic history is obtained, including menopausal status and exogenous hormone use. The surgeon obtains at least 1 gram of tumor tissue. This is placed on ice and immediately transferred to the pathology department. Then, part of the tissue is used for routine histology, and at least 1 gram is frozen. The frozen specimen is sent (in dry ice) to a central laboratory for estrogen receptor analysis. Results are usually available in 2 weeks. Immunohistochemical methods of estrogen receptor assay are available on specimens weighing <1 gram.

Contraindications. None.

Nursing considerations

Nursing Diagnoses/Collaborative Problems

- Possible knowledge deficit related to test purpose, preparation, and procedure.
- Possible anxiety related to test results.

Nursing Implications with Rationale

- Explain the procedure to the patient. Answer any questions that she may have.
- Women are usually very anxious regarding breast surgery. Provide emotional support.

Progesterone receptor assay

(PRA, PRP, PgR)

Normal values:
Negative; ≤10 fmol/mg
Positive; >10 fmol/mg

Rationale. Progesterone receptor (PR) assays are useful in the prognosis and treatment of breast cancer. They determine whether or not a tumor is likely to respond to endocrine medical therapy or to removal of the ovaries or adrenal glands. Hormone receptor assays should be done on all primary or recurrent breast carcinomas. This test is used in conjunction with estrogen receptor assays (see previous study) to increase predictability of tumor response to hormonal therapy in patients with breast carcinoma. PR levels tend to be higher in postmenopausal women. PR+ tumors probably have a better prognosis than PR− tumors.

Tumor response rate to medical or surgical hormonal manipulation is potentiated if estrogen receptor assay is also positive. Response rates are as follows:

ER+ PR+ = 75%
ER− PR+ = 60%
ER+ PR− = 35%
ER− PR− = 25%

Exogenous hormones should be discontinued before breast tumor biopsy. Any hormones taken during the past 2 months can cause false-negative results.

Procedure. Before biopsy, a gynecologic history is obtained including menopausal status and exogenous hormone use. The surgeon obtains at least 1 g of tumor tissue. This is placed on ice and immediately transferred to the pathology department. Then part of the tissue is used for routine histology and at least 1 g is frozen. The frozen specimen is sent (in dry ice) to a central laboratory for progesterone receptor analysis. Results are usually available in 2 weeks. Immunohistochemical methods of progesterone receptor assay are available on specimens weighing <1 g.

Contraindications. None.

Nursing considerations

Nursing Diagnoses/Collaborative Problems

- Possible knowledge deficit related to test purpose, preparation, and procedure.
- Possible anxiety related to test results.

Nursing Implications with Rationale

- Explain the procedure to the patient.
- Women are usually very anxious regarding breast surgery. Provide emotional support.

SUPPLEMENTAL INFORMATION

Breast sonogram

(ultrasound mammography)

Normal values: No evidence of abnormality

Rationale. Ultrasound mammography is a useful test for differentiating cystic and solid breast lesions, for diagnosing disease in women with very dense breasts, and in the follow-up of women with fibrocystic disease. In diagnostic ultrasound, harmless high-frequency sound waves are emitted and penetrate the breast. The sound waves are bounced back to the sensor and are arranged in a pictorial image by electronic conversion. A realistic Polaroid or x-ray film–like picture of the breast tissue is then obtained. Ultrasound of the breast is also useful in the examination of pregnant women who have a newly palpable breast mass and in whom radiation is to be avoided. Ultrasound may also be used to evaluate women who have silicone-prosthesis augmented breasts. The prosthesis can be penetrated by the ultrasound beam. Ordinarily, these prostheses would obscure residual tissue on physical examination and mammography.

Diagnostic accuracy is improved when breast ultrasound is combined with x-ray mammography. Ultrasound examination is a viable alternative for women who refuse to have x-ray mammography for fear of the diagnostic radiation. Ultrasound is especially useful in patients who have an abnormal mass on mammogram. The intrinsic nature (cystic versus solid) can be determined. Most cysts are benign.

Procedure. No fasting or sedation is required before this test. The patient lies in the prone position on the examining table, which contains a tank that holds heated water. One breast at a time is immersed into the water. The transducer that produces the ultrasound waves and detects their echoes is positioned at the bottom of the water tank. Total examining time takes about 15 minutes. Some laboratories use a hand-held transducer that can be placed on the skin overlying the breast after using a conductive paste.

There is no discomfort associated with a breast sonogram. Women with back problems or those with limited flexibility may have difficulty maintaining the position for this procedure.

Contraindications. None.

Nursing considerations

Nursing Diagnoses/Collaborative Problems

See Ultrasound Studies, p. 6.

Nursing Implications with Rationale

- Explain the procedure to the patient, assure the patient that no discomfort is associated with the study.
- Instruct the patient not to apply any lotions, powders or cosmetics to the breast area on the day of the examination.
- After the test is completed, the breasts are dried or the conductive paste is removed.

CASE STUDY 2: SERUM TUMOR MARKERS

Ms. T.G., 52 years old, had a 2-week history of abdominal discomfort associated with rapid onset of abdominal distention, weight gain, anorexia, and mild nausea. She had also noted marked shortness of breath and weakness.

Her physical examination indicated that she had decreased breath sounds bilaterally. Her abdomen was distended and obviously ascitic. She was mildly edematous in both lower extremities.

Studies	Results
Chest x-ray examination	Bilateral effusion
Routine laboratory studies	Within normal limits
Computed tomographic scan of the abdomen (see Chapter 4)	Diffuse ascites and nodular peritoneal tumor implantation
Serum tumor markers	
CA 15-3	20 U/ml (normal: <22 U/ml)
CA 125	859 U/ml (normal: 0-35 U/ml)
CA 19-9	18 units/ml (normal: <37 U/ml)
CEA (see Chapter 4)	1 ng/ml (normal: <2 ng/ml)

The patient's presenting symptoms were diffuse ascites and a pleural effusion apparently from a neoplastic cause. The tests supported the clinical findings. Possible neoplasms that might have caused the above findings included metastatic bowel cancer, pancreatic cancer, breast cancer, or ovarian cancer. The normal CEA did not support the bowel as a potential primary cancer site. Likewise, the normal CA 19-9 excluded pancreatic cancer, and the normal CA 15-3 made it unlikely that the primary cancer site was the breast. The markedly elevated CA 125 provided strong supportive evidence that the primary site of cancer was the ovaries. The results reflect the typical tumor marker profile of an ovarian cancer patient. The patient underwent a diagnostic laparotomy and a tumor debulking. She subsequently underwent chemotherapy, and on a second-look operation 1 year later, she was found to be free of disease.

DISCUSSION OF TESTS

CA 15-3 Serum tumor marker

Normal values: <22 U/ml

Rationale. CA 15-3 is a tumor-associated serum marker available for diagnosis and monitoring of treatment of breast cancer. Until now, no other good tumor marker has been available for breast cancer patients. The CEA, which is the most widely used tumor marker, is limited by poor sensitivity and specificity for patients with breast cancer. Most recently the monoclonal antibody technology has permitted the development of CA 15-3 antigen. CA 15-3 is not as sensitive in the diagnosis of primary breast cancer as other tumor markers are for their respective tumors. That is, CA 15-3 levels are not high in patients whose presenting symptoms are limited, localized, breast cancers or those with small tumor burden. On the other hand, patients with metastatic breast cancer do have markedly elevated levels. Therefore, its usefulness as a screening technique in early breast cancers, the most common cancer of women, does not exist.

Benign breast or ovarian disease and other nonbreast malignancies can cause elevated CA 15-3 levels. However, CA 15-3 is useful in monitoring the patient's response to therapy in the setting of metastatic breast cancer. A partial or complete response to treatment will be confirmed by declining levels. Likewise, a persistent rise of CA 15-3 levels despite therapy strongly suggests progressive disease.

CA 15-3 levels cannot be used in the surveillance of patients who have had a complete response to breast cancer as a result of surgery, radiation therapy, or chemotherapy. This marker's high sensitivity but lack of specificity often inappropriately suggests recurrent disease when indeed other benign processes exist.

Procedure. Seven to 10 ml of blood are drawn from the antecubital fossa, placed in a red-top tube, and sent to a major diagnostic laboratory for CA 15-3 determination. Results are made available in 7 to 10 days. CA 15-3 is a circulating tumor-associated antigen that is shed from mammary epithelial tumor cells into the circulation. It is measured by complexing with radiolabeled monoclonal antibodies to the CA 15-3 antigen. These antigen antibodies are usually created in serum. No preparatory steps are required.

Contraindications. None.

Nursing considerations

Nursing Diagnoses/Collaborative Problems

See Blood studies, p. 2.

Nursing Implications with Rationale

- After venipuncture is performed, assess the site for bleeding.

CA-125 Serum tumor marker

Normal values: 0-35 U/ml

Rationale. The detection, extent of disease, and response to the treatment of ovarian cancer can be determined with the use of CA-125. This tumor marker has a high degree of sensitivity and specificity for ovarian cancer and has proven to be of great benefit for clinicians. While $alpha_1$ fetoprotein (AFP) and human chorionic gonadotropin (HCG) are accurate tumor markers for germ cell tumors of the ovary, CA-125 is an extremely accurate tumor marker for epithelial tumors of the ovary.

CA-125 can be used in many ways. It is helpful in making the diagnosis of ovarian cancer. For example, CA-125 can be used in women whose presenting symptoms are a sudden onset of abdominal distention, ascites, and palpable pelvic masses. In these patients, a markedly elevated CA-125 is strong confirmatory evidence that the underlying etiology represents epithelial ovarian malignancy.

CA-125 serum tumor marker is also used to determine response to therapy. Serial comparative testing shows a progressive decline in CA-125 levels for patients having a response to treatment. Also, CA-125 tumor markers can predict whether or not a second-look diagnostic laparotomy will be positive. In 97% of patients whose CA-125 level is above 35 U/ml, a residual tumor is detected at a second-look laparotomy, whereas only 56% of ovarian cancer patients whose CA-125 level is below 35 have a positive second-look laparotomy.

Finally, CA-125 determinations can be used in post-treatment surveillance of ovarian cancer patients. If a patient has had complete tumor response as a result of radiation therapy, chemotherapy, or surgery, a delayed rise in CA-125 level may be an early predictor of a recurrent tumor. CA-125 serum tumor marker has not yet been used as a screening test for the asymptomatic population; however, it is presently being studied.

Other tumors and benign processes can cause elevation of CA-125. In 20% of patients with colon cancer and in 60% of patients with upper GI cancers, CA-125 levels exceed 35. Endometrial, fallopian tube, lung, and breast cancers also can cause elevations of this protein. It is interesting to note that patients with benign peritoneal diseases such as cirrhosis and endometriosis have mild elevations. Pregnancy and normal menstruation may also cause mild elevations of CA-125. Increased levels occur in 2% of healthy people and 6% of patients with nonmalignant diseases.

Procedure. Serum from the female patient is obtained in a red-top tube by a laboratory technician. No fasting or other preparatory steps are required. Although the blood can be drawn in any local hospital, it is usually sent to one of the few central diagnostic laboratories for determination of CA-125 level. CA-125 is an antigen that exists in the serum of patients with ovarian carcinoma.

A radiolabeled monoclonal antibody developed in mice that have been immunized to an epithelial cell line of tumor (cultured from the acidic fluid of a patient with ovarian carcinoma) acts as the antibody. By radioimmunoassay technique, the quantity of CA-125 in the patient's serum can be determined accurately by combining the patient's serum with the radiolabeled monoclonal antibody to CA-125. The results are available to the local hospital within 7 to 10 days.

Contraindications. None.

Nursing considerations

Nursing Diagnoses/Collaborative Problems

See Blood studies, p. 2.

Nursing Implications with Rationale

- Assess the venipuncture site for signs of bleeding.

CA 19-9 Serum tumor marker

Normal values: <37 U/ml

Rationale. CA 19-9 is a tumor marker used in diagnosis, evaluation of response to treatment, and surveillance of patients with pancreatic or hepatobiliary cancer. It is used primarily in the diagnosis of pancreatic carcinoma. For example, in a patient whose presenting symptoms are pancreatic mass or biliary obstruction, markedly elevated levels of CA 19-9 would be confirmatory evidence that pancreatic cancer exists. Likewise, patients whose presenting symptoms are ascites, jaundice, and an elevated CA 19-9 may have a hepatobiliary cancer. CA 19-9 levels, however, may not be elevated in all patients with pancreatic carcinoma. Approximately 70% with pancreatic carcinoma and 65% with hepatobiliary cancer have elevated levels.

CA 19-9 serum tumor marker is also used to determine response to treatment. In the few patients with pancreatic-biliary cancer who have a good tumor response to surgery, chemotherapy, or radiation therapy, a decline in serum levels of CA 19-9 confirm this response. CA 19-9 levels are used in the post-treatment surveillance of those who have had pancreatic-hepatobiliary cancers. A rapid rise in CA 19-9 levels can be associated with a recurrent or progressive tumor growth. Mildly elevated levels may exist in patients with gastric cancer, colorectal cancer, and even in 6% to 7% of patients with nongastrointestinal malignancies (e.g., of the lung). Patients who have pancreatitis, gallstones, cirrhosis, and cystic fibrosis may have minimally elevated levels of CA 19-9.

Procedure. CA 19-9 is performed on the serum of patients with suspected hepatobiliary neoplasms. Seven to 10 ml of blood are withdrawn from the patient into a red-top tube. No pretesting preparation is required. The blood is usually sent to a central diagnostic laboratory that performs this test in greater volumes. The results are returned to the local hospital in 7 to 10 days. CA 19-9 is an antigen that exists in exaggerated levels in patients having pancreatic cancers. Like CA 125, it is performed by radioimmunoassay using monoclonal antibodies. The monoclonal antibody is derived from an animal that has been immunized against a unique colon carcinoma cell line. The antibody is then radiolabeled and mixed with the patient's serum. It will then complex with CA 19-9 antigens, and the accurate serum level can be determined.

Contraindications. None.

Nursing considerations

Nursing Diagnoses/Collaborative Problems

See Blood studies, p. 2.

Nursing Implications with Rationale

- Assess the venipuncture site for signs of bleeding.

SUPPLEMENTAL INFORMATION

Gallium scan

Normal value: gallium uptake in the liver, spleen, bone, and colon; no other concentration noted

Rationale. Gallium scan is a total body scan usually performed 24, 48, and 72 hours after an intravenous injection of radioactive gallium (^{67}Ga). Gallium is a radionuclide that is concentrated by areas of inflammation, infection, or abscess and by benign and malignant tumors. However, not all types of tumors concentrate gallium. Tumors that can be detected by gallium scans include sarcomas, lymphomas, hepatomas, and carcinomas of the colon, kidney, uterus, stomach, and testicle.

This test is useful in detecting primary or metastatic tumors in patients whom cancer is suspected but cannot be located by other diagnostic techniques. It is also very useful in demonstrating the source of infection in patients who have fever of unknown origin. Unfortunately, this test is not capable of differentiating tumor from infection, inflammation, or abscess.

The radionuclide is normally taken up by the liver, spleen, bones, and large bowel. As a result, one can make a statement about the uniformity of uptake by the liver and spleen similar to that described by a technetium liver scan (p. 117). A normal total body gallium scan study would demonstrate some uptake of gallium in the liver, spleen, bone, and colon; there would be no marked concentration of the gallium elsewhere.

Procedure. The unsedated patient is injected with gallium citrate. A total body scan may be performed 4 to 6 hours later by slowly passing a radionuclide detector over the body. Additional scans are taken 24, 48, and 72 hours later. During the scanning process, the patient is positioned in the supine, prone, and lateral positions. Because the bowel can take up the gallium, suppositories or enemas are sometimes given a few hours before scanning. This is especially important when accurate imaging of the abdomen or pelvis is required. The patient is asked to lie very still during the actual scanning, which takes about 30 to 60 minutes each time. It is usually performed by a nuclear medicine technician and interpreted by the nuclear medicine physician. It is performed in the nuclear medicine department.

Contraindications. The test is contraindicated when a 72-hour delay in obtaining information is not possible before initiating therapy. Often a therapeutic modality must be started sooner.

Nursing considerations

Nursing Diagnoses/Collaborative Problems

See Nuclear scanning, p. 5.

Nursing Implications with Rationale

- Explain the procedure to the patient. Reassure the patient that the test is painless and that the dose of radionuclide is safe.
- Administer enemas or suppositories, as ordered, before scanning is performed to wash out the gallium secreted in the bowel. This eliminates the possibility that increased uptake in the sigmoid colon would be misread as a pathologic process.
- Be sure the patient is instructed to return for subsequent scanning.

Lymphangiography

(lymphangiogram, lymphography)

Normal values: normal lymph nodes and vessels

Rationale. Lymphangiography provides an x-ray examination of the lymphatic system after the injection of contrast medium into a lymphatic vessel in each foot or in each hand. The lymphatic system consists of lymph vessels and lymph nodes. Assessment of this system is important because cancer often spreads via the lymphatic system. When the lymph vessels become obstructed, edema usually results. Lymphangiography aids in evaluating unexplained swelling of an extremity.

Lymphangiography is indicated in patients with edema or signs of tumor (such as unexplained fever, weight loss, or enlarged lymph nodes) or to evaluate the spread of cancer within the body. Lymphangiography is useful in staging a lymphoma to determine appropriate therapy and in evaluating the results of chemotherapy or radiation therapy. Because the contrast medium remains in the lymph nodes for 6 months to 1 year, repeat plain film x-ray examinations may be done for follow-up of disease progression or response to treatment.

Lipid pneumonia may be a complication of lymphangiography if the contrast medium flows into the thoracic duct and causes microemboli in the lungs. These small emboli usually disappear after several weeks or months.

Procedure. No fasting or sedation is usually required for lymphangiography. This procedure is performed in the radiology department with the patient lying on his or her back. A blue dye is injected between each of the first three toes in each foot to outline the lymphatic vessels. (The dye can also be injected into the web of skin between the fingers.) A local anesthetic is then injected before a small incision is made in each foot. A lymphatic vessel is identified, and a cannula is inserted to infuse the iodine contrast agent. The dye is infused into the vessels for approximately 1½ hours. The infusion is usually done using an infusion pump to inject the dye at a slow continuous rate. The patient must lie very still during the dye injection. The flow of iodine dye throughout the body is followed by fluoroscopy (moving x-ray pictures on a television monitor). When the contrast medium reaches a certain level of the lumbar vertebrae, the dye is discontinued. Films are then taken of the stomach, the pelvis, and the upper body to demonstrate the filling of the lymphatic vessels. The patient must return in 24 hours to have additional x-ray studies taken to visualize the lymph nodes. When the injection is given in the hand, the axillary and supraclavicular lymph nodes are evaluated. When the injection is completed, the cannula is removed and the incision is sutured closed.

This procedure is performed by a radiologist in approximately 3 hours. Additional x-ray films must be taken again at 24 hours, but these take $<$30 minutes to perform. Discomfort may be felt when the toes are locally anesthetized. The injection of the dye between the toes or the fingers causes transient discomfort. However, the hardest part of this procedure may be lying still on the hard x-ray table.

Contraindications. Lymphangiography is contraindicated in patients allergic to iodine dye or those with severe chronic lung disease, cardiac disease, or advanced kidney or liver disease.

Nursing considerations

Nursing Diagnoses/Collaborative Problems

See X-ray studies, p. 4.

Nursing Implications with Rationale

- Explain the procedure to the patient. Inform the patient that remaining still during the test is essential. Before the study ensure that the patient has signed a consent form.
- Before the study is performed, the patient should be assessed for allergies to iodine, seafood, or any of the dyes used in diagnostic studies (such as intravenous pyelography).
- Inform the patient that the blue dye gives the skin a bluish tinge and may discolor the urine and stool for 2 days.
- After the study the vital signs are taken according to the physician's routine. The patient is checked for any signs of shortness of breath, chest pain, fever, or hypotension,

which could be caused by microemboli from spillage of the contrast dye into the thoracic duct.

- Be aware that usually after this test bed rest is prescribed for about 24 hours.
- After this procedure elevate the patient's affected extremity to help prevent edema.
- After lymphangiography the incision site may be sore for several days. Administer mild analgesics for pain after the local anesthetic wears off. Apply warm compresses as ordered, to reduce discomfort from inflammation.
- The sutures are removed in approximately 1 week. Until this time keep the incision site clean and dry. Examine the site for signs of infection (such as redness, swelling, and oozing). Report any numbness in the extremity immediately to the physician because of the possibility of nerve damage.

Alpha$_1$ fetoprotein

(AFP)

Rationale. AFP is discussed on p. 373 in regard to its evaluation of the patient with a high-risk pregnancy. AFP also has a role in the evaluation of patients with cancer. Normally, AFP exists in the embryonic liver and is secreted into the blood during normal gestation. AFP levels become undetectable in the blood soon after birth. However, neoplasms of the liver and germ cell tumors of the testicle and ovaries may secrete this protein into the blood. As a result, AFP can be used to detect and follow the clinical course of patients with tumors such as hepatomas, hepatoblastomas, teratoblastomas, and other embryonic tumors of the gonads. AFP levels are also useful in differentiating neonatal hepatitis from biliary atresia in the newborn. Other uses are described in Chapter 9.

Procedure. See p. 373.

Contraindications. See p. 373.

Nursing considerations

Nursing Diagnoses/Collaborative Problems

See Blood studies, p. 2.

Nursing Implications with Rationale

- See p. 373.

5-Hydroxyindoleacetic acid

(5-HIAA)

Normal values: 2-9 mg/24 hours (women's levels are lower than men's)

Rationale. Qualitative analysis of urine levels of 5-hydroxyindoleacetic acid (5-HIAA) is used to detect and follow the clinical course of patients with carcinoid tumors. Carcinoid tumors are serotonin-secreting tumors that may grow in the appendix, intestine, pancreas, ovaries, lung, or any tumor derived from the neuroectoderm. These tumors contain argentaffin cells, which produce serotonin and other powerful vasopressors that are metabolized by the liver to 5-HIAA and excreted in the urine. These powerful vasopressors are responsible for the clinical presentation of the carcinoid syndrome (bronchospasm, flushing, and diarrhea).

This test is used to evaluate the possibility of carcinoid tumor in patients who present with bronchospasm, diarrhea, and flushing. Also, patients with known carcinoid tumor may be evaluated by serial levels of urinary 5-HIAA. Rising levels of 5-HIAA indicate worsening of tumor; falling levels of 5-HIAA indicate a response to antineoplastic therapy. Foods high in serotonin (e.g., avocados, bananas, tomatoes, walnuts, and eggplant) can fictitiously raise 5-HIAA levels.

Procedure. Urine is collected for 24 hours in a large urine container that contains a preservative to keep the specimen at an appropriate pH level. The specimen is kept refrigerated during the collection period. After the 24-hour collection has been completed, the specimen is taken to the chemistry laboratory. Many medications may interfere with this test, including tricyclic antidepressants, monoamine oxidase inhibitors, methyldopa, phenacetin, acetaminophen, aspirin, phenothiazines, and any products containing phenylalanine and alcohol.

Contraindications. None.

Nursing considerations

Nursing Diagnoses/Collaborative Problems
See Urine studies, p. 3.

Nursing Implications with Rationale

- Explain the importance of accurately obtaining all urine during the 24-hour collection period. See Creatinine clearance, p. 231 (all but the first and last nursing implications) for the correct method of obtaining a 24-hour urine specimen.
- Instruct the patient to refrain from eating foods containing serotonin (such as plums, pineapples, bananas, eggplant, tomatoes, avocados, or walnuts) for several days (usually 3) before and during the testing period.
- Ensure that the patient has not been ingesting any of the previously mentioned drugs that affect 5-HIAA levels. If any of these medications have been or are being taken, list them on the lab slip and record them on the patient's chart.
- Instruct the patient to preserve the specimen in the refrigerator during the collection period.

Human chorionic gonadotropin

(HCG)

Normal value: negative

Rationale. HCG can be used to determine fetal or placental function as described on p. 355 in Chapter 9. However, it is also useful in determining the clinical course of patients with germ cell tumors.

As described previously (p. 355), HCG is produced by trophoblastic cells in the fetal placental unit. HCG provides the basis of all pregnancy tests. Gestational tumors (such as hydatidiform moles and uterine choriocarcinomas) and gonadal tumors can be detected by increased levels of HCG in patients who have clinical pictures suspicious for those tumors. Once these tumors have been diagnosed, HCG measurements can act as guidelines for evaluation of the success of the instituted therapy. Elevated levels of HCG are suspicious for tumor progression; decreased levels indicate effective antitumor treatment. Cancers of the GI tract, lung, and liver are also occasionally associated with elevated HCG levels.

Procedure. See p. 357.

Contraindications. See p. 357.

Nursing considerations

Nursing Diagnoses/Collaborative Problems
See HCG, p. 357.

Nursing Implications with Rationale

- See p. 357.

Urine test for Bence Jones protein

Normal value: No Bence Jones protein present.

Rationale. Bence Jones proteins are lightweight immunoglobulins that are commonly found in patients who have multiple myelomas. They may also be associated with tumor metastases to the bone, chronic lymphocytic leukemias, and amyloidosis. These proteins are most notably made by the plasma cell in patients with multiple myeloma. These immunoglobulins are rapidly cleared by the kidney and are excreted into the urine. Because the Bence Jones protein is rapidly cleared from the blood by the kidney, it is very difficult to detect in the blood; therefore, only urine is used for this study. Normally the urine should contain no Bence Jones proteins.

Procedure. An early morning urine specimen of at least 50 ml of uncontaminated urine is collected in a container. It is then taken to the laboratory where immunoelectrophoresis is carried out on the specimen. Less accurate thermal coagulation methods are also used. It is important to avoid contamination of the specimen with stool, menstrual blood, prostatic excretions, or semen. If the specimen cannot be taken to the laboratory immediately, it should be refrigerated because heat-coagulable proteins can decompose, causing a false-positive test.

Contraindications. None.

Nursing considerations

Nursing Diagnoses/Collaborative Problems

See Urine studies, p. 3.

Nursing Implications with Rationale

- Make sure the patient understands how to obtain a noncontaminated urine specimen. Assist the patient as needed.
- Ensure that the specimen is taken to the laboratory as soon as possible; if there is any delay refrigerate the specimen.

QUESTIONS AND ANSWERS

1. **QUESTION:** Your patient, who is having a routine evaluation, is found to have a suspicious lesion during mammography. Her physical examination results are negative, and she has no palpable masses. Should a biopsy of this mass be performed?

   ANSWER: With the wide-spread routine use of mammography, early nonpalpable cancers are being found more often. It is not unusual for a small cancer to be clinically undetectable. Therefore, if the mammography is suspicious, a biopsy should be performed so that the cancer can be treated at the earliest stage if the results are positive.
2. **QUESTION:** Your patient is a 56-year-old woman who has had a colon cancer removed 2 years ago. Her CEA level is now 4.2. Is this significant?

   ANSWER: This patient's CEA level (see Chapter 3) is clearly elevated. However, without knowing previous CEA levels, one cannot say with certainty that the level is representative of recurrent disease. Some patients persistently have a mildly elevated CEA level without evidence of recurrent disease. A rising CEA level is of clinical significance. If the CEA level is found to be rising monthly on three successive tests, one should strongly consider the possibility of recurrent colon cancer in this patient. Remember, however, many causes other than recurrent cancer can produce an elevated CEA level. These are listed in the chapter.
3. **QUESTION:** Your 36-year-old patient has had a routine screening thermogram of the breast. A "hot" area has been identified in the upper outer quadrant of the left breast. Should a biopsy be performed in that area?

   ANSWER: Thermography is far too unreliable to warrant a biopsy based on an abnormal result. Thermograms are quite sensitive and can pick up tumors, fibrocystic disease, and infection earlier than other tests can. However, thermograms cannot differentiate between these three abnormalities. The mammogram is a more specific test, yet less sensitive. The combination of a good physical examination and a mammogram can determine much more adequately the need of a breast biopsy. If the mammogram result is suspicious or the physical examination indicates a suspicious lump, biopsy should be performed. Biopsy, however, should not be performed on the basis of the thermogram alone.
4. **QUESTION:** Your 62-year-old patient is admitted to the hospital for melanoma. During his staging workup, he has a bone scan performed. The bone scan is normal except for a "hot spot" in the right rib. What might cause this abnormality?

   ANSWER: Increased uptake on a bone scan (hot spot) can be caused by many things. Obviously, metastatic tumor to the bone is one. Other possibilities would include an old, healed fracture, arthritis, or benign bone disease. In this case an x-ray examination of the rib was performed, and an old, healed rib fracture was identified. On obtaining a more accurate history from the patient, it was noted that he fell several years ago and had severe pain in that area for over 2 weeks. This history is compatible with a previous fractured rib.
5. **QUESTION:** Your 22-year-old female patient has been complaining of right upper quadrant abdominal pain. A gallbladder series and upper gastrointestinal study have been performed, and were found to be negative. A liver-spleen scan has indicated a filling defect in the anterior surface of the liver. Does this indicate a liver tumor?

   ANSWER: No. Many diseases can produce an abnormal liver scan such as this. Benign tumors, such as adenomas, cysts, or congenital abnormalities, can cause such an appearance. A CT scan should be performed to eliminate the possibility of a cyst. Also CT-guided liver biopsies can be performed to elucidate more clearly the cause of this abnormal liver scan. If these fail to resolve the problem, peritonoscopy with actual visualization of that portion of the liver can be performed.
6. **QUESTION:** Your patient has recently been admitted to the hospital with a rapid onset of ascites.

She is extremely uncomfortable and very anxious to institute treatment for this symptom. You are aware that tumor markers have been performed. The patient's family is frustrated with the delay in her diagnosis and treatment. What explanation can you give the family for the delay?

ANSWER: The nurse must explain to the family that because many of these serum tumor markers require radioimmunoassay testing for accurate results, they must be sent to a major diagnostic laboratory. Therefore, the test results may take 7 to 10 days. If these results are required before the institution of therapy, indicate that all efforts will be made to provide comfort to the patient until this information is available.

BIBLIOGRAPHY

Bischof P and others: Peripheral CA 125 levels in patients with uterine fibroids, Human Reprod 7(1):35-38, Jan 1992.

Bunn PA: Tumor markers. In Wyngaarden JB and others, editors: Cecil textbook of medicine, ed 19, Philadelphia, 1992, WB Saunders.

Cruickshank DJ and others: An independent evaluation of the potential clinical usefulness of proposed CA-125 indices previously shown to be of prognostic significance in epithelial ovarian cancer, Br J Cancer 65(4):597-600, April 1992.

Cruickshank DJ and others: CA 125–response assessment in epithelial ovarian cancer, Int J Cancer 51(1):58-61, April 1992.

Frohman LA: Endocrine manifestations for neoplasia. In Wilson J and others, editors: Harrison's principles of internal medicine, ed 12, New York, McGraw-Hill.

Garnick MB: Testicular cancer and other trophoblastic diseases. In Wilson J and others, editors: Harrison's principles of internal medicine, ed 12, New York, 1991, McGraw-Hill.

Glenn J and others: Evaluation of the utility of a radioimmunoassay for serum CA 19-9 levels in patients before and after treatment of carcinoma of the pancreas, J Clin Oncol 6(3):462-468, 1988.

Grover S and others: Factors influencing serum CA 125 levels in normal women, Obstet Gynecol 79(4):511-514, April 1992.

Halila H and others: Ovarian cancer antigen CA-125 levels in pelvic inflammatory disease and pregnancy, Cancer 57(7):1327-1329, 1988.

Henderson C: Breast cancer. In Wilson J and others, editors: Harrison's principles of internal medicine, ed 12, New York, 1991, McGraw-Hill.

Lewis BJ: Breast cancer. In Wyngaarden JB and others, editors: Cecil textbook of medicine, ed 19, Philadelphia, 1992, WB Saunders.

Liu L and others: Evaluation of second-look laparotomy for ovarian cancer: second-look versus serum CA 125, Clin Med Sci J 6(2):96-99, June 1991.

Mendelsohn J: Principles of neoplasia. In Wilson J and others, editors: Harrison's principles of internal medicine, ed 12, New York, 1991, McGraw-Hill.

Mija J and others: Analysis of cytosel CA 15-3, carcinoembryonic antigen, estrogens, and progesterone receptors in breast cancer tissues, Jpn Cancer Res 83(2):171-177, Feb 1992.

Rustin GJ and others: Savings obtained by CA-125 measurement during therapy for ovarian carcinoma, Eur J Cancer 28(1):79-82.

Salmon SE: Principles of cancer therapy. In Wyngaarden JB and others, editors: Cecil textbook of medicine, ed 19, Philadelphia, 1992, WB Saunders.

Tian F and others: Prognostic value of serum CA 19-9 levels in pancreatic adenocarcinoma, Ann Surg 215(4):350-355, April 1992.

Chapter 14

DIAGNOSTIC STUDIES USED IN ROUTINE LABORATORY TESTING AND MISCELLANEOUS TESTING

ROUTINE LABORATORY TESTING

Although a complete and thorough history and physical examination are essential to an adequate patient evaluation, they cannot detect many serious imbalances that may afflict a patient. Today, with the availability of multiphasic laboratory testing machines, the patient can be more completely screened for the presence of disease. Nearly every hospital clinical laboratory has multiphasic serum-screening machines capable of rapidly and inexpensively measuring calcium, phosphorus, triglycerides, protein, bilirubin, transaminases, alkaline phosphatase, lactic dehydrogenase (LDH), blood urea nitrogen (BUN), creatinine, electrolytes, and glucose. Also, the complete blood count (CBC) can be performed easily with the help of automation. Because many unsuspected diseases can be detected by the use of chest x-ray studies and electrocardiography (EKG), the performance of these tests has now also been standardized so that they, too, can be performed rapidly and easily. All of these studies are essential components of a complete medical evaluation of most patients.

Because multiple simultaneous testing techniques permit an easily performed and inexpensive evaluation of numerous patient samples at the same time, coagulation studies have become part of routine testing. Furthermore, the development of multiple dipstick testing (as with Multistix) has greatly increased the ease and availability of routine urine evaluation.

Routine testing, coupled with a thorough history and physical examination, allows one to screen for a large number of diseases that might otherwise go undetected. Also, many diseases can be detected at an early stage before symptoms become apparent and can therefore be treated more easily and effectively. The cost of routine testing is relatively small in comparison to its effectiveness.

When serum evaluations are performed singly, they are both costly and time-consuming, and, as a result, they cannot be performed frequently (such as for monitoring therapy). However, multiphasic automation has made these single serum tests inexpensive and easily available as a part of the multiphasic test. Examples of multiphasic testing include the SMA 6, SMA 12, and Astra 7. The numeral indicates the number of different laboratory tests performed in that series. Many combinations are available and can be obtained from the laboratory in one's institution. An inexpensive and practical method for monitoring electrolyte abnormalities and diseases such as gout and diabetes effectively is thus available.

Routine laboratory admission testing is usually done at a designated admission center in the hospital or in the patient's room by a technician or a nurse. Collecting the blood in the appropriate color-coded test tube is important. The rubber stoppers of the test tubes are coded by color to indicate the presence or absence of different additives in the collection tube. The most common additives are preservatives, which prevent chemical or physical changes in the specimen, and anticoagulants, which inhibit clot formation. Institutional procedure manuals should be consulted to determine the appropriate number and color of the specimen tubes that are required.

In addition to collecting the correct number of properly color-coded tubes of blood, the nurse or technician should prevent hemolysis of the blood sample. A hemolyzed sample is unsuitable for many tests and usually necessitates repeated venipuncture. Hemolysis can be prevented by avoiding the use of a small venipuncture needle. Usually a 20-, 21- or 22-gauge needle is used. If a syringe is used in contrast to a Vacutainer holder, the plunger should not be pulled back too forcefully. After the needle is removed, the blood should be slowly injected into the side of the glass test tube. The collected specimens should not be agitated. Gentle inversion of the container is sufficient to allow mixture of the additive with the blood.

Since more of these tests have been discussed in previous chapters, only those that have not been discussed properly will be mentioned here.

CASE STUDY 1: ROUTINE ADMISSION WORKUP

Mrs. A., 51 years old, developed an umbilical hernia after her last pregnancy at age 41. She had no other medical problems, and the results of her physical examination were normal. She was admitted to the hospital for repair of her hernia.

Studies	Results
CBC (see Chapter 10)	
Hemoglobin concentration	14 g/dl (normal: 12-16 g/dl)
Hematocrit	43% (normal: 37%-47%)
White blood cells (WBCs)	5300 (normal: 5,000-10,000)
Differential count	
Neutrophils	60% (normal: 55%-70%)
Lymphocytes	30% (normal: 20%-40%)
Monocytes	7% (normal: 2%-8%)
Eosinophils	2% (normal: 1%-4%)
Basophils	1% (normal: 0.5%-1%)
Red blood cells (RBCs)	4.8 million/mm^3 (normal: 4.2-5.4 million/mm^3)
Mean corpuscular volume (MCV)	88 μ^3 (normal: 80-95 μ^3)
Mean corpuscular hemoglobin concentration (MCHC)	34 g/dl (normal: 32-36 g/dl)
Mean corpuscular hemoglobin (MCH)	30 pg (normal: 27-31 pg)
Platelet count	350,000/mm^3 (normal: 150,000-400,000/mm^3)
Sequential multiple analyzer, 12-item test (SMA 12)	
Calcium (see Chapter 8)	9.9 mg/dl (normal: 9-10.5 mg/dl)
Phosphorus (see Chapter 8)	3.2 mg/dl (normal: 2.5-4.5 mg/dl)
Triglycerides (see Chapter 2)	100 mg/dl (normal: 40-150 mg/dl)
Uric acid (see Chapter 11)	6.1 mg/dl (normal: 2.5-8.5 mg/dl)

Studies	Results
Creatinine (see Chapter 7)	1 mg/dl (normal: 0.7-1.5 mg/dl)
BUN (see Chapter 7)	9 mg/dl (normal: 5-20 mg/dl)
Total bilirubin (see Chapter 4)	0.8 mg/dl (normal: 0.1-1.0 mg/dl)
Alkaline phosphate (see Chapter 4)	45 ImU/ml (normal: 30-85 ImU/ml)
SGOT (see Chapters 2 and 4)	25 IU/L (normal: 5-40 IU/L)
Lactate dehydrogenase (see Chapters 2 and 4)	125 ImU/ml (normal: 90-200 ImU/ml)
Total protein (see Chapter 4)	7.2 mg/dl (normal: 6-8 mg/dl)
Albumin (see Chapter 4)	3.8 g/dl (normal: 3.2-4.5 g/dl)
Serologic test for syphilis (VDRL) (see Chapter 9)	Negative, nonreactive (normal: negative, nonreactive)
Sequential multiple analyzer, 6-item test (SMA 6)	
Sodium	138 mEq/L (normal: 136-145 mEq/L)
Potassium	4.1 mEq/L (normal: 3.5-5.0 mEq/L)
Chloride	103 mEq/L (normal: 90-110 mEq/L)
Total CO_2	24 mEq/L (normal: 23-30 mEq/L)
Glucose (see Chapter 8)	90 mg/dl (normal: 60-120 mg/dl)
BUN (see Chapter 7)	9 mg/dl (normal: 5-20 mg/dl)
Erythrocyte sedimentation rate (sed rate)	14 mm/hour (normal: up to 20mm/hour)
Urinalysis (see Chapter 7)	
pH	6.2 (normal: 4.6-8.0)
Specific gravity	1.020 (normal: 1.010-1.025)
Color	Yellow (normal: amber-yellow)
Glucose	0 (normal: negative)
Protein	0 (normal: negative)
Blood	0 (normal: up to 2 RBCs)
Casts	
RBC	0-1 (normal: negative)
WBC	0-1 (normal: negative)
Crystals	0 (normal: negative)
Coagulation profile (see Chapter 10)	
Prothrombin time (PT)	90% (normal: 11-12.5 sec or 85%-100%)
Activated partial thromboplastin time (APTT)	32 sec (normal: 30-40 sec)
EKG (see Chapter 2)	Normal sinus rhythm: no ischemic changes
Chest x-ray study (see Chapter 5)	No active disease seen
Tuberculin skin test (see Chapter 5)	Negative
Mammography (see Chapter 13)	Negative

In light of the completely negative routine laboratory evaluation, the patient underwent herniorrhaphy. Unfortunately, a high fever developed 4 days after the operation. Specimens were obtained for culture and sensitivity testing.

Studies	Results
Throat culture	Negative
Sputum culture	Normal throat flora
Urine culture	No bacteria
Blood culture	No bacteria
Wound culture	*Staphylococcus aureus;* resistant to penicillin, sensitive to oxacillin

The wound was drained, and the patient was treated with oxacillin for a 10-day period. The patient did well and had no further problems.

DISCUSSION OF TESTS

Serum electrolyte concentration test

(sodium, potassium, chloride, and carbon dioxide content)

Sodium (Na)
- Adult/elderly: 136-145 mEq/L or 136-145 mmol/L (SI units)
- Child: 136-145 mEq/L
- Infant: 134-150 mEq/L
- Newborn: 134-144 mEq/L
- *Possible critical values:* <120 or >160 mEq/L

Potassium (K)
- Normal values:
  - Adults/elderly: 3.5-5.0 mEq/L, or 3.5-5.0 mmol/L (SI units)
  - Children: 3.4-4.7 mEq/L
  - Infants: 4.1-5.3 mEq/L
  - Newborns: 3.9-5.9 mEq/L
- *Possible critical values:*
  - Adults: <2.5 or >6.5 mEq/L
  - Newborns: <2.5 or >8.0 mEq/L

Chloride (Cl)
- Normal values:
  - Adults/elderly: 90-110 mEq/L, or 90-110 mmol/L (SI units)
  - Children: 90-110 mEq/L
  - Newborns: 96-106 mEq/L
  - Premature infants: 95-110 mEq/L
- *Possible critical values:* <80 or >115 mEq/L

Carbon dioxide (CO_2)
- Normal values:
  - Adults/elderly: 23-30 mEq/L, or 23-30 mmol/L (SI units)
  - Children: 20-28 mEq/L
  - Infants: 20-28 mEq/L
  - Newborns: 13-22 mEq/L
- *Possible critical values:* ≤6 mEq/L

Rationale

Sodium. The sodium content of the blood is a result of a balance between dietary sodium intake and renal excretion. In the healthy individual, nonrenal sodium losses are minimal. Many factors assist in this homeostatic sodium balance. The role of aldosterone is described on p. 222 (see Figure 7-3). Aldosterone tends to conserve sodium by decreasing renal losses. "Natriuretic hormone" tends to encourage renal losses of sodium. Water and sodium are physiologically very closely interrelated. As free body water is increased, serum sodium is diluted and the concentration may decrease. The kidney compensates by conserving sodium and excreting water. If free body water were to decrease, the serum sodium concentration would rise. The kidney would then respond by conserving free water.

Sodium is the major cation in the extracellular space, where serum levels of approximately 140 mEq/L exist. The concentration of sodium intracellularly is only 5 mEq/L. Sodium salts therefore are the major determinants of extracellular osmolality.

The following outline shows the causes of hypernatremia (increased serum sodium concentration) and hyponatremia (decreased serum sodium concentration).

A. Hypernatremia
   1. Increased sodium intake (without access to water)
      a. Excessive dietary intake
      b. Excessive sodium in intravenous fluid
   2. Decreased sodium loss
      a. Cushing's syndrome
      b. Hyperaldosteronism
   3. Excessive free body water loss (hypernatremic dehydration)
      a. Excessive sweating
      b. Extensive thermal burns
      c. Diabetes insipidus
      d. Osmotic diuresis (as in glycosuria and overzealous mannitol administration)
      e. Prolonged hyperpnea
      f. Severe water loss from diarrhea or vomiting
   4. Inadequate water intake
   5. Drugs such as steroids, carbenicillin, diazoxide, and sodium bicarbonate

B. Hyponatremia
   1. Decreased sodium intake
      a. Deficient dietary intake
      b. Deficient sodium in intravenous fluid
   2. Increased sodium loss
      a. Addison's disease

b. Diarrhea
c. Vomiting or nasogastric aspiration
d. Diuretic administration
e. Chronic renal insufficiency (inadequate tubular reabsorption of sodium)
3. Increased free body water (dilutional)
a. Excessive oral water intake
b. Excessive intravenous water intake
c. Congestive heart failure
d. Inappropriate secretion of antidiuretic hormone
e. Osmotic dilution (as in hyperglycemia and hyperproteinemia)
4. Third-space losses of sodium
a. Ascites
b. Peripheral edema
c. Pleural effusion
d. Intraluminal bowel loss (ileus or mechanical obstruction)
5. Drugs such as captopril, amitriptyline, diuretics, and antiinflammatory agents

Symptoms of hypernatremia may include dry mucus membranes, thirst, agitation, restlessness, hyperreflexia, mania, and convulsions. Hyponatremia's symptoms are weakness, confusion, lethargy, stupor, and coma.

Potassium. Potassium is the major cation within the cell. The intracellular potassium concentration is approximately 150 mEq/L, whereas normal serum potassium concentration is about 4 mEq/L. This ratio is the most important determinant in maintaining membrane potential in excitable neuromuscular tissue. Because the serum concentration of potassium is so small, minor changes in concentration have significant consequences.

Serum potassium concentration is dependent on many factors, including:

1. Aldosterone. This hormone tends to increase renal losses of potassium.
2. Sodium reabsorption. As sodium is reabsorbed, potassium is lost.
3. Acid-base balance. Alkalotic states tend to lower serum potassium levels causing a shift of potassium into the cell. Acidotic states tend to raise serum potassium levels by reversing the shift.

The following outline shows the causes of hyperkalemia (increased serum potassium concentration) and hypokalemia (decreased serum potassium concentration).

A. Hyperkalemia
1. Increased potassium intake
a. Excessive dietary intake
b. Excessive intravenous intake
2. Decreased potassium loss
a. Acute or chronic renal failure
b. Addison's disease
c. Hypoaldosteronism
d. Aldosterone-inhibiting diuretics (such as spironolactone and triamterene)
3. Shift from intracellular space
a. Acidosis
b. Infection
c. Crush injury to tissues
d. Malignant hyperthermia
4. Pseudohyperkalemia
a. Poor venipuncture technique
b. Transfusion of hemolyzed blood
5. Drugs such as arginine, ibuprofen, indomethacin

B. Hypokalemia
1. Decreased potassium intake
a. Deficient dietary intake
b. Deficient intravenous intake
2. Excessive potassium loss
a. Gastrointestinal disorders (diarrhea, vomiting, and villous adenomas)
b. Diuretics
c. Hyperaldosteronism
d. Cushing's syndrome
e. Renal tubular acidosis
f. Licorice ingestion
3. Shift to intracellular space
a. Alkalosis
b. Insulin or glucose administration
c. Calcium administration
4. Drugs such as albuterol, bisacodyl, steroids, and diuretics

Symptoms of hyperkalemia include irritability, nausea, vomiting, intestinal colic, and diarrhea. The EKG may demonstrate peaked T waves, a widened QRS complex, and depressed S-T segments. Signs of hypokalemia are related to a decrease in contractility of smooth, skeletal, and cardiac muscles, which results in weakness, paralysis, hyporeflexia, ileus, increased cardiac sensitivity to digoxin, cardiac arrhythmias, flattened T waves, and prominent U waves.

Chloride. Chloride is the major extracellular anion, whose major purpose is to maintain electrical neutrality, mostly as a salt with sodium. It follows sodium losses and accompanies sodium excesses. Chloride also serves as a buffer to assist in acid-base balance. As CO_2 increases, bicarbonate moves from intracellular space to the extracellular space. To maintain electrical neutrality, chloride shifts back into the cell.

Hypochloremia and hyperchloremia rarely occur by themselves and usually parallel shifts in sodium levels, the causes of which are listed in the outline under the discussion of sodium.

Carbon dioxide content. As discussed in Chapter 5 (see p. 150), CO_2 content is a measure of the bicarbonate ion (HCO_3^-) that exists in the serum. This anion is of secondary importance in electrical neutrality of extracellular and intracellular fluid. Its major role is in acid-base balance, as discussed on p. 150. Increases occur with alkalosis, and decreases occur with acidosis.

Procedure. Seven milliliters of peripheral venous blood are obtained and placed in a red-top tube (without any anticoagulants). Using at least a 20-gauge needle to obtain the blood is important in preventing hemolysis, which may cause pseudohyperkalemia. If the patient has an intravenous line, the venipuncture should be performed in the contralateral extremity to avoid artificial results caused by the fluid infusion.

The blood is then sent to the chemistry laboratory where a multiphasic machine performs the electrolyte concentration determinations. Results can frequently be reported in approximately 30 minutes. The only discomfort associated with this study is that of the venipuncture.

Contraindications. None.

Nursing considerations

Nursing Diagnoses/Collaborative Problems

See Blood studies, p. 2.

Nursing Implications with Rationale

- Explain the procedure to the patient.
- Obtain the blood by peripheral venipuncture. Avoid hemolysis by using a 20-gauge needle. Do not aspirate very strongly or push the plunger into the vacutainer tube too forcefully. This action can cause hemolysis and affect results.
- Apply a pressure dressing to the site. Assess the site for bleeding.
- If the patient is receiving an intravenous infusion, obtain the blood from the opposite arm.
- Because this study is usually performed with a glucose level determination, mark the time that the test was performed to avoid confusion in the glucose reading.
- If the results are abnormal, notify the physician. If the results are unexpectedly abnormal, the physician will occasionally repeat the test because the chance of laboratory error is great since many specimens are tested at the same time. The machine that performs the determinations may malfunction.

Culture and sensitivity testing

(C & S of the throat, sputum, urine, stool, blood, wound, cervix, and urethra)

Normal values (for all cultures): negative

Rationale. When a patient develops a fever of unknown origin (FUO), all of the major potential causes of infection must be investigated. This investigation includes a thorough history and physical examination along with the obtaining of appropriate specimens for culture and sensitivity (C & S) testing. When a patient has an obvious site of infection, this too should be cultured to identify the agent. Knowledge about the organism's sensitivity to commonly used antibiotics allows the physician to accurately determine the appropriate antibiotic therapy. If the organisms are not sensitive to an antibiotic being administered, no improvement in the disease occurs. In addition, when more than one organism is causing the infection, the sensitivity report assists the physician in choosing one drug to which all of the involved organisms will be sensitive. In cases of epidemics of a particular type of infection, the sensitivity report can be used as a rough guide to the common source. All similar organisms should have the same degree of sensitivity to the same antibiotics.

Culture media may vary according to the type of organism suspected to be causing the infection. Blood agar is used to grow most routine aerobic organisms (such as *Staphylococcus* and *Escherichia coli*). Anaerobic bacteria (such as *Bacteroides* and *Clostridium* organisms) do not grow in the presence of oxygen and thus require an anoxic environment. Chocolate (denatured blood) agar is best used for *Neisseria gonorrheae* growth. Fungi grow best on Sabourand agar.

All cultures should be performed before antibiotic therapy is initiated. Otherwise, the antibiotic may interrupt the growth of the organism in the laboratory. More often than not, however, the physician wants to institute antibiotic therapy before the culture results are reported. In these instances a *gram stain* of the specimen smeared on a slide is most helpful and can be reported in less than 10 minutes. All forms of bacteria are grossly classified as gram-positive (blue staining) or gram-negative (red staining). Knowledge of the shape of the organism (that is, spherical or rod-shaped, for example) can also be very helpful in the tentative identification of the infecting organism. With knowledge of the gram-stain results, the physician can institute a reasonable antibiotic regimen based on past experience as to what the organism might be. Most organisms take about 24 hours to grow in the laboratory, and a preliminary report can be given at that time. Occasionally 48 to 72 hours are required for growth and identification of the organism. Cultures may be repeated after appropriate antibiotic therapy to assess for complete resolution of the infection (especially in urinary tract infections).

Procedure. In general, all culture specimens should be delivered to the microbiology (bacteriology) laboratory and cultured as soon as they are obtained; otherwise, overgrowth of the bacteria occurs. If the specimen is obtained at night or on weekends and the bacteriology laboratory is closed, the specimen should be refrigerated until it can be placed on the culture medium. When an anaerobic infection is suspected, the specimen should be aspirated into a sterile syringe and "topped" until it can be cultured in anaerobic conditions.

Throat culture. Because the throat culture is normally colonized by many organisms, culture technique of this area serves only to isolate and identify a few particular pathogens (such as streptococci, meningococci, gonococci, *Bordetella pertussis,* or *Corynebacterium diphtheriae*). Recognition of these organisms requires treatment. Streptococci are most commonly looked for because a beta-hemolytic streptococcal pharyngitis may be followed by rheumatic fever or glomerulonephritis. This type of streptococcal infection most commonly affects children between the ages of 3 and 15 years. Therefore, all children who have a sore throat and fever should have a throat culture done to attempt to identify streptococcal infections. In adults, however, fewer than 5% of patients with pharyngitis have a streptococcal infection. Therefore, throat cultures in adults are only indicated when the patient has severe sore throat, fever, and palpable lymphadenopathy. All other adults with a severe sore throat usually do not receive throat cultures.

A throat culture specimen can best be obtained by depressing the tongue with a wooden blade (tongue blade) and touching the posterior wall of the throat with a sterile cotton swab. One must avoid touching any other part of the mouth. The swab is placed in a sterile container and sent to the microbiology laboratory.

Sputum culture. Sputum cultures aid in the identification of the organisms causing a pulmonary infection. However, because the specimen is usually obtained through the pharyngeal cavity, which is normally heavily colonized with bacteria, sputum culture results are frequently inaccurate.

When an overabundance of one type of organism is mixed in with microscopic evidence of WBCs, one can be relatively certain that bacteria is the pathogen. Deep pulmonary secretions are routinely obtained by having the patient cough when he or she awakens (see Chapter 5, p. 141). The cough may be induced by nasotracheal aspiration, nebulizers, or pulmonary physical therapy. Sputum can also be obtained by transtracheal needle aspiration or bronchoscopic aspiration. The specimen is placed in a sterile container and transported to the bacteriology laboratory.

Urine culture. The urine culture specimen must be a clean catch, midstream collection. The patient is asked to wipe the distal urethra with an antiseptic in a front-to-back direction. Voiding is initiated. Then, during midstream, the sterile container is placed into the urine stream to collect between 5 and 50 ml of urine. The container is removed from the stream, and voiding is completed. The urine can also be collected by suprapubic aspiration or directly from an indwelling catheter (see p. 228). The specimen container is covered, labeled, and transported to the bacteriology laboratory as soon as possible.

Frequently it is beneficial to culture the urine of a patient who has an indwelling Foley catheter immediately before the removal of the catheter. This procedure is called a "terminal urine for C & S" and is usually more accurate than culturing the tip of the catheter.

Stool culture. The stool (feces) can be cultured to detect bacteria and ova and parasites (see p. 80). Bacterial cultures are usually done to detect enteropathogens (such as *Staphylococcus aureus, Salmonella, Shigella*). When the patient is suspected of having a parasitic infection, the stool is examined for ova and parasite (O & P). The major intestinal parasites of clinical significance in the United States are described on p. 80. Stools for bacteria or parasites are collected in a clean, wide-mouthed, plastic or glass container with a tight-fitting lid. The patient usually defecates into a clean bedpan and transfers either a walnut-size piece of the feces or the entire specimen (as directed by the laboratory) into the specimen container. Urine and toilet paper should not be mixed with the specimen. Since parasites or bacteria are often found in mucus or blood streaks, some of this material, if present, should be included with the sample. Cultures can also be detected by the "tape test" or by a rectal swab, which are described on p. 81.

Blood culture. Bacteremia (bacteria in the blood) is usually intermittent and transient, except in endocarditis or suppurative thrombophlebitis. Bacteremia is usually marked by chills and fever. For this reason, blood for blood culture should be drawn at the time the patient manifests the chills and fever. At least two culture specimens should be obtained from two different sites. The two culture specimens are important because if one produces a bacteria and the other does not, it is safe to assume that the bacteria in the first culture is a contaminant and not the infecting agent. When both cultures produce the infecting agent, bacteremia exists. If the patient is receiving antibiotics, the laboratory should be notified; and the blood culture specimen should be taken shortly before the next dose of the antibiotic is administered.

In the taking of the blood specimens, two different peripheral venous sites are carefully prepared with povidone-iodine (Betadine). The tops of the vacutainer tubes or culture bottles are cleaned with povidone-iodine and allowed to dry. The venipuncture is then performed aseptically, and enough blood is aspirated (approximately 8 ml) to allow a dilution ratio of blood to culture broth of about 1:10. The culture bottles should be transported to the laboratory immediately. Culture specimens drawn through an intravenous catheter are frequently contaminated, and tests using them should not be performed unless catheter sepsis is suspected. In these situations, blood culture specimens drawn through the catheter indicate the causative agent more accurately than a culture specimen from the catheter tip.

Wound culture. Wound infections are most commonly caused by pus-forming organisms. The specimen for a wound culture can best be obtained by aseptically placing a sterile cotton swab into the pus and then putting the swab into a sterile, covered test tube. The specimen is transported to the laboratory as soon as possible. Culturing specimens taken from the skin edge is much less accurate than culturing the suppurative material. If an anaerobic organism is suspected, obtain an anaerobic culture tube from the microbiology laboratory. Routine wound cultures are also done at the same time.

Cervical culture. Cervical cultures are most commonly done to detect gonorrhea (see p. 350) or other sexually transmitted diseases. The female patient should refrain from douching and tub-bathing before a cervical culture is performed. The patient is placed in the lithotomy position, and a nonlubricated vaginal speculum is inserted to expose the cervix. Cervical mucus is removed with a cotton ball held in ring forceps. A sterile-tipped swab is then inserted into the endocervical canal and moved from side to side.

Urethral culture. Urethral cultures are most commonly performed on men in whom gonorrhea or other sexually transmitted diseases are suspected (see p. 350). The urethral specimen should be obtained before voiding. This is done by inserting a sterile swab gently into the anterior urethra.

Contraindications. None.

Nursing considerations

Nursing Diagnoses/Collaborative Problems

- Possible knowledge deficit related to test purpose, preparation, and procedure
- Possible anxiety related to unknown sensations of the procedure
- Possible anxiety related to test results
- Possible alteration in comfort related to test procedure

Nursing Implications with Rationale

- Explain the purpose and procedure to the patient. Thoroughly explain the instructions if the patient is to obtain the specimen. Be certain that the patient has the appropriate cleansing agents and sterile supplies available. If the patient cannot obtain the specimen, provide nursing assistance. Drape the patient appropriately during the procedure to prevent unnecessary exposure.
- Obtain the specimens in a sterile manner. Handle all specimens as though they were capable of transmitting disease. Specimens should be transported to the laboratory immediately (at least within 30 minutes).
- Obtain the specimens before initiating the prescribed antibiotic therapy. Antibiotics alter the growth of organisms in culture media.
- Carefully label all the specimens. Include the precise time at which the specimen was collected. Also indicate any medication the patient may be taking that could affect the results.
- Notify the physician of any positive results so that appropriate antibiotic therapy can be initiated.
- If wound cultures are to be obtained on a patient requiring wound irrigation, obtain the culture *before* the wound is irrigated.

MISCELLANEOUS TESTING

Sialography

Normal values: no evidence of pathology in salivary ducts and related structures

Rationale. Sialography is an x-ray procedure used to examine the salivary ducts (parotid, submaxillary, submandibular, and sublingual) and related glandular structures after the injection of a contrast medium into the desired duct. This procedure is used to detect calculi, strictures, tumors, or inflammatory disease in patients who complain of pain, tenderness, or swelling in these areas.

Procedure. No special preparation is required before sialography. However, the patient is instructed to rinse his or her mouth with an antiseptic solution before the dye is injected. X-ray studies are taken before the injection is given to ensure that stones are not present in the salivary ducts, which could prevent the contrast material from entering the ducts. After the patient is placed in a supine position on an x-ray table, the contrast medium is injected directly into the desired orifice via a cannula or a special catheter. X-ray films are then taken with the patient in various positions.

The patient is then given a sour substance (such as lemon juice) orally to stimulate salivary excretion. Another set of x-ray studies are taken to evaluate ductal drainage. A radiologist performs this procedure in less than 30 minutes. The patient may feel a little pressure as the contrast medium is injected into the ducts.

Contraindications. None.

Nursing considerations

Nursing Diagnoses/Collaborative Problems

See X-ray studies, p. 5.

Nursing Implications with Rationale

- Explain the procedure to the patient. Instruct the patient to remove jewelry, hairpins, and dentures, which could obscure x-ray visualization.
- Instruct the patient to rinse his or her mouth before the procedure with an antiseptic solution to reduce the possibility of introducing bacteria into the ductal structures.

Therapeutic drug monitoring

Normal values: see Table 14-1

Rationale. Therapeutic drug monitoring entails taking measurements of blood drug levels to determine effective drug dosages and to prevent toxicity. Drug monitoring is especially important in patients taking medications (such as antiarrhythmics, bronchodilators, antibiotics, anticonvulsants, and cardiotonics), where the margin of safety between therapeutic and toxic levels is narrow.

Table 14-1 lists the therapeutic and toxic ranges for most patients. One should note, however, that these ranges may not apply to all patients because clinical response is influenced by many factors (such as noncompliance, concurrent drug use, other clinical conditions, age, size, extent and rate of drug absorption, and metabolism). Also, one should be aware that different laboratories use different units for reporting test results and normal ranges. It is important that sufficient time pass between the administration of the medication and the collection of the blood sample to allow for therapeutic levels to occur.

Blood samples can be taken at the drug's *peak* level (the highest therapeutic concentration) or at the *trough* level (the lowest therapeutic concentration). Peak levels are useful when testing for toxicity, and trough levels are useful for demonstrating a satisfactory therapeutic level. (Trough levels are often referred to as residual levels.)

Procedure. Generally no fluid or food restrictions are needed for therapeutic drug monitoring. A peripheral venipuncture is performed, and a specimen of blood is collected in a tube as designated by the laboratory. The blood samples can be taken at the drug's peak level or at the trough (residual) level; one of the most important laboratory problems with drug monitoring is obtaining the specimen at the proper time. Drug blood levels should have reached a steady state or equilibrium, which as a rule of

TABLE 14-1. Therapeutic Drug Monitoring Data

Drug	Use	Therapeutic level	Toxic level
Acetaminophen	Analgesic, antipyretic	Depends on use	>250 μg/ml
Amikacin	Antibiotic	15-25 μg/ml	>25 μg/ml
Aminophylline	Bronchodilator	10-20 μg/ml	>20 μg/ml
Amitriptyline	Antidepressant	120-250 ng/ml	>500 ng/ml
Carbamazepine	Anticonvulsant	5-12 μg/ml	>12 μg/ml
Chloramphenicol	Antiinfective	10-20 μg/ml	>25 μg/ml
Desipramine	Antidepressant	150-300 ng/ml	>500 ng/ml
Digitoxin	Cardiac glycoside	15-25 ng/ml	>25 ng/ml
Digoxin	Cardiac glycoside	0.8-2.0 ng/ml	>2.4 ng/ml
Disopyramide	Antiarrhythmic	2-5 μg/ml	>5 μg/ml
Ethosuximide	Anticonvulsant	40-100 μg/ml	>100 μg/ml
Gentamycin	Antibiotic	5-10 μg/ml	>12 μg/ml
Imipramine	Antidepressant	150-300 ng/ml	>500 μg/ml
Kanamycin	Antibiotic	20-25 μg/ml	>35 μg/ml
Lidocaine	Antiarrhythmic	1.5-5.0 μg/ml	>5 μg/ml
Lithium	Bipolar disorder	0.8-1.2 mEq/L	>2.0 mEq/L
Methotrexate	Antitumor	>0.01 μmol	>10 μmol/24 hours
Nortriptyline	Antidepressant	50-150 ng/ml	>500 ng/ml
Phenobarbital	Anticonvulsant	10-30 μg/ml	>40 μg/ml
Phenytoin	Anticonvulsant	10-20 μg/ml	>30 μg/ml
Primidone	Anticonvulsant	5-12 μg/ml	>15 μg/ml
Procainamide	Antiarrhythmic	4-10 μg/ml	>16 μg/ml
Propranolol	Antiarrhythmic	50-100 ng/ml	>150 ng/ml
Quinidine	Antiarrhythmic	2-5 μg/ml	>10 μg/ml
Salicylate	Antipyretic, antiinflammatory, analgesic	100-250 μg/ml	>300 μg/ml
Theophylline	Bronchodilator	10-20 μg/ml	>20 μg/ml
Tobramycin	Antibiotic	5-10 μg/ml	>12 μg/ml
Valproic acid	Anticonvulsant	50-100 μg/ml	>100 μg/mlM

thumb takes five drug half-lives. *Half-life* (biologic half-life) refers to the time required to decrease the drug blood concentration by 50% and is usually measured after absorption has been completed. *Steady state* refers to drug blood level equilibrium between drug intake and elimination. Loading doses can decrease this time span considerably. Also, the blood level should be drawn at the true peak or residual level. Peak levels are usually obtained about 1 to 2 hours after oral intake, about 1 hour after intramuscular administration, and about ½ hour after intravenous administration. Residual levels are usually obtained shortly before (0 to 15 min) the next scheduled dose.

All blood samples should be clearly marked with the following information: patient's name, diagnosis, name of drug, time of last drug ingestion, time of sample, and any other medications the patient is currently taking. The specimen should be sent to the laboratory immediately after the venipuncture.

Contraindications. None.

Nursing considerations

Nursing Diagnoses/Collaborative Problems

See Blood studies, p. 2.

Nursing Implications with Rationale

- Explain the purpose of therapeutic drug monitoring to the patient. Tell the patient that monitoring ensures appropriate drug levels in the blood thereby preventing toxicity from overdosage.
- Ensure that the drug blood level is drawn at the appropriate peak or trough level. If a *peak* level is needed, record the exact time at which the drug was administered and then either draw the blood at the appropriate time or notify the lab technologist to obtain the specimen. If a *residual* level is needed, the next dose of the drug is usually held until the blood specimen is drawn, approximately 15 minutes before the scheduled dose. After the blood is drawn, the dose can then be administered. Unless the exact times that the specimen was obtained and the last dose was given are both known, drug blood levels cannot be properly interpreted and may be grossly misleading.
- Before drawing the blood specimen, be certain that appropriate blood concentrations have been reached. This can be determined by information about the half-life of the drug, which can be obtained by consulting with the pharmacist.
- Observe the patient for signs of toxicity related to the appropriate drug. Record all observations and notify the physician as needed.
- After the venipuncture has been obtained, assess the site for bleeding and hematoma formation.

Toxicology screening

Normal values: see Tables 14-2 and 14-3

Rationale. Toxicology screening is done to determine the cause of acute drug toxicity, to help monitor drug dependency, and to detect the presence of narcotics in the body for medical-legal purposes. Toxicology screening is especially important in patients with a drug overdose or poisoning.

Procedure. Generally peripheral venipuncture is performed and the blood is collected in a tube as designated by the laboratory. The blood is usually drawn immediately after admission to the emergency room. Random urine specimens can be collected, and gastric contents can be aspirated for analysis. The hair and nails are used for detecting or documenting long-term exposure to arsenic or mercury.

Contraindications. None.

Nursing considerations

Nursing Diagnoses/Collaborative Problems

- Possible knowledge deficit related to test purpose, preparation, and procedure
- Possible anxiety related to test results

Nursing Implications with Rationale

- Explain the procedure to the patient's significant others. Obtain as much information as possible about the type, amount, and ingestion time of the consumed drug.
- Carefully assess the patient for respiratory distress, which is a common side effect of drug overdosage.
- Perform gastric lavage as indicated.
- If the specimen is obtained for medical-legal testing, ensure that the patient or the family member has signed a consent form.
- Approach the patient in a nonjudgmental fashion. Refer the patient for appropriate drug or psychiatric counseling.

Carboxyhemoglobin test

(COHb, carbon monoxide)

Normal values:
Nonsmoker: less than 3%
Smoker: up to 12%
Newborn: up to 12%
Possible critical values >20%
20%-30%: dizziness, headache, disturbances in judgment
30%-40%: tachycardia, hyperpnea, hypotension, confusion
50%-60%: coma
>60%: death

TABLE 14-2. Blood Toxicology Screening

Drug	Type	Therapeutic level	Toxic level
Acetaminophen	Analgesic, antipyretic	Depends on the use	>250 μg/ml
Alcohol	—	None	80-200 mg/dl (mild to moderate intoxication) 250-400 mg/dl (marked intoxication) >400 mg/dl (severe intoxication)
Amobarbital	Sedative, hypnotic	0.5-3.0 μg/ml	>10 μg/ml
Butabarbital	Sedative, hypnotic	0.5-3.0 μg/ml	>10 μg/ml
Carboxyhemoglobin (COHb, carbon monoxide)	Gas	None	>30% COHb (beginning of coma)
Dilantin	Anticonvulsant	10-20 μg/ml	>20 μg/ml
Glutethmide	Sedative	0.5-3.0 μg/ml	>10 μg/ml
Lead	—	None	>40 μg/dl
Lithium	Manic episodes of manic-depression psychosis	0.8-1.2 mEq/L	>2.0 mEq/L
Meprobamate	Antianxiety agent	0.5-3.0 μg/ml	>10 μg/ml
Methyprylon	Hypnotic	0.5-3.0 μg/ml	>10 μg/ml
Phenobarbital	Anticonvulsant	15-30 μg/ml	>40 μg/ml
Salicylate	Antipyretic, antiinflammatory, analgesic	100-250 μg/ml	>300 μg/ml

TABLE 14-3. Urine Toxicology Screening for Amphetamines

Drug	Therapeutic level	Toxic level
Amphetamine	2-3 μg/ml	>3 μg/ml
Dextroamphetamine	0.1-1.5 μg/ml	>15 μg/ml
Methamphetamine	3-5 μg/ml	>40 μg/ml
Phenmetrazine	5-30 μg/ml	>50 μg/ml

Rationale. The carboxyhemoglobin test measures the amount of serum carboxyhemoglobin (COHb), which is formed by the combination of carbon monoxide (CO) and hemoglobin (Hb). CO combines with Hb (oxyhemoglobin) 200 times more readily than oxygen. This greater affinity of CO to Hb results in less Hb bonds available to bind oxygen and causes the patient to become hypoxic.

Principal sources of CO include tobacco smoke, petroleum and natural gas fuels, automobile exhaust, unvented natural gas heaters, and defective gas stoves. Continuous exposure to CO can lead to coma and death. The treatment of carbon monoxide toxicity is administration of high concentrations of O_2.

Procedure. CO poisoning is detected by Hb analysis for COHb. A specimen should be drawn as soon as possible after exposure, since CO is rapidly cleared from the Hb by breathing normal air. Approximately 5 to 10 ml of venous blood is collected in a lavender-top tube. CO poisoning is detected by an instrument called a CO-oximeter.

Contraindications. None.

Nursing considerations

Nursing Diagnoses/Collaborative Problems

See Blood studies, p. 2.

Nursing Implications with Rationale

- Explain the procedure to the patient or the family. Obtain a patient history related to any possible source of CO inhalation.
- Assess the venipuncture site for bleeding or hematoma formation.
- Assess the patient for signs and symptoms of mild CO toxicity (such as headache, weakness, dizziness, malaise, and dyspnea) and moderate to severe CO toxicity (such as severe headache, bright red mucous membranes, and cherry red blood).
- Treat the patient as indicated by the physician. Usually the patient is treated with high concentrations of O_2. Encourage respirations to allow the patient to clear CO from the Hb by breathing.

Positron-emission tomography

(PET)

Normal values: dependent on purpose of procedure.

Rationale. PET, or positron-emission tomography, is a unique technique that combines the biochemical assessment of pathology achieved by nuclear medicine with the precise localization achieved by computed tomography. PET is able to penetrate the body's metabolism by recording tracers of nuclear annihilations in body tissue. The selected tracers are chemically designed to measure bodily processes (such as blood flow and volume, and oxygen and protein metabolism).

A chemical compound with the desired biologic activity is labeled with a radioactive isotope that decays by emitting a positron (or positive electron). The positron combines with an electron, and the two are mutually annihilated with emission of two gamma rays. The gamma rays penetrate the surrounding tissue and are recorded outside the body by a circular array of detectors. Because the gamma rays travel in almost exactly opposite directions, their source can be established with a high degree of accuracy. A computer reconstructs the spatial distribution of the radioactivity for a selected plane within the patient and displays the resulting image on a cathode-ray screen. PET provides noninvasive regional assessment of many biochemical processes that are essential to the functioning of the organ being studied.

The technology of PET is now well developed, and both its capabilities and its limitations are being increasingly understood. Many PET studies are being carried out with results that cannot be obtained by other techniques. These include:

1. Determination of regional metabolism in the heart and brain. For example, radioactive glucose can be used to map biochemical activity in the brain. Abnormal results are seen in patients with epilepsy, Huntington's disease, Alzheimer's disease, Parkinson's disease, etc.
2. Studies of permeability of tissues.
3. Measurement of size of infarcts left in the heart by a coronary attack.
4. Investigation into the physiology of psychosis.
5. Assessment of the effects of drugs on tissues that are diseased or malfunctioning.
6. The possibility of measuring the effect of cancer treatment by changes in malignant tissues and by biochemical reactions in the normal tissues around it.

The dose of radioactive material given to the patient in either a gas or injectable form produces a radiation exposure comparable to exposure in other types of nuclear medicine studies. PET is now being implemented in many major medical centers throughout the world. The price of PET technology is high. It includes the presence of a cyclotron, appropriate chemical facilities, computer equipment, and effective group work by physicians, chemists, mathematicians, physiologists, and physicists. This procedure, which was once regarded as exotic, is now on the threshold of becoming a tool of fundamental importance in diagnostic medicine.

Procedure. Food or fluids are not restricted on the day of the test. However, the patient should refrain from alcohol, caffeine, and tobacco for 24 hours. Diabetics should take their pretest dose of insulin at a meal 3 to 4 hours before the test. The patient should empty his or her bladder before the test for comfort reasons. No sedatives or tranquilizers should be given because the patient needs to perform certain mental activities during the test.

The patient is positioned in a comfortable, reclining chair. Two IV lines are inserted, one to infuse the radioisotope and the other for serial blood samples. The radioactive material can also be inhaled as a radioactive gas. If the brain is being scanned, the patient may be asked to perform different cognitive activities such as reciting the Pledge of Allegiance to measure brain activity changes during reasoning or remembering. Extraneous auditory and visual stimuli are minimized by blindfolds and earplugs.

The only discomfort associated with this study is that of inserting the two IV lines. This procedure is performed in approximately 1 to 1½ hours. After the procedure, the patient is instructed to change positions slowly to avoid postural hypotension. Fluids are encouraged to aid in removing the radioisotope from the bladder.

Contraindications. This test is contraindicated in the uncooperative patient and in the pregnant patient because of the possibility of the radiopaque dye causing damage to the fetus.

Nursing considerations

Nursing Diagnoses/Collaborative Problems

See Nuclear scanning, p. 5.

- High risk for anxiety related to unknown sensations of the procedure
- Possible alteration in comfort related to test procedure

Nursing Implications with Rationale

- Explain the procedure to the patient. Prepare him or her for the insertion of two IVs and for the applications of earplugs and a blindfold. Tell the patient not to use imagery as a relaxation technique because this mental activity can interfere with test results.
- Be sure the patient refrains from alcohol, tobacco, and caffeine for 24 hours before the test. Do not give any sedatives or tranquilizers before the test because the patient needs to perform certain mental activities.
- After the procedure, monitor the patient for postural hypotension. Instruct the patient to change positions slowly.
- After the procedure, encourage fluids and frequent urination to aid in removal of the radioisotope from the bladder.

QUESTIONS AND ANSWERS

1. **QUESTION:** Your patient is admitted to the hospital for routine surgery. On routine admission testing, her potassium level was found to be 7 (normal: 3.5-5.0). Should the surgery be canceled?
   ANSWER: The elevated potassium level is most probably the result of RBC hemolysis caused by poor venipuncture technique in obtaining the specimen. Therefore, the electrolytes test should be repeated, using good technique. (The repeat potassium level in this patient was 4.)
2. **QUESTION:** Your patient is suspected of having a urinary tract infection. The urine culture report indicates that three bacterial species are present. Should antibiotic therapy be initiated based on the culture results?
   ANSWER: No. It is very rare for any nongastrointestinal infection to involve more than one bacterial specimen. Culture reports with more than one species usually indicate contamination of the specimen. Therefore, the specimen should be carefully obtained a second time, and the culture should be repeated.
3. **QUESTION:** Your patient has been admitted for eye surgery and is found to have a positive VDRL test result on routine testing. Should this patient be given antibiotic therapy?
   ANSWER: Because of the high incidence of false-positive results (20%) associated with the VDRL test, a positive result does not necessarily indicate syphilitic infection. A more accurate and specific test, such as the FTA test, should be performed. If the FTA test result is positive, appropriate an-

tibiotic therapy should be given (4.8 million units of procaine penicillin administered intramuscularly). If the FTA test is negative, the patient does not have syphilis and therapy is not indicated.

4. **QUESTION:** Your 48-year-old patient was admitted for a delayed repair of a nerve laceration. Eight weeks earlier, at the time of the original injury, a complete routine evaluation was performed, and its results were negative. Should the routine testing be repeated?

   ANSWER: The final decision, of course, rests with the attending anesthesiologist. However, as a rule, most anesthesiology departments request that all tests be performed not less than 14 days before the day of surgery. During longer time intervals, much can happen to the patient that could possibly increase the risk of general anesthesia. Therefore, the workup should be repeated.

5. **QUESTION:** Your 28-year-old patient was admitted for incision and drainage (I & D) of an infected pilonidal cyst. Should the routine evaluation include a chest x-ray study and EKG?

   ANSWER: A chest x-ray study should certainly be included, because serious pulmonary disease, which increases the risk of anesthesia, can occur at any age. The chance that EKG will demonstrate unsuspected cardiac disease is minimal. Therefore, in this age group, routine performance of EKG would not be worthwhile for clinical purposes or from a cost-benefit standpoint.

BIBLIOGRAPHY

Bryson PD: Comprehensive review in toxicology, Rockville, MD, 1989, Aspen.

Davis KR, Marin JB: Imaging of the nervous system. In Wilson J and others, editors: Harrison's principles of internal medicine, ed 12, New York, 1991, McGraw-Hill.

Ellenhorn MJ, Barceloux DG: Medical toxicology: diagnosis and treatment of human poisoning, New York, 1988, Elsevier.

Graef JW, Lovejoy FH: Heavy metal poisoning. In Wilson J and others, editors: Harrison's principles of internal medicine, ed 12, New York, 1991, McGraw-Hill.

Koepke JA: Practical laboratory hematology, New York, 1991, Churchill-Livingstone.

Lovejoy FH, Linden CH: Acute poison and drug overdose. In Wilson J and others, editors: Harrison's principles of internal medicine, ed 12, New York, 1991, McGraw-Hill.

Margulis AR: Overview of imaging techniques and projection for the future. In Wyngaarden JB and others, editors: Cecil textbook of medicine, ed 19, Philadelphia, 1992, WB Saunders.

Wyngaarden JB: The use and interpretation of laboratory derived data. In Wyngaarden JB and others, editors: Cecil textbook of medicine, ed 19, Philadelphia, 1992, WB Saunders.

Appendix 1

ABBREVIATIONS AND SYMBOLS FOR UNITS OF MEASUREMENT

$<$	Less than
$\le$	Less than or equal to
$>$	Greater than
$\ge$	Greater than or equal to
C	Celsius
cc	Cubic centimeter
cg	Centigram
cm	Centimeter
cm H_2O	Centimeter of water
cu	Cubic
dl	Deciliter (100 ml)
g	Gram
IU	International unit
ImU	International milliunit
IμU	International microunit
K	Kilo
kg	Kilogram
L	Liter
m	Meter
m^2	Square meter
m^3	Cubic meter
mEq	Milliequivalent
mEq/L	Milliequivalent per liter
mg	Milligram
min	Minute
ml	Milliliter
mm	Millimeter
mm^3	Cubic millimeter
mM	Millimole
mmHg	Millimeter of mercury
mm H_2O	Millimeter of water
mol	Mole
mmol	Millimole
mOsm	Milliosmole
mμ	Millimicron
mU	Milliunit
mV	Millivolt
ng	Nanogram
nmol	Nanomole
Pa	Pascal
pg	Picogram (or micromicrogram)
pl	Picoliter
pm	Picomole
S	Second (SI)
sec	Second
SI units	International System of Units
μ	Micron
μ^3	Cubic micron
μg	Microgram
μIU	Microinternational unit
μmol	Micromole
μU	Microunit
U	Unit
yr	Year

Appendix 2

COMMONLY USED ABBREVIATIONS FOR DIAGNOSTIC AND LABORATORY TESTS

ABEP	Auditory brainstem evoked potentials
ABG	Arterial blood gases
ACE	Angiotension converting enzyme
ACTH	Adrenocorticotropic hormone
ADH	Antidiuretic hormone
AFB	Acid-fast bacilli
AFP	Alpha fetoprotein
A/G ratio	Albumin/globulin ratio
AIDS	Acquired immunodeficiency syndrome
AIT	Agglutination inhibition test
ALA	Aminolevulinic acid
ALP	Alkaline phosphatase
ALT	Alanine aminotransferase
ANA	Antinuclear antibodies
APTT	Activated partial thromboplastin time
ARC	AIDS-related complex
ASO	Antistreptolysin O titer
AST	Aspartate aminotransferase
BE	Barium enema
BE	Base excess
BUN	Blood urea nitrogen
C & S	Culture and sensitivity
CATT	Computerized axial transverse tomography
CBC	Complete blood count
CDE	Common duct exploration
CEA	Carcinoembryonic antigen
CI	Cardiac index
CK	Creatinine kinase
Cl	Chloride
CMV	Cytomegalovirus
CO	Cardiac output
CO	Carbon monoxide
CO_2	Carbon dioxide
COHb	Carboxyhemoglobin test
CPK	Creatinine phosphokinase
CRF	Corticotropin-releasing factor
CRP	C-reactive protein
CSF	Cerebrospinal fluid
CST	Contraction stress test
CT	Computed tomography
Cu	Copper
CVB	Chorionic villi biopsy
CVS	Chorionic villi sampling
CXR	Chest x-ray
D & C	Dilation and curettage
DIC	Disseminated intravascular coagulation
DSA	Digital subtraction angiography
DST	Dexamethasone suppression test
EBV	Epstein-Barr virus
ECG	Electrocardiogram
ECHO	Echocardiography
EEG	Electroencephalogram
EF	Ejection fraction
EGD	Esophagogastroduodenoscopy
EKG	Electrocardiogram
ELISA	Enzyme-linked immunosorbent assay
EMG	Electromyography
ENG	Electroneurography
EP	Evoked potentials
ERCP	Endoscopic retrograde cholangio-pancreatography
ERP	Estrogen receptor positive
ERV	Expiratory reserve volume
ESR	Erythrocyte sedimentation rate
ESV	End systolic volume
EUG	Excretory urography
FBS	Fasting blood sugar
FDP	Fibrin degradation products
Fe	Iron
FEV	Forced expiratory volume
FSH	Follicle-stimulating hormone
FTA-ABS	Fluorescent treponemal antibody absorption test
FTI	Free thyroxine index
FUT	Fibrinogen uptake test
FVC	Forced vital capacity
G-6-PD	Glucose-6-phosphate dehydro-genase

GB series	Gallbladder series
GE reflux	Gastroesophageal reflux scan
GFR	Glomerular filtration rate
GGT	Gamma-glutamyl transferase
GGTP	Gamma-glutamyl transpeptidase
GH	Growth hormone
GHb, GHB	Glycosylated hemoglobin
GI series	Gastrointestinal series
GTT	Glucose tolerance test
HAA	Hepatitis-associated antigen
HAI	Hemagglutination inhibition test
HAT	Heterophile antibody titer
HAV	Hepatitis A virus
HbA	Glycohemoglobin
HBcAb	Hepatitis B core antibody
HBcAg	Hepatitis B core antigen
HBeAb	Hepatitis B e-antibody
HBeAg	Hepatitis B e-antigen
HBsAb	Hepatitis B surface antibody
HBsAg	Hepatitis B surface antigen
HBV	Hepatitis B virus
HCG	Human chorionic gonadotropin
HCO_3^-	Bicarbonate
HCS	Human chorionic somatomammotropin
Hct	Hematocrit
HDL	High-density lipoprotein
Hgb	Hemoglobin
5-HIAA	5-Hydroxyindoleacetic acid
HPL	Human placental lactogen
HTLV-III	Human T-lymphotropic virus, type III
IFA	Indirect fluorescent antibody test
Ig	Immunoglobulin
IRV	Inspiratory reserve volume
IVC	Intravenous cholangiography
IV-GTT	Intravenous glucose tolerance test
IVP	Intravenous pyelography
K	Potassium
KS	Ketosteroid
KUB	Kidney, ureters, and bladder x-ray
LAP	Leucine aminopeptidase
LATS	Long-acting thyroid hormone
LDH	Lactic dehydrogenase
LDL	Low-density lipoprotein
LE	Lupus erythematosus test
LES	Lower esophageal sphincter
LFT	Liver function tests
LH	Leutinizing hormone
Li	Lithium
LP	Lumbar puncture
L/S ratio	Lecithin/sphingomyelin ratio
LS spine	Lumbosacral spine
MAC	Midarm circumference
MAMC	Midarm muscle circumference
MCH	Mean corpuscular hemoglobin
MCHC	Mean corpuscular hemoglobin concentration
MCV	Mean corpuscular volume
Mg	Magnesium
MMEF	Maximal midexpiratory flow
MRI	Magnetic resonance imaging
MV	Minute volume
MVV	Maximal volume ventilation
Na	Sodium
NMR	Nuclear magnetic resonance
NST	Nonstress test
O & P	Ova and parasites
OB	Occult blood
OCT	Oxytocin challenge test
OGTT	Oral glucose tolerance test
17-OHCH	17-hydroxycorticosteroid
OPG	Oculoplethysmography
P	Phosphorus
PAP	Prostatic acid phosphatase
Pb	Lead
PBI	Protein bound iodine
Pco_2	Partial pressure of CO_2
PEG	Pneumoencephalography
PET	Positron-emission tomography
PFT	Pulmonary function tests
pH	Hydrogen ion concentration
PKU	Phenylketonuria test
PMN	Polymorphonuclear (type of WBC)
Po_2	Partial pressure of O_2
PPBS	Postprandial blood sugar
PPD	Purified protein derivative
PPG	Postprandial glucose
PRA	Plasma renin activity
PSA	Prostate-specific antigen
PT	Prothrombin time
PTH	Parathormone or parathyroid hormone
PTHC	Percutaneous transhepatic cholangiography
PTT	Partial thromboplastin time
RAIU	Radioactive iodine uptake
RBC	Red blood cell
RDW	Red cell distribution width
RF	Rheumatoid factor
RIA	Radioimmunoassay
RPR	Rapid plasma reagin test
RRA	Radio receptor test
RV	Residual volume
S & A	Sugar and acetone
SACE	Serum angiotensin-converting enzyme
SBF	Small bowel followthrough
SER	Somatosensory evoked responses
SGOT	Serum glutamic oxaloacetic transaminase

SGPT	Serum glutamic pyruvic transaminase
SLE	Systemic lupus erythematosus
STS	Serologic test for syphilis
SMA	Sequential multiple analyzer
SV	Stroke volume
T_3	Triiodothyronine
T_4	Thyroxine
T & CM	Type and cross match
T & S	Type and screen
TBG	Thyroxine-binding globulin
TDM	Therapeutic drug monitoring
TEE	Transesophageal echocardiography
TIBC	Total iron-binding capacity
TLC	Total lung capacity
TPI	*Treponema pallidium* immobilization
TPR	Tubular phosphate reabsorption
TSF	Triceps skin-fold thickness
TSH	Thyroid-stimulating hormone
TTE	Transthoracic echocardiography
TV	Tidal volume
UA	Urinalysis
UGI series	Upper gastrointestinal series
UPP	Urethral pressure profile
US	Ultrasound
VDRL	Venereal disease research laboratory
VER	Visual evoked response
VLDL	Very low-density lipoprotein
VMA	Vanillylmandelic acid
WBC	White blood cell

Appendix 3

BLOOD, PLASMA, OR SERUM VALUES

Test	Reference range: Conventional values	Reference range: SI units*	Discussion
Acetoacetate plus acetone	0.30-2.0 mg/dl	3-20 mg/l	
Acetone	Negative	Negative	
Acid phosphatase	Adults: 0.10-0.63 U/ml (Bessey-Lowry) 0.5-2.0 U/ml (Bodansky) 1.0-4.0 U/ml (King-Armstrong) Children: 6.4-15.2 U/L	28-175 nmol/s/L	Chapter 7
Activated partial thromboplastin time (APTT)	30-40 sec	30-40 sec	Chapter 10
Adrenocorticotropic hormone (ACTH)	6 AM 15-100 pg/ml 6 PM <50 pg/ml	10-80 ng/L <50 ng/L	Chapter 8
Alanine aminotransferase (ALT)	5-35 IU/L	5-35 U/L	Chapter 4
Albumin	3.2-4.5 g/dl	35-55 g/L	Chapter 4
Alcohol	Negative	Negative	Chapter 14
Aldolase	Adults: 3.0-8.2 Sibley-Lehninger units/dl Children: approximately 2 × adult values Newborns: approximately 4 × adult values	22-59 mU/L at 37° C	Chapter 12
Aldosterone	Peripheral blood: Supine: 7.4 ± 4.2 ng/dl Upright: 1-21 ng/dl Adrenal vein: 200-800 ng/dl	 0.08-0.3 nmol/L 0.14-0.8 nmol/L	Chapter 7

*The use of the System of International Units (SI) was recommended at the 30th World Health Assembly in 1977 to implement an international language of measurement. Because this system is being adopted by numerous laboratories, many of the common values are expressed in both conventional and SI units. SI units are calculated by multiplying the conventional unit by a number factor. The SI measurement system uses *moles* as the basic unit for the amount of a substance, *kilograms* for its mass, and *meter* for its length.

Test	Reference range		Discussion
	Conventional values	SI units	
Alkaline phosphatase	Adults: 30-85 ImU/ml Children and adolescents: <2 years: 85-235 ImU/ml 2-8 years: 65-210 ImU/ml 9-15 years: 60-300 ImU/ml (active bone growth) 16-21 years: 30-200 ImU/ml		Chapter 4
Alpha-aminonitrogen	3-6 mg/dl	2.1-3.9 mmol/L	
Alpha-1-antitrypsin	>250 mg/dl		Chapter 5
Alpha fetoprotein (AFP)	<25 ng/ml		Chapters 9, 13
Ammonia	Adults: 15-110 μg/dl Children: 40-80 μg/dl Newborns: 90-150 μg/dl	47-65 μmol/L	Chapter 4
Amylase	56-190 IU/L 80-150 Somogyi units/ml	25-125 U/L	Chapter 4
Angiotensin-converting enzyme (ACE)	23-57 U/ml		Chapter 7
Antinuclear antibodies (ANA)	Negative		Chapter 12
Antistreptolysin O (ASO)	Adults: ≤160 Todd units/ml Children: Newborns: similar to mother's value 6 months-2 years: ≤50 Todd units/ml 2-4 years: ≤160 Todd units/ml 5-12 years: ≤200 Todd units/ml		Chapter 7
Antithyroid microsomal antibody	Titer <1:100		Chapter 8
Antithyroglobulin antibody	Titer <1:100		Chapter 8
Ascorbic acid (vitamin C)	0.6-1.6 mg/dl	23-57 μmol/L	
Aspartate aminotransferase (AST, SGOT)	12-36 U/ml 5-40 IU/L	0.10-0.30 μmol/s/L 5-40 U/L	Chapters 2, 4
Australian antigen (hepatitis-associated antigen, HAA)	Negative	Negative	Chapter 4
Barbiturates	Negative	Negative	Chapter 14
Base excess	Men: −3.3 to +1.2 Women: −2.4 to +2.3	0 ± 2 mmol/L 0 ± 2 mmol/L	
Bicarbonate (HCO_3^-)	22-26 mEq/L	22-26 mmol/L	Chapter 5
Bilirubin			
Direct (conjugated)	0.1-0.3 mg/dl	1.7-5.1 μmol/L	Chapter 4
Indirect (unconjugated)	0.2-0.8 mg/dl	3.4-12.0 μmol/L	
Total	Adults and children: 0.1-1.0 mg/dl Newborns: 1-12 mg/dl	5.1-17.0 μmol/L	

Test	Reference range: Conventional values	Reference range: SI units	Discussion
Bleeding time (Ivy method)	1-9 min		Chapter 10
Blood count (see complete blood count)			Chapter 10
Blood gases (arterial)			
pH	7.35-7.45		Chapter 5
Pco_2	35-45 mm Hg	4.7-6.0 kPa	
HCO_3^-	22-26 mEq/L	21-28 nmol/L	
Po_2	80-100 mm Hg	11-13 kPa	
O_2 saturation	95%-100%		
Blood urea nitrogen (BUN)	5-20 mg/dl	3.6-7.1 mmol/L	Chapter 7
Bromide	Up to 5 mg/dl	0-63 mmol/L	
Bromosulfophthalein (BSP)	<5% retention after 45 min		
CA 15-3	<22 U/ml		Chapter 13
CA-125	0-35 U/ml		Chapter 13
CA 19-9	<37 U/ml		Chapter 13
C-reactive protein (CRP)	<6 μg/ml		Chapter 12
Calcitonin	<50 pg/ml	<50 pmol/L	Chapter 8
Calcium (Ca)	9.0-10.5 mg/dl (total) 3.9-4.6 mg/dl (ionized)	2.25-2.75 mmol/L 1.05-1.30 mmol/L	Chapter 8
Carbon dioxide (CO_2) content	23-30 mEq/L	21-30 mmol/L	Chapter 14
Carboxyhemoglobin (COHb)	3% of total hemoglobin		Chapter 14
Carcinoembryonic antigen (CEA)	<2 ng/ml	0.2-5 μg/L	Chapter 3
Carotene	50-200 μg/dl	0.74-3.72 μmol/L	
Chloride (Cl)	90-110 mEq/L	98-106 mmol/L	Chapter 14
Cholesterol	150-250 mg/dl	3.90-6.50 mmol/L	Chapter 2
Clot retraction	50%-100% clot retraction in 1-2 hours, complete retraction within 24 hours		Chapter 10
Complement	C_3: 70-176 mg/dl C_4: 16-45 mg/dl	0.55-1.20 g/L 0.20-0.50 g/L	Chapter 12
Complete blood count (CBC)			
Red blood cell (RBC) count	Men: 4.7-6.1 million/mm^3 Women: 4.2-5.4 million/mm^3 Infants and children: 3.8-5.5 million/mm^3 Newborns: 4.8-7.1 million/mm^3		Chapter 10
Hemoglobin (Hgb)	Men: 14-18 g/dl Women: 12-16 g/dl (pregnancy: >11 g/dl) Children: 11-16 g/dl Infants: 10-15 g/dl Newborns: 14-24 g/dl	8.7-11.2 mmol/L 7.4-9.9 mmol/L 1.74-2.56 mmol/L 2.56-3.02 mmol/L	Chapter 10

Test	Reference range: Conventional values	Reference range: SI units	Discussion
Hematocrit (Hct)	Men: 42%-52% Women: 37%-47% (pregnancy: >33%) Children: 31%-43% Infants: 30%-40% Newborns: 44%-64%		Chapter 10
Mean corpuscular volume (MCV)	Adults and children: 80-95 μ^3 Newborns: 96-108 μ^3	80-95 fl	Chapter 10
Mean corpuscular hemoglobin (MCH)	Adults and children: 27-31 pg Newborns: 32-34 pg	0.42-0.48 fmol	Chapter 10
Mean corpuscular hemoglobin concentration (MCHC)	Adults and children: 32-36 g/dl Newborns: 32-33 g/dl	0.32-0.36	
White blood cell (WBC) count	Adults and children >2 years: 5,000-10,000/mm^3 Children ≤2 years: 6,200-17,000/mm^3 Newborns: 9000-30,000/mm^3		Chapter 10
Differential count			Chapter 10
Neutrophils	55%-70%		
Lymphocytes	20%-40%		
Monocytes	2%-8%		
Eosinophils	1%-4%		
Basophils	0.5%-1%		
Platelet count	150,000-400,000/mm^3		Chapter 10
Coombs' test			
Direct	Negative	Negative	Chapter 10
Indirect	Negative	Negative	Chapter 10
Copper (Cu)	70-140 μg/dl	11.0-24.3 μmol/L	
Cortisol	6-28 μg/dl (A.M.) 2-12 μg/dl (P.M.)	170-635 nmol/L 82-413 nmol/L	Chapter 8
CPK isoenzyme (MB)	<5% total		Chapter 2
Creatinine	0.7-1.5 mg/dl	<133 μmol/L	Chapter 7
Creatinine clearance	Men: 95-104 ml/min Women: 95-125 ml/min	<133 μmol/L	Chapter 7
Creatinine phosphokinase (CPK)	5-75 mU/ml	12-80 units/L	Chapter 2
Cryoglobulin	Negative	Negative	Chapter 12
Differential (WBC) count (see CBC)			Chapter 10
Digoxin	Therapeutic level: 0.5-2.0 ng/ml Toxic level: >2.4 ng/ml	40-79 μmol/L >119 μmol/L	Chapter 14
Erythrocyte count (see complete blood count)			

Test	Reference range: Conventional values	Reference range: SI units	Discussion
Erythrocyte sedimentation rate (ESR)	Men: up to 15 mm/hour Women: up to 20 mm/hour Children: up to 10 mm/hour		Chapter 12
Ethanol	80-200 mg/dl (mild to moderate intoxication) 250-400 mg/dl (marked intoxication) >400 mg/dl (severe intoxication)	17-43 mmol/L 54-87 mmol/L >87 mmol/L	Chapter 14
Euglobulin lysis test	90 min-6 hours		Chapter 10
Fats	Up to 200 mg/dl		
Ferritin	15-200 ng/ml	15-200 μg/L	
Fibrin degradation products (FDP)	<10 μg/ml		Chapter 10
Fibrinogen (factor I)	200-400 mg/dl	5.9-11.7 μmol/L	Chapter 10
Fibrinolysis/euglobulin lysis test	90 min-6 hours		Chapter 10
Fluorescent treponemal antibody (FTA)	Negative	Negative	Chapter 9
Fluoride	<0.05 mg/dl	<0.027 mmol/L	
Folic acid (Folate)	5-20 μg/ml	14-34 mmol/L	Chapter 10
Follicle-stimulating hormone (FSH)	Men: 0.1-15.0 ImU/ml Women: 6-30 ImU/ml Children: 0.1-12.0 ImU/ml Castrate and postmenopausal: 30-200 ImU/ml		
Free thyroxine index (FTI)	0.9-2.3 ng/dl		Chapter 8
Galactose-1-phosphate uridyl transferase	18.5-28.5 U/g hemoglobin		Chapter 9
Gammaglobulin	0.5-1.6 g/dl		
Gamma-glutamyl transpeptidase (GGTP)	Men: 8-38 U/L Women: <45 years: 5-27 U/L	5-40 U/L at 37°C	Chapter 4
Gastrin	40-150 pg/ml	40-150 ng/L	Chapter 3
Glucagon	50-200 pg/ml	14-56 pmol/L	Chapter 8
Glucose, fasting (FBS)	Adults: 70-115 mg/dl Children: 60-100 mg/dl Newborns: 30-80 mg/dl	3.89-6.38 mmol/L	Chapter 8
Glucose, 2-hour postprandial (2-hour PPG)	<140 mg/dl		Chapter 8
Glucose-6-phosphate dehydrogenase (G-6-PD)	8.6-18.6 IU/g of hemoglobin		Chapter 10
Glucose tolerance test (GTT)	Fasting: 70-115 mg/dl 30 min: <200 mg/dl 1 hour: <200 mg/dl 2 hours: <140 mg/dl 3 hours: 70-115 mg/dl 4 hours: 70-115 mg/dl		Chapter 8

Test	Reference range		Discussion
	Conventional values	SI units	
Glycosylated hemoglobin	Adults: 2.2%-4.8% Children: 1.8%-4.0% Good diabetic control: 2.5%-6% Fair diabetic control: 6.1%-8% Poor diabetic control: >8%		Chapter 8
Growth hormone	<10 ng/ml	<10 μg/L	Chapter 8
Haptoglobin	100-150 mg/dl	16-31 μmol/L	Chapter 10
Hematocrit (Hct)	Men: 42%-52% Women: 37%-47% (pregnancy: >33%) Children: 31%-43% Infants: 30%-40% Newborns: 44%-64%		Chapter 10
Hemoglobin (HgB)	Men: 14-18 g/dl Women: 12-16 g/dl (pregnancy: >11 g/dl) Children: 11-16 g/dl Infants: 10-15 g/dl Newborns: 14-24 g/dl	8.7-11.2 mmol/L 7.4-9.9 mmol/L	Chapter 10
Hemoglobin electrophoresis	Hgb A_1: 95%-98% Hgb A_2: 2%-3% Hgb F: 0.8%-2% Hgb S: 0 Hgb C: 0		Chapter 10
Hepatitis B surface antigen (HB_sAG)	Nonreactive	Nonreactive	Chapter 4
Heterophil antibody	Negative	Negative	Chapter 12
HLA-B27	None	None	Chapter 12
Human chorionic gonadotropin (HCG)	Negative	Negative	Chapter 13
Human placental lactogen (HPL)	Rise during pregnancy		Chapter 9
5-Hydroxyindoleacetic acid (5-HIAA)	2.8-8.0 mg/24 hours		Chapter 13
Immunoglobulin quantification	IgG: 550-1900 mg/dl IgA: 60-333 mg/dl IgM: 45-145 mg/dl	5.5-19.0 g/L 0.6-3.3 g/L 0.45-1.5 g/L	Chapter 12
Insulin	4-20 μU/ml	36-179 pmol/L	Chapter 8
Iron (Fe)	60-190 μg/dl	13-31 μmol/L	Chapter 10
Iron-binding capacity, total (TIBC)	250-420 μg/dl	45-73 μmol/L	Chapter 10
Iron (transferrin) saturation	30%-40%		Chapter 10
Ketone bodies	Negative	Negative	
Lactic acid	0.6-1.8 mEq/L		
Lactic dehydrogenase (LDH) isoenzymes	90-200 ImU/ml LDH-1: 17%-27% LDH-2: 28%-38% LDH-3: 19%-27% LDH-4: 5%-16% LDH-5: 6%-16%	0.4-1.7 μmol/s/L	Chapters 2, 4

Test	Reference range: Conventional values	Reference range: SI units	Discussion
Lead	120 μg/dl or less	<1.0 μmol/L	Chapter 14
Leucine aminopeptidase (LAP)	Men: 80-200 U/ml Women: 75-185 U/ml		Chapter 4
Leukocyte count (see Complete blood count)			
Lipase	Up to 1.5 units/ml	0-417 U/L	Chapter 4
Lipids			
Total	400-1000 mg/dl	4-8 g/L	Chapter 2
Cholesterol	150-250 mg/dl	3.9-6.5 mmol/L	
Triglycerides	40-150 mg/dl	0.4-1.5 g/L	
Phospholipids	150-380 mg/dl	1.9-3.9 mmol/L	
Lithium (see Table 14-2)			Chapter 14
Long-acting thyroid-stimulating hormone (LATS)	Negative	Negative	Chapter 8
Magnesium (Mg)	1.6-3.0 mEq/L	0.8-1.3 mm/L	
Methanol	Negative	Negative	
Mononucleosis spot test	Negative	Negative	Chapter 12
Nitrogen, nonprotein	15-35 mg/dl	10.7-25.0 mmol/L	
Nuclear antibody (ANA)	Negative	Negative	Chapter 12
5′-Nucleotidase	Up to 1.6 units	27-233 nmol/s/L	Chapter 4
Osmolality	275-300 mOsm/kg		Chapter 8
Oxygen saturation (arterial)	95%-100%	0.95-1.00 of capacity	Chapter 5
Parathormone (PTH)	<2000 pg/ml		Chapter 8
Partial thromboplastin time, activated (APTT)	30-40 sec		Chapter 10
P_{CO_2}	35-45 mm Hg		Chapter 5
pH	7.35-7.45	7.35-7.45	Chapter 5
Phenylalanine	Up to 2 mg/dl	<0.18 mmol/L	
Phenylketonuria (PKU)	Negative	Negative	Chapter 9
Phenytoin (Dilantin)	Therapeutic level: 10-20 μg/ml		Chapter 14
Phosphatase (acid)	0.10-0.63 U/ml (Bessey-Lowry) 0.5-2.0 U/ml (Bodansky) 1.0-4.0 U/ml (King-Armstrong)	0.11-0.60 U/L	
Phosphatase (alkaline)	Adults: 30-85 ImU/ml Children and adolescents: <2 years: 85-235 ImU/ml 2-8 years: 65-210 ImU/ml 9-15 years: 60-300 ImU/ml (active bone growth) 16-21 years: 30-200 ImU/ml	20-90 units/L	Chapter 4
Phospholipids (see Lipids)			
Phosphorus (P, PO_4)	Adults: 2.5-4.5 mg/dl Children: 3.5-5.8 mg/dl	0.78-1.52 mmol/L 1.29-2.26 mmol/L	Chapter 8

Test	Reference range: Conventional values	Reference range: SI units	Discussion
Platelet count	150,000-400,000/mm^3		Chapter 10
Po_2	80-100 mm Hg		Chapter 5
Potassium (K)	3.5-5.0 mEq/L	3.5-5.0 mmol/L	Chapter 14
Progesterone	Men, prepubertal girls, and postmenopausal women: <2 ng/ml	6 nmol/L	
	Women, luteal: peak >5 ng/ml	>16 nmol/L	
Prolactin	2-15 ng/ml	2-15 μg/L	
Prostate-specific antigen (PSA)	<4 ng/ml		Chapter 7
Protein (total)	6-8 g/dl	55-80 g/L	Chapter 4
Albumin	3.2-4.5 g/dl	35-55 g/L	
Globulin	2.3-3.4 g/dl	20-35 g/L	
Prothrombin time (PT)	11.0-12.5 sec	11.0-12.5 sec	Chapter 10
Pyruvate	0.3-0.9 mg/dl	34-103 μmol/L	
Red blood cell count (see Complete blood count)			
Red blood cell indexes (see Complete blood count)			
Renin			Chapter 7
Reticulocyte count	Adults and children: 0.5%-2% of total erythrocytes Infants: 0.5%-3.1% of total erythrocytes Newborns: 2.5%-6.5% of total erythrocytes		Chapter 10
Rheumatoid factor	Negative	Negative	Chapter 12
Rubella antibody test			Chapter 9
Salicylates	Negative		Chapter 14
	Therapeutic: 20-25 mg/dl (to age 10: 25-30 mg/dl)	1.4-1.8 mmol/L	
	Toxic: >30 mg/dl (after age 60: >20 mg/dl)	>2.2 mmol/L	
Schilling test (vitamin B_{12} absorption)	8%-40% excretion/24 hours		Chapter 9
Serologic test for syphilis (STS)	Negative (nonreactive)		Chapter 9
Serum glutamic oxaloacetic transaminase (SGOT, AST)	12-36 U/ml 5-40 IU/L	0.10-0.30 μmol/s/L	Chapters 2, 4
Serum glutamic-pyruvic transaminase (SGPT, ALT)	5-35 IU/L	0.05-0.43 μmol/s/L	Chapter 4
Sickle cell	Negative		Chapter 10
Sodium (Na^+)	136-145 mEq/L	136-145 mmol/L	Chapter 14
Sugar (see glucose)			

Test	Reference range: Conventional values	Reference range: SI units	Discussion
Syphilis (see Serologic test for syphilis, Fluorescent treponemal antibody, Venereal Disease Research Laboratory)			Chapter 9
Testosterone	Men: 300-1200 ng/dl Women: 30-95 ng/dl Prepubertal boys and girls: 5-20 ng/dl	10-42 nmol/L 1.1-3.3 nmol/L 0.165-0.70 nmol/L	
Thymol flocculation	Up to 5 units		
Thyroglubulin antibody (see Antithyroglobulin antibody)			
Thyroid-stimulating hormone (TSH)	1-4 μU/ml Neonates: <25 μIU/ml by 3 days	5 m U/L	Chapter 8
Thyroxine (T_4)	Murphy-Pattee: neonates: 10.1-20.1 μg/dl 1-6 years: 5.6-12.6 μg/dl 6-10 years: 4.9-11.7 μg/dl >10 years: 4-11 μg/dl Radioimmunoassay: 5-10 μg/dl	50-154 nmol/L	Chapter 8
Thyroxine-binding globulin (TBG)	12-28 μg/ml	129-335 nmol/L	Chapter 8
Toxoplasmosis antibody titer	See Chapter 9		Chapter 9
Transaminase (see Serum glutamic-oxaloacetic transaminase, Serum glutamic pyruvic transaminase)			
Triglycerides	40-150 mg/dl	0.4-1.5 g/L	Chapter 2
Triiodothyronine (T_3)	110-230 ng/dl	1.2-1.5 nmol/L	Chapter 8
Triiodothyronine (T_3) resin uptake	25%-35%		Chapter 8
Tubular phosphate reabsorption (TPR)	80%-90%		Chapter 8
Urea nitrogen (see Blood urea nitrogen)			
Uric acid	Men: 2.1-8.5 mg/dl Women: 2.0-6.6 mg/dl Children: 2.5-5.5 mg/dl	0.15-0.48 mmol/L 0.09-0.36 mmol/L	Chapter 11
Venereal Disease Research Laboratory (VDRL)	Negative	Negative	Chapter 9
Vitamin A	20-100 g/dl	0.7-3.5 μmol/L	
Vitamin B_{12}	200-600 pg/ml	148-443 pmol/L	
Vitamin C	0.6-1.6 mg/dl	23-57 μmol/L	
Whole blood clot retraction (see Clot retraction)			Chapter 10
Zinc	50-150 μg/dl		

Appendix 4

URINE VALUES

Test	Reference range: Conventional values	Reference range: SI units*	Discussion
Acetone plus acetoacetate (ketone bodies)	Negative	Negative	Chapter 8
Addis count (12-hour)	Adults: WBCs and epithelial cells: 1.8 million/12 hours RBCs: 500,000/12 hours Hyaline casts: Up to 5000/12 hours Children: WBCs: <1 million/12 hours RBCs: <250,000/12 hours Casts: >5000/12 hours Protein: <20 mg/12 hours	Negative	Chapter 8
Albumin	Random: ≤8 mg/dl 24-hour: 10-100 mg/24 hours	Negative 10-100 mg/24 hr	
Aldosterone	2-16 μg/24 hours	5.5-72 nmol/24 hours	Chapter 7
Alpha-aminonitrogen	0.4-1.0 g/24 hours	28-71 nmol/24 hours	
Amino acid	50-200 mg/24 hours		
Ammonia (24-hour)	30-50 mEq/24 hours 500-1200 mg/24 hours	30-50 nmol/24 hours	Chapter 4
Amylase	≤5000 Somogyi units/24 hours 3-35 IU/hour	6.5-48.1 U/hr	Chapter 4
Arsenic (24-hour)	<50 μg/L	<0.65 mol/L	
Ascorbic acid (vitamin C)	Random: 1-7 ng/dl 24-hour: >50 mg/24 hours	0.06-0.40 mmol/L >0.29 mmol/24 hours	
Bacteria	None	None	Chapter 7
Bence Jones protein	Negative	Negative	Chapter 13
Bilirubin	Negative	Negative	Chapter 4
Blood or hemoglobin	Negative	Negative	Chapter 7
Borate (24-hour)	<2 mg/L	<32 μmol/L	

*The use of the System of International Units (SI) was recommended at the 30th World Health Assembly in 1977 to implement an international language of measurement. Because this system is being adopted by numerous laboratories, many of the common values are expressed in both conventional and SI units. SI units are calculated by multiplying the conventional unit by a number factor. The SI measurement system uses *moles* as the basic unit for the amount of a substance, *kilograms* for its mass, and *meter* for its length.

Test	Reference range: Conventional values	Reference range: SI units	Discussion
Calcium	Random: 1 + turbidity 24-hour: 1-300 mg (diet dependent)	1 + tubidity	Chapter 8
Catecholamines (24-hour)	Epinephrine: 5-40 μg/24 hours Norepinephrine: 10-80 μg/24 hours Metanephrine: 24-96 μg/24 hours Normetanephrine: 75-375 μg/24 hours	<55 nmol/24 hours <590 nmol/24 hours 0.5-8.1 μmol/24 hours	Chapter 7
Chloride (24-hour)	140-250 mEq/24 hours	140-250 mmol/24 hours	
Color	Amber-yellow	Amber-yellow	Chapter 7
Concentration test (Fishberg test)	Specific gravity: >1.025 Osmolality: 850 mOsm/L	>1.025 >850 mOsm/L	
Copper (CU) (24-hour)	Up to 25 μg/24 hours	0-0.4 μmol/24 hours	
Coproporphyrin (24-hour)	100-300 μg/24 hours	150-460 nmol/24 hours	
Creatine	Adults: <100 mg/24 hours or <6% creatinine Pregnant women: ≤12% Infants <1 year: equal to creatinine Older children: ≤30% of creatinine		
Creatinine (24-hour)	15-25 mg/kg body wt/24 hours	0.13-0.22 nmol/kg^{-1} body wt/24 hours	
Creatinine clearance (24-hour)	Men: 90-140 ml/min Women: 85-125 ml/min	90-140 ml/min 85-125 ml/min	Chapter 7
Crystals	Negative	Negative	Chapter 7
Cystine or cysteine	Negative	Negative	
Delta-aminolevulinic acid (ΔALA)	1-7 mg/24 hours	10-53 μmol/24 hours	Chapter 10
Epinephrine (24-hour)	5-40 μg/24 hours		Chapter 7
Epithelial cells and casts	Occasional	Occasional	Chapter 7
Estriol (24-hour)	>12 mg/24 hours		Chapter 9
Fat	Negative	Negative	
Fluoride (24-hour)	<1 mg/24 hours	0.053 mmol/24 hours	Chapter 9
Follicle-stimulating hormone (FSH) (24-hour)	Men: 2-12 IU/24 hours Women: During menses: 8-60 IU/24 hours During ovulation: 30-60 IU/24 hours During menopause: >50 IU/24 hours		
Glucose	Negative	Negative	Chapter 8
Granular casts	Occasional	Occasional	Chapter 7
Hemoglobin and myoglobin	Negative	Negative	Chapter 7

Test	Reference range: Conventional values	Reference range: SI units	Discussion
Homogentisic acid	Negative	Negative	
Human chorionic gonadotropin (HCG)	Negative	Negative	Chapter 13
Human placental lactogen (HPL)			Chapter 9
Hyaline casts	Occasional	Occasional	Chapter 7
17-Hydroxycorticosteroids (17-OCHS) (24-hour)	Men: 5.5-15.0 mg/24 hours Women: 5.0-13.5 mg/24 hours Children: lower than adult values	8.3-25 μmol/24 hours 5.5-22 μmol/24 hours	Chapter 8
5-Hydroxyindoleacetic acid (5-HIAA, serotonin) (24-hour)	Men: 2-9 mg/24 hours Women: lower than men	10-47 μmol/24 hours	Chapter 13
Ketones (see acetone plus acetoacetate)			
17-Ketosteroids (17-KS) (24-hour)	Men: 8-15 mg/24 hours Women: 6-12 mg/24 hours Children: 12-15 yr: 5-12 mg/24 hours <12 yr: <5 mg/24 hours	21-62 μmol/24 hours 14-45 μmol/24 hours	Chapter 8
Lactose (24-hour)	14-40 mg/24 hours	41-116 μm	
Lead	<0.08 g/ml or <120 g/24 hours	0.39 μmol/L	Chapter 14
Leucine aminopeptidase (LAP)	2-18 U/24 hours		Chapter 4
Magnesium (24-hour)	6.8-8.5 mEq/24 hours	3.0-4.3 mmol/24 hours	
Melanin	Negative	Negative	Chapter 13
Odor	Aromatic	Aromatic	Chapter 7
Osmolality	500-800 mOsm/L	38-1400 mmol/kg water	
pH	4.6-8.0	4.6-8.0	Chapter 7
Phenolsulfonphthalein (PSP)	15 min: at least 25% 30 min: at least 40% 120 min: at least 60%	At least 0.25 At least 0.40 At least 0.60	
Phenylketonuria (PKU)	Negative	Negative	Chapter 9
Phenylpyruvic acid	Negative	Negative	
Phosphorus (24-hour)	0.9-1.3 g/24 hours	29-42 mmol/24 hours	
Porphobilinogen	Random: negative 24-hour: up to 2 mg/24 hours	Negative	Chapter 10
Porphyrin (24-hour)	50-300 mg/24 hours		Chapter 10
Potassium (K^+) (24-hour)	25-100 mEq/24 hours	25-100 nmol/24 hours	
Pregnancy test	Positive in normal pregnancy or with tumors producing HCG	Positive in normal pregnancy or with tumors producing HCG	Chapters 9, 13
Pregnanediol	After ovulation: >1 mg/24 hours		Chapter 9
Protein (albumin)	Random: ≤8 mg/dl 10-100 mg/24 hours	>0.05 g/24 hours	Chapter 7
Sodium (Na^+) (24-hour)	100-260 mEq/24 hours	100-260 nmol/24 hours	
Specific gravity	1.010-1.025	1.010-1.025	Chapter 7
Steroids (see 17-Hydroxycorticosteroids, 17-Ketosteroids)			Chapter 8

Test	Reference range: Conventional values	Reference range: SI units	Discussion
Sugar (see Glucose)			Chapter 8
Titratable acidity (24-hour)	20-50 mEq/24 hours	20-50 mmol/24 hours	
Turbidity	Clear	Clear	Chapter 7
Urea nitrogen (24-hour)	6-17 g/24 hours	0.21-0.60 mol/24 hours	
Uric acid (24-hour)	250-750 mg/24 hours	1.48-4.43 mmol/24 hours	Chapter 11
Urobilinogen	0.1-1.0 Ehrlich U/dl	0.1-1.0 Ehrlich U/dl	Chapter 4
Uroporphyrin	Negative	Negative	Chapter 10
Vanillylmandelic acid (VMA) (24-hour)	1-9 mg/24 hours	<40 μmol/day	Chapter 7
Zinc (24-hour)	0.20-0.75 mg/24 hours		

INDEX

B

C

D

E

F

G

M

P

Q

R

T

W

X

Y

Z